ANNUAL PROGRESS IN CHILD PSYCHIATRY AND CHILD DEVELOPMENT 1988

ANNUAL PROGRESS IN CHILD PSYCHIATRY AND CHILD DEVELOPMENT 1988

Edited by

STELLA CHESS, M.D.

Professor of Child Psychiatry
New York University Medical Center

ALEXANDER THOMAS, M.D.

Professor of Psychiatry
New York University Medical Center

and

MARGARET E. HERTZIG, M.D.

Associate Professor of Psychiatry
Cornell University Medical College

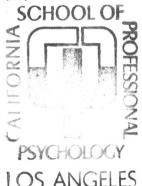

BRUNNER/MAZEL, *Publishers* • **New York**

Library of Congress Card No. 68-23452
ISBN 0-87630-538-9
ISSN 0066-4030

MANUFACTURED IN THE UNITED STATES OF AMERICA
10 9 8 7 6 5 4 3 2 1

CONTENTS

v

ANNUAL PROGRESS IN CHILD PSYCHIATRY AND CHILD DEVELOPMENT 1988

Part I

DEVELOPMENTAL STUDIES

The wide range of subjects in this section attests to the diversity of interests of those concerned with the study of developmental processes. The first paper by Hinde and Stevenson-Hinde draws attention to the fact that the growing and developing child is not an isolated unit, but a social being, forming part of a network of relationships. Interactions, relationships, social groups, and the sociocultural structure form successive levels of social complexity. To assess simultaneously the nature, dynamics, and mutual influences between relationships is a difficult task, but is, in the authors' view, a crucial step in understanding the development of an individual. The paper reviews the current state of the art with respect to the description of interactions, relationships, and groups; ways of generalizing from interactions; the characterization of the roles of various participants; the definition of levels of social complexity; the nature of explanatory concepts; and the dynamics of consistency/inconsistency. This approach, with its roots in ethology, is compatible with "systems theory." However, the development of methods for the study of different levels of complexity, ranging from individuals to interaction, relationships, and social structure, is still in its infancy, and as Hinde and Stevenson-Hinde indicate, it is essential at this stage to remain eclectic.

Rapid advances in the neurosciences in recent years have enhanced dramatically our knowledge and concepts of the relationships between brain function and developmental psychology. These new possibilities for integrating brain and behavior are reflected in a special section in the June 1987 issue of *Child Development*.

In this special section six neuroscientists review the present status of our knowledge in fields that are directly pertinent to behavioral scientists, such as memory, language, cognition, emotion, and the effects of experience. Each review is followed by a commentary written by a child developmentalist. It is impossible for us to reprint the entire section, for it would constitute a volume of 200 pages by itself. Instead, we have selected one of the commentaries, by Bertenthal and Campos, which discusses clearly and concisely the implica-

1

tions of a number of neuroscience findings in the study of early experience. They cover such topics as a proposed mechanism for the explanation of sensitive-period phenomena and their generalizability and the role of experience in human development. Beyond this, we strongly recommend the entire series of articles in the special section to all of our readers. Even the pure clinician can gain fresh insight into the meaning of his or her patients' behavior with the new perspectives on brain functioning that these review articles provide.

Homosexual gender identity and psychoneuroendocrinology is the subject of John Money's comprehensive review of the data of both devised animal experiments and human experiments in nature—clinical intersexual (hermaphroditic) syndromes. The two sources of data supplement one another in indicating that prenatal hormonalization of the brain influences the subsequent sexual orientation as bisexual, heterosexual, or homosexual. However, among humans, there is no evidence that prenatal hormonalization alone, independent of postnatal history, inexorably preordains sexual orientation. Rather, neonatal antecedents may facilitate a homosexual or bisexual orientation, provided the postnatal determinants in social and communicational history are also facilitative. In Money's view it is counterproductive to characterize prenatal determinants of sexual orientation as biological and postnatal determinants as not. Postnatal determinants that enter the brain through the senses by way of social communication and learning are also biological, for there is a biology of learning and remembering. He goes on to suggest that when nature and nurture interact during critical developmental periods, the residual products may persist immutably. Full specification of such interactive products must await the development of appropriate methods for study. However, potential utility of the approach extends beyond the study of the origins of sexual orientation.

In his review of the role of cognition in child development and disorder, Michael Rutter provides a conceptual framework for considering a subject that has long been of central concern to students of normal development as well as developmental psychopathology. Cognition is considered under two broad headings: cognitive processing and cognitive deficits. Research on the emergence of the self-system; the effects of psychosocial experiences; risk, vulnerability, and protective mechanisms; the etiology and treatment of depression; the socioemotional consequences of language delay and reading difficulties; hyperkinetic/attentional deficit syndromes; schizophrenia; and autism are discussed. In concluding this far-ranging survey, Rutter suggests that the ways in which we appraise our life circumstances and the ways in which we react to experiences of all kinds are greatly influenced by how we think about ourselves and our environment. Biases and distortions in cognitive processing may be associated with social and emotional malfunction. Such biases may reflect deficits in the ability to process incoming information, but temperamental styles and earlier life experiences also affect the ways in which individuals perceive and respond to environmental stimuli.

In the next paper Kagen and co-workers examine the biological correlates of individual differences in the behavioral reactions of young children to unfamiliar and cognitively challenging events. Longitudinal study of two groups of children, selected in the second or third year of life to be extremely cautious and shy, or fearless and outgoing in unfamiliar situations, revealed preservation of these two behavioral qualities through the sixth year of life. The behavior of the children characterized as "inhibited" in this study appears similar to that of children characterized as "slow to warm up" in the New York Longitudinal Study. More of the shy or inhibited children were found to show signs of activation in one or more of the physiological circuits that usually respond to novelty or challenge: the hypothalamic-pituitary-adrenal axis, the reticular activating system, and the sympathetic arm of the autonomic nervous system. The data are the first to demonstrate a correlation between physiological characteristics and a temperamental trait. Although there may be an inherited biological contribution to the profile of behaviors characterized as inhibited, the authors emphasize that there is also an important role for learning. A thoughtful discussion further examines factors influencing the choice between continuous quantities or discrete qualities in characterizing both the behavior and the physiological attributes of the subjects. If the research focus is on environmental contributions to the formation of and change in inhibited and uninhibited behavior, experiential dimensions, which imply continuity, will be selected for study. If attention is to be directed toward the examination of the possibility of a biological contribution to behavioral profiles, and especially genetic influences, the dimensions selected will emphasize qualities. Each perspective has validity, given the investigator's initial assumptions and intentions.

Colombo and Horowitz advance an interesting and intriguing proposition for the consideration of infant researchers—that neonatal state be studied as an important functional variable in its own right. They note that progress in documenting the perceptual and cognitive capacities of the human newborn has been accomplished with much difficulty. The very young human infant is not the most cooperative of subjects, and in most research on neonatal stimulus processing, many more subjects are tested than actually provide data. The reason for this high rate of attrition appears to lie in the fact that state variables typically interfere with or override the neonate's attentional and stimulus processing tendencies. The authors review of the relevant literature leads them to conclude that neonatal state measures in and of themselves might well provide good predictive indicators of later developmental status. The study of state maturation and control in combination with the development of information processing abilities in very young infants integrates understanding of both the neonate's behavioral competence and behavioral limitations in responding to the environment. In the author's view, such a strategy should yield a more accurate characterization of early postnatal human development and a more precise understanding of the mechanisms that underlie changes in behavioral organization during the first days and weeks of life.

1

Interpersonal Relationships and Child Development

Robert A. Hinde and Joan Stevenson-Hinde

MRC Unit on the Development and Integration of Behaviour, Madingley, Cambridge, United Kingdom

In studies of psychological development, the child must be seen not as an isolated unit, but as a social being, forming part of a network of relationships. Interactions, relationships, social groups, and the sociocultural structure form successive levels of social complexity, each level involving properties not relevant to lower levels. The levels are connected by dialectical relations and are to be seen not as entities but as processes in continuous creation through the agency of the dialectics. It is rarely possible to study one level in isolation; the dialectics almost always obtrude. A relationships approach must be integrated with others in the field, and especially with that of family systems theorists.

The nature and dynamics of interpersonal relationships impinge on many branches of psychology, but until relatively recently they have not been the focus of systematic study. During the last decade the necessity for a concerted effort in this area has been recognized by a number of authors (e.g., Duck & Gilmour, 1981; Hinde, 1979; Kelley, 1979; Kelley et al., 1983). However, the implications of a relationships approach are not yet widely recognized. The purpose of this article is to spell out some of those implications, especially as they apply to the field of child development.

In our society, most children grow up in a nuclear family, interacting daily with one or two parents, with siblings, and from time to time with relatives

Reprinted with permission from *Developmental Review,* 1987, Vol. 7, 1–21. Copyright 1987 by Academic Press, Inc.

This work was supported by the Royal Society and the Medical Research Council.

and friends. In due course, through schools and peer groups, the range and variety of their interactions increase (e.g., Foot, Chapman, & Smith, 1980; Rubin & Ross, 1982). In other societies the details differ (e.g., Whiting & Whiting, 1975), but the general pattern of a network of relationships expanding from one or more with blood relatives (including nearly always the mother) is ubiquitous. Indeed, something similar occurs in many nonhuman primates (Berman, 1983) and was almost certainly present in, to use Bowlby's (1969) term, our "environment of evolutionary adaptedness" (Alexander, 1974; Mellen, 1981; Short, 1979).

This network of interpersonal relationships, of which the growing child forms part, constitutes a crucially important part of his or her environment. In studying psychological development, therefore, it is necessary to treat the child not as an isolated entity but as a social being, formed by and forming part of a network of relationships which are crucial to its integrity (see e.g., Bronfenbrenner, 1979; Clarke-Stewart, 1978; Parke, Power, & Gottman, 1979). This view is now becoming widely accepted, and *Child Development* (1985), 56(2)) recently devoted nearly a whole issue to studies of children in a family context. Thus it seems timely to focus on the special problems posed by relationships to the developmental psychologist.

SOME GENERAL ISSUES—INTERACTIONS, RELATIONSHIPS, AND GROUPS

It is necessary first to consider the nature of relationships in general terms. Most data on social behavior concern interactions between individuals. The developmental psychologist, though focusing on a particular child, is recording behavior generated by two or more individuals—peers, parent and child, teacher and child, and so on. Even in a test situation, the behavior observed is in part a product of interaction with the experimenter (Perret-Clermont & Brossard, 1985).

When two individuals interact on successive occasions over time, each interaction may affect subsequent ones, and we speak of them as having a relationship. Their relationship includes not only what they do together, but the perceptions, fears, expectations, and so on that each has about the other and about the future course of the relationship, based in part on the individual histories of the two interactants and the past history of their relationship with each other. For instance, a mother's behavior may depend not just on her child's behavior at the moment, but also on their past interactions (Halverson & Waldrop, 1970) and on her hopes for the future.

The nature of any interaction depends on the characteristics of both (or all) of the individuals involved. For example, Elder, Van Nguyen, and Caspi

(1985) found that drastic income loss was associated with rejecting behavior of fathers (but not mothers) to daughters (but not sons). However, the extent of the effect was influenced by a characteristic of the other partner in the relationship, namely the unattractiveness of the daughter. Since interactions and relationships depend on both participants, data obtained from observation of interactions cannot be ascribed solely to the characteristics of one or the other participant. Thus how quickly a mother goes to a crying baby is not solely a measure of her sensitivity, but depends in part on how often the baby has cried recently. And how often a baby cries depends in part on how quickly the mother goes to it when it does so.

While the nature of an interaction depends in part on the individuals involved, it is affected also by the relationship in which it is embedded. Thus the behavior each individual shows depends in part on his or her feelings and expectations about the relationship of which the interaction forms part. The extent to which each placates the other, demands, displays affection, and so on, will be partially influenced by his hopes for the future. In the longer run the behavior an individual *can* show depends in part on the relationships he or she has experienced in the past. While early relationships may have a crucial importance, it is probable that current relationships continue to affect future responsiveness throughout life. And the nature of the relationship, and the participants feelings and predictions about it, depend on the nature of the interactions. Thus we must come to terms with two dialectics—between the characteristics of individuals and interactions on the one hand, and between interactions and relationships on the other, with two-way cause-effect influences in each case.

However, that is not all (see Fig. 1). Each relationship is influenced by the social nexus of other relationships in which it is embedded: A's relationship with B is affected by B's relationship with C, and so on. Conversely the characteristics of the social group are determined by the dyadic and higher

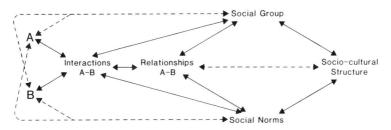

Figure 1. The dialectics between successive levels of social complexity (modified from Hinde, 1979).

order relationships within it. Relationships are affected also by the social norms and values current in the group: the dynamics of a marriage, or of a parent-child relationship, are affected by the expectations and goals of the participants and by the relations between those expectations and perceived reality (e.g., Andreyeva & Gozman, 1981). Those norms and values are transmitted and transmuted through the agency of dyadic relationships.

And the sociocultural structure, used here for the system of institutions and beliefs, and the relations between them, shared by the members of the group, in turn both influences and is influenced by the relationships between individuals (e.g., Hinde, 1984). To give but one example, individual attitudes toward males vs females is related to the presence of a female deity in the belief system of the group (Williams & Best, 1982). Beyond that, each group is juxtaposed with other groups, contact with which affects diverse aspects of the social behavior of its individuals. Finally each group is set in a physical environment, which affects and is affected by the group members. Social scientists must therefore come to terms with a series of dialectics between successive levels of complexity—the behavior of individuals, interactions, relationships, social structure, sociocultural structure, and intergroup relationships. At the same time they must remember that *each level represents not an entity but a process in continuous creation through the agency of the dialectics.*

Each of these levels has properties not relevant to the level below. For example, synchrony and meshing are relevant to interactions but not to the behavior of individuals; properties of relationships that depend on the relative frequency or patterning of different types of interactions (e.g., is maternal control associated with nurturance and warmth?) are not relevant to individual interactions; and a group may have characteristics of internal structure (hierarchical, centripetal, etc.) irrelevant to the component relationships. Furthermore, as we emphasize later, properties at more than one level may be important for understanding dynamics: for instance, the course of interactions may be affected by the participant's perceptions of the relationship.

While some of the social sciences seem to be concerned with one or another of these levels, in practice the dialectics always obtrude. It is rarely possible to study one level in isolation. Thus at the individual level, students of personality find that the cross-situational consistency of supposed "traits" tends to be low. While some of the weakness in the correlations is due to measurement error, and can be overcome by aggregation (Block, 1981; Rushton, Brainerd, & Pressley, 1983), it is necessary to recognize that behavior may be affected (to differing extents according to the nature of the individual and of the behavior) by the context (Bem & Funder, 1978; Endler

& Hunt, 1968, 1969; Endler & Magnusson, 1976; Kenrick & Stringfield, 1980; Mischel, 1973). And the most important aspect of the context is the interactional and relationship one, including the meaning that the individual attributes to his relationships according to his or her sociocultural scheme of reference and past experience.

Developmental psychologists are now well aware that, for instance, 12- to 18-month-olds may behave differently when with their mothers in the Ainsworth Strange Situation from when with their fathers (Grossmann, Grossmann, Huber, & Wartner, 1981; Main & Weston, 1981; see also Sroufe, 1985), and that 4-year-olds adjust the language they use according to whom they are with (Gelman & Shatz, 1977; Shatz & Gelman, 1973; Snow, 1972). They have had to come to terms with the interacting influences of parent on child and child on parent (e.g., Bell & Harper, 1977), and to consider the relative importance of parent-child and peer relationships in the development of personality (e.g., Bowlby, 1969; Sullivan, 1938; Youniss, 1980).

Among social psychologists, the same issue is implicit in the symbolic interactionists' description of individuals as having a number of "role identities" which emerge in interaction with a particular other and provide plans for action and criteria for evaluating action (Goffman, 1959; G. J. McCall, 1974; M. McCall, 1970). The interdependence theorist makes a related point in emphasizing that every relationship is in part a product of its own history and anticipated future and is thereby differentiated from every other relationship (Kelley, 1979).

Even cognitive psychologists find that the mathematics used in the market place may differ from those used in the schoolroom (Carraher, Carraher, & Schliemann, 1985), and that how an individual tackles an intellectual problem may change radically with the social situation (Doise & Mugny, 1984; Donaldson, 1978; Perret-Clermont & Brossard, 1985). And anthropologists and sociologists, concerned with sociocultural structure, seek to understand the ways in which beliefs, myths and legends affect the lives of individuals and reciprocally how those beliefs reflect the natures, desires, wishes, and frustrations of individuals (e.g., Herdt, 1981; Keesing, 1982).

THE TWO ROUTES FOR GENERALIZATIONS FROM INTERACTIONS

As we have seen, data about social behavior concern interactions. From data on interactions there are two principle routes to generalizations (Hinde & Stevenson-Hinde, 1976). These can be illustrated by reference to Fig. 2, which concerns data on two-parent, one-child families. In that figure, Rectangles 1, 2, and 3 represent specific instances of three types of interaction

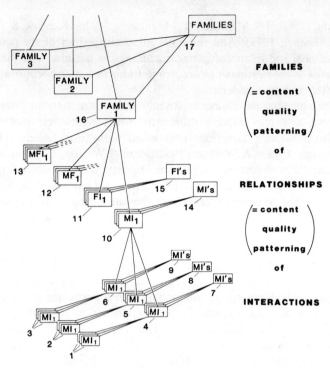

Figure 2. The relations between interactions, relationships, and families, illustrating the two routes for generalizations from data on interactions (modified from Hinde & Stevenson-Hinde, 1976).

between a particular mother and her infant—say mother inhibits and child complies, mother inhibits and child ignores, and mother speaks affectionately. Such are the basic data. From them we can make generalizations about the incidence of these three types of interaction in that mother-infant dyad (4, 5, and 6). The rectangles behind 4 represent comparable data on maternal inhibitions with child compliance for other mother-infant dyads, those behind 5 for maternal inhibition without compliance and those behind 6 for maternal affection. The usual route is to remain at the same level of social complexity, seeking for generalizations about *each type* of interaction *across dyads,* as at 7, 8, and 9. This is the procedure followed in most studies of the relations between particular independent variables (e.g., sex or age of child) and particular dependent variables (e.g., maternal affection). Comparable procedures could be followed for interactions between father and infant, between mother and father, and for triadic interactions.

A second route involves proceeding to the relationship level of social complexity, examining the incidence of and relations between *different types* of interaction in the *same dyad*. Thus in the figure, 10 represents aspects of this particular mother-infant relationship (and the rectangles behind it comparable aspects of other mother-infant relationships). These will include not only the frequencies of the different types of interactions, but also their relative frequencies (e.g., were expressions of affection more or less common than maternal inhibitions), the sequential relations between different types of interaction (e.g., were maternal inhibitions accompanied by expressions of affection, or were these two maternal modes always separated in time), and other properties (see below).

Comparable procedures allow generalizations about other relationships in that family, i.e., father-infant (11), mother-father (12), and their triadic relationship (13), and in other families.

From here we can again remain at the same level, seeking generalizations about mother-infant relationships for a number of dyads (14), father-infant relationships (15), etc.; or we can proceed to the group level, in this case examining the nature and structure of that particular family (16). The latter would include the relations between the intrafamilial relationships. This could lead in turn either to generalizations about families (17) or to descriptions of higher order groups within which the families were located (not shown).

It must be noted that although Fig. 2 portrays the task of description as proceeding from interactions to relationships and family structure, it can sometimes proceed in the opposite direction: that is, descriptions of relationships can permit deductions about the nature of interactions. More importantly, cause-effect relations proceed in both directions (see above and Fig. 1).

The diagram emphasizes that attempts to obtain generalizations about relationships (14, 15) from generalizations about specific interactions (7, 8, & 9) would lose information about some of the most important properties of relationships, namely those that depend upon the relative frequency and patterning of different types of interactions. The number and the proportions of maternal inhibitions complied with provide information about very different aspects of the mother-child relationship, and a given number of commands from a mother who also often expresses affection is unlikely to have the same meaning for the child as the same number of commands from a mother who never expresses affection would have. Such properties of the mother-child relationship would be lost if we examined merely the absolute frequencies of different types of interactions.

Similarly, attempts to obtain generalizations about families (17) from generalizations about relationships (14, 15) would lose crucial information about how relationships are patterned and affect each other within families. A mother-child relationship involving frequent inhibitions might have quite different impacts on the child, depending on whether or not the father-child relationship was also inhibitory. Furthermore the properties of the mother-child relationship may affect the father-child relationship, and the manner in which it does so may depend on the nature of the parental relationship. Such issues would be lost if we merely examined the properties of the several relationships.

Of course, which of the approaches represented in Fig. 2 is more appropriate depends upon the problem. For example, studies of the effects of given independent variables upon particular types of behavior often involve generalizations across dyads (7–9). Where dyadic differences are important or are the focus of study, and one type of interaction is salient, it may be adequate to use differences at the interaction level (e.g., 4, 5, or 6) as an index of the relationship. But interaction measures (e.g., frequency of maternal controls) may be less revealing than the relations between interactions (e.g., proportion of maternal controls that are successful, proportion of interactions that are positive). And where more than one aspect of the relationship, or the relations between different types of interaction within the relationship, are important, the comparisons are at the relationship level (e.g., 10). For instance, the distinctions between authoritarian, authoritative, and permissive parents depend upon assessments of several types of interaction concerned with parental control and acceptance (Baumrind, 1967, 1971). This type of approach (reviewed in Maccoby & Martin, 1983) has been more successful than those involving simple aspects of parent-child interaction.

This suggests that it is sometimes more accurate to think of personality as influenced by relationships than by specific types of interaction. This could be critically important in many ways. For instance, if a single mother attempts to fill two roles by indulging in rough-and-tumble play with her son as well as by behaving with maternal solicitude and sensitivity, are the consequences of rough-and-tumble play coming from the same person as she who provides maternal sensitivity the same as if it were part of a different relationship? We do not know the answer to this, but thinking in relationship terms at least forces us to put the question.

But we must recognize that relationships can never be adequately assessed along a single scale. Of course, the same is true of interactions: aggression must be assessed not only in terms of frequency, but also of quality, context dependence, and so on. But the problem is very much more severe with relationships. Relationships are measurable along many dimensions, and some of the most important may involve ratio measures (Hinde & Herrmann, 1977). The proportion of occasions on which a baby cries in which the mother picks it up tells us something different about their relationship from the absolute frequencies of crying or picking up. At best we can categorize relationships according to where they stand along a limited number of dimensions that we deem to be important.

THE DESCRIPTION OF RELATIONSHIPS

Although difficult, the task of describing relevant features of relationships must not be bypassed. The generalizations we make, or the explanatory concepts we use, will depend upon the sort of relationship with which we are concerned.

Major decisions implicit in any system for describing relationships concern the level of analysis at which to proceed and the sort of categories likely to be useful. One approach is to select initially the level of analysis at which we habitually talk about relationships, and aspects of relationships that appear to be important in everyday life. Such an approach can be justified by the view that we have been shaped, culturally and/or biologically, to be reasonably efficient prognosticians about relationships (e.g., Jolly, 1966; Humphrey, 1976; Osgood, 1969). Thus, as a way of ordering the almost limitless data about relationships, it has been suggested (Hinde, 1979) that the more important dimensions fall into eight categories. These categories proceed from those concerned primarily with individual interactions to those concerned with more global properties of the relationship, and from its more behavioral to its more subjective aspects.

   i. The content of the interactions (what do the participants do together?);

  ii. The diversity of the interactions (how many different things do they do together?);

 iii. The qualities of the several types of interaction;

 iv. Qualities that emerge from the relative frequency and patterning of the interactions (e.g., not *how often* does the child do what it is told, but on *what proportion* of the occasions on which it receives an instruction does it comply);

  v. The reciprocity vs complementarity of the various types of interactions (i.e., do the partners behave similarly to each other, or do they behave in differing but complementary fashions? This includes the question of relative power);

 vi. Intimacy (how much do they reveal themselves to each other?);

vii. Interpersonal perception (does A perceive B as B is, as B perceives B, as close to A's ideal partner, etc.);

viii. Commitment to continuing the relationship and/or to maintaining or improving its quality.

Not all these categories of dimensions will be relevant to any one problem: complete descriptions of a relationship is impracticable and unnecessary. But they may provide convenient pigeonholes for ordering data on relationships.

However, as emphasized already, a relationship is not a static entity but a process in continuous creation through time. Thus any description must refer to a limited span of time, and we must not forget that the future course of a relationship may be affected by events before the period in which is was studied. Indeed *changes* in dimensions within these categories may be as important for prognosis as the dimensions themselves.

The categories listed above are concerned with dimensions that are seen as important in everyday life. Although in large part based on data referring to a finer level of analysis (e.g., interactions, perceptions), they involve also higher level properties emergent from their patterning (Hinde, 1979). Another approach, that of Kelley et al. (1983), rests more exclusively on the interaction level of analysis. Picturing a relationship as the interconnections between the temporal chains of two individuals' affect, thought, and action, they suggest analysis of relationships in terms of (i) the kinds of events in each chain that are interconnected and (ii) the pattern; (iii) strength, (iv) frequency, and (v) diversity of interconnections; (vi) the extent to which the interconnections facilitate or interfere with the chains of action etc; (vii) their symmetry vs asymmetry (i.e., whether the effects of each chain on the other are similar or different); and (viii) the duration of interactions and/or the relationship.

These two approaches to description are not incompatible: that of Kelley et al. (1983), attempts to specify the events upon which some of the more global properties, described in the first approach, depend. Discussion at the interaction level may often be necessary to explain the dynamic importance of some of the more global properties of relationships. However, the interaction level cannot be sufficient by itself because, apart from anything else, we evaluate relationships in terms of global properties, and the evaluations by the participants affect their relationship's future course.

TEASING APART THE ROLES OF THE TWO PARTNERS

We have seen that the nature of an interaction depends on both (or all) participants. We must also ask how far it is meaningful, and how far it is possible, to tease apart their roles. Some discussions of this issue by developmental psychologists fall into the trap of causal chain thinking: one must never forget that the links in a supposed causal chain are in reality spiders' webs (Hanson, 1955).

Just because at least two individuals participate in every interaction or relationship, and each is continuously influencing the other, simple answers to questions of the type, "Who is influencing whom?" are seldom meaningful. Many of the flaws in attempts to answer such questions have been reviewed by Maccoby and Martin (1983). In addition, behavior within a relationship usually involves long sequences of interactions, so that specifying the initiation may be arbitrary.

However, we can ask hard questions about differences or changes: the crucial issue is that the questions must be specified precisely. Given groups of dyads, one approach involves the use of cross-lagged analyses (e.g., Clarke-Stewart, 1973). This can perhaps tell us something about the relative extent to which interactions type A and interactions type B at Time 1 affect interactions at Time 2, but its shortcomings are now well-known (Eron, Huesmann, Lefkowitz, & Walder, 1972; Kenny, 1975; Rogosa, 1980). In any case it must be emphasized that the conclusions usually properly refer to influences of properties of the interactions or relationship at Time 1 and not, as is often implied, to those of the individual participants.

As another approach, given certain assumptions about how one type of interaction affects another within the relationship, some progress can be made in teasing apart the roles of the partners if we examine changes or differences in the relative frequencies of interactions of different types. For example, we might be interested in whether a change in time spent together by a mother and toddler was due primarily to a change in the mother or to a change in the toddler. If the time together increased, but a smaller proportion of approaches between mother and toddler (and a higher proportion of leavings) were due to the mother, and if the importance of long-distance signaling, etc., can be disregarded, we could deduce that the change was due more to a change in the toddler than to a change in the mother (see Table 1). In this way we can answer questions of the type, "Is a given *change* in A_1's relationship with B_1 due more to a *change* in A_1 or to *change* in B_1," or, "Is the *difference* between A_1's relationship with B_1 and A_2's relationship with B_2 due more to *differences* between A_1 and A_2 or between B_1 and B_2?" The answers in each case are, it will be noted, in relative terms. Furthermore, this approach demonstrates the crucial importance of distinguishing questions about responsibility for the nature of the relationship over a limited span of time, from those concerning changes in the relationship over time, and each from those concerning differences between relationships at one time. The

Table 1. Assessing the Extent to Which Changes in Time Spent Together by a Mother and Toddler Are Due to Changes in the Mother or Changes in the Child

	Behavioral measures	
Types of change	Time together	Proportion of approaches by mother
Mother–child $\rightarrow$	+	+
Mother–child $\leftarrow$	−	−
Mother–child $\leftarrow$	+	−
Mother–child $\rightarrow$	−	+

Note. The four rows concern four possible types of change (mother becomes more possessive; mother becomes less possessive; child becomes more dependent; child becomes less dependent). The symbols $(+, -)$ indicate the direction of change in these two measures. If the change is due to a change in the mother, these two measures should change in the same direction; if due to the child, the measures should change in opposite directions. A precisely similar argument can be applied to *differences* between mother–toddler dyads: If the difference is primarily due to a difference between mothers, the dyad spending more time together would have a higher proportion of approaches by the mother. If the difference is due primarily to a difference between the toddlers, the reverse would be the case.

method has been discussed in more detail elsewhere (Hinde, 1969, 1979), and can be extended to the triadic situation (Hinde, 1977), but has so far been applied only to nonhuman species.

Concerned not with particular cases but with generalizations, a more direct route for the developmental psychologist is to study the extent to which differences between relationships are associated with differences in the characteristics of the participating individuals. This is, of course, the route followed in studies of sex differences—for instance, in comparisons between mother-child and father-child relationships (Lamb, 1976), or between the friendships of boys and those of girls (Hartup, 1983). However, most such studies involve comparisons between measures of particular types of interaction—for instance, comparisons of father-child with mother-child relationships show that the former involve more physical play and less tender care, and the play of boy—boy dyads differs in many ways from that of girl—girl dyads (e.g., Clarke-Stewart, 1978; Hartup, 1983; Parke, 1979).

However, the sex of one or another participant may be associated not merely with differences in frequencies between particular types of interactions, but also with the relations between interactions, or what we may call the structure of the relationship. Thus in a recent study of preschoolers, most correlations between items of mother-child interaction were broadly similar for boys and girls. However, the item *mother strong controls* was associated with other negative items (e.g., *mother and child hostile, mother and child noncomply with requests, mother inhibits*) in boys but not in girls. This is in harmony with the view that strong controls were used by mothers of boys mainly in relationships that were generally tensionfilled, whereas with mothers of girls there was no such restriction (and even some opposite tendency) (Hinde & Stevenson-Hinde, in preparation).

If the sex of one or both participants has a dramatic effect on the nature of a relationship, other characteristics are likely also to do so. Thus the developmental psychologist can compare mother-child relationships between depressed and nondepressed mothers (Pound, 1982), or assess the associations between dimensions of child temperament and mother-child interactions (e.g., Lee & Bates, 1985). In addition one characteristic of one or the other partner may affect the influence of another characteristic on an outcome measure. For instance, in a study of preschool children we found virtually no sex differences in the temperamental characteristics of the children in the sample and very few sex differences between measures of mother-child interaction. Nevertheless there were some differences in the correlations between temperamental characteristics and measures of mother-child interaction. These involved particularly the characteristic *shy*, assessed by maternal interview questions about initial withdrawal from strangers and not settling into strange situations. Interview data indicated that, whereas shy boys tended to have more behavior problems and worse family interactions than nonshy boys, for shy girls the opposite was the case. A similar picture was provided from observational data on mother-child interaction, obtained on different days by a different observer. Thus the characteristic "shy," as measured by the instruments we used, interacts with sex to affect the mother-child relationship. Comments made by a number of mothers in the interviews suggested that this difference was a consequence of social norms—for these mothers it was appropriate for a little girl to be shy, but not for a little boy (Simpson & Stevenson-Hinde, 1985). Thus maternal values appear to affect many aspects of the mother-child relationship, and perhaps they have ramifying effects throughout the family (Fig. 1).

CROSSING THE LEVELS OF SOCIAL COMPLEXITY

Awareness of the dialectics between successive levels of social complexity (Fig. 1) brings recognition of the need to cross levels in order to understand the dynamics of changes or differences in relationships, or to understand mutual influences between relationships. The differences between the correlations between "shy" ratings and measures of mother-child interactions between boys and girls is a case in point: the relationship differences appear to be due to differences in social norms for boys vs girls. A more interesting example is provided in the study by Sroufe, Jacobvitz, Mangelsdorf, De Angelo, and Ward (1985) of mothers showing a "seductive" pattern with their 2-year-old sons. Such mothers tended to be not seductive but hostile (deriding) toward their daughters. Thus the "seductive" pattern cannot be viewed in maternal trait terms, but depends critically on the relationship. However, this mother-son/mother-daughter difference was understandable in terms of psychological processes in the mothers related to a history of emotional exploitation by their own fathers, and the resulting dissolution of "generational boundaries." And these psychological processes in the mothers appeared to involve reconstructing relationship patterns that they had known in their own families.

Similarly, Belsky and Isabella (1985) found that recollected experiences as a child in the family of origin predicted changes in marital quality following the birth and rearing of a baby: they suggest that a warm upbringing enhances communicative competence which in turn facilitates the maintenance of the marital relationship in spite of the changes in routine that inevitably accompany the birth of a baby.

THE NATURE OF EXPLANATORY CONCEPTS

The fact that the behavior shown in an interaction depends on both participants forces us to consider carefully the nature of the explanatory concepts that we use. For instance, the categories of attachment derived from the Ainsworth Strange Situation (Ainsworth, Blehar, Waters, & Wall, 1978) reflect aspects of a relationship more than individual characteristics: children may be categorized differently according to the parent who is present (Grossmann et al., 1981; Main & Weston, 1981). But what about supposed measures of child characteristics, such as temperament? In so far as temperament assessments are based on the child's behavior in particular relationships or social situations, they may reflect aspects of relationships as well as individuals. While the moderate nature of the correlations usually obtained between assessments of temperament by fathers and mothers (reviewed in Bates, in press) could be ascribed to error, they may also reflect differences between the father-child and mother-child relationships. These might include differences in what father and mother do with the child, the quality of their interactions, the extent to which their relationships with the child are nurturant/succorant, authoritarian/permissive, etc., their differing

Belsky, J., & Isabella, R. A. (1985). Marital and parent-child relationships in family of origin and marital change following the birth of a baby: A retrospective analysis. *Child Development,* 56, 342–349.

Bell, R. Q., & Harper, L. V. (1977), *Child effects on adults.* Hillsdale, NJ: Erlbaum.

Bem, D. J., & Funder, D. C. (1978). Predicting more of the people more of the time. *Psychological Review,* 85, 485–501.

Berman, C. (1983). Differentiation of relationships among rhesus monkey infants. In R. A. Hinde (Ed.), *Primate social relationships.* Oxford: Blackwell.

Block, J. (1981). Some enduring and consequential structures of personality. In A. Robin, J. Aronoff, A. M. Barclay, & R. A. Zucker (Eds.), *Further explanations in personality.* New York: Wiley.

Bowlby, J. (1969). *Attachment and loss.* New York: Basic Books.

Bronfenbrenner, U. (1979). *The ecology of human development.* Cambridge, MA: Harvard Univ. Press.

Carraher, T. N., Carraher, D. W., & Schliemann, A. D. (1985). Mathematics in the streets and in schools. *British Journal of Developmental Psychology,* 3, 21–30.

Clarke-Stewart, K. A. (1973). Interactions between mothers and their young children: Characteristics and consequences. *Monographs of the Society for Research in Child Development,* 38(6 & 7, Serial No. 153).

Clarke-Stewart, K. A. (1978). And daddy makes three: The father's impact on mother and young child. *Child Development,* 49, 466–478.

Daniels, D., & Plomin, R. (1985). Origins of individual differences in infant shyness. *Developmental Psychology,* 21, 118–121.

Doise, W., & Mugny, G. (1984). *The social development of the intellect.* Oxford: Pergamon.

Donaldson, M. (1978). *Children's minds.* London: Fontana.

Duck, S., & Gilmour, R. (1981, et seq.) *Personal relationships* (Vols 1–5). Orlando/London: Academic Press.

Dunn, J. (1983). Sibling relationships in early childhood. *Child Development,* 54, 787–811.

Elder, G. H., Van Nguyen, T., & Caspi, A. (1985) *Child Development,* 56, 361–375.

Endler, N. S., & Hunt, J. McV. (1968). Inventories of hostility and comparisons of the proportions of variance from persons, responses, and situations for hostility and anxiousness. *Journal of Personality and Social Psychology,* 9, 309–315.

Endler, N. S., & Hunt, J. McV. (1969). Generalizability of contributions from sources of variance in the S—R inventories of anxiousness, *Journal of Personality,* 37, 1–24.

Endler, N. S., & Magnusson, D. (1976). Toward an interactional psychology of personality. *Psychological Bulletin,* 83, 956–997.

Eron, L. D., Huesmann, L. R., Lefkowitz, M. M., & Walder, L. O. (1972). Does television violence cause aggression? *American Psychologist,* 27, 253–263.

Foot, H. C., Chapman, A. J., & Smith, J. R. (1980). *Friendship and social relations in children.* New York: Wiley.

Gelman, R., & Shatz, M. (1977). Speech adjustments in talk to 2-year-olds. In M. Lewis & L. A. Rosenblum (Eds.), *Interaction, conversation and the development of language.* New York: Academic Press.

Goffman, E. (1959). *The presentation of self in everyday life.* New York: Doubleday/Anchor.

Grossmann, K. E., Grossmann, K., Huber, F., & Wartner, U. (1981). German children's behaviour towards their mothers at 12 months and their fathers at 18 months in Ainsworth's Strange Situation. *International Journal of Behavioral Development,* 4, 157–181.

Halverson, C. F., & Waldrop, M. F. (1970). Maternal behavior toward own and other preschool children: The problem of "owness." *Child Development,* 41, 838–845.

Hanson, N. R. (1955). Causal chains. *Mind,* 255, 289–311.

Hartup, W. W. (1983). Peer relations. In P. H. Mussen (Ed.), *Child psychology* (Vol. 4, pp. 103–197). New York: Wiley.

Herdt, G. H. (1981). *Guardians of the flute: Idioms of masculinity.* New York: McGraw-Hill.

Hinde, R. A. (1969). Analysing the roles of the partners in a behaviour interaction— mother-infant relations in rhesus macaques. *Ann. N.Y. Acad. Sci.,* 159, 651–667.

Hinde, R. A. (1972). *Social behavior and its development in subhuman primates.* Condon Lectures, Eugene, OR.

Hinde, R. A. (1976). Interactions, relationships and social structure. *Man,* 11, 1–17.

Hinde, R. A. (1977). On assessing the bases of partner preferences. *Behaviour,* LXII(102), 1–9.

Hinde, R. A. (1979). *Toward understanding relationships.* Ontario/London: Academic Press.

Hinde, R. A. (1984). Why do the sexes behave differently in close relationships? *Journal of Social and Personal Relationships,* 1, 471–501.

Hinde, R. A., & Bateson, P. P. G. (1984). Discontinuities versus continuities in behavioural development and the neglect of process. *International Journal of Behavioral Development,* 7, 129–143.

Hinde, R. A., & Dennis, A. (1986). Categorizing individuals: An alternative to linear analysis. *International Journal of Behavioral Development,* 9, 105–119.

Hinde, R. A., & Herrmann, J. (1977). Frequencies, durations, derived measures, and their correlations in studying dyadic and triadic relationships. In H. R. Schaffer (Ed.), *Studies in mother-infant interaction.* Orlando/London: Academic Press.

Hinde, R. A. & Stevenson-Hinde, J. (1976). Towards understanding relationships: Dynamic stability. In P. P. G. Bateson & R. A. Hinde (Eds.), *Growing points in ethology* (pp. 451–479). Cambridge: Cambridge Univ. Press.

Hinde, R. A., Stevenson-Hinde, J., & Tamplin, A. (1985). Characteristics of 3- to 4-year-olds assessed at home and their interactions in preschool. *Developmental Psychology,* 21(1), 130–140.

Hinde, R. A., & Stevenson-Hinde, J., (in preparation). Varieties of sex-differences in the mother-child relationships of 42–50 months olds.

Hinde, R. A., & Tamplin, A. (1983). Relations between mother-child interaction and behaviour in preschool. *British Journal of Developmental Psychology,* 1, 231–257.

Humphrey, N. K. (1976). The social function of intellect. In P. P. G. Bateson & R. A. Hinde (Eds.) *Growing points in ethology.* London/New York: Cambridge Univ. Press.

Jolly, A. (1966). Lemur social behavior and primate intelligence. *Science,* 153, 501–506.

Kagan, J., Reznick, J. S., Clarke, C., Snidman, N., & Garcia-Coll, C. (1984). Behavioral inhibition to the unfamiliar. *Child Development,* 55, 2212–2225.

Keesing, R. M. (1982). Introduction. In G. H., Herdt (Ed.), *Rituals of manhood.* Berkeley: Univ. of California Press.

Kelley, H. H. (1979). *Personal relationships: Their structures and processes.* Hillsdale, NJ: Erlbaum.

Kelley, H. H., Berscheid, E., Christensen, A., Harvey, J. H., Huston, T. L., Levinger, G., McClintock, E., Peplau, L. A., & Peterson, D. R. (1983). *Close relationships.* New York: Freeman.

Kenny, D. A. (1975). Cross-lagged panel correlation: A test for spuriousness. *Psychological Bulletin,* 82, 887–903.

Kenrick, D. T., & Stringfield, D. O. (1980). Personality traits and the eye of the beholder. *Psychological Review,* 87, 88–104.

Lamb, M. E. (1976). *The role of the father in child development.* New York: Wiley.

Lee, C. L., & Bates, J. E. (1985). Mother-child interaction at age two years and perceived difficult temperament. *Child Development,* 56, 1314–1325.

Maccoby, E. E., & Martin, J. A. (1983). Socialization in the context of the family: Parent-child interaction. In P. H. Mussen (Ed.), *Child psychology* (Vol. 4, pp. 1–103). New York: Wiley.

Main, M., & Weston, D. (1981). The quality of the toddler's relationship to mother and to father: Related to conflict behavior and the readiness to establish new relationships. *Child Development,* 52, 932–940.

McCall, G. J. (1974). A symbolic interactionist approach to attraction. In T. L. Huston (Ed.) *Foundations of Interpersonal Attraction.* New York, Academic Press.

McCall, M. (1970). Boundary rules in relationships and encounters. In G. J. McCall et al., (Eds.), *Social relationships.* Chicago: Aldine.

McFarland, D. J. (1974). *Motivational control systems analysis.* Orlando/London: Academic Press.

Mellen, S. L. W. (1981). *The evolution of love.* Oxford: Freeman.

Minuchin, P. (1985). Families and individual development: Provocations from the field of family therapy. *Child Development,* 56, 289–302.

Mischel, W. (1973). Toward a cognitive social learning reconceptualization of personality. *Psychological Review,* 80, 252–283.

Osgood, C. E. (1969). On the whys and wherefores of E, P, and A. *Journal of Personal and Social Psychology,* 12, 194–199.

Parke, R. D. (1979). Perspectives of father-infant interaction. J. D. Osofsky (Ed.) *Handbook of infant development.* New York: Wiley.

Parke, R. D., Power, T. G., & Gottman, J. (1979). Conceptualizing and quantifying influence patterns in the family triad. In M. E. Lamb, S. J. Suomi, & G. R. Stephenson (Eds.), *Social interaction analysis.* Madison: Univ. of Wisconsin Press.

Perret-Clermont, A-N., & Brossard, A. (1985). On the interdigitation of social and cognitive processes. In R. A. Hinde, A-N. Perret-Clermont, & J. Stevenson-Hinde (Eds.), *Social relationships and cognitive development.* Oxford: Oxford Univ. Press (Clarendon).

Pound, A. (1982). Attachment and maternal depression. In C. M. Parkes, & J. Stevenson-Hinde (Eds.), *The place of attachment in human behavior.* London/New York: Tavistock/Basic Books.

Rogosa, D. (1980). A critique of cross-lagged correlation. *Psychological Bulletin,* 88, 245–258.

Rubin, K. H., & Ross, H. S. (1982). *Peer relationships and social skills in childhood.* New York: Springer-Verlag.

Rushton, J. P., Brainerd, C. J., & Pressley, M. (1983). Behavioral development and construct validity: The principle of aggregation. *Psychological Bulletin,* 94, 18–38.

Rutter, M. D., Quinton, D., & Liddle, C. (1983). Parenting in two generations: Looking backwards and looking forwards. In N. Madge (Ed.), *Families at risk.* London: Heinemann.

Shatz, M., & Gelman, R. (1973). The development of communication skills: modifications in the speech of young children as a function of the listener. *Monog. Soc. Res. Child Devel.,* 38,(5).

Short, R. (1979). Sexual selection and its component parts, somatic and genital selection, as illustrated by man and the great apes. *Advances in the Study of Behaviour,* 9, 131–158.

Simpson, A. E., & Stevenson-Hinde, J. (1985). Temperamental characteristics of three- to four-year-old boys and girls and child-family interactions. *Journal of Child Psychology and Psychiatry,* 26, 43–53.

Snow, C. (1972). Mother's speech to children learning language. *Child Development,* 43, 549–564.

Sroufe, L. A. (1979). The coherence of individual development. *American Psychologist,* 34, 834–841.

Sroufe, L. A. (1985). Attachment classification from the perspective of infant-caregiver relationships and infant temperament. *Child Development,* 56, 1–14.

Sroufe, L. A., Jacobvitz, D., Mangelsdorf, S., DeAngelo, E., & Ward, M. J. (1985). Generational boundary dissolution between mothers and their preschool children: A relationship systems approach. *Child Development,* 56, 317–325.

Stevenson-Hinde, J., & Hinde, R. A. (1986). Changes in associations between characteristics and interactions. In R. Plomin and J. Dunn (Eds.), *The study of temperament: changes, continuities and challenges.* Hillsdale, NJ: Erlbaum.

Stevenson-Hinde, J. (in press). Towards a more open construct. In D. Kohnstamm (Ed.), *Temperament discussed.* Holland: Swets & Zeitlinger.

Sullivan, H. S. (1938). The data of psychiatry. *Psychiatry,* 1, 121–134.

Tinbergen, N. (1951). *The study of instinct.* Oxford: Oxford Univ. Press (Clarendon).

Whiting, B. B., & Whiting, J. W. M. (1975). *Children of six cultures.* Cambridge, MA: Harvard Univ. Press.

Williams, J. E., & Best, D. L. (1982). *Measuring sex stereotypes.* Beverly Hills, CA: Sage.

Youniss, J. (1980). *Parents and peers in social development.* Chicago: Univ. of Chicago Press.

PART I: DEVELOPMENTAL STUDIES

2

New Directions in the Study of Early Experience

Bennett I. Bertenthal
University of Virginia, Charlottesville
Joseph J. Campos
University of Denver, Colorado

In this commentary, we review Greenough, Black, and Wallace's conceptual framework for understanding the effects of early experience, and illustrate the applicability of their model with recent data on the consequences for animals and human infants of the acquisition of self-produced locomotion.

The purpose of this paper is threefold: First, we evaluate how the proposal by Greenough, Black, and Wallace (1987, in this issue) provides a new level of understanding about sensitive periods in development. Second, we consider the generalizability of their conceptualization to other examples of sensitive periods during human development. And third, we comment on the more general implications of their position for understanding the role of experience in human development.

Reprinted with permission from *Child Development,* 1987, Vol. 58, 560–567. Copyright 1987 by the Society for Research in Child Development, Inc.

Preparation of this paper was supported by NICHD grant HD-16195 and NICHD Career Development Award HD-00065 to the first author, and NIMH grant 22803 and a grant from the John D. and Catherine T. MacArthur Foundation to the second author. Reprint requests should be addressed to Bennett Bertenthal, Department of Psychology, Gilmer Hall, University of Virginia, Charlottesville, VA 22903.

A PROPOSED MECHANISM FOR THE EXPLANATION
OF SENSITIVE-PERIOD PHENOMENA

The concept of sensitive period is widely considered to be fundamental to understanding the effects of early experience on biobehavioral development (Aslin, 1981). In essence, this concept covers both the age ranges during which the developing organism is especially subject to the effects of specific forms of experience, and outcomes in the form of significant structural and functional changes that are resistant to change at later ages. The concept has had a long and venerable history, dating back at least to the embryologists of the late nineteenth century (Hubel, 1972), but the concept is poorly understood both because there has been little systematic inquiry into the mechanisms underlying it, and because traditional behavioral criteria of age-dependency and irreversibility are less clear-cut than once thought (Colombo, 1982). As with many other concepts in the behavioral and neurosciences, the processes underlying sensitive periods are subject to very subtle endogenous (biological) and exogenous (environmental) variations.

We believe that Greenough et al. have made very significant progress toward advancing our understanding of the underlying mechanisms of sensitive-period phenomena. They relegate to secondary importance the behavioral and functional criteria of age-dependency and irreversibility. In their place, they propose a *neurophysiological* mechanism organized around the concept of *experience-expectancy.*

The neurophysiological process they believe to be basic to sensitive periods is the intrinsic generation of an excess number of synaptic connections among neurons. With development, some of these synaptic connections survive, while others do not. What determines the survival of synaptic connections is the principle of use: Those synapses activated by sensory or motor experience survive; the remainder are lost through disuse. For Greenough et al., then, experience does not create tracings on a blank tablet; rather, experience erases some of them.

The basic logic for synaptic proliferation is that it creates a tendency to anticipate certain types of experiences—those that are ubiquitous in the life of all members of the species. Among ubiquitous experiences, the authors list exposure to contours, orientation, speech, binocular input, and, more generally, stimuli generated by the organism's own activity. From an adaptive standpoint, we find this argument quite compelling since it suggests a mechanism for reducing the demands on genotypic specification of a phenotype without sacrificing necessary constraints on behavioral development.

There is a second category of neural plasticity which the authors call experience-dependent. This type of plasticity takes into account that certain experiences will not occur in any fixed order; hence, the nervous system must be prepared to incorporate the information whenever it occurs. In contrast to experience-expectant events, experience-dependent processes initiate the generation of new synapses, continue throughout the life span, and are specific to the individual experiences of the organism.

In the case of experience-expectant processes, it is not only the nature of the experiential input but the timing of that input that determines which synaptic organization emerges. Although the authors are somewhat vague about the temporal parameters of this process, we assume that the *onset* of the sensitive period is determined by the point when intrinsic synaptic proliferation is complete, the *decline* of this period starts when selective competitive success of some synapses over others has begun, and the *end* of the period occurs when synapses involved in a particular process have been reduced beyond a point adequate to compete for the control of a behavioral function. The principles of synaptic proliferation and selective survival thus not only replace the behavioral criteria for the sensitive period (i.e., age-dependency and irreversibility) but also provide the beginnings of a theory of sensitive-period phenomena.

Two caveats are in order before we discuss this proposal further. First, we are not experts in neurophysiology and therefore do not feel that we can adequately evaluate the interpretations of the data referred to in this proposal. As a consequence, we accept the proposal at face value and defer the task of critical evaluation to those more knowledgeable in the field. Second, it is often argued that explaining a behavioral phenomenon at the neurophysiological level does not constitute true explanation but rather a description at a different level of analysis. This criticism, however, seems less applicable to the current phenomenon because, by definition, sensitive periods are presumed to reflect changes in susceptibility to experience at the neural level. We thus feel that, in this case, it is appropriate to seek explanations of behavior in neurophysiological structures and functions.

Proceeding with these caveats in mind, we believe that Greenough et al.'s neural mechanism advances our understanding of sensitive-period phenomena in two very important ways. First, and most important, this formulation provides compelling evidence that the effects of experience during a sensitive period are *qualitatively different* from other experiential effects. There is growing evidence that plasticity continues throughout the life span (Lerner, 1984), and we know that many outcomes attributable to experiences during a sensitive period are reversible (Colombo, 1982; Ganz, 1978). The Greenough et al. formulation permits one to hypothesize precisely as to which phenomena will be expectably changeable during the early part of an organism's life, and which phenomena may involve the compensatory overlay of experience-dependent effects on experience-expectant ones. Their proposal requires that we abandon monistic conceptualizations of neural plasticity and that we devise methods of measuring underlying neurophysiological processes at the synaptic level.

The second contribution of the Greenough et al. proposal is that it sheds new light on why the traditional criteria for the sensitive period are much less rigid than originally conceived. They propose that a relative reduction in synaptic activity, as occurs during visual deprivation, may prolong the neural competition process, which, in turn, prolongs the sensitive period. They also present pharmacological evidence that substances that interfere with the effects of brain neurotransmitters can prevent some of the effects of visual deprivation during a sensitive period. Their approach thus draws attention to the underlying neurophysiological processes involved in preventing synaptic competitive success.

GENERALIZABILITY OF THE PROPOSED FORMULATION

Although Greenough et al. propose a fundamentally different conceptualization of the sensitive-period concept, and although they recognize that this proposal may not apply to all sensitive-period phenomena, their discussion fails to make clear the boundaries for their conceptualization, that is, the conditions under which they expect their proposal to apply and those under which they do not. It thus becomes an empirical issue when to expect synaptic proliferation to peak, how to determine when synaptic competition is complete, which experience-dependent processes can compensate or substitute for experience-expectant ones, and how to evaluate the generalizability of these mechanisms to human behavioral development.

Since the last issue is the one of greatest immediate relevance to developmental psychologists, we shall examine a select set of examples of sensitive periods in human development in order to determine whether they readily fit the Greenough et al. model. The examples suggest that phenomena of sensory or motor function better fit the model than do phenomena involving more complex aspects of behavior.

Nicely fitting the Greenough et al. conceptualization is one of the best-known examples of a sensitive period in human infancy. This example concerns the development of binocularity and stereopsis. Two different groups of researchers (Banks, Aslin, & Letson, 1975; Hohmann & Creutz-feldt, 1975) investigated binocular functioning in children and adults who had anomalous visual experiences early in life (e.g., because of misalignment of the two eyes). The principle finding was that binocular visual performance was found to vary as a function of the age when corrective surgery was conducted. In particular, those individuals who did not experience concordant visual information during the first 3 years of life showed dramatic deficits in binocular function. These findings suggest that a sensitive period exists for binocular vision in humans just as Greenough et al. report is the case for cats and monkeys.

Another example possibly fitting the Greenough et al. model involves a sensitive period for language acquisition. There are a number of different sources of evidence suggesting that during the period between 2 and 5 years of age, the child is especially primed for acquiring language. For example, Lenneberg (1967) reported that children who became deaf prior to 2 years of age had greater difficulty learning to speak than children who became deaf at later ages. Also, there is evidence showing that preschoolers who have suffered damage to the language portions of the brain quickly regain much of their capacity for language, whereas older children and adults recover much more slowly and not always completely (Hecaen, 1976; Lenneberg, 1967). It is our impression that these findings, at least at a general level, are consistent with the predictions of the proposed neural model. We must admit, however, that our confidence in the generalizability of the Greenough et al. model to this behavior is less secure than was true for the first example, since there is much less known about the neurophysiological underpinnings of language development. As a consequence, it is difficult to establish whether or not the predicted neural changes actually occur in the appropriate cortical areas during this sensitive period.

In contrast to the others, the third example does not neatly fit the proposed conceptualization. The example involves a proposed sensitive period for psychosexual development. Money and Ehrhardt (1972) studied prenatal hormonal anomalies that resulted in masculinizing female infants who were then assigned to the wrong gender category. Again, a sensitive period was reported to take place in human infants: If reassignment did not occur by 3–4 years of age, inadequate sex typing and poor psychological adjustment ensued.

The point of this last example is that the mechanisms responsible for the occurrence of this sensitive period must necessarily be far more complex than those proposed by Greenough et al. In contrast to the preceding two examples, the behavior in question is neither primarily sensory nor motor, but rather involves some level of conceptual understanding. This example underscores the much greater complexity of many of the human behaviors that undergo a sensitive period. Consistent with recent theorizing about human plasticity (Lerner, 1984), the mechanism for a sensitive period for such complex phenomena as gender identity may involve mechanisms at multiple levels of the organism, from neural to conceptual, that are integrated together in some hierarchical fashion. It is not clear how Greenough et al.'s approach can deal with such complex sensitive-period phenomena. To reiterate: The approach may be better suited to explain simpler sensory and motoric processes than more complex ones.

ROLE OF EXPERIENCE IN HUMAN DEVELOPMENT

Although the Greenough et al. article is largely concerned with terms of sensitive-period phenomena, its major implication may be in once again calling the attention of developmental psychologists to the role of experience in development. Too often, even today, developmental psychologists often interpret the outcomes of complex interactions between experience and endogenous biological changes as "the unfolding of a maturational blueprint." These views on genetic blueprinting have been called *predetermined epigenesis* by Gottlieb (1983) to capture the assumptions of such theorists that developmental changes (epigenesis) indeed take place, but that these changes occur with no variation as a function of differential experiences.

Like Greenough et al., Gottlieb (1983) stresses an opposing viewpoint—one called probabilistic epigenesis—to call attention to the possibility that the final form of a phenotype is a function of a complex set of endogenous and exogenous factors.

A number of phenomena are often cited in support of predetermined epigenesis. Among them are processes that (1) are essential to the survival of the species (Bowlby, 1973; Freedman, 1974), (2) codevelop jointly with many other processes during times of rapid developmental transition (Emde, Gaensbauer, & Harmon, 1976), and (3) are invariant across members of the species because of their evolutionary adaptedness (Kagan, 1976). The large number of phenomena that fit one or more of these criteria has reinforced predetermined epigenetic views.

In recent years, however, evidence has begun to mount against predetermined epigenesis. Phenomena once thought to be predetermined have been shown to result from interactions with experiences. Some of these experiences are so ubiquitous that their impact has been overlooked. This discovery is consistent, of course, with the notions of Greenough et al. that the organism does not develop in an experiential vacuum, and that infants of various species appear programmed to benefit from selected experiences in the development of virtually all behavior systems.

One phenomenon inconsistent with predetermined epigenesis has already been discussed—the development of binocularity. We shall now discuss another—the development of spatial understanding in the third quarter year of life. We will show how a neglected but nearly universal experience, the acquisition of self-produced locomotion, results in widespread changes often assumed to be under maturational control (Kagan, Kearsley, & Zelazo, 1978).

First, we will discuss the well-known phenomenon of avoidance of heights by infants on the visual cliff (Walk & Gibson, 1961). Avoidance of heights was until recently considered a prototype of predetermined epigenesis, with most textbooks and many authorities claiming that this behavior is present in the infant animal from the earliest testing opportunity (Bowlby, 1973; Freedman, 1974).

It is now clear from the work of many researchers that this view is wrong and that avoidance of heights develops between 7 and 9 months of age (Campos, Hiatt, Ramsay, Henderson, & Svejda, 1978; Richards & Rader, 1981; Scarr & Salapatek, 1970). Nevertheless, many still argue for a maturational interpretation of the development of avoidance of heights. For instance, Richards and Rader (1981) attributed the origins of avoidance of heights to a maturational unfolding of a visuomotor program that permits vision to guide where the infant steps. In the absence of such a program, depth perception does not mediate avoidance of heights, and the infant crosses the visual cliff. When the program develops, the infant begins to show avoidance.

The principal evidence for this claim was that the age of onset of locomotion, and not locomotor experience itself, was the best predictor of visual cliff performance (see also Richards & Rader, 1983). We have argued elsewhere that the Richards and Rader data are subject to alternative interpretations (Bertenthal & Campos, 1984). However, the more important point for this discussion is that Richards and Rader were wrong in attributing developmental changes in avoidance of heights to maturational factors alone. It is now clear that the development of wariness of heights is the outcome of experiences made possible by self-produced locomotion (Bertenthal, Campos, & Barrett, 1984), and interpretation consistent with the animal work on the "kitten carousel" by Held and Hein (1963).

As with other studies of the effects of early experience, there are a number of procedures that can be used to test for the effects of certain experiences. One method involves *environmental enrichment*, whereby experience is provided to subjects who otherwise would not encounter it at that time. In the case of self-produced locomotion, enrichment takes the form of providing "artificial" locomotor experience to infants who are otherwise endogenously prelocomotor (i.e., they cannot move about without assistance). This can be done by giving infants many hours of experience in walkers (a seat that is attached to a frame on wheels, permitting the infant to propel him/herself voluntarily around the room by pushing on the floor with his or her feet). When one compares infants with "enriched" locomotor experience to age-matched controls who are also endogenously prelocomotor, the walker infants show evidence of wariness of heights (heart-rate accelerations) as they are lowered to the deep side of the cliff, whereas the control infants do not (Bertenthal et al., 1984). Interestingly, infants with *both* artificial *and* endogenous locomotor experience show the most reliable evidence for wariness of heights, as if a "double dose" of locomotor experience compounds the consequences of locomotion (see Fig. 1). Enrichment of the experience of locomoting thus facilitates the developmental transition involving wariness of heights.

A second method used to test for the effects of environmental experiences involves *deprivation of experience.* The subject is experimentally prevented from obtaining the experience in question. Although deprivation studies are ordinarily limited to investigations using animals because of ethical considerations with humans, deprivation sometimes occurs "naturally" in human infants who, for orthopedic or other reasons, are prevented from locomotion. A deprivation study concerned with fear of heights involves two predictions: (1) that the development of wariness of heights will be delayed relative to the performance of infants not impeded from locomotion, and (2) that, albeit delayed, the developmental onset of wariness of heights will follow the acquisition of locomotion.

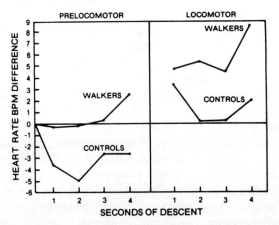

Figure 1. Heart-rate reactions to being lowered toward the deep side of the visual cliff in infants with at least 40 hours of artificial ("walker") locomotor experience compared to age- and sex-matched controls. Left panel shows data from infants tested when unable to move about without assistance. Right panel shows data from infants tested 5 days after beginning to crawl spontaneously. (From Bertenthal et al., 1984; reprinted by permission.)

Both of these predictions were tested, and confirmed, in a case study of an orthopedically handicapped infant whose locomotion was delayed by the imposition of a heavy cast that prevented normal locomotion until 9.5 months of age. Locomotion onset was 10 weeks later than developmental norms for onset of crawling, and took place at an age at which some 90% of infants are crawling spontaneously. Beginning at 6 months of age, this infant, whose Bayley DQ score was 126, showed no cardiac differentiation upon being lowered to the deep or the shallow side of the visual cliff. In contrast, at 10 months of age, after self-produced locomotor experience had begun, clear cardiac accelerations accompanied lowering the baby onto the deep side of the cliff, while cardiac responses to the shallow side became deceleratory. As predicted, deprivation seemed to retard the expectable performance of this infant until after crawling developed (see Fig. 2).

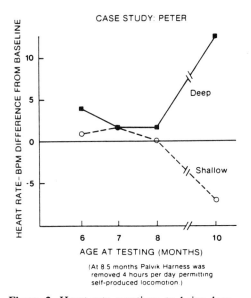

Figure 2. Heart-rate reactions to being lowered toward the deep and shallow side of the visual cliff in an orthopedically handicapped infant. Heart-rate levels during the 3 sec of descent and first second of contact with cliff surface were averaged and subtracted from base-level heart rate. (Reprinted by permission as in Fig. 1.)

A third method of studying the effects of experience involves dissociating the separate effects of age and locomotor experience on avoidance of heights. This can be done by testing infants who start crawling at different ages and determining the probability of avoidance of crossing the deep side of the cliff as a function of (a) the age when the infant began to crawl, and (b) the duration of locomotor experience when tested. As with the enrichment and deprivation paradigms, results obtained with this approach supported the importance of locomotor experience; moreover, there was no evidence that the age when the infant began to crawl was a significant factor. As can be seen in Figure 3, about 35% of the infants at each age of locomotion onset avoided crossing the deep side if they had 11 days of locomotor experience. In contrast, the percent of avoidance jumped to about 75% after 41 days of locomotor experience. Taken as a whole, there seems little doubt that the development of avoidance of heights follows a probabilistic epigenetic pathway, and not one of either predetermined epigenesis or nativism, as so frequently assumed.

Self-produced locomotion accounts for other developmental changes attributed to maturation as well. Kagan et al. (1978) speculated that memory for locations showed a developmental onset between 7 and 9 months of age because of endogenous factors probably linked to frontal lobe maturation. Empirical support for this contention was presumably provided by the results from a newly developed test of memory for locations. Recently, however, Kermoian (1986) showed that performance on this test, like that on the visual cliff, is powerfully affected by self-produced locomotion. Figure 4 presents the data from Kermoian's study, which involved three groups of 8.5-month-old infants (plus or minus 1 week): One group was endogenously locomotor, one was prelocomotor but the infants had varying amounts of walker experience, and one was prelocomotor and had no experience locomoting of any kind.

As can be observed, these findings revealed clear effects of locomotor experience on the memory-for-locations task. In particular, infants with 6 or more weeks of locomotor experience (whether endogenous or artificial) were significantly superior in spatial search performance than prelocomotor infants or infants with 3 weeks or less of locomotor experience. More recent data from a follow-up study using experimenters unaware of the locomotor status of the infants replicated these findings, and moreover, linked them to the *quality* of locomotor experience: Infants locomoting on their hands and knees performed significantly better on the memory-for-locations task than did infants locomoting on their bellies. The effort involved in belly crawling may have left little capacity for the infant to deploy attentional resources to note self-generated changes in environmental stimulation.

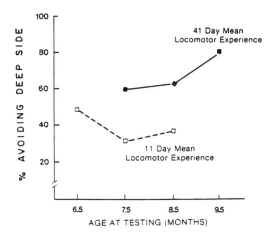

Figure 3. Proportion of infants failing to cross to the mother over the deep side of the visual cliff in a 120 sec period as a function of both age and locomotor experience. (Reprinted by permission as in Fig. 1.)

There are a number of other lines of evidence showing that the development of self-produced locomotion facilitates developmental shifts in spatial cognition. For instance, prelocomotor infants localize the position of objects in a predominantly egocentric way (i.e., to their right or left), while locomotor and walker infants localize objects in a predominantly objective fashion (i.e., by reference to external landmarks; Bertenthal, Campos, Benson, & Rudy, in preparation). Also, prelocomotor infants faced with a two-position object-hiding task show great difficulty searching correctly, whereas same-age infants with locomotor experience do not (Campos, Benson, & Rudy, 1986). Lastly, infants with menyngomyelocele (a neural tube defect that impedes locomotion) show 5- and 6-month delays in searching correctly for a hidden object in a two-position hiding task, but begin to search correctly once they start moving about spontaneously (Telzrow, Campos, & Bertenthal, 1986). The effects of self-produced locomotion are thus not paradigm-specific nor issue-specific but are both broad and, until recently, unrecognized.

In sum, the recent work on the relation between the development of self-produced locomotion and the development of spatial understanding fits a probabilistic epigenetic perspective in paradigmatic fashion. Moreover, it provides strong support for Greenough et al.'s view that many of the

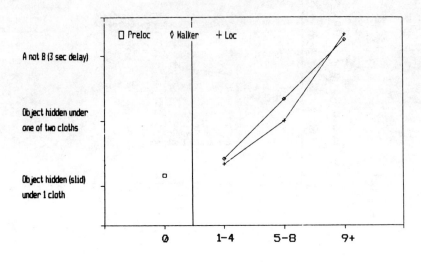

Figure 4. Memory for locations performance of prelocomotor infants with no artificially induced locomotor experience, prelocomotor infants with different number of weeks of artificially induced locomotor experience, and locomotor infants with different number of weeks of spontaneous locomotor experience. Task items have been ordinally scaled, and were adapted from Kagan et al. (1978).

experiences that will prove crucial to synaptic development will be those that are ubiquitous and are linked to the animal's own activity. Whether the experiences provided through self-produced locomotion are categorized as experience-expectant or experience-dependent may, at this time, be less crucial for the behavioral scientist than that they represent the role of environmental experiences in facilitating developmental changes.

REFERENCES

Aslin, R. (1981). Experiential influences and sensitive periods in development. In R. Aslin, J. Alberts, & M. Peterson (Eds.), *Development of perception* (Vol. 2, pp. 45–93). New York: Academic Press.

Banks, M., Aslin, R., & Letson, R. (1975). Sensitive period for the development of human binocular vision. *Science, 190*, 675–677.

Bertenthal, B., & Campos, J. (1984). A reexamination of fear and its determinants on the visual cliff. *Psychophysiology, 21*, 413–417.

Bertenthal, B., Campos, J., & Barrett, K. (1984). Self-produced locomotion: An organizer of emotional, cognitive, and social development in infancy. In R. Emde & R. Harmon (Eds.), *Continuities and discontinuities in development* (pp. 175–210). New York: Plenum.

Bowlby, J. (1973). *Attachment and loss: Vol. 2. Separation.* New York: Basic.

Campos, J., Benson, J., & Rudy, L. (1986). *The role of self-produced locomotion in spatial behavior.* Paper read at the meetings of the International Conference on Infant Studies, Beverly Hills, CA.

Campos, J., Hiatt, S., Ramsay, D., Henderson, C., & Svejda, M. (1978). The emergence of fear on the visual cliff. In M. Lewis & L. Rosenblum (Eds.), *The development of affect* (pp. 149–182). New York: Plenum.

Colombo, J. (1982). The critical period concept: Research, methodology, and theoretical issues. *Psychological Bulletin, 91,* 260–275.

Emde, R., Gaensbauer, T., & Harmon, R. (1976). Emotional expression in infancy: A biobehavioral study. *Psychological Issues* (Vol. 10, No. 37). New York: International Universities Press.

Freedman, D. (1974). *Human infancy: An evolutionary perspective.* Hillsdale, NJ: Erlbaum.

Ganz, L. (1978). Sensory deprivation and visual discrimination. In R. Held, H. Leibowitz, & H. Teuber (Eds.), *Handbook of sensory physiology: Vol. 8. Perception* (pp. 437–488). Berlin: Springer-Verlag.

Gottlieb, G. (1983). The psychobiological approach to developmental issues. In M. Haith & J. Campos (Eds.), *Infancy and developmental psychobiology* (pp. 1–26). New York: Wiley.

Greenough, W., Black, J., & Wallace, C. (1987). Experience and brain development. *Child Development, 58,* 539–559.

Hecaen, H. (1976). Acquired aphasia in children and the ontogenesis of hemispheric functional specialization. *Brain and Language, 3,* 114–134.

Held, R., & Hein, A. (1963). Movement-produced stimulation in the development of visually guided behavior. *Journal of Comparative and Physiological Psychology, 81,* 394–398.

Hohmann, A., & Creutzfeldt, O. (1975). Squint and the development of binocularity in humans. *Nature, 254,* 613–614.

Hubel, D. (1972). Effects of distortion of sensory input on the visual system of kittens. In D. Singh & C. Morgan (Eds.), *Current status of physiological psychology: Readings* (pp. 296–315). Monterey, CA: Brooks-Cole.

Kagan, J. (1976). Emergent themes in human development. *American Scientist, 64,* 186–196.

Kagan, J., Kearsley, R., & Zelazo, P. (1978). *Infancy: Its place in human development.* Cambridge, MA: Harvard University Press.

Kermoian, R. (1986). *Locomotor experience and spatial search.* Paper read at the biennial meetings of the Developmental Psychobiology Research Group, Estes Park, CO.

Lenneberg, E. (1967). *The biological foundations of language.* New York: Wiley.

Lerner, R. (1984). *On the nature of human plasticity.* Cambridge: Cambridge University Press.

Money, J., & Ehrhardt, A. (1972). *Man and woman, boy and girl.* Baltimore: Johns Hopkins University Press.

Richards, J., & Rader, N. (1981). Crawling-onset age predicts visual-cliff avoidance in human infants. *Child Development,* 51, 61–68.

Richards, J., & Rader, N. (1983). Affective, behavioral, and avoidance responses on the visual cliff: Effects of crawling onset age, crawling experience, and testing age. *Psychophysiology,* 20, 633–642.

Scarr, S., & Salapatek, P. (1970). Patterns of fear development during infancy. *Merrill-Palmer Quarterly,* 16, 53–90.

Telzrow, R., Campos, J., & Bertenthal, B. (1986). *Spatial search follows the acquisition of self-produced locomotion in motorically delayed meningomyelocele infants.* Paper read at the meetings of the MacArthur Network on the Transition from Infancy to Early Childhood, Chatham, MA.

Walk, R., & Gibson, E. (1961). A comparative and analytical study of visual depth perception. *Psychological Monographs,* 75 (Whole No. 519).

3

Sin, Sickness, or Status? Homosexual Gender Identity and Psychoneuroendocrinology

John Money

Johns Hopkins University and Hospital, Baltimore, Maryland

Devised animal experiments show conclusively that sex hormones influence the male/female dimorphism of the brain, prenatally, in four possible ways, namely, masculinizing, demasculinizing, feminizing, and defeminizing. The human counterparts of devised animal experiments are clinical intersexual (hermaphroditic) syndromes that occur spontaneously as experiments of nature. The two sources of data supplement one another. Both lead to the conclusion that prenatal hormonalization of the brain influences the subsequent sexual status or orientation as bisexual, heterosexual, or homosexual. This effect is more robot-like in subprimate than in primate species. As in subhuman primates, in the human species sexuoerotic status is dependent not only on prenatal hormonalization, but also on postnatal socialization effects. There are several different human hermaphroditic syndromes, each of which makes its own specific contribution to the science of homosexology and to

Reprinted with permission from *American Psychologist,* 1987, Vol. 42, No. 4, 384–399. Copyright 1987 by the American Psychological Association, Inc.

Editor's note. This article was originally presented as a Distinguished Scientific Award for the Applications of Psychology award address at the meeting of the American Psychological Association in Washington, DC, August 1986.

Award addresses, submitted by award recipients, are published as received except for minor editorial changes designed to maintain *American Psychologist* format. This reflects a policy of recognizing distinguished award recipients by eliminating the usual editorial review process to provide a forum consistent with that employed in delivering the award address.

Research on which the award was based was supported by U.S. Public Health Service Grant HD00325 and by Grant 830–86900 from the William T. Grant Foundation.

the understanding of genetic, prenatal-hormonal, pubertal-hormonal, and socialization determinants of being gay, straight, or bisexual. In combination, they indicate that sexual orientation is not under the direct governance of chromosomes and genes, and that, whereas it is not foreordained by prenatal brain hormonalization, it is influenced thereby, and is also strongly dependent on postnatal socialization. The latter is, like native language, programmed into the brain through the senses. Postnatal programming may become incorporated into the brain's immutable biology.

HISTORICAL AND CULTURAL RELATIVITY

The phenomenon that is today named homosexuality did not have that name until it was coined by K. M. Benkert, writing under the pseudonym of Kertbeny, in 1869. Though he applied the term *homosexuality* to both males and females, he defined it on the criterion of erectile failure:

> In addition to the normal sexual urge in men and women, Nature in her sovereign mood has endowed at birth certain male and female individuals with the homosexual urge, thus placing them in a sexual bondage which renders them physically and psychically incapable—even with the best intention—of normal erection. This urge creates in advance a direct horror of the opposite sex, and the victim of this passion finds it impossible to suppress the feeling which individuals of his own sex exercise upon him. (Benkert, 1869, quoted in Bullough, 1976, p. 637)

Instead of the criterion of genital sexuality, as in homo*sexual*, Benkert could have used the criterion of falling in love, as in homo*philic*, or the criterion of being attracted to those of the same sex, as in homo*genic*. Both terms were proposed by others, but homosexual won the day, probably because it was taken up in the early years of the 20th century by Havelock Ellis and Magnus Hirschfeld (Ellis, 1942; Hirschfeld, 1948). Neither of these two writers recognized that the ethnocentricity of Benkert's definition of homosexuality as a sickness, though freeing it from being a sin or a crime, confines it too narrowly to pathological deviancy. It leaves no place for homosexuality as a status that is culturally ordained to be normal and healthy, as it is in societies that have, since time immemorial, institutionalized bisexuality. In bisexuality, homosexuality and heterosexuality may coexist concurrently, or they may be sequential, with a homosexual phase of development antecedent to heterosexuality and marriage. Concurrent bisexuality was exemplified in classical Athenian culture (Bullough, 1976). Sequential bisexuality is exemplified in various tribal Melanesian and related cultures.

There is vast area of the world, stretching from the northwestern tip of Sumatra through Papua-New Guinea to the outlying islands of Melanesia in the Pacific, in which the social institutionalization of homosexuality is shared by various ethnic and tribal people (Herdt, 1984; Money & Ehrhardt, 1972). More precisely, it is sequential bisexuality that is institutionalized in these societies. Their cultural tradition dictates that males between the ages of 9 and 19 reside no longer with their families but in the single long-house in the village center where males congregate. Until the age of 19, the prescribed age of marriage, they all participate in homosexual activities. After marriage, homosexual activity either ceases or is sporadic.

The Sambia people (Herdt, 1981) of the eastern highlands of New Guinea are among those whose traditional folk wisdom provided a rationale for the policy of prepubertal homosexuality. According to this wisdom, a prepubertal boy must leave the society of his mother and sisters and enter the secret society of men in order to achieve the fierce manhood of a head hunter. Whereas in infancy he must have been fed woman's milk in order to grow, in the secret society of men he must be fed men's milk—that is, the semen of mature youths and unmarried men—in order to become pubertal and grow mature himself. It is the duty of the young bachelors to feed him their semen. They are obliged to practice institutionalized pedophilia. For them to give their semen to another who could already ejaculate his own is forbidden, for it robs a prepubertal boy of the substance he requires to become an adult. When a bachelor reaches the marrying age, his family negotiates the procurement of a wife and arranges the marriage. He then embarks on the heterosexual phase of his career. He could not, however, have become a complete man on the basis of heterosexual experience alone. Full manhood necessitates a prior phase of exclusively homosexual experience. Thus, homosexuality is universalized and is a defining characteristic of head-hunting, macho manhood.

In Sambia culture, omission of, rather than participation in, the homosexual development phase would be classified as sporadic in occurrence, if it occurred at all, and would stigmatize a man as deviant. In our own culture, by contrast, it is homosexual participation that is classified as sporadic and stigmatized as a deviancy in need of explanation. For us, heterosexuality, like health, is taken as a verity that needs no explanation, other than being attributed to the immutability of the natural order of things. Because heterosexuality needs no explanation, then in bisexuality the homosexual component alone needs explanation. Consequently, there has been no satisfactory place for bisexuality in theoretical sexology. The universalization of sequential bisexuality, as in the Sambia tradition, is unexplainable in homosexual theory that is based exclusively on the concept of homosexuality as sporadic in occurrence and pathologically deviant (Stoller & Herdt, 1985).

Institutionalized homosexuality, in serial sequence with institutionalized heterosexuality and marriage, as among the Sambia and other tribal peoples, must be taken into account in any theory that proposes to explain homosexuality. The theory will be deficient unless it takes heterosexuality into account also. Culturally institutionalized bisexuality signifies either that bisexuality is a universal potential to which any member of the human species can be acculturated or that bisexuality is a unique potential of those cultures whose members have become selectively inbred for it. There are no data that give conclusive and absolute support to either alternative. However, genetically pure inbred strains are an ideal of animal husbandry, not of human social and sexual interaction. Therefore, it is likely that acculturation to bisexuality is less a concomitant of inbreeding than it is of the bisexual plasticity of all members of the human species. It is possible that bisexual plasticity may vary over the life span. Later in life it may give way to exclusive monosexuality—or it may not.

PREFERENCE VERSUS STATUS OR ORIENTATION

In the human species, a person does not prefer to be homosexual instead of heterosexual, nor to be bisexual instead of monosexual. *Sexual preference* is a moral and political term. Conceptually it implies voluntary choice, that is, that one chooses, or prefers, to be homosexual instead of heterosexual or bisexual, and vice versa. Politically, sexual preference is a dangerous term, for it implies that if homosexuals choose their preference, then they can be legally forced, under threat of punishment, to choose to be heterosexual.

The concept of voluntary choice is as much in error here as in its application to handedness or to native language. You do not choose your native language as a preference, even though you are born without it. You assimilate it into a brain prenatally made ready to receive a native language from those who constitute your primate troop and who speak it to you and listen to you when you speak it. Once assimilated through the ears into the brain, a native language becomes securely locked in—as securely as if it had been phylogenetically preordained to be locked in prenatally by a process of genetic determinism or by the determinism of fetal hormonal or other brain chemistries. So also, sexual status or orientation, whatever its genesis, may become assimilated and locked into the brain as monosexually homosexual or heterosexual or as bisexually a mixture of both.

A sexual status (or orientation) is not the same as a sexual act. It is possible to participate in, or be subjected to, a homosexual act or acts without, thereby, becoming predestined to have, as a consequence, a homosexual status, and vice versa with heterosexuality. The Skyscraper Test exemplifies the difference between act and status. One of the versions of this test applies to a person with a homosexual status who is atop the Empire State Building or other high building and is pushed to the edge of the parapet by a gun-toting, crazed sex terrorist with a heterosexual status. Suppose the homosexual is a man and the terrorist a woman who demands that he perform oral sex with her or go over the edge. To save his life, he might do it. If so, he would have performed a heterosexual act, but he would not have changed to have a heterosexual status. The same would apply, vice versa, if the tourist was a straight man and the terrorist a gay man, and so on.

This Skyscraper Test, by dramatizing the difference between act and status, points to the criterion of falling in love as the definitive criterion of homosexual, heterosexual, and bisexual status. A person with a homosexual status is one who has the potential to fall in love only with someone who has the same genital and bodily morphology as the self. For a heterosexual, the morphology must be that of a person of the other sex. For the bisexual it may be either.

It is not necessary for the masculine or feminine bodily morphology of the partner to be concordant with the chromosomal sex, the gonadal sex, or the sex of the internal reproductive anatomy. For example, a male-to-female, sex-reassigned transsexual with the body morphology transformed to be female in appearance is responded to as a woman—and vice versa in female-to-male transsexualism.

Discordance between the body morphology and other variables of sex occurs also in some cases of intersexuality. For example, it is possible to be born with a penis and empty scrotum and to grow up with a fully virilized body and mentality, both discordant with the genetic sex (46,XX), the gonadal sex (two normal ovaries), and the internal sexual structures (uterus and oviducts). Conversely, it is possible to be born with a female vulva and to grow up with a fully feminized body and mentality, both discordant with the genetic sex (46,XY), the gonadal sex (two testes), and the internal sexual structures (vestigated feminine mullerian-duct structures and differentiated masculine wolffian-duct structures). Clinical photographic examples of these syndromes, and many others, are reproduced in Money (1986b, 1974).

The 46,XX intersexed man who falls in love with and has a sex life with a 46,XX normal woman is regarded by everyone as heterosexual, and so is his partner. The criterion of their heterosexuality is the sexual morphology of their bodies and the masculinity or femininity of their mentality and behavior, not the sex of their chromosomes, gonads, or internal organs. The same principle applies conversely in the case of the feminized 46,XY intersexed woman whose sex life is with a normal 46,XY man.

EVOLUTIONARY BISEXUALITY

Any theory of the genesis of either exclusive homosexuality or exclusive heterosexuality must address primarily the genesis of bisexuality. Monosexuality, whether homosexual or heterosexual, is secondary and a derivative of the primary bisexual or ambisexual potential. Ambisexuality has its origins in evolutionary biology and in the embryology of sexual differentiation.

Ambisexuality has many manifestations in evolutionary biology. Oysters, garden worms, and snails, for example, are ambisexual. They are also classified as bisexual and as hermaphroditic. There are many species of fish capable of changing their sex from female to male, or from male to female, in some species more than once (Chan, 1977). The change is so complete that the fish spends part of its life breeding as a male with testicles that make sperms and part as a female with ovaries that make eggs—an exceptionally thorough degree of sequential bisexuality.

There is a species of whiptail lizard from the Southwest, *Cnemedophorus uniparens,* that offers a unique contribution to bisexual theory (Crews, 1982, in press). This species has neither males nor females but is monecious and parthenogenic. Nonetheless, as judged by comparison with closely related two-sexed whiptail species, each individual lizard is able at different times to behave as if a male and as if a female in mating. The one in whom a clutch of eggs is ripening, ready to be laid in the sand for sun-hatching, is mounted by a mate whose ovaries are in a dormant, nonovulatory phase. This enactment is believed to affect the hormonal function of the pituitary of the ovulating lizard and to facilitate reproduction. At a later date, their roles reverse.

In this parthenogenic reptilian species, the brain is bisexual or ambisexual, even though the pelvic reproductive anatomy is not. According to MacLean's evolutionary theory of the triune brain, the mammalian brain is made up of an evolutionary ancient reptilian brain overlaid by a paleocortex that is shared by all mammals, and that in turn is overlaid by the neocortex, which is most highly evolved in the human species (MacLean, 1972). Thus, the behavorial bisexuality of parthenogenic whiptail lizards may provide a key to understanding the bisexual potential of mammalian species.

It has long been known that the mammalian embryo, in the early stages of its development, is sexually bipotential. The undifferentiated gonads differentiate into either testes or ovaries. Thereafter, the Eve principle triumphs over the Adam principle: Sexual differentiation proceeds to be that of a female unless masculinizing hormones are added, normally by being secreted by the fetal testes. One of the two masculinizing hormones from the fetal testes is actually a defeminizing hormone, MIH (mullerian inhibiting hormone). It has a brief life span during which it vestigiates the two mullerian ducts and prevents them from developing into a uterus and fallopian tubes (oviducts). The other hormone masculinizes. It is testosterone (or one of its metabolites). It presides over the two wolffian ducts and directs their development into the male internal accessory organs, including the prostate gland and seminal vesicles.

Differentiation of the internal genitalia is ambitypic. That is, the male and female anlagen are both present to begin with, after which one set vestigiates while the other set proliferates (Figure 1). By contrast, differentiation of the external genitalia is unitypic. That is, there is a single set of anlagen which have two possible destinies, namely, to become either male or female (Figure 2). Thus, the clitoris and the penis are homologues of one another, as are the clitoral hood and the penile foreskin. The tissues that become the labia minora in the female wrap around the penis in the male and fuse along the midline of the underside to form the tubular urethra. The swellings that otherwise form the divided labia majora of the female fuse in the midline to form the scrotum of the male.

The Adam principle as applied to hormonal induction of sexual dimorphism of the genitalia applies also to dimorphism of the brain and its governance of the genitalia and their functioning. According to present evidence, hormone-induced brain dimorphism takes place later than that of the genitalia, and, dependent on the species, may extend into the first few days or weeks of postnatal life. The primary masculinizing hormone is testosterone, though it is not necessarily used in all parts of the brain as such. Within brain cells themselves, as within cells of the pelvic genitalia, it may be reduced to dihydrotestosterone. Paradoxically, it may also exert its masculinizing action only if first aromatized into estradiol, one of the sex steroids that received its name when it was considered to be exclusively an estrogenic, feminizing hormone. In both sexes, estradiol is metabolized from testosterone, which, in turn, is metabolized from progesterone, of which the antecedent is the steroidal substance, cholesterol, from which all of the steroidal hormones are derived.

On the basis of animal experimental studies of the effects of the prenatal brain hormonalization on subsequent sexually dimorphic behavior, it is now generally acknowledged that the converse of brain masculinization is not feminization but demasculinization. The converse of feminization is defeminization. It is possible for masculinization to take place with defeminization, and for feminization to take place without demasculinization (Baum, 1979;

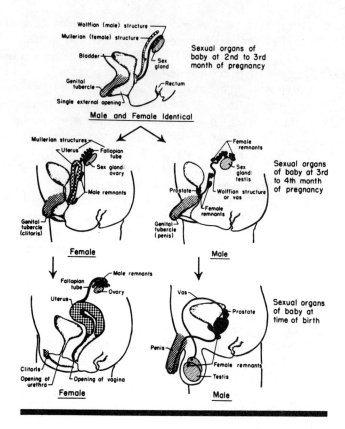

Figure 1. Cross-sectional diagrams to illustrate internal, ambi-typic genital differentiation in the human fetus.

Baum, Gallagher, Martin, & Damassa, 1982; Beach, 1975; Ward, 1972, 1984; Ward & Weisz, 1980; Whalen & Edwards, 1967). That means that the differentiation of sexual dimorphism in the brain is not unitypic, like that of the external genitalia, but ambitypic, like that of the internal genitalia. Ambitypic differentiation allows for the possible coexistence of both masculine and feminine nuclei and pathways, and the behavior they govern, in some if not all parts of the brain. The two need not necessarily have equality. One may be more dominant than the other. To illustrate, when cows in a herd are in season, the central nervous system functions in such a way as to permit cow to mount cow, whereas when a bull is present, the cow is receptive and the bull does the mounting. Mounting is traditionally defined as

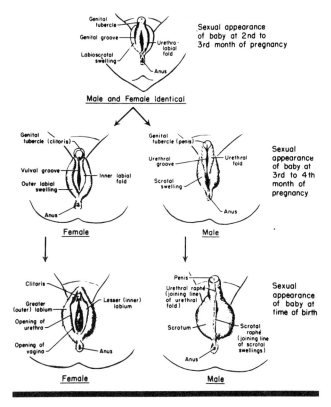

Figure 2. Diagrams to illustrate external, unitypic genital differentiation in the human fetus.

masculine behavior, but it would be more accurately defined as ambisexual, because it is shared by both sexes. On the criterion of mounting, cows are bisexual insofar as they mount and are mounted. Bulls are less so, insofar as they are seldom mounted.

The first evidence of the hormonal induction of sexual dimorphism in the brain was inferred from its effects on behavior. The first experiment was done by Eugen Steinach early in the 20th century (Steinach, 1940). He demonstrated that the mating behavior of female guinea pigs would be masculinized if, in fetal life, they had been exposed to male hormone injected into the pregnant mother. The theoretical implications of Steinach's finding were too advanced for their time. They lay dormant until William C. Young replicated the experiment in the 1950s (Young, Goy, & Phoenix, 1964). Since then, there has developed a whole new science of hormone-brain-behavior dimorphism.

By the 1970s it had become evident that hormone-mediated dimorphism of the brain was no longer an inference based on sexually dimorphic behavior, but an actuality that could be neuroanatomically demonstrated directly in brain tissue. In 1969, Dörner and Staudt reported that the nuclear volume of nerve cells in the preoptic area and ventromedial nucleus in the rat hypothalamus was larger in females than in males and that androgen administered in late prenatal and early neonatal life would reduce the volume of these cells in females and castrated males. In 1971, Raisman and Field reported their discovery of sexual dimorphism in the dendritic synapses of the preoptic area of the rat brain. Thus began a new era of research into the prenatal hormone determinants of sex differences in the neuroanatomy of those regions of the brain that mediate mating behavior (see reviews by Arnold & Gorski, 1984; De Voogd, 1986; De Vries, De Brun, Uylings, & Corner, 1984).

Confirmatory findings followed in quick succession. In rats, Gorski and his research colleagues found and named the sexually dimorphic nucleus of the preoptic area (SDN-POA; Gorski, Gordon, Shryne, & Southam, 1978). Corresponding sexually dimorphic tissues in the human brain Gorski referred to as interstitial nuclei of the anterior hypothalamus. The SDN-POA of male rats is bigger than that of females and becomes so under the influence of steroid hormone from the testes (testosterone or its metabolite, estradiol) during the critical period of the first few days after birth (Döhler et al., 1982). Also in rats, Breedlove and Arnold (1980) discovered sexual dimorphism in the number of motor neurons innervating the perineal muscles and that it is during the critical period of the first few days after birth that the larger number of these motor neurons in males is produced by the presence of steroid hormone from the testes (Breedlove, 1986).

In songbirds, as well as in rats, the presence of testicular hormone during a brief critical period proved to be the determinant in the male brain of the neuroanatomy that governs song (Nottebohm & Arnold, 1976). In the zebra finch, testicular hormone exerts its masculinizing effect once and forever during the early critical period. There is no backtracking. The song pattern of the first spring singing season persists unchanged in subsequent years. In the canary, by contrast, the entire process is reactivated each spring, which allows the male to change his song and learn a new one each year instead of having only the one that he learned in the first year of life. An adult female, provided she is treated with steroid hormone, is able to learn a song for the first time as an adult. Learning the song first as a newly hatched nestling is not imperative. Male songbirds copy the song they hear in the nest even though they do not sing it until weeks later.

The findings with respect to canary song demonstrate a type of sexual dimorphism in which the ambisexual window is not forever closed after the neonatal critical period, but it reopened annually. Thus a canary of either sex may sing one year but not the next, depending on the degree of steroidal hormonalization of the sexually dimorphic brain in the springtime of each year. As songsters, canaries thus have the possibility of being serially, rather than concurrently, bisexual.

Concurrent bisexuality would require two coexistent, dimorphic neuroanatomical systems, one subserving masculine and one feminine dimorphism of behavior—for example, mounting and lordosing, respectively. In rat experiments, Nordeen and Yahr (1982) found such a duality in the form of hemispheric asymmetry in the neighborhood of the sexually dimorphic nucleus of the preoptic area of the hypothalamus. They implanted pellets of the steroid hormone estradiol separately into the left and right sides of the hypothalamus of newborn female rat pups. The subsequent effect of the hormone on the left side was to defeminize—that is, to suppress lordosis— and on the right side to masculinize—that is, to facilitate mounting behavior—after the rats became mature.

The lateral distribution in the brain of masculine to the right and feminine to the left means that the two sides may develop to be either concordant (one masculinized and the other defeminized, or one feminized and the other demasculinized) or discordant (one masculinized and the other feminized, or one demasculinized and the other defeminized). Disparities may come into being on the basis of the amount of hormone needed by and available to each side; the timing of its availability to each side; the synchrony or dissynchrony of the hormonal programming on each side; and the pulsatility or continuity of the hormonal supply on each side. Thus, there are alternative ways in which one side could be rendered masculine and the other feminine to a sufficient degree to constitute bisexuality. Likewise, there are alternative ways in which the brain may be masculinized when the genitals are feminized, or vice versa, so as to constitute homosexuality.

These alternative ways of predisposing the brain to be either bisexual or homosexual can, of course, be manipulated experimentally. They may also occur adventitiously as an unrecognized side effect of hormone imbalance secondary to nutritional, medicinal, or endocrine changes, including stress-derived changes, in the pregnant mother's bloodstream. Sleeping pills containing barbiturate, for example, may have a demasculinizing effect on the brain of the human fetus, because the drug has been shown to have such an effect on male rat pups (reviewed in Reinisch & Saunders, 1982). Also in rats, maternal stress that alters maternal adrenocortical hormones may exert a prenatal demasculinizing effect on male pups, subsequently evident in their bisexual and homosexual mating behavior (Ward, 1984).

The dramatic power of the steroid hormones in prenatal life to foreordain the sexual orientation and mating behavior of adult life has been illustrated in several laboratory species in experiments in which fetal females are hormonally masculinized or males demasculinized. The hormonal intervention may be timed so as to change the sex first of the external genitalia and then of the brain or to spare the external genitalia and change the brain only.

There is remarkable film (Short & Clarke, undated; see Clarke, 1977) that shows how the brains and behavior of ewe lambs, independently of their bodies, can be masculinized in utero by injecting the pregnant mother with testosterone at the critical period of gestation, Day 50 and thereafter. The lamb grows up to be a lesbian ewe. Its brain is so effectively masculinized that its mating behavior (and its urinating behavior also), including mating rivalry and the proceptive courtship ritual, is exactly like that of a ram, even though, at the same time, its own ovaries are secreting estrogen, not androgen. Moreover, the normal rams and ewes of the flock respond to the lesbian ewe's masculinized mating behavior as if it were that of a normal ram.

Sheep, cattle, and swine (reviewed by D'Occhio & Ford, in press) and other four-legged species are, more or less, hormonal robots insofar as a masculine or a feminine mating pattern can be foreordained on the basis of regulating the prenatal hormonalization of the brain. Even among sheep, however, the final outcome will be influenced by whether the lamb grew up in a normal flock of ewes and rams or in a sex-segregated herd. Primates are even more influenced by the social conditions of growing up and are less subject to hormonal robotization.

In the now well-known hermaphrodite experiments from the primate centers in Oregon and Wisconsin, female rhesus monkeys were masculinized prenatally so that they were born with a penis and empty scrotum. Though they engaged in tomboyish play in childhood, unlike the sheep they did not grow up to mature sexually as lesbians. According to the evidence available, the postpubertal sexological outcome of prenatal hormonalization was modulated, in some degree, by the social conditions of their rearing in a coeducational as opposed to an all-male or all-female group of age mates (Goldfoot, 1977; Goldfoot & Neff, in press; Goldfoot & Wallen, 1978; Goldfoot, Wallen, Neff, McBrair, & Goy, 1984).

Social rearing was not, however, the only factor that influenced the sexological outcome. Other factors proved to be age at testing; whether intact or castrated; if castrated, whether primed with estradiol or testosterone as a replacement hormone; hormonal dosage; and sex of the partner (Phoenix &

Chambers, 1982; Phoenix, Jensen, & Chambers, 1983). Taking into consideration these different variables, it has become evident that masculinized mating behavior, with an estrus female partner, may be a sequel to prenatal hormonal masculinization but is far from being an inevitable one, irrespective of whether the hermaphroditic animals had their own ovaries intact or had been ovariectomized and treated with replacement estradiol or with replacement testosterone. On testosterone, the younger they were, the more they were likely to get an erection, but the prevalence of intromission and of the movements of ejaculation (without semen) was, though not zero, very low.

There were no youthful tests of the effect of prenatal masculinizing on the effect of pairing the hermaphrodite with a male partner. The hermaphrodites had no external vaginal opening and could not be given one by plastic surgery because they would have mutilated the postsurgical wound. Themselves aggressive, the hermaphrodites were at risk of attacking and of being attacked by a male partner. At a later age, this risk was circumvented by using partners of proven gentleness, namely, aged monkey eunuchs treated with testosterone. The hermaphrodites and the control females were treated with estradiol, because both groups had a history of having been ovariectomized. In this experiment, the hermaphrodites were sexologically not different from the controls in responding to the males as females. The males mounted them both but were able to achieve intromission and ejaculation only with the control females, in view of the fact that the hermaphrodites had no vaginal opening.

The conclusion from the foregoing is that, in a primate species, prenatal hormonal masculinization (a) although it is compatible with subsequent masculinized mating, does not ensure it, and (b) although it does not guarantee feminized mating, does not obliterate it. Masculinized and feminized mating responses may coexist in an experimentally manipulated manifestation of monkey bisexuality.

INTERSEXUALITY AND BISEXUALITY

Although the sequential influence of prenatal hormonal and postnatal rearing effects cannot be studied experimentally by inducing intersexuality in human beings, it can be studied in the so-called experiments of nature, namely, the syndromes of intersexual and other birth defects of the sex organs. These are the syndromes that are known collectively by the term *hermaphroditism* as well as by its synonym, *intersexuality.* They are augmented by syndromes of agenesis of the sex organs, as in congenital absence of the penis and in congenital micropenis, and by syndromes of traumatic or surgical loss of the genitalia.

By definition, intersexuality, and likewise its synonym, hermaphroditism, signifies ambiguity as to whether an individual is male or female. In the human species, as in all mammals, it is not possible to be both male and female, either simultaneously or sequentially. Intersexual ambiguity means, therefore, that the multiple criteria of sex are not consistently either all male or all female, but that there is some degree of inconsistency or incongruity among them. The criteria of sex are as follows (Money, 1955; Money, Hampson, & Hampson, 1955): chromosomal sex, H-Y antigenic sex, gonadal sex, prenatal hormonal sex, internal genital sex, external genital sex, pubertal hormonal sex, assigned sex and rearing, and gender-identity/role (G-I/R; see also *Dorland's Illustrated Medical Dictionary,* 1981).

In some instances, intersexuality is concealed: The external genitalia appear to conform to the criterion of being either male or female but are inconsistent with all or part of the internal reproductive anatomy. In other instances, intersexuality is visible as ambiguity of the external genitals: What might be a penile clitoris might also be a clitoridic penis, and what might be labial fusion might also be a labioscrotum. Internally, the reproductive structures may be predominantly either male or female.

Discordances among the criteria of sex, as manifest in intersex syndromes, can be explained embryologically in terms of the Adam/Eve principle, as mentioned earlier. Incomplete or partial masculinization of the external genitalia leaves a protuberant penoclitoris (or clitoropenis) with an open gutter on its underside and a urogenital opening or funnel at its base. This ambiguous condition is named hypospadias if the individual is designated as a male and surgically corrected as a male. Correspondingly, the same condition is named partial urogenital fusion with clitoromegaly if the individual is designated as a female and surgically corrected as a female. In such cases among the newborn, the final intersexual (or hermaphroditic) diagnosis cannot be established by visually inspecting the "unfinished," birth-defective genitalia. The diagnosis is not necessarily the final criterion of the sex to which the baby would best be assigned, reared, and clinically habilitated. It is on this account, and because, historically, medical opinion has not been unanimous regarding the sex of assignment in cases of birth defect of the sex organs, that science has serendipitously been provided with matched pairs of two or more cases that are concordant for prenatal history and diagnosis but discordant for postnatal history and treatment.

There are two grand strategies for utilizing intersexual cases to investigate the genesis of homosexual, bisexual, or heterosexual status. One is the group-comparison method. The other is the matched-pair method.

The group-comparison strategy requires a sufficient number of individuals with the same diagnosis to constitute a diagnostically homogeneous sample—

homogeneous for intersexual diagnosis. It is compared with either a matched clinical control group or a matched normal control group, or both. The clinical control group is homogeneous for its own diagnosis, which is specifically selected because of either its similarity to or divergence from the primary research sample. The investigative design allows status (or orientation) in adulthood as homosexual, bisexual, or heterosexual to be the dependent variable. It is compared with the other variables or determinants of sex from conception onward, namely, chromosomal sex, H-Y antigen, gonadal sex, prenatal hormonal sex, internal morphologic sex, external morphologic sex, assigned sex and rearing, and pubertal hormonal sex.

The paired-comparison strategy matches pairs or sets of pairs of individuals who are intersexually concordant for prenatal etiology and diagnosis but discordant for sex of assignment and rearing, and compares them with respect to adult homosexual, bisexual, or heterosexual status. The paired-comparison strategy may also be applied to intersexed individuals who are concordant for sex of rearing and for some, though not all, of the other variables of sex—for example, genetic sex and gonadal sex may be male in one case (androgen-insensitivity syndrome) and female in another (Rokitansky syndrome), with the other variables of sex in both cases being female.

In the 19th century, the nomenclature of intersexuality was assigned on the criterion of the gonads (Klebs, 1876). When both ovarian and testicular tissues were found, either separately or combined in an ovotestis, the diagnosis was true hermaphroditism. If both gonads were ovarian, the diagnosis was female pseudohermaphroditism, and if both were testicular, male pseudohermaphroditism. Today the prefix pseudo- is falling into disuse because it is redundant and also incorrectly implies that the condition is not authentically intersexual. Today it is also know that intersexuality may exist in the presence of vestigial gonads that are neither ovarian nor testicular. Contemporary classification of intersexuality tends increasingly to reflect advances in etiological knowledge of inborn errors of hormonal synthesis (21-hydroxylase deficiency in female hermaphroditism, and 5 α-reductase deficiency in male hermaphroditism, for example) or hormonal metabolism (intracellular inability to use androgen in the androgen-insensitivity syndrome of male hermaphroditism, for example).

A diagnosis on the basis of endocrine etiology is currently more readily established in the case of female than male hermaphroditism, true hermaphroditism, or agonadal hermaphroditism. Especially in the case of male hermaphroditism, the method of establishing an etiological diagnosis today is not a routine procedure, but a research laboratory one. In addition, there are some cases of male hermaphroditism for which an etiological diagnosis has not yet been established. Thus, for a given etiological diagnosis, the available sample may be small, in which case the paired-comparison strategy takes precedence over the group-comparison strategy. In female hermaphroditism, by contrast, there are fewer limitations on assembling a larger sample group, specifically in the case of the adrenogenital syndrome, the most prevalent form of female hermaphroditism. However, there are also some less common varieties of female hermaphroditism, as discussed in the following sections.

ANDROGEN-INDUCED HERMAPHRODITISM

The least commonly recorded variety of female hermaphroditism is that in which an embryonically normal female is hormonally masculinized prenatally in fetal life by an excess of androgen that passes through the placenta from the mother's bloodstream. The excess androgen has its most likely source in an androgen-secreting ovarian or adrenocortical tumor that becomes hormonally active in the mother during the course of the pregnancy. In the fetus, embryonic differentiation of fertile ovaries is not affected. Unlike testes, ovaries make no mullerian-inhibiting hormone, so the mullerian ducts do not vestigiate but differentiate into a uterus and oviducts. Differentiation of the external genitalia, by contrast, is profoundly altered by the excess of androgen. The clitoris becomes hypertrophied so as to become a penile clitoris with incomplete fusion and a urogenital sinus or, if fusion is complete, a penis with urethra and an empty scrotum.

According to the principle of the statistics of extremes, only one case of this type would be needed to break the stranglehold of the traditional dogma that sexual orientation and erotic status in adulthood are innately and genetically preordained by the gonads and their hormonal functioning at puberty. To break the stranglehold, it would be necessary to have a case in which, at birth, the baby was assigned, reared, and clinically habilitated as a boy. The latter would entail surgery to masculinize the external genitalia. To prevent hormonal feminization (breasts and menses) at puberty would require either surgical removal of the ovaries or treatment with testosterone to suppress their secretion of female hormones. Testosterone treatment would induce pubertal virilization. It would then be necessary to follow the case to adulthood in order to establish that the erotosexual status and sex life were those of a man.

That was, indeed, the outcome not only in one such case (Money, 1967; Money et al., 1955) but in two, the second unpublished. In each case, the individual grew up to be an adult who was universally accepted by his professional peers and friends as a man, by his wife as a husband, and by his adopted children as a father, not notably different from other fathers in the kinship or the community. Absolutely no one ever thought of either of these individuals as being lesbian, or even as bisexual.

Their lives have great value for homosexological theory. With a different postnatal social and clinical history, they could have grown up, as others like them have done, to become women, wives, and mothers who carried their own pregnancies. Instead, they grew to adulthood with a heterosexual orientation or status as men. Their masculine orientation may have been facilitated by some degree of prenatal hormonal masculinization of the brain in parallel with the prenatal hormonal masculinization of the external genitals. It may also have been facilitated by the clinical intervention, at the time of the spontaneous onset of ovarian puberty, to arrest breast enlargement and put an end to menstruation through the penis. Hormones and surgery notwithstanding, their adult status as men was certainly not only facilitated by but developmentally engendered by the cumulative influences of their having been reared and socialized as boys.

Cases like these two demonstrate that both prenatal hormonal and postnatal social factors contribute to adult erotosexual status; but they do not spell out the details as they might apply to nonintersexed, morphologically normal girls who grow up, in the absence of hormonal masculinization, to be lesbians. No one yet knows what, if any, covert prenatal hormonal influences may predispose to lesbianism in anatomically normal girls. In addition, no one yet knows the social-learning formula, if there is one, that will unfailingly guarantee lesbianism as the outcome, with or without a predisposition. Conjectures and hypotheses that have been put forward have not been confirmed. They exist only as doctrines and dogmas.

PROGESTIN-INDUCED HERMAPHRODITISM

There is one form of human intersexuality that resembles an experiment of nature but is actually an experiment of iatrogenic trial and error. The error in this instance occurred when in the 1940s newly synthesized steroid hormones came on the market (McGary, 1987). Though they eventually proved to share both adrogenic and progestinic properties, as well as chemical structure, they were initially prescribed as a progesterone substitute in the belief, false as it turned out, that they would prevent threatened miscarriage. In a small minority of unexplained cases, the external sex organs of a female fetus were masculinized, so that they had an intersexual external genital appearance. With very rare exceptions, the babies were assigned and surgically corrected as girls. They needed no hormonal treatment to develop at puberty as females. During childhood they had a penchant for tomboyism (Ehrhardt & Money, 1967), which suggested the possibility (wrongly as it turned out) of a sufficient degree of brain masculinization that they might, in adolescence, have bisexual imagery, ideation, and experience.

It was possible to obtain a follow-up on 11 of these individuals in adulthood (Money & Matthews, 1982). The finding at this time was that their earlier tomboyism had not persisted and that they had only heterosexual imagery, ideation, and practice, with no homosexual inclinations. They were more interested in marriage and motherhood than in a nonmaternal career.

Evidently, the synthetic hormone that masculinized their external genitalia did not have a lasting masculinizing effect on that part of the brain that, at puberty and thereafter, governs sexuality. Possibly the prenatal hormonal effect was too weak or did not persist long enough to have an enduring effect on the brain. Another possibility is that hormonally sensitive brain cells did not recognize and were unable to respond to the synthetic hormone, whereas the cells of the developing external sex organs were able to do so. Whatever the explanation, the heterosexual outcome in the progestin-induced syndrome of female hermaphroditism was not replicated in the adrenocortical-induced syndrome (adrenogenital syndrome) of female hermaphroditism.

ADRENOGENITAL SYNDROME

The adrenogenital syndrome is also known as congenital adrenal hyperplasia (CAH) and congenital virilizing adrenal hyperplasia (CVAH). Inclusion of the term *virilizing* denotes the fact that, if left untreated, the syndrome induces the onset of puberty as early as the age of 18 months and that it is invariably masculinizing in both sexes. During fetal life and continuously thereafter, unless corrected, the masculinizing hormone is secreted instead of cortisol by the affected individual's own adrenocortices in response to a recessively transmitted genetic error of cortisol synthesis. The error takes various forms, of which the most common is the 21-hydroxylase deficiency.

In fetal life, 21-hydroxylase deficiency does not alter the masculine differentiation of the chromosomally (46,XY) and gonadally (testicular) male fetus. By contrast, 21-hydroxylase deficiency has a profound effect in altering the feminizing differentiation of the chromosomally (46,XX) and gonadally (ovarian) female fetus—namely, by inducing masculinization of the external genitalia. The internal genitalia, which differentiate earlier, escape alteration. Masculinization of the external genitalia may be so extreme that the clitoris and its hood and labia minora become a normal penis with foreskin and covered urethra opening at the tip of the glans. The divided labia majora fuse and they do so completely, so as to become an empty scrotum when the formation of the penis is complete, thus producing normal appearing external genitalia except for the missing testes. In the least extreme degree of masculinization, the sole evidence may be clitoral enlargement. Between the two extremes are various degrees of clitoromegaly plus external urogenital closure, with resultant ambiguity as to the sex of the newborn baby. On the basis of visual inspection alone it cannot be decided whether the surgical correction should be designed to make the ambiguous organs more feminine or more masculine. At different times and places, and for different reasons, each decision has been made. Here as in other syndromes, the outcome is of great relevance to the theory of homosexology.

The 21-hydroxylase deficiency in a chromosomally 46,XX, gonadal female born with a penis and empty scrotum is one of the intersexual conditions that holds a key to the very definition of homosexuality. Some such individuals have been assigned and reared as boys, either because they were given a diagnosis of undescended testes, or because, in the era prior to 1950, there was no known treatment to prevent the relentless and precocious progress of pubertal virilization (Money & Daléry, 1977). Such a boy encounters no unusual hazards in growing up to have an adolescent romantic and erotosexual life with a female partner and in adulthood to become a husband and father by either donor insemination or adoption. Yet, like his wife, he was born as a genetic female with two ovaries and female reproductive organs internally. Had his case been differently managed endocrinologically and surgically, he could have become pregnant and delivered a live baby by Caesarian section. Hence the question: Are he and his wife both lesbians?

The answer is that they are not. This is another of the cases that confirm the proposition that, in general usage, homosexuality is not defined on the basis of the chromosomal sex, nor of any of the internal and concealed variables of sex. Instead, it is defined on the basis of the external sexual anatomy and the sexual characteristics of the body in general. Two people are identified as having a homosexual encounter or relationship provided that their external sex organs are anatomically of the same sex, regardless of how different they may be in secondary sexual characteristics. The 46,XX gonadal female with a penis and empty scrotum assigned and reared as a boy would be classified as homosexual if he had an affair with another person with a penis. However, if he did something so far unheard of, namely undergo surgical sex reassignment and then continue the affair with the same lover, then the relationship would be redefined as heterosexual. Hormonal treatment alone, even if it brought about breast growth and menstruation through the penis, would not suffice to change the definition of the relationship from homosexual to heterosexual. Only one partner should have a penis to permit a relationship to be defined as heterosexual, and vice versa, only one should have a vulva.

Social conformity to the cultural criterion of femininity (or, vice versa, masculinity) does not, per se, override the genital criterion of homosexuality. To illustrate: In the case of a morphologically normal male who is a female impersonator, no matter how ladylike the appearance, or how hormonally feminized the body, the impersonator who is a lady with a penis is still regarded morally and legally as a homosexual (or perhaps as a preoperative transsexual) if she has a sexual partner who also has a penis. Her syndrome is gynemimesis—the miming of a female by a person who has a penis (Money & Lamacz, 1984).

The syndrome of gynemimesis, otherwise known as syndrome of the lady with a penis, has not yet been known to have occurred in association with a diagnosis of 46,XX, CVAH with a penis. Quite to the contrary, congenital virilizing adrenal hyperplasia seems to blockade, utterly, the possibility of gynemimesis (Money & Lewis, 1982). The responsible blocking factor is, presumably, the high degree of prenatal androgenization which, by inference, masculinizes the sexual brain as well as the external genitalia. The effect of prenatal androgenization may completely override the effect of pubertal feminization, according to the evidence of a unique case of the 46,XX adrenogenital syndrome (Money, 1974).

In this case the baby was one of those born with a fully formed penis and empty scrotum. The diagnosis was not changed from male with undescended testes until age 10, when it was established as congenital virilizing adrenal hyperplasia in a genetic and gonadal female hermaphrodite. On the basis of an erroneous belief that hormones would feminize the mind as well as the body, and without his own consent, the boy's local physician gave him hormonal treatment with cortisol, thus releasing his ovaries to secrete their own feminizing hormones of puberty. His breasts developed and heralded the approach of first menstruation, through the penis. He was mortified.

Behaviorally he was very much a macho boy. His parents said he was the very antithesis of his sister. His mother discovered a love letter he had written to his girlfriend. She and his father agreed that to convert him to a girl (despite the fact that he had two ovaries and no testes) would be the equivalent of forcing him to be a lesbian, with a girlfriend as a lover. They saw no point in forcing him to have his penis amputated as the first step in surgical feminization, nor in forcing him to take hormonal treatments that would enlarge his breasts and induce menstruation but would not demasculinize his voice or body hair. They decided, instead, to seek a second opinion regarding masculinizing treatment. They were, of course, correct. They had a son, not a daughter, irrespective of his clinical diagnosis as a female hermaphrodite with two ovaries and 46,XX chromosomes. He had the sexual orientation of a heterosexual boy. It was too late to change it by edict or by any known method of intervention.

This particular boy had missed being diagnosed neonatally because his life was not threatened by the salt-losing symptom associated with one variant of adrenal hyperplasia. Babies who are salt-losers are diagnosed. Otherwise they die. Some of them have had a penis and empty scrotum, and some an enlarged clitoris, variable in size, with incomplete labioscrotal fusion. In either case, today's standard pediatric recommendation is to assign the child as a girl or, in some instances, to make a reassignment if the child had initially been announced as a boy. Assignment as a girl entails surgical feminization of the genitalia. It entails also antimasculinizing hormonal treatment with a substitute for the missing adrenal glucocorticoid, cortisol, throughout life. This treatment, which arrests the continuation of masculinization, postnatally, and permits puberty to be feminizing, was discovered only in 1950. Thus, the first generation of babies to be treated with cortisol now constitute the first generation of young adults whose prenatal history of masculinization was not followed by a history of postnatal virilization. With respect to homosexology, they provide an opportunity to investigate the role of hormonal masculinization that is prenatal only, and not also postnatal, relative to sexual orientation as homosexual, bisexual, or heterosexual.

On the basis of longitudinal follow-up findings (Money, Schwartz, & Lewis, 1984), it does appear that prenatal hormonal masculinization may have the same long-term sexological effect on 46,XX, adrenogenital babies who are clinically habilitated as girls as it does on those who are clinically habilitated as boys. That is, both are able to grow up to be romantically and sexually attracted to girls. In the case of those who grow up as boys, this predisposition is unhindered. It is incorporated into the postnatal effects of clinical and social masculinization, so that the ultimate outcome is socially approved heterosexuality as a male.

By contrast, in the case of those who grow up as girls, the predisposition set by prenatal hormonal masculinization is at odds with postnatal effects of clinical and social feminization. In adulthood, the ultimate outcome is heterogenously distributed between heterosexuality, bisexuality, or homosexuality as a female. In a sample of 30 follow-up cases, the actual percentages were heterosexual, 40% ($n = 12$); bisexual, 20% ($n = 6$); homosexual, 17% ($n = 5$); and noncommittal, 23% ($n = 7$)—all grossly different from the control group ($n = 27$), $x^2 (1, n = 57) = 18.5; p < .001$. If the noncommittal group is omitted and the percentages recalculated, then 48% ($n = 11$) classified themselves as bisexual on the basis of imagery and/or activity, of whom 5 classified themselves as predominantly or exclusively lesbian as adults. This proportion, 48%, is similar to that obtained in an earlier study

(Ehrhardt, Evers, & Money, 1968) of 23 women who grew up in the pre-1950, precortisol era and who were therefore, highly masculinized in physique. Evidently the high degree of masculinization that these 23 women underwent postnatally did not argument the predisposition set by prenatal masculinization. In CVAH syndrome, prenatal brain masculinization alone is sufficient to predispose to a bisexual or lesbian orientation.

One young woman in this CVAH follow-up study who did develop a lesbian orientation said, after having had two different boyfriends with whom she attempted in vain to relate in sexual intercourse, that she had to admit that she could fall in love only with a chick, not a guy. She became lovesick over a girlfriend who, though her close companion, was unable to fall in love homosexually, only heterosexually. Driven to the despair of love unrequited, worsened by adversarial parents, the CVAH girl drove her car into isolated swamp country, and there was found, two weeks later, dead of self-inflicted gunshot wounds.

In the target tissues of the brain, the site where prenatal hormonal masculinization is translated into a predisposition toward subsequent bisexuality or homosexuality has not been demonstrated in the human species. One must infer, on the basis of studies of laboratory animals that the site of masculinization is in the limbic system or paleocortex, intimately connected with the hypothalamus. In the adrenogenital syndrome, there is as yet no way of identifying either a timing or a dose-response effect that would distinguish those who eventually become bisexual from those who become monosexual as either homosexual or heterosexual. The difference might not prove to be exclusively prenatal, but postnatal also, in the overlay of developmental events and experiences that augment a prenatally established disposition that, by itself alone, would be too weak to preordain the status of adult sexual orientation.

ADOLESCENT GYNECOMASTIA

The adrenogenital syndrome occurs in 46,XY, gonadal males as well as in 46,XX, gonadal females. Since 1950, the year when treatment became available, CVAH boys have been hormonally regulated with cortisol so that they do not undergo a precociously virilizing puberty which, in older texts, was termed the infant Hercules syndrome. Before birth, however, their own bodies made a flood of male hormone of adrenocortical origin, which exposed the brain to a supramasculinizing level of the hormone.

Youths with a history of the treated adrenogenital syndrome ($N = 8$) were selected in late teenage or early adulthood as suitable for a contrast group of controls for youths ($N = 10$) who at puberty developed breast enlargement like that of a girl (Money & Lewis, 1982). The latter condition, idiopathic adolescent gynecomastia, is of unknown etiology. One possibility is that the glandular tissue behind the nipple is unduly sensitive to estrogen in the amount normally secreted by the male's testicles. An alternative possibility is that the same tissue is unduly resistant to the effect of testosterone in overriding the effect of estrogen. Before puberty, there are no signs of unusual body development. Retrospectively, no evidence has been obtained that would point to unusual hormonal functioning in prenatal life, and no cases have turned up in prospective studies. Thus, there is no evidence, one way or the other, of the possibility of deficient brain masculinization, nor of a demasculinizing process, prenatally. Similarly, because there is no evidence for or against brain feminization, prenatally, there is no evidence for or against brain ambisexualization.

The 10 boys with adolescent gynecomastia constituted an unbiased and geographically available sample from a larger clinic list. Three of them proved to have a homosexual status, about which they talked openly. Long before puberty they had been stigmatized as sissy by their peers and recognized as atypical by adults. Their boyhood lives had been marked by family adversity. Some of the CVAH boys also experienced family adversity. Nonetheless, there was no evidence of either a homosexual or bisexual status in any CVAH boys.

Thus, one may assume that with a history of hormonal supramasculinization prenatally, the CVAH syndrome boys had no leeway to develop other than heterosexually, no matter what. By contrast, one may assume that the boys who were destined to develop breasts were destined also to have leeway to veer toward homosexuality, provided other circumstances so conspired. It is possible that in prenatal life their brains were insufficiently responsive to androgen or in some other way were suboptimally masculinized hormonally. It will require a new and advanced research technology before this issue can be addressed.

It may be argued that the sample size in this study, being small, may have produced a fortuitous finding that will fail to be replicated. That argument is refuted by the data from the full list of patients from which the study sample was drawn. Among the 33 CVAH males, there was only one known instance of a homosexual status. The patient had a rare, asymptomatic case of CVAH and would not have been ascertained except for the fact that he was a cousin of two CVAH brothers and participated in a pedigree study. Among the 41 adolescent gynecomastia males, there were 8 who had homosexual (or bisexual) imagery and ideation. One of them was explicit in disclosing details of actual homosexual participation. One youth, struggling to resolve his dilemma, declared that if he could not become heterosexual, he would become either a priest with an abstinent sex life or a male-to-female transsexual. Instead, he became reconciled to being a practicing gay.

ANDROGEN-INSENSITIVITY SYNDROME

Whereas the adrenogenital syndrome is characterized by prenatal supramasculinization, the reverse applies to the androgen-insensitivity syndrome (AIS), formerly known as the testicular-feminizing syndrome. Inframasculinization characterizes partial androgen insensitivity, whereas complete antimasculinization characterizes complete androgen insensitivity. It is for this reason that patients with the complete syndrome of androgen insensitivity were selected to constitute the clinical contrast group of controls for the women with the 46,XX adrenogenital syndrome mentioned earlier.

The complete androgen-insensitivity syndrome occurs in girls and women who, paradoxically, are chromosomally 46,XY and whose gonads are histologically testicular, though without spermatogenesis and without the capacity to do the work of testes. Their incapacitation stems from a genetically transmitted, X-linked recessive error that blocks, in all cells of the body, either the uptake or the utilization of the hormone, testosterone, secreted by the testes. Unable to use testosterone in both prenatal and postnatal life, the body fails to masculinize. Confronted with that failure, nature reverts to her primal template which is to construct not Adam, but Eve. In fetal life, this reversion takes place after the gonads have formed and secreted their antimullerian hormone, which blocks the growth of the mullerian ducts into a uterus and fallopian tubes. Thereafter, no further masculinization occurs, so that the baby is born as Eve, but without Eve's internal reproductive organs. The vagina is present, but lacks depth until dilated. The vulva appears normally female except that, in adulthood, pubic hair is sparse or absent. Pubic and axillary hair follicles, unable to utilize androgen, are unable to grow hair. At puberty, the breasts develop and the body feminizes in contour under the influence of the amount of testicular estrogen that normally circulates in the bloodstream of all males.

Two characteristics of the syndrome most commonly responsible for bringing the individual to medical attention are the shallow or atresic vagina and the failure to menstruate. These same two characteristics, vaginal atresia and amenorrhea, secondary to congenital absence of the uterus and fallopian tubes, are found also in women who are chromosomally 46,XX and gonadally female with a diagnosis of Rokitansky syndrome (or Mayer-Rokitansky-Küster [MRK] syndrome).

The two syndromes, AIS and MRK, are admirably suited to be clinical contrast or control groups for one another, because they are similar on all counts except chromosomal sex, gonadal sex, and hormonal cyclicity. A comparative study of an unbiased sample of 18 women (Lewis & Money, 1983); Money & Lewis, 1983), 9 in each diagnostic group, showed the two groups to be identical on a range of erotosexual variables.

All 18 were exclusively heterosexual as women in imagery, ideation, and practice. The significance of this finding for homosexology is that it rules out three of the criteria of female sex—namely, chromosomal status, gonadal status, and hormonal cyclicity—as essential to the development of a feminine sexual orientation, because the two groups were antithetical on these three variables. The variables that they shared in common as heterosexual women were female external genital anatomy and body build, spontaneous hormonal feminization of the body at puberty, and a history of having been assigned and reared as girls.

Androgen insensitivity is another of the syndromes that points to the definition of homosexuality as sexual and erotic expression between two people who have the same external genital anatomy and body morphology. No one would ever consider a married androgen-insensitive mother with two adopted children a male homosexual simply because her husband had the same chromosomal sex as she has and the same gonadal sex as she had preoperatively. Common sense demands that she be accorded the same heterosexual status as her Rokitansky-woman counterpart.

The similarity between the two syndromes proved to be so perfect that it was, in fact, quite in order to combine the two diagnoses in order to get a sufficiently large control group for the aforementioned study of 30 adrenogenital women.

MALE HERMAPHRODITISM

Partial androgen insensitivity in a 46,XY fetus allows the Eve principle to take over partially. So also does partial androgen insufficiency. In both instances, the baby is born with a birth defect of the external sex organs, so that the genital appearance is ambiguously hermaphroditic or intersexed. Some such babies have been assigned and reared as boys, and some as girls. At puberty, irrespective of their sex of rearing, some have undergone spontaneous hormonal feminization and developed breasts. They do not menstruate, as they lack a uterus. The masculinizing puberty of those who do not feminize is likely to be partial or eunuchoidal, rather than complete.

In androgen-insensitivity cases, when the individual's own hormonal puberty is inadequate, hormonal treatment to bring about feminization is successful, whereas treatment to bring about masculinization is unsatisfactory. The consequences are dire if the partially androgen-insensitive individual has been assigned and reared to live as a boy, because he forever fails to gain the bodily appearance of masculine maturity. If he has grown up to the age of puberty self-identified as a boy, and if his imagery and ideation are heterosexually masculine, then it is impossible for him to espouse the rational logic of becoming hormonally and surgically reassigned to live as a woman, even if, untreated, he has already developed breasts and a feminine body morphology. To impose feminizing surgery of his genitalia would be totally incompatible with the history of the multiple operations to which his penis had already been subjected in order to affirm genital masculinity and to permit urination as a male.

In the annals of male hermaphroditism, cases of sex reassignment from male to female are rare, even in cases of impaired masculine bodily maturation on the basis of partial androgen insensitivity (Money & Norman, in press), whereas sex reassignment from female to male is not so rare (Money, Devore, & Norman, 1986). The parallel phenomenon occurs in female hermaphroditism insofar as a sex reassignment from female to male is virtually unheard of, no matter how extensive the degree of masculinization (Money, 1968a). However, there is no corresponding parallel in female hermaphroditism with respect to the prevalence of reassignment from male to female, the explanation being that only a very few female hermaphrodites are reared as boys. Even if they are announced as boys neonatally, a reannouncement is likely to follow very soon thereafter. The explanation lies in the fact that female hermaphroditism is almost always associated with the adrenogenital syndrome, which produces a sufficiency of complicating symptoms— especially severe salt loss, which is lethal if not neonatally detected and treated—to lead to the neonatal diagnosis of gonadal sex (ovarian) and chromosomal sex (46,XX).

There is absolutely no doubt that in the traditional wisdom of most parents and their religious advisors, as well as of many doctors, primacy is attributed to chromosomal and gonadal sex, and to the prospect of fertility, as the criteria on which to decide the sex of assignment. Surgically, it is technically more feasible to demasculinize and feminize the external genitalia than it is to defeminize and masculinize them. Thus, the greater simplicity of feminizing corrective surgery also is a criterion in announcing the sex of a female hermaphrodite as female. This criterion is quite often disregarded in announcing or reannouncing the sex of a chromosomally and gonadally diagnosed male hermaphrodite as a boy. In consequence he may be nosocomially traumatized by multiple surgical admissions in childhood, only to have, in adulthood, a small and deformed penis inadequate for copulation (Money & Lamacz, 1986) and possibly for urination as well.

The primacy accorded the chromosomal sex and, more especially, the gonadal sex as the ultimate criteria by which to decide the sex of a hermaphrodite child influences the destiny of the male hermaphroditic child at any age. For the baby assigned and reared as a girl and not diagnosed as gonadally and chromosomally male until later in life, the diagnosis may lead to an imposed sex reassignment. Or, if in childhood or adolescence, the male hermaphrodite living as a girl is ambivalent about or rejects her status as a girl, the covert if not the overt influence of the primacy of the chromosomal and gonadal criteria tips the scales in favor of permitting a sex reassignment that would otherwise be vetoed. Sex reassignment would be vetoed in the corresponding case of a male hermaphrodite living as a boy and ambivalent about or rejecting his status as a boy. In the same way, sex reassignment from girl to boy would be vetoed for a female hermaphrodite (Jones, 1979; Money, 1968a).

Sex is a binary system: male and female. A hermaphroditic child who grows up ambivalent about his or her status in the sex of assignment has effectively only one alternative, namely, to change to the other sex. If this alternative is congruous with the criteria of the agents of society, including parents and professionals, who set the rules as to who may change, then sex reassignment is more likely to be permitted or endorsed.

A hermaphroditic individual's nonconformity with respect to his or her status in the sex of assignment and rearing manifests itself in nonconformity regarding social and legal stereotypes with respect to the male-female division of labor, play, education, dress, adornment, wealth, and so forth, but more specifically with respect to the imagery, ideation, and practices of falling in love and having a sex life. In the love life and in the sex life, nonconformity may be manifested as bisexuality, or as homosexuality defined on the criterion of assigned sex, or as a change of sexual status through sex reassignment.

With respect to homosexology, it is of major theoretical significance not that some male hermaphrodites, assigned and clinically habilitated as girls, grow up to be bisexual, homosexual, or sex reassigned, but that others grow up with a heterosexual status as women who have men as romantic partners and husbands. Unless informed of the clinical history and intersex diagnosis of these women, other people do not suspect anything amiss, nor do they have reason to do so. Socially and in bodily appearance, as well as romantically and in the sex life, the male hermaphrodite successfully habilitated as a woman is not conspicuous and identifiable among other women. The same applies also to the related birth defect of micropenis (Money, 1984). Both types of cases further substantiate the principle, aforementioned, that homosexuality is defined in terms of the genital and body morphology of the two partners, not in terms of the chromosomal sex, nor of the sex of the gonads. Correspondingly, of course, heterosexuality is also defined on the criterion that the two partners do not have the same kind of genital and overall body conformation. Thus, the woman with a history of having been treated for either male hermaphroditism or micropenis is defined as heterosexual, regardless of her chromosomal or gonadal status, provided her habilitation has been to develop from girlhood to womanhood with a romantic and erotic life shared with at least one boyfriend or husband. By contrast, this same woman, with her history of having been reared as a girl, would be defined as homosexual and a lesbian if she had grown up to be attracted erotically only to another woman and to be repelled by the advances of a would-be boyfriend whose attraction to her she would personally equate, in her own case, with the homosexuality of two men being together. She might resolve her dilemma by changing to live as a man with a woman lover, or she might continue to live as a woman with a woman lover and be known in society as a lesbian, or with both a man and a woman lover and be known as bisexual. Each outcome would qualify as a manifestation of some degree of gender transposition away from the ideological norm of femininity toward the ideological norm of masculinity. The criterion standard is the ideological, not the statistical, norm. The extreme degree of transposition is sex reassignment. Living as a lesbian is a lesser degree of transposition, and as a bisexual lesser still.

The prevalence of gender transposition was the object of a study (Money et al., 1986) of adult patients ($N = 32$) with a history of having been diagnosed as male hermaphrodites, assigned as girls, reared as girls, and clinically habilitated to live as girls and women. In this study, sex reassignment from female to male was classified as a gender transposition phenomenon, as were imagery and ideation or actual experience of attraction to a female either exclusively, as a lesbian, or bisexually.

The high proportion of patients ($n = 15$) who were classified as manifesting a transposition phenomenon is in part an artifact of sampling, because one reason for a patient's referral to Johns Hopkins was the presence of a transposition dilemma. Thus, the ratio of 15:17 exaggerates the prevalence of transposition in the syndromes of male hermaphroditism at large. That proved to be an advantage for present purposes, as it provides a nice balance of cases among which to search for correlates or determinants of the phenomenon of transposition.

The only variable that proved to be significantly correlated (χ^2 (1, $N = 32$) $= 10.98$, $p < .001$) with transposition phenomena was a history of stigmatization during the childhood years. Stigmatization at home took the form of never mentioning the unspeakable birth defect, never explaining frequent clinic checkups or anything else connected with the defect, and never allowing the genitalia to be exposed except medically. Among peers it took the form of being teased as a sexual freak on the basis of a leakage of information about either the genital condition or the neonatal history of indeterminacy regarding the sex of announcement or reannouncement.

The stigmatization effect proved to be prepubertal in origin and not related to the incongruity of undergoing a masculinizing or eunuchoidal puberty instead of a feminizing one. Those children who would masculinize at puberty are presumed to have been more likely than the pubertal feminizers to have undergone stronger hormonal brain masculinization, prenatally. However, childhood stigmatization did not happen exclusively to the future pubertal masculinizers. This finding seems to rule out the possibility that prenatal brain masculinization might somehow or other have preordained an early behavioral manifestation of a gender transposition, such as uncompromising tomboyism of behavior, that would provoke teasing and stigmatization during childhood. Moreover, if a girl is tomboyish in behavior and a winner in athletics, her success builds self-esteem and inures her against the otherwise deleterious effects of teasing and stigmatization.

A male hermaphrodite with a history of having been assigned as a girl, and of subsequently having subjectively sensed the prospect or realization of a sexual relationship with a man as homosexual, is cited as a triumph of nature over nurture by those who label themselves as biological determinists. To maintain the triumph, however, they neglect or discard the converse evidence of cases in which nurture may be said to triumph over nature.

The example most quoted by the naturists is that of a pedigree of male hermaphrodites in an inbred population inhabiting three isolated mountain villages in the Dominican Republic (Imperato-McGinley, Guerrero, Gautier, & Peterson, 1974; Imperato-McGinley & Peterson, 1976; Imperato-McGinley, Peterson, Gautier & Sturla, 1979). The biochemical error responsible for the intersexed condition is 5 α-reductase deficiency. At birth the defective sex organs resemble those of a female more than those of a male.

In the first generation of intersexed births, affected babies were assigned as girls. When they reached the age of puberty they failed to feminize, but developed in a eunuchoid, masculine way instead. The clitoridic organ enlarged and protruded sufficiently so as to qualify in some instances as a small, hypospadiac penis that would require surgery to release it for copulatory use.

Because all of the intersexed children had the same condition, they all developed in the same nonfeminine way. Subsequently, therefore, newborn intersex babies were assigned as boys. Those who had already grown up were more readily tolerated in the village if they changed to live and earn a living as men, and perhaps to try to have the sex life of a man. In the absence of local hospital facilities, there was no hormonal treatment available either to feminize or to better masculinize the body, and there was no available corrective surgery for the deformed sex organs.

Imperato-McGinley and her coauthors proposed the hypothesis that the testosterone of puberty had a masculinizing effect not only on the body, including the sex organs, but also on the mind, including the sex drive. Hence the changing of sex.

There is a flaw in the biological reductionism of this hypothesis: It ignores the nonhormonal variables that affected the intersexed children's lives. Though assigned to live as girls, they were stigmatized as freaks by being known pejoratively as *guevodoces,* translated literally as "eggs at twelve," for which the idiomatic English is "balls (testicles) at twelve." They were also known as *machi hembra,* which translates as "macho miss" with its strong implication of half-girl, half-boy freakishness as well as of being tomboyish. There was no possibility in a traditional Hispanic village culture for such a person to be a wife and mother, and there was no other role for a woman except to be an economic liability as an unmarriageable freak supported by her family. The alternative was to adapt as well as possible to being a man.

A consideration of the sociological variables in these cases of 5 α-reductase deficiency does not exclude the possibility that they were superimposed on a substrate somehow made compliantly masculine by reason of the 5 α-reductase deficiency. The ideal test, in the best of all possible experimental designs, would be to have as a control group another pedigree, in another location, where all cases would be clinically and socially habilitated as girls from birth onward, beginning with surgical feminization of the genitalia in early infancy. The onset of puberty would be clinically regulated and would be exclusively feminine. Vaginoplasty, if required, would be available on an elective basis as soon as the body was adolescently mature. There are individual cases of 5 α-reductase deficiency that have been treated in this way. The outcome is not as in the Dominican pedigree. The girl becomes a woman and has a heterosexual status as a woman, even though it is contradictory to her chromosomal and gonadal sexual status.

The Dominican Republic pedigree does not stand up to the claim of being unique in demonstrating the triumph of nature over nurture. On the contrary, it demonstrates, as do all other examples of intersexuality, that the status of sexual orientation in adulthood cannot be attributed to any variable that is either exclusively nature or exclusively nurture. By itself alone, testosterone at puberty cannot be held responsible for male heterosexuality in 5 α-reductase deficient hermaphroditism. That would be tantamount to claiming that testosterone is responsible for all male heterosexuality. If that were so, then the vast majority of homosexual men would be heterosexual, because they have a normal level of testosterone. Similarly, the vast majority of male-to-female transsexuals would be heterosexually normal men, because they also have a normal level of testosterone prior to reassignment.

It is a basic requirement of any theory that it cannot be used to explain one set of data if that explanation is inconsistent with, or totally contradicted by, a related set of data. Imperato-McGinley's theory fails to satisfy this requirement. It fails to take into account gender transpositions not associated with the 5 α-reductase syndrome.

EPILOGUE AND SYNOPSIS

In the culture of the West, we characterize homosexuality as sporadic and pathological in occurrence. Elsewhere, as among the Sambia of New Guinea, homosexuality is characterized as a phase of universalized sequential bisexuality, the absence of which is sporadic and pathological in occurrence. A theory of homosexuality must encompass both manifestations.

Human sexological syndromes in the clinic represent experiments of nature that are the counterpart of animal sexological syndromes induced experimentally in the laboratory. Despite species differences and variations, data from these two sources are mutually compatible. They indicate that, in all species, the differentiation of sexual orientation or status as either bisexual or monosexual (i.e., exclusively heterosexual or homosexual) is sequential. Prenatally and with a possible brief neonatal extension, differentiation begins under the aegis not of genetics but of brain hormonalization and continues postnatally under the aegis of the senses and social communication and learning.

Dimorphic hormonalization of the brain prenatally takes place under the influence of a steroidal hormone. Normally it is testosterone, secreted by the fetal testes. Some target cells receive testosterone and change it into one of its metabolites, notably estradiol and dihydrotestosterone. Steroidal hormone masculinizes and defeminizes. Its lack or insufficiency demasculinizes and feminizes. It is possible for masculinization and feminization both to coexist to some degree, with consequent bisexual rather than monosexual manifestations of behavior.

Whereas brain dimorphism formerly was inferred from its effects in producing male/female dimorphism of behavior, in recent years it has been directly demonstrated in neuroanatomical structures that differ in the brains of males and females, especially in the region of the hypothalamus.

In subprimate species, prenatal hormonal differentiation of the brain preordains subsequent mating behavior as male or female more inexorably than is the case in primate species, especially the human species. Even in subprimates, however, the final outcome is not immune to postnatal modulation by variations in the circumstances of infant care and social contact. In primates, as compared with subprimates, the influence of prenatal and neonatal hormonalization is more susceptible to subsequent superimposed variations in social communication and learning. In particular, juvenile sexual rehearsal play is prerequisite to both masculinized and feminized proficiency in adult mating skill.

In the human species, there are only a few, infrequently occurring clinical syndromes in which it is possible to reconstruct the prenatal and neonatal hormonal history and relate it to subsequent orientation as heterosexual, bisexual, or homosexual. In other homosexual and bisexual people, one may conjecture the possibility of unsuspected nutritional, medicinal, or hormonal changes, including stress-derived changes in the chemistries of the pregnant mother's bloodstream—changes that may induce a masculinizing or demasculinizing, feminizing or defeminizing effect on sexual differentiation of the baby's brain. Prenatal maternal stress, for example, is known to have a demasculinizing effect on rat pups; and, likewise, barbiturates ingested by the mother are demasculinizing.

With respect to orientation as homosexual or bisexual, there is no human evidence that prenatal hormonalization alone, independently of postnatal history, inexorably preordains either orientation. Rather, neonatal antecedents may facilitate a homosexual or bisexual orientation, provided the postnatal determinants in the social and communicational history are also facilitative.

Logically, there is a possibility that the postnatal determinants may need no facilitation from prenatal ones. Defense of this proposition precipitates, yet once again, the obsolete nature-nurture debate, with no resolution. On the issue of the determinants of sexual orientation as homosexual, bisexual, or heterosexual, the only scholarly position is to allow that prenatal and postnatal determinants are not mutually exclusive. When nature and nurture interact at critical developmental periods, the residual products may persist immutably. It will require new methodology and new increments of empirical data before the full catalogue of these residuals can be specified.

Meanwhile, it is counterproductive to characterize prenatal determinants of sexual orientation as biological, and postnatal determinants as not. The postnatal determinants that enter the brain through the senses by way of social communication and learning also are biological, for there is a biology of learning and remembering. That which is not biological is occult, mystical, or, to coin a term, "spookological." Homosexology, the science of orientation or status as homosexual or bisexual rather than heterosexual, is not a science of spooks.

REFERENCES

Arnold, A. P., & Gorski, R. A. (1984). Gonadal steroid induction of structural sex differences in the central nervous system. *Annual Review of Neuroscience, 7,* 413–442.

Baum, M. J. (1979). Differentiation of coital behavior in mammals: A comparative analysis. *Neuroscience and Biobehavioral Reviews, 3,* 265–284.

Baum, M. J., Gallagher, C. A., Martin, J. T., & Damassa, D. A. (1982). Effects of testosterone, dihydrotestosterone, or estradiol administered neonatally on sexual behavior of female ferrets. *Endocrinology, 111,* 773–780.

Beach, F. A. (1975). Hormonal modification of sexually dimorphic behavior. *Psychoneuroendocrinology, 1,* 3–23.

Breedlove, S.M. (1986). Cellular analyses of hormone influence on motoneuronal development and function. *Journal of Neurobiology, 17,* 157–176.

Breedlove, S.M., & Arnold, A. P. (1980). Hormone accumulation in a sexually dimorphic motor nucleus of the rat spinal cord. *Science, 210,* 564–566.

Bullough, V. L. (1976). *Sexual variance in society and history.* New York: Wiley.

Chan, S. T. H. (1977). Spontaneous sex reversal in fishes. In J. Money & H. Musaph (Eds.), *Handbook of sexology* (pp. 91–105). Amsterdam: Excerpta Medica.

Clarke, I. J. (1977). The sexual behavior of prenatally androgenized ewes observed in the field. *Journal of Reproduction and Fertility, 49,* 311–315.

Crews, D. (1982). On the origin of sexual behavior. *Psychoneuroendocrinology, 7,* 259–270.

Crews, D. (in press). Functional associations in behavioral endocrinology. In J. M. Reinisch, L. A. Rosenblum, & S. A. Sanders (Eds.), *Masculinity/femininity: Concepts and definitions.* New York: Oxford University Press.

DeVoogd, T. J. (1986). Steroid interactions with structure and function of avian song control regions. *Journal of Neurobiology, 17,* 177–201.

De Vries, G. J., De Brun, J. P. C., Uylings, H. B. M., & Corner, M. A. (Eds.). (1984). *Sex differences in the brain: Relation between structure and function.* Amsterdam: Elsevier.

D'Occhio, M. J., & Ford, J. J. (in press). Contribution of studies in cattle, sheep and swine to our understanding of the role of gonadal hormones in processes of sexual differentiation and adult sexual behavior. In J. M. A. Sitsen (Ed.), *Handbook of sexology* (Vol. 7). Amsterdam: Elsevier.

Dörner, G., & Staudt, J. (1969). Perinatal structural sex differentiation of the hypothalamus in rats. *Neuroendocrinology, 5,* 103–106.

Döhler, K. D., Coquelin, A., Davis, F., Hines, M., Shryne, J. E., & Gorski, R. A. (1982). Differentiation of the sexually dimorphic nucleus in the preoptic area of the rat brain is determined by the perinatal hormone environment. *Neuroscience Letters, 33,* 295–298.

Dorland's illustrated medical dictionary (26th ed.). (1981). Philadelphia: Saunders.

Ellis, H. (1942). *Studies in the psychology of sex* (Vols. 1 and 2). New York: Random House.

Ehrhardt, A. A., Evers, K., & Money, J. (1968). Influence of androgen and some aspects of sexually dimorphic behavior in women with late-treated adrenogenital syndrome. *Johns Hopkins Medical Journal, 123,* 115–122.

Ehrhardt, A. A,. & Money, J. (1967). Progestin-induced hermaphroditism: IQ and psychosexual identity in a study of ten girls. *Journal of Sex Research, 3,* 83–100.

Goldfoot, D. A. (1977). Sociosexual behaviors of nonhuman primates during development and maturity: Social and hormonal relationships. In A. M. Schrier (Ed.), *Behavioral primatology: Advances in Research and Theory* (Vol. 1, pp. 139–184). Hillsdale, NJ: Erlbaum.

Goldfoot, D. A., & Neff, D. A. (in press). On measuring behavioral sex differences in social contexts. In J. M. Reinisch, L. A. Rosenblum, & S. A. Sanders (Eds.), *Masculinity/femininity: Basic perspectives.* New York: Oxford University Press.

Goldfoot, D. A., & Wallen, K. (1978). Development of gender role behaviors in heterosexual and isosexual groups of infant rhesus monkeys. In D. J. Chivers & J. Herbert (Eds.), *Recent advances in primatology: Vol. 1. Behaviour* (pp. 155–159). London: Academic Press.

Goldfoot, D. A., Wallen, K., Neff, D. A., McBrair, M. C., and Goy, R. W. (1984). Social influences upon the display of sexually dimorphic behavior in rhesus monkeys: Isosexual rearing. *Archives of Sexual Behavior, 13,* 395–412.

Gorski, R. A., Gordon, J. H., Shryne, J. E., & Southam, A. M. (1978). Evidence for a morphological sex difference within the medial preoptic area of the rat brain. *Brain Research, 148,* 333–346.

Herdt, G. H. (1981). *Guardians of the flutes: Idioms of masculinity.* New York: McGraw-Hill.

Herdt, G. H. (Ed.). (1984). *Ritualized homosexuality in Melanesia.* Berkeley: University of California Press.

Hirschfeld, M. (1948). *Sexual anomalies: The origins, nature and treatment of sexual disorders.* New York: Emerson Books.

Imperato-McGinley, J., Guerrero, L., Gautier, T., & Peterson, R. E. (1974). Steroid 5 α-reductase deficiency in man: An inherited form of male pseudohermaphroditism. *Science, 186,* 1213–1215.

Imperato-McGinley, J., & Peterson, R. E. (1976). Male pseudohermaphroditism: The complexities of male phenotypic development. *American Journal of Medicine, 61,* 251–272.

Imperato-McGinley, J., Peterson, R. E., Gautier, T., & Sturla, E. (1979). Androgens and the evolution of male-gender identity among male pseudohermaphrodites with 5 α-reductase deficiency. *New England Journal of Medicine, 300,* 1233–1237.

Jones, H. W., Jr. (1979). A long look at the adrenogenital syndrome. *Johns Hopkins Medical Journal, 145,* 143–149.

Klebs, E. (1876). *Handbuch der Pathologischen Anatomie.* Berlin: A. Herschwald.

Lewis, V. G., & Money, J. (1983). Gender-identity/role: G-I/R Part A: XY (androgen-insensitivity) syndrome and XX (Rokitansky) syndrome of vaginal atresia compared. In L. Dennerstein and G. Burrows, (Eds.), *Handbook of psychosomatic obstetrics and gynaecology* (pp. 51–60). Amsterdam/New York/Oxford: Elsevier Biomedical Press.

MacLean, P. D. (1972). A triune concept of the brain and behavior. In T. Boag (Ed.), *The Hincks Memorial Lectures.* Toronto: Toronto University Press.

McGarry, J. M. (1987). The discovery of the contraceptive pill. *British Journal of Sexual Medicine, 14,* 6–8.

Money, J. (1955). Hermaphroditism, gender and precocity in hyperadrenocorticism: Psychologic findings. *Bulletin of The Johns Hopkins Hospital, 96,* 253–264.

Money, J. (1967). *Hermaphroditism: An inquiry into the nature of a human paradox.* (Doctoral dissertation, Harvard University, 1952, University Microfilms No. 65–6698).

Money, J. (1968a). Psychologic approach to psychosexual misidentity with elective mutism: Sex reassignment in two cases of hyperadrenocortical hermaphroditism. *Clinical Pediatrics, 7,* 331–339.

Money, J. (1968b). *Sex errors of the body: Dilemmas, education, counseling.* Baltimore: Johns Hopkins University Press.

Money, J. (1974). Prenatal hormones and postnatal socialization in gender identity differentiation. *Nebraska Symposium on Motivation* (Vol. 21, pp. 221–295). Lincoln: University of Nebraska Press.

Money, J. (1984). Family and gender-identity/role. Parts I, II and III. *International Journal of Family Psychiatry, 5,* 317–381.

Money, J., & Daléry, J. (1977). Hyperadrenocortical 46,XX hermaphroditism with penile urethra. Psychological studies in seven cases, three reared as boys, four as girls. In P. A. Lee, L. P. Plotnick, A. A. Kowarski, & C. J. Migeon (Eds.), *Congenital adrenal hyperplasia* (pp. 433–446). Baltimore: University Park Press.

Money, J., Devore, H., & Normal, B. F. (1986). Gender identity and gender transposition: Longitudinal study of 32 male hermaphrodites assigned as girls. *Journal of Sex and Marital Therapy, 12,* 165–181.

Money, J., & Ehrhardt, A. A. (1972). Gender-dimorphic behavior and fetal sex hormones. In E. B. Astwood (Ed.), *Recent progress in hormone research* (Vol. 28, pp. 735–754). New York: Academic Press.

Money, J., Hampson, J. G., & Hampson, J. L. (1955). An examination of some basic sexual concepts: The evidence of human hermaphroditism. *Bulletin of The Johns Hopkins Hospital, 97,* 301–319.

Money, J., & Lamacz, M. (1984). Gynemimesis and gynemimetophilia: Individual and cross-cultural manifestations of a gender coping strategy hitherto unnamed. *Comprehensive Psychiatry, 25,* 392–403.

Money, J., & Lamacz, M. (1986). Nosocomial stress and abuse exemplified in a case of male hermaphroditism from infancy through adulthood. Coping strategies and prevention. *International Journal of Family Psychiatry, 7,* 71–105.

Money, J., & Lewis, V. G. (1982). Homosexual/heterosexual status in boys at puberty: Idiopathic adolescent gynecomastia and congenital virilizing adrenocorticism compared. *Psychoneuroendocrinology, 7,* 339–346.

Money, J., & Lewis, V. G. (1983). Gender-identity/role: G-I/R Part B: A multiple sequential model of differentiation. In L. Dennerstein & G. Burrows (Eds.), *Handbook of psychosomatic obstetrics and gynaecology* (pp. 61–67). Amsterdam/New York/Oxford, England: Elsevier Biomedical Press.

Money, J., & Mathews, D. (1982). Prenatal exposure to virilizing progestins: An adult follow-up study of twelve women. *Archives of Sexual Behavior, 11,* 73–83.

Money, J., & Norman, B. F. (in press). Gender identity and gender transposition: Longitudinal outcome study of 24 male hermaphrodites assigned as boys. *Journal of Sex and Marital Therapy, 13.*

Money, J., Schwartz, M., & Lewis, V. G. (1984). Adult erotosexual status and fetal hormonal masculinization and demasculinization: 46,XX cogenital virilizing adrenal hyperplasia and 46,XY androgen-insensitivity syndrome compared. *Psychoneuroendocrinology, 9,* 405–414.

Nordeen, E. J., & Yahr, P. (1982). Hemispheric asymmetries in the behavioral and hormonal effects of sexually differentiating mammalian brain. *Science, 218,* 391.

Nottebohm, F., & Arnold, A. P. (1976). Sexual dimorphism in vocal control areas of the song-bird brain. *Science, 194,* 211–213.

Phoenix, C. H., & Chambers, K. C. (1982). Sexual behavior in adult gonadectomized female pseudohermaphrodite, female, and male rhesus macaques (*Macaca mulatta*) treated with estradiol benzoate and testosterone propionate. *Journal of Comprehensive Physiology, 96* 823–833.

Phoenix, C. H., Jensen, J. N., & Chambers, K. C. (1983). Female sexual behavior displayed by androgenized female rhesus monkeys. *Hormones and Behavior, 17,* 146–151.

Raisman, C., & Field, P. M. (1971). Sexual dimorphism in the preoptic area of the rat. *Science, 173,* 731–733.

Reinisch, J. M., & Sanders, S. A. (1982). Early barbiturate exposure: The brain, sexually dimorphic behavior, and learning. *Neuroscience and Biobehavioral Reviews, 6,* 311–319.

Short, R. V., & Clarke, I. J. (undated). *Masculinization of the female sheep* [Film]. (Distributed by MRC Reproductive Biology Unit, 2 Forrest Road, Edinburgh, EHI 2QW, U.K.)

Steinach, E. (1940). *Sex and life. Forty years of biological and medical experiments.* New York: Viking Press.

Stoller, R. J., & Herdt, G. H. (1985). Theories of origins of male homosexuality. *Archives of General Psychiatry, 42,* 399–404.

Ward, I. L. (1972). Prenatal stress feminizes and demasculinizes the behavior of males. *Science, 175,* 82–84.

Ward, I. L. (1984). The prenatal stress syndrome: Current status. *Psychoneuroendocrinology, 9,* 3–11.

Ward, I. L., & Weisz, J. (1980). Maternal stress alters plasma testosterone in fetal males. *Science, 207,* 328–329.

Whalen, R. E. & Edwards, D. A. (1967). Hormonal determinants of the development of masculine and feminine behavior in male and female rats. *Anatomical Record, 157,* 173–180.

Young, W. C., Goy, R. W., & Phoenix, C. H. (1964). Hormones and sexual behavior. *Science, 143,* 212–218.

PART I: DEVELOPMENTAL STUDIES

4

The Role of Cognition in Child Development and Disorder

Michael Rutter

Institute of Psychiatry, De Crespigny Park, London, United Kingdom

The role of cognition in child development is reviewed with respect to the role of cognitive processing and cognitive deficits. Cognitive processing is discussed with respect to the self-system; the effects of psychosocial experiences; risk, vulnerability and protective mechanisms; vulnerability to depression; aetiology and treatment of depression. Cognitive deficits are discussed with respect to the socio-emotional consequences of language delay and reading difficulties; hyperkinetic/attentional deficit syndromes; schizophrenia; and autism. It is concluded that the ways in which we appraise our life circumstances and the ways in which we react to experiences of all kinds are greatly influenced by how we think about ourselves and our environment. Biases and distortions in such cognitive processing may be associated with social and emotional malfunction. These biases may derive from earlier experiences, from intensive temperamental styles, or from deficits in the ability to process incoming information. The further study of cognitive processing and cognitive deficits is likely to be rewarding and helpful for clinical practice.

The study of thought processes has always been a central feature of psychiatry in all its branches. Thus, abnormalities of thinking, as reflected in delusions and hallucinations, constituted the bread and butter of Kraepelinian nosology and Jasperian psychopathology. Equally, intrapsychic defence mechanisms have been one of the central pillars of psychoanalysis from Freud's very first writings. There is nothing new in the notion that cognition

Reprinted with permission from the *British Journal of Medical Psychology,* 1987, Vol. 60, 1–16: Copyright 1987 by The British Psychological Society.

plays a crucial role in both child development and child psychiatric disorder. Yet there have been important changes in the ways in which the role of cognition has been conceptualized.

It is convenient to consider cognition under two broad headings, cognitive processing and cognitive deficits, although the two cannot be regarded as wholly separate. Cognitive processing has to be invoked in four main domains. First, the last decade or so has seen a major upsurge of interest in the development of what has been called the 'self-system' (Harter, 1983), a term applied to the set of beliefs that we all develop about ourselves and about our environment. Developmentalists have become interested in the mediating role of qualities such as self-esteem, self-efficacy, and locus of control. Second, child psychologists have come to emphasize the extent to which children's cognitive capacities regulate their susceptibility to the influence of different life experiences. For example, very young infants are less affected by separations from their parents because they have yet to develop the capacity to form enduring selective attachments; conversely older children are less vulnerable to the ill-effects of separation because they have acquired the capacity to maintain relationships over the course of a period of absence (Rutter, 1981 *a*). Third, increasing attention has come to be paid to the importance of people's cognitive interpretation of their experiences. Thus, Kagan (1980, 1984) has argued that experiences have long-term effects only by virtue of their cognitive transduction. He suggested that infants' limited abilities to process experiences in this way is the main reason why experiences in infancy so rarely lead to lasting psychological sequelae. In rather different fashion, Bowlby (1969, 1973, 1980), followed by Brown & Harris (1978), argued that parental loss in childhood creates a negative cognitive set that provides a vulnerability to respond with depression to later loss events. The suggestion is, that it is not the immediate pain of the loss itself that is damaging, but rather the lasting impairment to a person's sense of self-esteem or self-efficacy that may be a consequence of the loss. Fourth, cognitions have been postulated as important causal factors in the genesis and the prolongation of psychiatric disorders, especially depression. Beck (1967) and others have emphasized that depression is not just a state of profoundly dysphoric mood; also it is a cognitive state characterized by a negative view of the self, of the life situation and of the future. Moreover, it is hypothesized that this belief that one is powerless to influence the bad things happening to oneself prevents coping actions that could bring the depressive state to an end. The negative mood is prolonged by the thought processes that accompany, or form part of, the abnormal mood disorder.

It is evident in all four domains that there has been a coming together of developmental and clinical perspectives (Rutter & Garmezy, 1983; Sroufe &

Rutter, 1984; Rutter & Sandberg, 1985; Rutter, 1986 *a*). There is an assumption that there are likely to be continuities, as well as discontinuities, in the span of behavioural variation from normality to psychopathology. Equally it is presumed that events and happenings at one phase of development are likely to have implications for those in later phases. Once more, there is nothing particularly novel in those suggestions but the ways in which clinical and developmental perspectives have been cojoined do have some components that differ from those that have been traditional in psychiatry, psychoanalysis and child development.

The second aspect of cognition, cognitive deficits, appears at first glance to refer to an entirely different set of mechanisms and concepts, although in reality the differences may not be as great as they appear. Such deficits have been thought to operate in both direct and indirect ways. Autism constitutes an example of hypothesized direct effects (Rutter, 1983). Autistic individuals' failure to engage in normal reciprocal responsive social interchanges and their failure to make and maintain love relationships constitute the social incapacity that defines the disorder (Fein *et al.*, 1986). However, it is known that autism is accompanied by a variety of cognitive deficits and it has been suggested that these may underlie the social deviance and social impairment (Rutter, 1983). Similarly, it has been argued that attentional deficits may constitute the core of both hyperkinetic disorders (Douglas, 1983) and schizophrenia (Nuechterlein & Dawson, 1984), with the specific type of attentional problem not quite the same in the two conditions (Nuechterlein, 1983). Possible indirect effects are exemplified by the relatively strong and well-documented associations between language retardation and psychiatric disorder (Howlin & Rutter, 1987) and between reading disabilities and conduct disorders (Rutter & Giller, 1983; Yule & Rutter, 1985). The mechanisms involved in these associations remain ill-understood but it is generally presumed that in some manner the language and reading difficulties predispose to psychiatric disorder.

The evidence on these various links between cognition and development or disorder has been extensively reviewed by several different writers and I will make no attempt to provide a critique of the mass of relevant empirical findings. Instead I shall seek briefly to summarize the current state of the art in order to discuss the theoretical and clinical implications that derive from the research.

COGNITIVE PROCESSING

The Self-System

Let me begin with the complex composite of ideas encompassed by the concept of the self-system (Harter, 1983). The central notion is that personality involves, amongst other things, a set of cognitions about ourselves, our relationships and our interactions with the environment. We see ourselves as having a coherence of functioning that is related to our concept of ourselves as witty or incompetent, as pushed around by external forces or as firmly in control of our destinies. The counterpart of our self-image is our tendency to respond to others on the basis of their reputations or our perceptions of what sort of person they are. That we *do* so respond to such precepts, and not just to people's immediate behaviours, has been well demonstrated both experimentally and naturalistically with respect, for example, to gender and aggressivity. In other words, it has been shown that to an important extent we respond to people on the basis of the label 'male' or 'female' and not just to their tendency to behave in male or female ways. The studies of ambiguously dressed toddlers given names that are the opposite of their biological sex illustrate this tendency (Smith & Lloyd, 1978; Condry & Ross, 1985). In similar fashion it has been found that we respond negatively to people regarded as aggressive on the basis of their previous behaviour, even when at the moment they are behaving in a prosocial or compliant fashion (Dodge, 1980; Asher, 1983; Brunk & Hengeller, 1984).

In the same sort of way, it has been demonstrated that our allocated social roles influence our concepts and ideas about ourselves, which in turn influence our behaviour. For instance, longitudinal studies have shown that factory workers' attitudes change when they are promoted to charge hands or when they join the management (see Kelvin, 1969). Children who are treated as if they have certain qualities tend to live up (or down) to their reputations (see Maccoby & Martin, 1983). There is an abundance of evidence that people vary greatly in their levels of self-esteem (Harter, 1983) or self-efficacy (Bandura, 1977), and there is a more limited body of data suggesting that these self-concepts influence how they respond to life situations. Clearly, people *do* respond differently to, for example, task failure. Some react to failure by increasing their efforts to succeed whereas others are more likely to give up trying. Thus, this contrast has been shown to differentiate secure and insecure infants (Lütkenhaus *et al.,* 1985), and adolescent boys and girls in certain task situations (see Dweck & Elliott, 1983). Even when no mediating self-concept has been demonstrated, there seems a need to impute some such intervening mechanism.

It is obvious that there is still an immense amount to learn about the self-system but we *can* infer that it exists in some form. Several consequences flow from that inference. Firstly, it has implications for views on personality and personality development. Some theorists suppose that personality comprises a collection of constitutionally determined traits or temperamental attributes such as neuroticism (Eysenck, 1953, 1967) or behavioural inhibition (Kagan,

1984; Reznick *et al.,* 1986). That such traits exist, that they show modest stability over time and that, to a limited extent, they predict people's behaviour in various situations can be accepted. But the evidence on the role of cognitive concepts in the self-system argues strongly against this being the whole of personality. Indeed, it seems preferable to refer to the traits as *temperament* in order to retain the concept of personality for the coherence of functioning that derives from how people react to their given attributes, how they think about themselves, and how they put these concepts together into some form of conceptual whole (Rutter, 1987 *d)*. The need to reject the view of personality as just a collection of traits is shown by the evidence that people's behaviour is often predictable in terms of an understandable psychological coherence rather than a generalization of behaviour (Rutter, 1984). Indeed, the coherence may be shown by people behaving in *opposite* ways in different situations, an opposite that is predictable and understandable in terms of the contrasting meaning of the situations. But thought processes have to be invoked; functioning is *not* explicable solely on the basis of generalized tendencies to be inhibited or outgoing, emotionally stable or unstable.

The view that personality development involves the operation of intrapsychic thought processes of which we may lack awareness is, of course, central to psychoanalytic theory. Nevertheless, it is important for psychoanalysts to recognize that the specifics of their theory do *not* fit the facts as demonstrated and that many of the mechanisms postulated in traditional Freudian views have *not* stood up to empirical test. It is right that those within psychoanalysis have drawn attention to the very wide range of psychoanalytic concepts that have had to be abandoned (such as the energy flow of libidinal energies or some of the specifics of psychosexual stages)—a range so wide that necessarily it raises the question of whether it would not be better to start anew rather than to pretend that the original tenets still remain (Eagle, 1984). Psychiatry and psychology have been greatly enhanced by the immense contributions of psychoanalysis in opening our ideas to the richness of the workings of the human mind, to the crucial importance of the meanings attached to experiences, to the influence on development of early family relationships, and to the process of psychosocial development itself. But the very success of psychoanalysis lies in the extent to which many of its ideas have become so part of the currency of other theories that they are no longer distinctively psychoanalytic. Some of the differences that remain are seriously blocking progress because they serve to prevent people from seeing the need to change their ways of looking at personality development and personality functioning.

Psychosocial Experiences and Their Effects

It is not necessary to dwell on the importance of children's growing cognitive capacities for their ability to perceive and respond to different life experiences, as it is obvious and well accepted. Thus, young babies fail to show the separation anxiety and fear of strangers that is characteristic of toddlers. Probably, this is because they lack the necessary cognitive skills to appreciate differences between people, to maintain schemata in active memory and to remember the past (Kagan, 1984). The capacity of anticipation, which arises towards the end of the first year, is important for both pleasurable emotions (as in the peek-a-boo game—Sroufe, 1979 *a*) and unpleasant ones (as in the anticipatory fear associated with previous experience of the inoculation needle—Izard, 1978). Cognitive factors also influence the *salience* of experiences (Maccoby & Martin, 1983). For example, three-year-olds are deterred from touching a forbidden object if its fragility is stressed but they are relatively impervious to appeals to property rights. By contrast, five-year-olds are responsive to being told that the object belongs to someone else (Parke, 1974). Similarly, imagination plays little part in the fears of infants but a major role in those of older children (Rutter, 1980). Concepts of moral rights and of external control also come to influence children's reactions to external pressures (Lepper, 1982). Children who are rewarded for doing something that they want to do tend to lose spontaneous interest in the activity; conversely, if children perceive threats or punishments as excessive they are less likely to comply than if the pressure is mild but sufficient. Punishment reduces disruptive behaviour but unduly severe punishment may actually increase it—presumably because the ill-effects of the resentment so induced predominate (Rutter & Giller, 1983).

These cognitive effects on children's responsivity to particular experiences are clearly evident. What requires more discussion, however, is the role of cognitive processing in the changes brought about by psychosocial experiences and, more especially, in the maintenance or otherwise of the effects of those experiences. Two rather separate questions are involved here. The first is 'what happens to the organism as a result of experiences, good or bad?' (Rutter, 1984). Curiously, this is a question that has received very little attention so far from either developmentalists or social researchers. Yet, surely, we have to pose the query? The answer could be that nothing happens to the organism other than the acquisition of conditioned emotions or learned skills or habits or styles of responding. However, already we know that that is not a sufficient answer, although undoubtedly it is part of the explanation. Thus, for example, altered neuroendocrine responses play a role in the process of adaptation to both physical and psychosocial acute stressors (see

Rutter, 1981 *a)*. The suggestion put forward in recent times is that cognitive attributions and other forms of cognitive processing must be added to the list of mechanisms. The need, it must be emphasized, is to find mechanisms to account for both continuities and discontinuities in development and especially in the long-term effects of early life experiences (Rutter, 1987 *a)*.

The overall pattern of findings is complex and fascinating, but not easy to account for in terms of any single process, cognitive or non-cognitive. Let me take selective attachments as an example. Initially stimulated by the writings of Bowlby (1969, 1973, 1980) and Ainsworth (1969; Ainsworth *et al,*. 1978), the concept of attachment as a crucial aspect of personal relationships and as a major mediator in the process of psychosocial development has become firmly established (Sroufe, 1979 *a,* 1985; Emde *&* Harmon, 1982; Parkes *&* Stevenson-Hinde, 1982; Bretherton *&* Waters, 1985). The main findings and ideas are too well known to need any review here. But let me point out a few of the apparent paradoxes that require explanation. Firstly, although the security of a child's relationship with one parent does not predict to the relationship with the other parent at the *same* time (i.e. it is a dyadic measure and not an individual attribute) it *does* predict peer relationships several years later (Bretherton *&* Waters, 1985). In part this may be a function of the demonstrated responsivity to varying social circumstances, but also it seems necessary to invoke some mechanism by which a dyadic quality leads to some characteristic in the individual that endures over time and situation to some degree. What is that quality? Secondly, although children's first selective attachments ordinarily develop in the first couple of years, Tizard *&* Hodges (1978) found that institution-reared children who were adopted as late as four, five, six or even seven years developed close intimate ties with their adoptive parents even at that relatively late age. Changed social circumstances led to a changed pattern of attachments. Yet, in spite of that change, follow-up to 16 years of age showed that there were persisting differences in the children's pattern of peer relationships and in their tendency to confide in others (Hodges *&* Tizard, in press *a, b)*. Why? Something had endured from the experiences in infancy in spite of a radical change in the later social environment. Yet why did that show in peer relationships when one might have expected it to be most apparent in parent-child relationships, and why did the secure adoptive parent-child relationship not enable the child to go on to a normal pattern of friendships? Thirdly, although the sequelae of poor parent-child relationships can sometimes be seen in adult life or even in the next generation, it is also the case that a good marital relationship in adult life can do much to remedy the ill-effects of early bad experiences (Rutter, in press *b)*. We have to explain both persistence and change.

The concept of an 'internal working model' of relationships has become a popular contender as an explanatory variable (Bretherton & Waters, 1985). The general idea is that children derive a set of expectations about their own relationship capacities and about other people's responses to their social overtures and interactions, these expectations being created on the basis of their early parent-child attachments. In other words, to some extent, children *shape* their later relationships as a result of cognitive concepts derived from earlier relationships. Nevertheless, later relationships are far from determined by such working models and if later relationships are markedly better, worse, or different from earlier ones, the working models may thereby change. It has been suggested that later relationships, or even later thoughts, may alter the meaning of earlier experiences and, by so doing, may alter their impact. Thus, Ricks (1985) suggested that it may be adaptive for someone to reconceptualize his earlier rejection by his mother as due to his mother's depression or social circumstances, rather than to dislike of him as a person. The reconceptualization thereby removes the connotation of personal failing and allows re-establishment of self-esteem. Some theorists, too, suggest that it is necessary to accept the reality of past bad experiences and to integrate them into a coherent whole (Main *et al.,* 1985). Thus, Epstein (cited by Ricks, 1985) argues that even an unpleasant concept of the world is preferable to a chaotic and inherently contradictory one.

The ideas are important and intuitively plausible but largely untested. Their importance lies in the need to develop ways of measuring attachment relationships after infancy and of measuring children's (and adults') concepts or models of relationships. The crucial role of relationships in personality development is obvious but it is nowhere near so obvious which processes in the organism mediate continuities and discontinuities. Internal working models provide a possibility but numerous questions remain. How early are such models within children's cognitive capacities? What are the differences in the types of models possible at, say, two years and 12 years? How complex and differentiated are the models for different types of relationships? How important is coherence, and why? What is necessary to bring about change and which features work against change? How can the models serve to account for contradictory and ambivalent patterns of relationships? The postulate of cognitive models seems helpful but it is apparent that the models must include affective as well as cognitive components.

Risk, Vulnerability and Protective Mechanisms

Numerous studies have attested to the immense variations in children's responses to stress and adversity, both in the short term and in the extent to which effects persist over time (Rutter, 1981 *a, b,* 1985). Numerous factors serve to determine these individual differences. Many of the factors are unconnected with cognitive mechanisms but some involve thought processes in crucial ways. To begin with, cognitive capacities necessarily define the salience of events for children. However, in addition, past experiences may alter the meaning of new ones or may change the way in which the happenings are appraised and understood. Thus, both previous happy separations and preventive programmes designed to prepare children for hospital admission have been shown to reduce the rate of distress reactions (Rutter, 1979 *a).* Conversely, a previous admission to hospital during the preschool years increases the likelihood that children will develop disorder following a later admission (Douglas, 1975; Quinton & Rutter, 1976). Clearly, something was changed that altered the later reaction but just what that something was remains obscure. It seems likely that part of the explanation may lie in the children's mental sets about hospital admission and about being separated from their families, but the suggestion has yet to be put to the critical test.

The observation, however, raises a more general issue—namely, that it is a common occurrence for people's responses to stress and adversity to be modified by prior experiences that either increase their vulnerability or protect them from ill-effects (Rutter, 1987 *a, c).* Research has followed several different approaches to the elucidation of the processes underlying resilience. First, there were attempts to identify the happenings or circumstances that seemed to increase the likelihood that people would escape unscathed. These were found to include harmonious close confiding relationships, a wide range of social support, successful task accomplishment, and effective coping with previous similar life hazards (Rutter, 1979 *b,* 1985; Garmezy, 1985; Masten & Garmezy, 1985). Secondly, investigators focused on the personal qualities that appeared to be protective. Some of these involved temperamental features that were likely to be at least partially constitutional in origin. However, others were described in terms of self-concepts. The implication was that people's cognitive sets made a difference to how they reacted to potentially negative life experiences. The evidence required to provide a crucial test of the postulated mediating role of cognitive sets is not yet available, but it seems likely they do indeed play a role. What is much less certain, however, is which aspect of the self-concept is most important in this connection.

One possibility is that what matters is a high sense of self-esteem or a global feeling of one's own worth as an individual. The suggestion is that it is easier to ride the psychosocial storm if you feel good about yourself as a person. However, even this apparently straightforward notion is more complicated than it appears at first sight (Harter, 1986). To begin with, a person's self-evaluation of their worth is not synonymous with their appraisal of their competence, although the two are likely to be interconnected. The extent to which poor competence leads to low self-esteem will be influenced by the value placed on that skill by the individual and by society (everyone is poor at some things but often that does not matter to them because it is not a domain of personal importance or investment). Also, it will be affected by the individual's social comparison group (other handicapped people, the general population, or high achievers), by the value placed on the balance between their skills and deficits, and by the gap between their performance and their aspirations. Finally, self-esteem may be at least as much a result of being loved and wanted, as being good at anything (other than personal relationships).

Self-esteem may not be the crucial dimension, however. Bandura (1977) has laid emphasis on the role of self-efficacy—the belief that one is able to control one's life and deal with life's challenges. The concept here is of a self-confidence that the individual is able to cope with whatever has to be faced. But this concept too is multifaceted. The reverse pole emphasized by Seligman (Abrahamson *et al.,* 1978; Peterson & Seligman, 1984) under the term 'learned helplessness' is similar but slightly different in its details. The central notion is that people tend to attribute bad experiences to global faults in themselves that are unalterable and lasting. The implication, as with self-efficacy, is that vulnerability resides in a tendency to assume that bad circumstances are outside one's control and that there is nothing that can be done to make things better. Conversely, protection comes from a belief that action is possible and likely to be effective.

The third hypothesized mediating factor, after self-esteem and self-efficacy, concerns social-problem-solving skills (Pellegrini, 1985). The suggestion, here, differs in proposing that what matters is the specific knowledge on *how* to deal with life crisis rather than a general belief in one's worth as a person or a concept of one's self as a capable individual who can take positive and effective action to overcome hazards and adversities. The factor sounds very different in its focus on specific skills but it is clear that what is involved is not only a repertoire of responses but also an approach to social problems that recognizes a need to take action to deal with them, and which reflects a self-concept that includes a belief that this is possible.

The data are not available to allow any decision on the relative importance of these three facets of self-concept. However, it seems reasonable to suppose that in varying degrees all play a part. First, there are effects on people's *appraisal* of life experiences; second, on their mental *reaction* to them in terms of the extent to which they can be controlled or modified, and third on their *action* to deal with their situation, an action that involves planning and coping strategies to deal with the real-life situation together with the rather different type of coping that is involved in dealing with one's internal emotional responses to the psychosocial stress or hazard.

There are several implications for theory and practice that follow from these views on the probable importance of cognitive mediation in vulnerability and protective mechanisms. The recent evidence on protective mechanisms (Rutter, 1987 *c*) is in keeping with cognitive processing concepts in its emphasis on the crucial role of turning points in people's lives in which new experiences bring about changes in people's views of themselves, of their environment and of their relationships with other people. Such experiences need not necessarily be pleasant; indeed, some positive reappraisals of self-concept come from successful coping with adversity rather than from happy events in the ordinary sense of the word. To be protective, probably the reappraisal must lead to active coping and not just passive acceptance. It is important that people feel in control of their lives and act on that belief. This belief may well be influenced by lasting personality qualities but also it may be changed (for the better or the worse) by new experiences in adult life as well as childhood.

Vulnerability to Depression

Let me turn now to a more directly clinical issue. At one time, psychiatrists tended to suppose that major depressive disorders could not occur in childhood because children lacked both a well-developed superego and also the necessary intrapsychic structures required to turn in anger against the self (Rie, 1966). There are doubts regarding the validity of the psychoanalytic ideas that constituted the basis for that view, but in any case, empirical observations have shown that, contrary to theoretical presuppositions, depressive conditions can and do occur in childhood (Rutter *et al.,* 1986). Nevertheless, the same evidence has shown that major affective disorders are decidedly less frequent in early childhood than they are in adult life, with the main rise in incidence occurring during the adolescent years. This has been shown for clinical cases of depression and of mania, for suicide and attempted suicide, and for depressive feelings as reported by young people in the general population. The question that has to be posed is why there is this very marked age trend.

Clearly, it is *not* that young children lack the ability to experience misery and unhappiness. Dysphoric mood occurs at all ages and some types of expression, for example crying, are actually more frequent in early life (Shepherd *et al.,* 1971). But depressive disorders consist of much more than sadness. The cognitive components of depression are a major part of the clinical picture (Beck, 1967). The depressive state is characterized as much by guilt, self-blame, self-depreciation, helplessness and hopelessness as by dysphoric mood. Emphasis has come to be placed on the cognitive triad of negative feelings about the self, the immediate life situation and the future. Could it be that young children are protected against depression because they lack the cognitive capacities to experience these thoughts, at least with the depth or extent that is required for depression?

There is indeed a certain amount of evidence in support of that proposition. If children are to experience feelings of unworthiness and a sense of failure, presumably they must appreciate the meaning of standards, be able to compare themselves with others and understand the concept of failure to meet expected standards. Kagan's (1981) data suggest that these self-concepts related to guilt do not arise until about two years of age. But, depressive feelings of hopelessness require more than a sense of failure; that sense must be experienced as generalized and projected into the future. Other evidence suggests that the tendency to do this does not become established until much later in childhood (Dweck & Elliot, 1983; Harter, 1983, 1986; Shantz, 1983; Cicchetti & Schneider-Rosen, 1986). Young children tend to view performance in specific task terms and it is only in middle childhood that they begin to see people's characteristics as stable psychological traits and to make general comparisons between themselves and other people. At first, children tend to have rather overoptimistic views of their own competence and they are less likely to respond to task failure with feelings of helplessness and of an inability to do better next time. Only at about eight years of age do children usually have any generalized concept about themselves as people. As they grow older, they come to have an increasing sense of their own responsibilities and power to act; moreover, there is a growing tendency to think about the future and to project feelings into it. Young children can feel guilty about what they have done already but they are less likely to experience anticipatory guilt.

It has to be said that our knowledge on depression-related social cognitions is quite limited. Nevertheless, it seems that the ability to experience shame and guilt arises during the late infancy period. At first such feelings tend to be tied strictly to the immediate; then during middle childhood there is an increasing tendency to generalize the cognitions to build up a view of the self in comparison with others and it becomes more likely that task failure will result in a general feeling of helplessness. Initially such negative cognitions tend to be confined to the present situation or to conceptually related circumstances but in later childhood there is an increasing tendency to think about the future, to project feelings of failure into the future (i.e. to proceed from helplessness to hopelessness), and to experience anticipatory guilt and shame.

If these age trends in cognition are confirmed, could they account for the relative lack of depressive disorders in early childhood and their frequency after adolescence? The possibility warrants serious study. However, there are both methodological and substantive problems. To begin with, we have to ask whether it is that children do not *experience* these thoughts or rather whether they do but that they lack the conceptual language to tell us about them. Also, however, we must beware of assuming cognitive primacy in depression. Although clearly depression is not just a mood disorder, equally obviously it is not just a cognitive disorder either, and we lack understanding of how the two interrelate. Moreover, there is no evidence that the few young children with major depression are at all cognitively advanced; in those cases the disorder seems to have allowed the expression of negative cognitions that would otherwise be unusual at that age. Maybe, the relevance of children's cognitive limitations concerns their response to threatening life events, rather than the existence of depression as such. In adult life, it seems that depressive disorders are often precipitated by negative life events that carry long-term threat that causes people to feel helpless and hopeless with a resulting depressive re-evaluation of themselves. Perhaps children are less likely to respond in this way. If so, one might expect children to be just as likely as adults to show acute distress following adverse life events but for there to be a lesser tendency in childhood for this to develop into a clinical disorder in which the negative cognitions and emotions persist long after the event has passed and been dealt with.

The implication is that greater attention should be paid to the possible role of cognitive processing in children's responses to life experiences as well as the development of affective disorders. It remains quite uncertain what answers will emerge from research into these issues but it is evident that it should be informative to ask questions about the meaning of age trends, with cognitive features as one possible mediating mechanism.

Aetiology and Treatment of Depression

Cognitive concepts have also played a key role in recent ideas on the genesis and perpetuation of depression. Various theorists, most notably Beck (1967, 1976), Brown & Harris (1978) and Seligman (Abrahamson *et al.,* 1978; Peterson & Seligman, 1984), have argued that negative cognitions are not only part of depressive symptomatology but also serve to bring about depression and to prevent its recovery. It has proved quite difficult to test the causal hypothesis but there is rather stronger evidence in support of the view that negative attributions involving feelings of helplessness serve to maintain depression (Brewin, 1985). These cognitive theories have led to the development of therapeutic interventions designed to alter the negative cognitions (so-called cognitive therapies). The evidence available so far from comparative evaluations suggests that cognitive therapy is roughly equivalent to tricyclic medication in effectiveness (Mathews, 1986) and that cognitive approaches may be particularly useful for preventing relapses (Simons *et al.,* 1986). Up to now these techniques have been little used with children but there is reason to suppose that they might prove to be similarly applicable. Although the field of inquiry is still in its infancy, already there are several implications for theory and practice. First, the findings cast doubt on the soma-psyche dichotomy. Just as cognitive therapies relieve mood, so also antidepressant drugs diminish dysfunctional cognitions (Murphy *et al.,* 1984). Environmentally induced disorders may be perpetuated by biological changes in the organism which respond to medication; conversely endogenous conditions may involve distorted thought processes which then serve to interfere with recovery. An integrated psychobiological approach to psychiatric disorder is required (Rutter, 1986 *b*). Psychotherapists cannot afford to ignore the biology of psychiatric disorder any more than biological psychiatrists can ignore its psychology.

Second, the efficacy of cognitive methods has implications for the content and strategies of psychological therapies. Traditional psychoanalytically oriented psychotherapies have focused on the meanings of past experiences, on intrapsychic conflicts and defences, and on analysis of the patient-therapist relationship. Work with children has required considerable modification of the techniques used but there has been less change in the principles employed. The implication from the cognitive approaches, as well as from many other developments in psychological therapies (Rutter, 1982) is that it is necessary to have a greater focus on the ways in which people think about themselves and their experiences and the ways in which they actually deal with their current real-life situations.

Thirdly, the findings force us to pay attention to the need in treatment to *maintain* therapeutic gains. There are several examples in psychiatry where the methods that are most successful in the short term are not those most effective in the long term (Rutter, 1986 *c)*. One of the key goals in treatment must be to help the patient acquire coping strategies that give the skills required to maintain adaptive functioning and to deal with the hazards and adversities that remain ahead.

Conclusions on Cognitive Processing

In this discussion of cognitive processing I have concentrated on the role of cognition in relation to socio-emotional development and disorders. There is much evidence that the role is an important one. However, it is crucial to emphasize that the interactions are two-way. Affective states also influence cognitive processing, as the evidence on the effects of mood on memory shows (Bower, 1981). It would be foolish to suppose that either cognition or affect was primary; development involves an integrated organization of the two (Sroufe, 1979 *a, b*). My purpose has simply been to point to some of the many ways in which cognitive processing needs to be taken into account in considering child development and disorder.

COGNITIVE DEFICITS

It seems reasonable to suppose that, if cognitive processing is so important in people's appraisal of and response to experiences, then abnormalities or limitations in the ability to undertake such cognitive processing might have profound implications for the risk of psychiatric disorder. The empirical evidence suggests that this is indeed the case, although the mechanisms by which the psychiatric risk comes about remain unclear.

Socio-emotional Consequences of Language Delay and Reading Difficulties

The issues are well illustrated by the findings on the socio-emotional consequences of language delay (Howlin & Rutter, 1987). General population follow-up studies of preschool children have been quite consistent in showing that those with language delay have a much increased incidence of emotional and behavioural disturbance (Fundudis *et al.,* 1979; Richman *et al.,* 1982; Drillien & Drummond, 1983; Silva *et al.,* 1983). Psychiatric problems are more frequent in those with a global intellectual deficit in addition to specific language problems (Cantwell & Baker, 1977; Silva *et al.,* 1983) but the psychiatric risk still applies to those who are not mentally retarded. The risk also tends to be greatest when the language deficit is severe and when it involves comprehension as well as expression, but even children with relatively mild speech defects tend to show a raised incidence of fear, anxieties and problems making friends (Baker *et al.,* 1980). The psychiatric problems associated with language delay tend to persist, at least into middle childhood, and indeed the presence of language delay at three years is predictive of an *increase* in the level of disturbance over the next five years (Stevenson *et al.,* 1985). Such disturbance does not conform to any one clinical picture; emotional and conduct problems are both common, social difficulties are frequently present and hyperactivity is often a feature.

A variety of cognitive and non-cognitive mechanisms have been proposed to account for the association between language delay and psychiatric disorder. First, there may be common background factors such as low IQ, adverse temperamental features, or family problems. Second, children with oddities of any kind tend to be more than usually prone to rejection by their peers, and children with a language disability are likely to be at a disadvantage in social interactions. Both mechanisms seem important but perhaps additional processes need to be invoked to account for the persistence of socio-emotional problems long after the children are fluent in spoken language. Possibly the language delay is associated with cognitive deficits that are more lasting than the inability to speak. Unfortunately, we know very little about the later cognitive functioning of children with language retardation, apart from the well-documented association with reading difficulties (Howlin & Rutter, 1987). There is a great need for a systematic study of the social and cognitive functioning in adolescence of young people who have experienced a serious delay in language acquisition but who now show a normal level of spoken language.

In the absence of such data, some clues are provided by the progression from language delay to reading retardation. It has long been known that reading difficulties are associated with a substantially increased risk of conduct disorders (Rutter & Yule, 1973; Rutter & Giller, 1983). To some extent this association may reflect a maladaptive response to educational failure (Rutter *et al.,* 1970) but this does not seem to be the main explanation, if only because the behavioural disturbances are often present at, or soon after, school entry, before reading failure can be manifest (McMichael, 1979; Stott, 1981).

The prior association with language delay suggests the probable role of either temperamental attributes or attentional/cognitive problems, both of which are linked with reading disabilities and conduct disturbance. On the face of it, temperament and cognition seem rather different concepts but in practice they have been difficult to separate. The difficulties are best illustrated by consideration of hyperkinetic/attentional deficit syndromes.

Hyperkinetic/Attentional Deficit Syndromes

In recent years clinicians have come to accept that problems in concentration constitute the core of what used to be called hyperkinetic disorder and which now tend to be called attention deficit syndromes. The suggestion is that a physiological deficit in the ability to process information coming into the brain underlies the disturbance of behaviour. The idea is an important one because, if it could be validated, it would have very important implications for our concepts of causation of psychiatric disorders. Unfortunately, as Taylor (1980, 1986) has pointed out, there are problems in testing the hypothesis because inattention is used both as a behavioural description (i.e. to describe the fact that children are not paying attention to some task allocated to them) and as an explanatory variable (i.e. an abnormality in the brain functions that deal with the processing of incoming sensory input). Moreover, the latter involves many processes, not one. People need to divide as well as concentrate their attention, and to shift as well as maintain the focus of their interest. Children may perform badly on any of these functions because they cannot process information efficiently, because they can but choose not to do so, or because the given task is less interesting than others that they would like to engage in. Furthermore, the behaviour of *looking* attentive (as by staring at the teacher or the textbook) may not be accompanied by any relevant cognitive processing; the child's eyes may be on the task while his mind is engaged on something entirely different. Conversely, children may appear not to be listening while still taking everything in (as well illustrated by the amount picked up by children seemingly engaged in play while the parents are talking about them to someone else).

The distinctions between these various physiological and psychological processes are difficult. Nevertheless, the empirical evidence suggests that there are important cognitive-behavioural connections. Studies on hyperactive children have shown them to be impaired on tests of cognitive performance. Furthermore, within clinic groups of children of normal IQ with disturbances of conduct, poor test performance is associated with hyperactivity but not with defiant aggressive behaviour (Taylor, 1986). There does seem to be a real connection between inattention and overactivity. There is also a further association between overactivity and conduct disturbance. The mechanisms involved in both sets of linkages remain uncertain. The inattention linkage is not specific in that there are also associations with low IQ, with clumsiness, and with developmental delays. It is not at all self-evident that the main process involved is a deficit in cognitive processing, although this may well form part of the problem. In addition, it is not known why hyperactivity is associated with conduct disturbance. It could be that the overactive behaviour is irritating to others and hence leads to maladaptive patterns of interaction. However, attributional factors may also be important. People interpret other people's behaviour according to their attribution of intention (Parke & Slaby, 1983). It seems relevant that aggressive boys are more likely to attribute hostile intentions to others. As a result they elicit, as well as initiate, more negative interactions (Dodge, 1980; Dodge *et al.*, 1984). Is this attributional bias a result of past experiences or does it reflect some kind of deficit in cognitive processing? A complex set of cognitive-behavioural associations is involved and treatment methods should be enhanced if the meaning of that tangle could be elucidated.

Schizophrenia

A word is necessary on attentional deficits in schizophrenia. There is a mass of evidence showing associations between the two (Nuechterlein & Dawson, 1984; Nuechterlein, 1986) and it has been suggested that a deficit in signal/noise discrimination may form part of the basis of schizophrenia. The suggestion is made plausible by the finding that similar attentional problems are found in the offspring of schizophrenics and that such deficits are predictive of psychopathology (not necessarily schizophrenic in form) within that group. Two main issues await resolution. First, do the attentional deficits specifically predict schizophrenia or is the association with a broader range of psychiatric problems? Second, is the deficit similar or different in type from that associated with hyperactivity or with other psychiatric syndromes? The evidence on both points is inconclusive as yet. A specific linkage for certain types of attentional deficit is possible but it has still to be established. As problems in information processing occur in a variety of psychiatric disorders, and as some measures do not differentiate the offspring of schizophrenics from the offspring of depressed parents, the need is to develop discriminating measures of different types of attentional problem. The ubiquity of cognitive-behavioural associations shows their importance but the meanings to be attached to them depend on the determination of specific mechanisms. That remains a task for the future.

Autism

The last topic to mention concerns the role of cognitive deficits in autism. There is now a mass of evidence to show that autistic children do indeed have serious cognitive deficits which tend to follow a distinctive pattern—with impairments in sequencing, abstraction, conceptualization and the use of meaning (Rutter, 1983). Moreover, these deficits are rather resistant to treatment and constitute the most important predictors of outcome. It has seemed plausible to suggest that they might underlie autistic children's social difficulties. The problem has been to know how this might operate. Hobson (1983, 1986) showed that autistic children were impaired in their ability to distinguish emotional cues and to discriminate age and gender features. The implication seemed to be that there was some type of cognitive deficit that applied to the processing of social and emotional stimuli. But what could that deficit be and how did it relate to autistic children's other cognitive problems? Recent research by Baron-Cohen and his colleagues (1985, 1986) suggests that the deficit may involve an inability to infer other people's intentions. Because of this, autistic children lack a theory of mind that might allow them to appreciate other people's feelings, beliefs and mental states. They suggest that the critical feature may not be turning away from social interactions as such but rather a specific dysfunction in conceiving of mental states. This comes nearest to a directly cognitive explanation for a social phenomenon but much further research is needed to put the hypothesis to critical tests. Of all psychiatric conditions, autism is the one in which there is the closest, and probably most direct, connection between cognitive deficits and social malfunction. Elucidation of the processes involved seems to be on the horizon and if that riddle can be solved it should throw light on aspects of development and disorder that extend beyond autism.

CONCLUSIONS

This, necessarily selective, overview of some of the ways in which cognition may play a role in child development and in psychiatric disorder indicates the richness of the territory. The associations between cognition and socio-emotional functioning are many and various. The ways in which we appraise our life circumstances and the ways in which we react to experiences of all kinds are greatly influenced by how we think about ourselves and our environment. Research has begun to suggest some of the mechanisms that may be involved in these cognitive processes. It is clear that biases and distortions in such processing may be associated with social and emotional malfunction. These biases may derive from earlier experiences, from intrinsic temperamental styles, or from deficits in the ability to process incoming information. The further study of cognitive processing and cognitive deficits is likely to be rewarding and helpful for clinical practice.

REFERENCES

Abrahamson, L. Y., Seligman, M. E. P. & Teasdale, J. D. 1978). Learned helplessness in humans: Critique and reformulation. *Journal of Abnormal Psychology, 87,* 49–74.

Ainsworth, M. (1969). Object relations, dependency and attachment: A theoretical review of the mother-infant relationship. *Child Development, 40,* 969–1025.

Ainsworth, M., Blehar, M., Waters, E. & Wall, S. (1978). *Strange-situation Behavior of One-Year-Olds: Its Relations to Mother-Infant Interaction in the First Year and to Qualitative Differences in the Infant-Mother Attachment Relationship.* New York: Erlbaum.

Asher, S. R. (1983). Social competence and peer status: Recent advances and future directions. *Child Development, 54,* 1427–1434.

Baker, L., Cantwell, D. & Mattison, R. (1980). Behavior problems in children with pure speech disorders and in children with combined speech and language disorders. *Journal of Abnormal Child Psychology, 8,* 245–250.

Bandura, A. (1977). *Social Learning Theory.* Englewood Cliffs, NJ: Prentice-Hall.

Baron-Cohen, S., Leslie, A. M. & Frith, U. (1985). Does the autistic child have a 'theory of mind'? *Cognition, 21,* 37–46.

Baron-Cohen, S., Leslie, A. M. & Frith, U. (1986). Mechanical, behavioural and intentional understanding of picture stories in autistic children. *British Journal of Developmental Psychology, 4,* 113–125.

Beck, A. T. (1967). *Depression: Causes and Treatment.* Philadelphia, PA: University of Pennsylvania Press.

Beck, A. T. (1976). *Cognitive Therapy and the Emotional Disorders.* New York: International Universities Press.

Bower, G. N. (1981). Mood and memory. *American Psychologist, 36,* 129–148.

Bowlby, J. (1969). *Attachment and Loss I: Attachment.* London: Hogarth Press.

Bowlby, J. (1973). *Attachment and Loss II: Separation Anxiety and Anger.* London: Hogarth Press.

Bowlby, J. (1980). *Attachment and Loss III: Loss, Sadness and Depression.* New York: Basic Books.

Bretherton, I. & Waters, E., (eds)(1985). Growing points of attachment theory and research. *Monographs for the Society for Research in Child Development,* Serial No. 209, *50,* 1, 2.

Brewin, C. (1985). Depression and causal attributions: What is their relation? *Psychological Bulletin, 98* (2), 297–309.

Brown, G. W. & Harris, T. O. (1978). *Social Origins of Depression: A Study of Psychiatric Disorders in Women.* London: Tavistock Publications.

Brunk, M. A. & Hengeller, S. W. (1984). Child influences on adult controls. An experimental investigation. *Developmental Psychology, 20* (6), 1074–1081.

Cantwell, D. & Baker, L. (1977). Psychiatric disorder in children with speech and language retardation: A critical review. *Archives of General Psychiatry, 34,* 583–591.

Cicchetti, D. & Schneider-Rosen, K. (1986). An organizational approach to childhood depression. In M. Rutter, C. Izard & P. Read (eds), *Depression in Young People: Developmental and Clinical Perspectives,* pp. 71–134. New York: Guilford Press.

Condry, J. C. & Ross, D. F. (1985). Sex and aggression: The influence of gender label on the perception of aggression in children. *Child Development, 56,* 225–233.

Dodge, K. A. (1980). Social cognition and children's aggressive behavior. *Child Development, 51,* 162–172.

Dodge, K. A., Murphy, R. R. & Buchsbaum, K. (1984). The assessment of intention and detection skills in children: Implications for developmental psychopathology. *Child Development, 55,* 163–173.

Douglas, J.W.B. (1975). Early hospital admissions and later disturbances of behaviour and learning. *Developmental Medicine and Child Neurology, 17,* 456–480.

Douglas, V. I. (1983). Attentional and cognitive problems. In M. Rutter (ed.), *Developmental Neuropsychiatry,* pp. 280–329. New York: Guilford Press.

Drillien, C. & Drummond, M. (1983). *Developmental Screening and the Child with Special Needs.* Clinics in Developmental Medicine 86. London: SIMP/Heinemann Medical.

Dweck, C. S. & Elliott, E. S. (1983). Achievement motivation. In E. M. Hetherington (ed.), *Socialization, Personality and Social Development,* vol. 4, *Mussen's Handbook of Child Psychology,* 4th ed. New York: Wiley.

Eagle, M. N. (1984). *Recent Developments in Psychoanalysis: A Critical Evaluation.* New York: McGraw–Hill.

Emde, R. N. & Harmon, R. J. (eds) (1982). *The Development of Attachment and Affiliative Systems.* New York: Plenum.

Eysenck, H. J. (1953). *The Structure of Human Personality.* New York: Wiley.

Eysenck, H. J. (1967). *The Biological Basis of Personality.* Springfield, IL: Thomas.

Fein, D., Pennington, B., Markowitz, P., Braverman, M. & Waterhouse, L. (1986). Toward a neuropsychological model of infantile autism: Are the social deficits primary? *Journal of the American Academy of Child Psychiatry, 25,* 198–212.

Fundudis, T., Kolvin, I. & Garside, R. (eds) (1979). *Speech Retarded and Deaf Children: Their Psychological Development.* London: Academic Press.

Garmezy, N. (1985). Stress resistant children: The search for protective factors. In J. Stevenson (ed.), *Recent Research in Developmental Psychopathology.* Book supplement to the *Journal of Child Psychology* No. 4. Oxford: Pergamon.

Harter, S. (1983). Developmental perspectives on the self-system. In E. M. Hetherington (ed.), *Socialization, Personality and Social Development,* vol. 4, *Mussen's Handbook of Child Psychology,* 4th ed. New York: Wiley.

Harter, S. (1986). Processes underlying the construction, maintenance and enhancement of the self-concept in children. In J. Suls & A. Greenwald (eds), *Psychological Perspectives on The Self,* vol. 3. New York: Erlbaum.

Hobson, R. P. (1983). The autistic child's recognition of age-related features of people, animals and things. *British Journal of Developmental Psychology, 1,* 343–352.

Hobson, R. P. (1986). The autistic child's appraisal of expressions of emotion. *Journal of Child Psychology and Psychiatry, 27,* 321–342.

Hodges, J. & Tizard, B. (in press *a).* IQ and behavioural adjustment of ex-institutional adolescents. *Journal of Child Psychology and Psychiatry.*

Hodges, J. & Tizard, B. (in press *b).* Social and family relationships of ex-institutional adolescents. *Journal of Child Psychology and Psychiatry.*

Howlin, P. & Rutter, M. (1987). The consequences of language delay for other aspects of development. In W. Yule & M. Rutter (eds), *Language Development and Disorders.* London: MacKeith/Blackwell.

Izard, C. E. (1978). On the ontogenesis of emotions and emotion-cognitive relationships in infancy. In M. Lewis & L. A. Rosenblum (eds), *The Development of Affect.* New York: Plenum Press.

Kagan, J. (1980). Perspectives on continuity. In O. Brim & J. Kagan (eds), *Constancy and Change in Human Development.* Cambridge, MA: Harvard University Press.

Kagan, J. (1981). *The Second Year: The Emergency of Self-awareness.* Cambridge, MA: Harvard University Press.

Kagan, J. (1984). *The Nature of the Child.* New York: Basic Books.

Kelvin, P. (1969). *The Bases of Social Behaviour: An Approach in Terms of Order and Value.* London: Holt, Rinehart & Winston.

Kepper, M. R. (1982). Social control processes, attributions of motivation and the internalization of social values. In E. T. Higgins, D. N. Ruble & W. W. Hartup (eds), *Social Cognition and Social Behavior: Developmental Perspectives.* Cambridge: Cambridge University Press.

Lütkenhaus, P., Grossman, K. E. & Grossman, K. (1985). Infant-mother attachment at twelve months and style of interaction with a stranger at age of three years. *Child Development, 56,* 1535–1542.

Maccoby, E. E. & Martin, J. A. (1983). Socialization in the context of the family: Parent-child interaction. In E. M. Hetherington (ed.), *Socialization, Personality and Social Development,* vol. 4, *Mussen's Handbook of Child Psychology,* 4th ed. New York: Wiley.

Main, M., Kaplan, N. & Cassidy, J. (1985). Security in infancy, childhood and adulthood. In I. Bretherton & E. Waters (eds), Growing points of attachment theory and research. *Monographs for the Society for Research in Child Development,* Serial No. 209, *50,* 1, 2, pp. 66–104.

Masten, A. S. & Garmezy, N. (1985). Risk, vulnerability and protective factors in developmental psychopathology. In B. B. Lahey & A. E. Kazdin (eds), *Advances in Clinical Child Psychology,* vol. 8. New York: Plenum.

Mathews, A. (1986). Cognitive processes in anxiety and depression: A discussion paper. *Journal of the Royal Society of Medicine, 79,* 158–161.

McMichael, P. (1979). The hen or the egg? Which comes first—Antisocial emotional disorders or reading disability? *British Journal of Educational Psychology, 49,* 226–238.

Murphy, G. E., Simons, A. D., Wetzel, R. D. & Lustman, P. J. (1984). Cognitive theory and pharmacotherapy: Single and together in the treatment of depression. *Archives of General Psychiatry, 41,* 33–41.

Nuechterlein, K. H. (1983). Signal detection in vigilance tasks and behavioural attributes among offspring of schizophrenic mothers and among hyperactive children. *Journal of Abnormal Psychology, 92,* 4–28.

Nuechterlein, K. H. (1986). Childhood precursors of adult schizophrenia: Annotation. *Journal of Child Psychology and Psychiatry, 27,* 133–144.

Nuechterlein, K. H. & Dawson, M. E. (1984). Information processing and attentional functioning in the developmental cause of schizophrenic disorders. *Schizophrenia Bulletin, 10,* 160–203.

Parke, R. D. (1974). Rules and roles and resistance to deviation. Recent advances in punishment, discipline and self-control. In A. D. Pick (ed.), *Minnesota Symposium on Child Psychology,* vol. 8. Minneapolis, MS: University of Minnesota Press.

Parke, R. D. & Slaby, R. G. (1983). The development of aggression. In E. M. Hetherington (ed.), *Socialization, Personality and Social Development,* vol. 4, *Mussen's Handbook of Child Psychology,* 4th ed., pp. 547–641, New York: Wiley.

Parkes, C. M. & Stevenson-Hinde, J. (eds) (1982). *The Place of Attachment in Human Behavior.* New York: Basic Books.

Pellegrini, D. (1985). Training in social problem-solving. In M. Rutter & L. Hersov (eds), *Child and Adolescent Psychiatry: Modern Approaches,* 2nd ed., pp. 839–850. Oxford: Blackwell Scientific.

Peterson, C. & Seligman, M. E. P. (1984). Causal explanation as a risk factor for depression. Theory and evidence. *Psychological Review, 91,* 347–374.

Quinton, D. & Rutter, M. (1976). Early hospital admissions and later disturbances of behaviour: An attempted replication of Douglas's finding. *Developmental Medicine and Child Neurology, 18,* 447–459.

Reznick, J. S., Kagan, J., Snidman, N., Gersten, M., Baak, K. & Rosenberg, A. (1986). Inhibited and uninhibited children: A follow-up study. *Child Development, 55,* 660–680.

Richman, N., Stevenson, J. & Graham, P. (1982). *Preschool to School: A Behavioural Study.* London: Academic Press.

Ricks, M. H. (1985). The social transmission of parental behaviour: Attachment across generations. In I. Bretherton & E. Waters (eds), Growing points of attachment theory and research. *Monographs for the Society for Research in Child Development,* Serial No. 209, *50,* 1, 2, pp. 211–227.

Rie, H. E. (1966). Depression in childhood: A survey of some pertinent contributions. *Journal of the American Academy of Child Psychiatry, 5,* 653–685.

Rutter, M. (1979 *a*). Separation experiences: A new look at an old topic. *Journal of Pediatrics, 95,* 147–154.

Rutter, M. (1979 *b*). Protective factors in children's responses to stress and disadvantage. In M. W. Kent & J. E. Rolf (eds), *Primary Prevention of Psychopathology,* vol. 3: *Social Competence in Children,* pp. 49–74. Hanover, NH: University Press of New England.

Rutter, M. (1980). Emotional development. In M. Rutter (ed.), *Scientific Foundations of Developmental Psychiatry.* London: Heinemann Medical.

Rutter, M. (1981 *a*). Stress, coping and development: Some issues and some questions. *Journal of Child Psychology and Psychiatry, 22,* 323–356.

Rutter, M. (1981 *b*). *Maternal Deprivation Reassessed,* 2nd ed. Harmondsworth, Middx.: Penguin Books.

Rutter, M. (1982). Psychological therapies: Issues and prospects. *Psychological Medicine, 12,* 723–740.

Rutter, M. (1983). Cognitive deficits in the pathogenesis of autism. *Journal of Child Psychology and Psychiatry, 24,* 513–531.

Rutter, M. (1984). Psychopathology and development. H. Childhood experiences and personality development. *Australian and New Zealand Journal of Psychiatry, 18,* 314–327.

Rutter, M. (1985). Resilience in the face of adversity: Protective factors and resistance to psychiatric disorder. *British Journal of Psychiatry, 147,* 598–611.

Rutter, M. (1986 *a*). Child psychiatry: The interface between clinical and developmental research. *Psychological Medicine, 16,* 151–169.

Rutter, M. (1986 *b*). Meyerian psychobiology, personality development and the role of life experiences. *American Journal of Psychiatry, 143,* 1077–1087.

Rutter, M. (1986 *c*). Child psychiatry: Looking 30 years ahead. *Journal of Child Psychology and Psychiatry, 27,* 803–840.

Rutter, M. (1987 *a*). Continuities and discontinuities from infancy. In J. Osofsky (ed.), *Handbook of Infant Development,* 2nd ed. New York: Wiley.

Rutter, M. (1987 *b*). Intergenerational continuities and discontinuities in serious parenting difficulties. In D. Cicchetti & V. Carlson (eds), *Research on the Consequences of Child Maltreatment.* New York: Cambridge University Press.

Rutter, M. (1987 *c*). Psychosocial resilience and protective mechanism. In J. Rolf, A. Masten, D. Cicchetti, K. Nuechterlein & S. Weintraub (eds), *Risk and Protective Factors in the Development of Psychopathology.* New York: Cambridge University Press.

Rutter, M. (1987 *d*). Temperament, personality and personality disorder. *British Journal of Psychiatry* (in press).

Rutter, M. & Garmezy, N. (1983). Developmental psychopathology. In E. M. Hetherington (ed.), *Socialization, Personality and Social Development,* vol. 4, *Mussen's Handbook of Child Psychology,* 4th ed. New York: Wiley.

Rutter, M. & Giller, H. (1983). *Juvenile Delinquency: Trends and Perspectives.* New York: Guilford Press.

Rutter, M., Izard, C. E. & Read, P. B. (eds) (1986). *Depression in Young People: Developmental and Clinical Perspectives.* New York: Guilford Press.

Rutter, M. & Sandberg, S. (1985). Epidemiology of child psychiatric disorder: Methodological issues and some substantive findings. *Child Psychiatry and Human Development, 15,* 209–233.

Rutter, M., Tizard, J. & Whitmore, K. (eds) (1970). *Education, Health and Behaviour.* London: Longmans (reprinted, 1981, New York: Krieger).

Rutter, M. & Yule, W. (1973). Specific reading retardation. In L. Mann & D. Sabatino (eds), *The First Review of Special Education.* Philadelphia, PA: Buttonwood Farms.

Shantz, C. E. (1983). Social cognition. In J. H. Flavell & E. M. Markman (eds), *Cognitive Development,* vol. 3, *Mussen's Handbook of Child Psychology,* 4th ed. pp. 485–555. New York: Wiley.

Shepherd, M., Oppenheim, B. & Mitchell, S. (1971). *Childhood Behaviour and Mental Health.* London: University of London Press.

Silva, P., McGee, R. & Williams, S. (1983). Developmental language delay from 3 to 7 years and its significance for low intelligence and reading difficulties at age seven. *Developmental Medicine and Child Neurology, 28,* 783–793.

Simons, A. D., Murphy, G. E., Levine, J. L. & Wetzel, R. D. (1986). Cognitive therapy and pharmacotherapy for depression: Sustained improvement over one year. *Archives of General Psychiatry, 43,* 43–48.

Smith, C. & Lloyd, B. (1978). Maternal behaviour and perceived sex of infant: Revisited. *Child Development, 40,* 1263–1265.

Sroufe, L. A. (1979 *a*). Socioemotional development. In J. D. Osofsky (ed.), *Handbook of Infant Development.* New York: Wiley.

Sroufe, L. A. (1979*b*). The coherence of individual development. *American Psychologist, 34,* 834–841.

Sroufe, L. A. (1985). Attachment classification from the perspective of infant temperament. *Child Development, 56,* 1–14.

Sroufe, L. A. & Rutter, M. (1984). The domain of developmental psychopathology. *Child Development, 55,* 17–29.

Stevenson, J., Richman, N. & Graham, P. (1985). Behaviour problems and language abilities at 3 years and behavioural deviance at 8 years. *Journal of Child Psychology and Psychiatry, 26,* 215–230.

Stott, D. H. (1981). Behaviour disturbance and failure to learn: A study of cause and effect. *Educational Research, 23,* 163–172.

Taylor, E. (1980). Development of attention. In M. Rutter (ed.), *Scientific Foundations of Developmental Psychiatry,* pp. 185–197. London: Heinemann Medical.

Taylor, E. (1986). *The Overactive Child.* Clinics in Developmental Medicine, 97. Oxford: SIMP/Blackwell Scientific.

Tizard, B. & Hodges, J. (1978). The effect of early institutional rearing on the development of eight-year-old children. *Journal of Child Psychology and Psychiatry, 19,* 99–118.

Winters, K. C., Stone, A. A., Weintraub, S. & Neale, J. M. (1981). Cognitive and attentional deficits in children vulnerable to psychopathology. *Journal of Abnormal Child Psychology, 9,* 435–453.

Yule, W. and Rutter, M. (1985). Reading and other learning difficulties. In M. Rutter & L. Hersov (eds), *Child and Adolescent Psychiatry: Modern Approaches,* 2nd ed. Oxford: Blackwell Scientific.

5

The Physiology and Psychology of Behavioral Inhibition in Children

Jerome Kagan, J. Steven Reznick, and Nancy Snidman
Harvard University, Cambridge, Massachusetts

Longitudinal study of 2 cohorts of children selected in the second or third year of life to be extremely cautious and shy (inhibited) or fearless and outgoing (uninhibited) to unfamiliar events revealed preservation of these 2 behavioral qualities through the sixth year of life. Additionally, more of the inhibited children showed signs of activation in 1 or more of the physiological circuits that usually respond to novelty and challenge, namely, the hypothalamic-pituitary-adrenal axis, the reticular activating system, and the sympathetic arm of the autonomic nervous system. It is suggested that the threshold of responsivity in limbic and hypothalamic structures to unfamiliarity and challenge is tonically lower for inhibited than for uninhibited children.

There are three important advantages of gathering information on both physiological and psychological qualities in developmental investigations. First, such information permits deeper understanding. For example, through investigations of separation of infant primates from their mothers one gains a richer appreciation of the phenomenon by describing changes in both behavior and cortisol secretion because some infants show no change in behavior following separation but display elevated cortisol levels (Coe, Wiener, Rosenberg, & Levine, 1985). If investigators coded only the infants'

Reprinted with permission from *Child Development*, 1987, Vol. 58, 1459–1473. Copyright 1987 by the Society for Research in Child Development, Inc.

This research was supported in part by grants from the John D. and Catherine T. MacArthur Foundation and NIMH. We thank Jane Gibbons, Maureen Johnson, and Katherine Baak for their contributions to this research.

behavior they might conclude that these monkeys were not distressed by the mother's absence. Most studies of separation from the caretaker in human infants, especially those that use the Strange Situation, record only behavior and do not gather any physiological evidence (Ainsworth, Blehar, Waters, & Wall, 1978).

Second, gathering both physiological and psychological information makes it possible to discover interactions between the inherent, biological characteristics of an organism and the nature of a class of incentive events with respect to some outcome variable of interest. Although most psychologists acknowledge the possibility of these interactions, and biologists continue to affirm them, most psychological investigations do not explicitly plan or search for such interactions. Third, when two very different sources of evidence relevant to a phenomenon are gathered, as is the case with psychological and physiological data, investigators have a clearer recognition of the choice between use of qualitative or quantitative descriptions. For example, if only a proportion of phobic adults show relevant physiological signs, one can view that group as qualitatively different from the phobic subjects with no signs, or regard all the subjects as varying on a continuum of vulnerability to fear.

This article presents data indicating a correlation in young children between selected peripheral physiological characteristics and behavioral reactions to unfamiliar and cognitively challenging events. We believe that the individual differences in behavioral reactions to unfamiliarity, threat, or challenge are due, in part, to tonic differences in the threshold of reactivity of parts of the limbic lobe, especially the amygdala and the hypothalamus, which result in enhanced activity of the pituitary-adrenal axis, reticular activating system, and sympathetic nervous system—three circuits that are influenced directly by hypothalamic activity. The Discussion section contains a more detailed rationale for this hypothesis.

Activity in the hypothalamic-pituitary-adrenal axis, which is usually increased following exposure to a novel event that cannot be assimilated or a threat that cannot be removed, leads to the production of cortisol by the adrenal cortex. Both infant primates removed from their mothers (Levine, Coe, Smotherman, & Kaplan, 1978) and phobic adults exposed to relevant incentives react with elevated cortisol levels (Fredrikson, Sundin, & Frankenhaeuser, 1985). The hypothalamus also affects skeletal motor tracts through its projection to the reticular activating system. One such tract in the brain stem involves the nucleus ambiguus, which monitors tension in the skeletal muscles of the larynx and vocal folds. These muscles contract under stress, producing changes in both the average fundamental frequency and variability of the pitch periods of vocal output (Stevens & Hirano, 1981). The third circuit involves the sympathetic nervous system and its many target organs.

Sympathetic activation, which usually follows encounter with unfamiliarity, threat, or challenge, is accompanied by increases in heart rate, blood pressure, and contractility of the heart, as well as dilation of the pupil and secretion of epinephrine from the adrenal medulla and norepinephrine from postglangionic synapses of the sympathetic nervous system (Ciarenello, 1983). The work to be reported reveals a correlation in children between signs of reactivity in one or more of these circuits and a tendency toward behavioral inhibition to unfamiliar events or situations that pose a psychological challenge that cannot be handled without effort.

LONGITUDINAL STUDY

Our laboratory has been following two independent groups of Caucasian children, middle and working class, who were selected at 21 or 31 months of age from larger samples to be either behaviorally inhibited or uninhibited when exposed to unfamiliar rooms, people, and objects. The original classification into one of the two temperamental groups required a child to show consistent withdrawal or approach to a variety of incentives. We had to screen over 400 children, by telephone and/or observation, to find groups of 60 consistently inhibited and 60 consistently uninhibited children with equal numbers of boys and girls in each group (see Garcia-Coll, Kagan, & Reznick, 1984; Snidman, 1984, for details). It may not be a coincidence that when German kindergarten teachers in Munich were asked to select only those children who were extremely shy, 15% of the total school population of 1,100 were chosen—a proportion similar to the one we found in our screening (Cranach et al., 1978).

The index of inhibited or uninhibited behavior in Cohort 1, which was seen initially at 21 months, was based on the child's behavior with an unfamiliar female examiner; unfamiliar toys; a woman displaying a trio of acts that was difficult to recall and to imitate; a talking robot; and temporary separation from the mother. The signs of behavioral inhibition were long latencies to interact with, or immediate retreat from, the unfamiliar people or objects; proximity to the mother; and cessation of play or vocalization. The uninhibited children showed the opposite profile.

The index of inhibited behavior in Cohort 2 seen first at 31 months was based primarily on behavior with an unfamiliar peer of the same sex and age and, second, on behavior with an unfamiliar woman. The behavioral indexes of inhibition were similar to those used with Cohort 1—long latencies to interact with the child, adult, or toys; retreat from the unfamiliar events; and long periods of time proximal to the mother. Each of these samples was seen on two additional occasions after the original selection, the latest being at 5½ years of age, with about 10% attrition in the samples (see Garcia-Coll et al., 1984; Kagan, Reznick, Clarke, Snidman, & Garcia-Coll, 1984; Reznick et al., 1986; Snidman, 1984).

On the second visit, at 4 years of age for Cohort 1 and at 3½ years for Cohort 2, the primary index of inhibition was based on behavior with an unfamiliar child of the same sex and age. At 5½ years of age the index was based more broadly on behavior with an unfamiliar peer in a laboratory setting, with classmates in a school setting, with an examiner during a 90-min testing situation, and in a room that contained unfamiliar objects mildly suggestive of risk (a balance beam, a black box with a hole). An aggregate index of inhibition for Cohort 1 at 5½ years of age represented a mean standard score across the correlated variables from the separate situations noted above. (Analyses of the data for Cohort 2 are not yet complete.)

Preservation of Behavior

The behaviors that characterize inhibited and uninhibited children were preserved to a significant degree from the original assessment to the two later assessments at 4 and 5½ years of age. (The adjectives inhibited and uninhibited refer to the original classifications at 21 or 31 months, unless stated otherwise.) The correlation, for Cohort 1, between the index of inhibition at 21 months and the aggregate index at 5½ years was .52 ($p <$ .001); the correlation between the indexes at age 4 and 5½ was .67 ($p < $.001). The correlation between the behavioral indexes of inhibition at 31 and 43 months for Cohort 2 was .59 ($p < $ .001).

The preservation of inhibited and uninhibited behavior also generalized to the school context. In her doctoral research, Gersten (1986) trained observers who did not know the child's prior classification to code the child's behavior in his or her kindergarten class during the first week of school in September, as well as during a day in the Spring of the same academic year. Each observer noted every 15 sec whether the target child was displaying one or more of a small number of responses, but especially whether the child was alone and isolated or in social interaction with the teacher or another peer. The children classified as inhibited at 21 months were more likely to be alone and less likely to be in social interaction on both the Fall and Spring visits ($r = .34, p < .05$, between the index of inhibition at 21 months and the index of inhibited behavior in the school setting across the two visits).

One of the most sensitive indexes of inhibition in a laboratory context at 5½ years was a reluctance to talk spontaneously to the female examiner during the 90-min testing battery. Videotapes of the testing session were scored by observers blind to the children's classification for the latency to the child's first two spontaneous comments to the examiner (a spontaneous comment was any remark that was not a direct reply to an examiner's question), as well as the total number of spontaneous comments. Although the latencies to the first and second comments yielded similar results, the latter variable was more sensitive; hence, we used it in the analyses. Figure 1 illustrates a scatter plot of these two conversation variables for the children in Cohort 2 who had been classified as inhibited or uninhibited at 2½ years of age. Not one inhibited child, but 14 uninhibited children, issued their second spontaneous comment within 3 min of entering the room and, in addition, made 40 or more comments. By contrast, 13 inhibited but only two uninhibited children failed to make their second spontaneous comment until at least 10 min had passed, and they spoke less than 10 times ($p < .01$ by the Exact Test).

There was more obvious preservation of uninhibited than inhibited behavior in both cohorts, which we believe is a result of socialization experiences. This asymmetry in the stability of the two profiles seems reasonable because American parents, reflecting the values of their society,

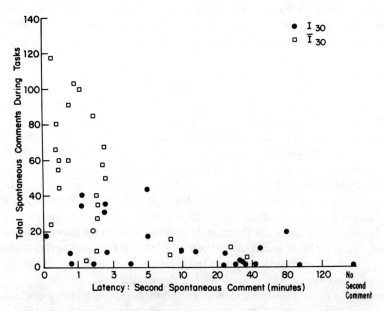

Figure 1. Scatter plot relating total spontaneous comments against latency to second spontaneous comment during testing session at 5½ years: Cohort 2.

regard outgoing, sociable behavior as much more desirable and adaptive than shy, timid behavior (Singer, 1984). About 40% of the original groups of inhibited children became less inhibited at 5½ years, while less than 10% of the uninhibited children became more inhibited. There is, however, a gender asymmetry in the direction of change. More boys than girls changed from inhibited to uninhibited. Maternal interviews suggested that more of the mothers of children who had become less inhibited, compared with those who remained inhibited, had self-consciously helped their children to overcome their inhibition by introducing peers into the home and by encouraging the child to cope with stressful situations. A much smaller group of originally uninhibited children, about 10% and typically girls from working-class families, became more inhibited at later ages. The interviews with these mothers suggested they wanted a more cautious child and encouraged such a profile.

There are more inhibited children who are later—rather than firstborn—about two-thirds—and more uninhibited children who are firstborn—a result affirmed by Snow, Jacklin, and Maccoby (1981). Interpretation of this finding is unclear. It may be due to the fact that firstborn children are encouraged to be more independent of the mother when the next child arrives and, as a result, gradually learn to control behavioral signs of fear, while the youngest child may have fewer incentives promoting uninhibited behavior. A second interpretation, biological in nature, assumes that fetal stress is less likely during the first than during subsequent pregnancies. A third interpretation is that later-born status is associated with more stressful experiences for the small group of infants who are born with a biological disposition to become inhibited as a result of a lower threshold of reactivity in the limbic lobe. An infant with a low threshold of responsivity in limbic structures might react with psychological uncertainty to the mild, but unexpected, intrusions of an older 3- or 4-year-old sibling who seizes a toy, pinches an arm, or pushes the young infant off a chair. Although these aggressive and predatory acts might have minimal effects on most infants, they could generate limbic arousal and development of a habit of withdrawal to intrusion and unfamiliarity in those infants who possess the more excitable limbic structures.

Because any behavioral surface can be the result of different mediating processes, the reasonableness of the assumption that extremely inhibited children are born biologically different from uninhibited ones depends upon evidence showing that more inhibited than uninhibited children display some of the physiological signs to be expected from a lower threshold of limbic excitability to events that are unfamiliar or pose a potential threat. The following sections describe the physiological variables we quantified.

Heart Period and Heart Period Variability

Because we measured the child's heart period and heart period variability to baseline and cognitive tasks on every assessment, we are able to make the firmest statements about these two autonomic parameters. Heart period variability was defined as the standard deviation of all the interbeat intervals during a particular episode. The mean heart period and variability for a multitrial episode was always the average of the values for the separate trials in that episode. Although we shall occasionally use the terms heart rate and heart rate variability in the text, the reader should understand that all statistical analyses were performed on the heart period values because that was the form of the original data. Average heart period and heart period variability in our data were always positively correlated under both relaxed conditions as well as under conditions of mild cognitive stress (correlations .6 and .7).

More inhibited than uninhibited children had high and stable (i.e., less variable) heart rates at every age of evaluation, with the magnitude of the correlation at 5½ years higher than the relation at 21 months. We suspect this is because of more effective sampling of heart rate under cognitive stress at the older age. At 21 months, heart rate was gathered while the child looked at slides or listened to auditory stimuli with no requirement for mental work. Individual differences in both heart rate and heart rate variability in Cohort 1 were preserved from 4 to 5½ years ($r = .58, p < .001; r = .64, p < .001$); differences in heart rate variability were preserved from 21 months to 5½ years ($r = .39, p < .01$). Further, the original index of inhibited behavior at 21 months predicted both a higher and a less variable heart rate at 5½ years ($r = .44, .39$) (see Table 1).

More important, the inhibited children in Cohort 1 who had higher and more stable heart rates over the first two assessments were more likely to remain inhibited than the inhibited children who had lower and more variable heart rates. The former children were significantly more inhibited with the unfamiliar peer at 5½ years, had a larger number of unusual fears, and were more likely to had symptoms suggestive of arousal of the sympathetic nervous system during the first year of life, especially chronic constipation, allergy, and sleeplessness (see Reznick et al., 1986).

Spectral Analysis of Heart Rate

Both heart rate and heart rate variability are under the joint influence of sympathetic and parasympathetic activity (Glick & Braunwald, 1965). Respiration exerts a major influence on heart rate variability, especially at

Table 1. Preservation of Behavior and Heart Rate Variables in Cohort 1 and Their Relation to Physiological Indexes.

PREDICTOR VARIABLES	BEHAVIOR AND CARDIAC VARIABLES AT 5½ YEARS			
	Inhibited Behavior	Heart Period	Heart Period Variability	MEAN PHYSIOLOGICAL INDEX
21 months:				
Inhibited behavior	.52***	−.44**	−.39**	.70***
Heart period	.03	.15	.11	−.18
Heart period variability	−.06	.19	.39**	−.10
4 years:				
Inhibited behavior	.67***	−.46**	−.44**	.66***
Heart period	−.39**	.58***	.44***	−.44**
Heart period variability	−.39**	.54***	.64***	−.36*

* $p < .05$.
** $p < .01$.
*** $p < .005$.

rest, and this variability, called respiratory sinus arrhythmia, is mediated primarily by vagal activity (Chess, Tam, & Calaresu, 1975; Katona & Jih, 1975; Porges, McCabe, & Yongue, 1982). Other cyclical sources of variability in heart rate are much less obvious on a polygraph tracing; however, spectral analysis can express the complex beat-to-beat variation in a subject's heart rate as a power spectrum describing the separate rhythms, with peaks at characteristic frequencies. The total area under all of the peaks accounts for the total variability in the heart rate data, while the magnitude of each peak represents the contribution of that particular frequency to the total variation. Peaks at particular frequencies are associated with different physiological processes, especially respiration, blood pressure, and temperature regulations (Akselrod et al., 1981, 1985; Pomeranz et al., 1985). In human subjects, peak frequency between 0.2 and 0.5 Hz is due primarily to respiration and is associated with parasympathetic activity; peaks at lower frequencies are due primarily, but not exclusively, to sympathetic activity. But it is possible to assess the relative contribution of parasympathetic and sympathetic activity to the total heart rate spectrum, as well as to shifts in the balance of the two systems over time. Analysis of the changes in the heart rate power spectrum of the children in Cohort 2 at 43 months revealed that more inhibited than uninhibited children shifted to greater sympathetic activity from a baseline period prior to cognitive testing to a subsequent baseline period following the stress of a series of cognitive procedures ($p < .05$ by the Exact Test).

Pupillary Dilation

Additional support for the hypothesis that the temperamentally inhibited children have a lower threshold for sympathetic activation comes from data on pupillary dilation gathered while the children were administered a series of cognitive tasks that included recall memory for words and digits, a mental comparison of the relative size of objects, inferring an object from its features, and listening to a story. The inhibited children had significantly larger pupillary diameters than uninhibited children under both baseline and task conditions, even though the differences between the two groups were less striking for pupil size than for heart rate or heart rate variability. Additionally, more inhibited than uninhibited children in Cohort 1 maintained a larger pupil across a series of cognitive episodes (67% vs. 36% of each group). The combination of a tonically large pupil together with a high and stable heart rate across a series of cognitive episodes invites the inference that sympathetic activity is greater in inhibited children, presumably because of a lower threshold in the circuit that links the limbic lobe and hypothalamus to the sympathetic nervous system and its target organs.

Muscle Tension

The stress circuit involving the reticular activating system and skeletal motor tracts also seems to be at a lower threshold in inhibited children. The reticular activating system, which is influenced by hypothalamic activity, sends axons to nuclei in skeletal motor tracts, one of which is the nucleus ambiguus serving the muscles of the larynx and the vocal folds. Increased tension in these skeletal muscles is usually accompanied by a decrease in the variability of the pitch periods of vocal utterances (Lieberman, 1961; Stevens & Hirano, 1981). The increased muscle tension can be due not only to discharge of the nucleus ambiguus but also, indirectly, to sympathetic activity that constricts arterioles serving the muscles of the larynx and vocal folds (Vallbo, Hagbarth, Torebjork, & Wallin, 1979).

In the production of human speech, the vocal cords of the larynx open and close at a rapid rate during the process of phonation to produce a sequence of puffs of air. The rate at which the vocal cords open and close defines the fundamental frequency of phonation (Fo). But the vocal cords do not maintain a steady rate as they open and close. The duration of each period of the successive phonatory cycles varies around a mean of 4 msec, even when a person is maintaining a steady average fundamental frequency. These perturbations in the rate at which the vocal cords open and close appear to be a consequence of the inherent interplay of aerostatic, aerodynamic, and tissue forces involved in phonation. The perturbations tend to decrease when the laryngeal muscles are under tension (Lieberman, 1961). If the expected increase in muscle tension in limbs and trunk that usually occurs under task demands also occurs in the vocal cords and laryngeal muscles, one consequence would be less variation in the duration of the successive cycles of the fundamental frequency of phonation (i.e., less variability in the duration of the pitch periods of a single utterance). The index of variability we used was the standard deviation of the normalized distribution of twice the difference between two successive periods divided by the sum of the periods (see Lieberman, 1961).

In her doctoral research, Coster (1986) has found that at 5½ years of age the inhibited, compared with the uninhibited, children in Cohort 1 showed less variability in the pitch periods of single word utterances spoken under psychological stress (the words were bed, cake, dog, goat, pipe, and tub). The child first spoke each of the six words singly (no stress) and then repeated the same words in a series of three to six words (mild stress due to requirement of recalling the words). Most children in both groups showed a marked decrease in variability of the pitch periods to this cognitive stress. In a second stressful condition, which followed immediately, the child was asked to guess which of the six words just repeated was the correct answer to a particular question (e.g., "Which one chases squirrels?" "Which one is a bad pet?"). Under this last condition, inhibited children not only showed significantly lower average variability ($r = -.43$, $p < .01$, with the classification of inhibition at 21 months) but more often showed a decrease in variability across the six questions, reflecting increasing muscle tension. Figure 2 illustrates this decrease in variability for a single, but typical, inhibited child.

Note in Figure 2 that this child's variability is smallest to the first word spoken under the initial nonstressful condition. The variability decreases to the four words that had to be recalled but increases to recall of the six-word series. On the final test condition—elicited—variability decreased across the questions, reaching its lowest value on the fourth question ("Which one chases squirrels?").

In addition, the inhibited children showed a smaller standard deviation across all the variability values gathered under both stressful and nonstressful conditions ($r = -.39$, $p < .05$, with the classification of inhibition at 21 months). Further, the standard deviation of all of the fundamental frequency values (about 22 values), which was unrelated to the variability of the pitch periods, was also smaller (but not significant) for inhibited than for uninhibited children. Similar data from Cohort 2 seen at 43 months revealed that inhibited children showed a significantly greater decrease in variability than uninhibited children when data based on speaking single words (minimal stress) were compared with data gathered when the child had to recall the words as part of a series of four, five, or six words—identical with conditions 2 and 3 for Cohort 1.*

Norepinephrine Level

Because norepinephrine is a primary neurotransmitter in the sympathetic nervous system, a urine sample collected from each child in Cohort 1 at the end of the test battery at 5½ years was assayed for norepinephrine and its derivatives using mass fragmentography (Karoum, 1983). The assays yielded values for norepinephrine, normetanephrine, 3-methoxy-4-hydroxyphenyglycol (MHPG), and vanillylmandelic acid (VMA). The concentrations of each compound were transformed into moles per gram of creatinine, and an index of total norepinephrine activity was computed by averaging the concentrations of the four products (in micromoles per gram of creatinine). This index reflected primarily peripheral norepinephrine activity, including the cardiac

---

*This work is part of a collaboration with Philip Lieberman, Department of Linguistics, Brown University.

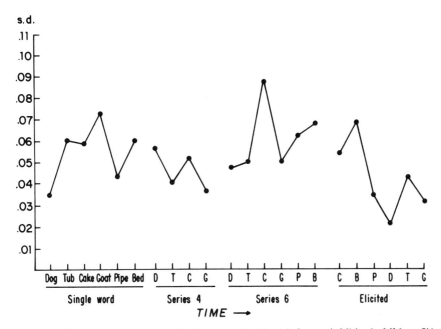

Figure 2. Sample of vocal perturbation index (ordinate) for an inhibited child at 5½ years: Cohort 1.

system. The relation between the index of norepinephrine activity and the original index of behavioral inhibition at 21 months was not significant ($r = .15$), but the correlations with the later indexes of inhibited behavior at age 4 and 5½ were significant ($r = .34$, $p < .05$, with the index at age 4 and $r = .31$, $p < .05$, with the index at age 5½). Although these correlations were modest, they imply greater sympathetic activity among the children who were behaviorally inhibited at 4 and 5½ years of age.*

Cortisol

Samples of saliva were gathered on the children in Cohort 1 at 5½ years before and after the 90-min laboratory session, as well as at home on 3 days during the early morning hours before the stress of the day had begun. These

_____

*This work is part of a collaboration with Richard J. Wyatt and Farouk Karoum of St. Elizabeth's Hospital, Washington, DC.

saliva samples were analyzed for unbound cortisol level using a modification of a standard radioimmunoassay method (Walker, Riad-Fahmy, & Read, 1978). Levels of salivary cortisol correlate highly with levels obtained from plasma (Walker, 1984). The inhibited children had significantly higher cortisol levels than uninhibited children in both home and laboratory (see Fig. 3). The correlation between the mean of the two laboratory values and the original index of behavioral inhibition at 21 months was .45 ($p < .01$); the correlation with the aggregate index of inhibition at 5½ years was .37 ($p < .05$). Further, the average cortisol level across the three morning samples at home was correlated with the index of inhibition at 5½ years ($r = .39, p < .05$).* This last result suggests that the hypothalamic-pituitary-adrenal axis of inhibited children is at a tonically higher level of activity, even in minimally stressful contexts.

High levels of cortisol in the laboratory saliva sample were more discriminating of the two behavioral groups than any of the other physiological variables, for laboratory cortisol values correctly predicted the original 21-month behavioral classifications for 78% of the Cohort 1 children. Although very high levels of cortisol (roughly the top quartile and over 2,000 pmol/l) were more characteristic of inhibited children (nine inhibited vs. one uninhibited for the home value; 10 inhibited vs. two uninhibited for the laboratory value), about one-half of the inhibited children had relatively low cortisol levels. Recall that the correlation between cortisol level and contemporary behavior at 5½ years was 0.37. However, nine inhibited children had high levels of cortisol (above the mean) for both the home and laboratory values. Most of these children differed in important ways from the remaining inhibited children, as well as all of the uninhibited children as described below.

One of the assessment situations at 5½ years was a 30-min play session with an unfamiliar child of the same sex and age but of the opposite behavioral style. Two- to 4-year-old inhibited children tend to remain proximal to the mother for the first few minutes. However, this particular behavioral sign is rare at 5½ years. Among the older, inhibited children, the usual signs of behavioral inhibition are more subtle; usually the children remain quiet, avoid the unfamiliar child, but stare at the unfamiliar peer frequently. Nonetheless, three of the nine children with cortisol levels above the mean for both home and laboratory assays remained proximal to their mother for the first 5–10 min of the session. This is atypical behavior for children at this age. One child sat passively in the middle of the room doing

---

*This work is part of a collaboration with Peter Ellison, Terrence Deacon, and Pamela Lutz of the Department of Anthropology, Harvard University.

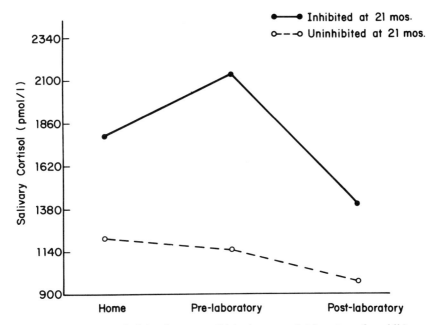

Figure 3. Mean cortisol levels at age 5½ in home and laboratory for children classified as inhibited or uninhibited at 21 months of age: Cohort 1.

nothing, and one glanced at her mother frequently throughout the 30-min play session. Only two of the nine children showed no obvious signs of inhibited behavior in this context. In a similar peer play situation at 4 years of age every one of these nine children had scores above the mean index of inhibition, and two had the highest indexes at that age.

Interviews with all of the mothers revealed that six of the nine inhibited children with high cortisol for both home and laboratory showed other signs of high physiological arousal and either intense or unusual fears. For example, one child was constipated during infancy, retained urine during the first 3 years of life, and showed many contemporary fears, including a fear of loud voices. Another child was extremely irritable during the first year and at age 4 had a fear of blood, bugs, and defecating. A third child had allergies, chronic constipation, and colic during infancy and was afraid of playing alone during the second and third years. Currently, this child woke up frequently during the night with nightmares. A fourth child had a spastic colon as an infant and currently had nightmares, a fear of heights, and was afraid of being alone. A fifth subject displayed extreme separation fear during infancy and currently was asthmatic and had a fear of taking a bath. A sixth child was constipated as an infant, showed a long-lasting fear of going to nursery school, and currently was afraid of leaving her backyard. None of the uninhibited children, even those with high cortisol levels, showed these kinds of symptoms; these children tend to be more active and vigorous than the uninhibited children with low cortisol levels.

It is of interest that a group of French investigators studying preschool and kindergarten children found higher urinary levels of a derivative of adrenocortical activity (17-hydroxycorticosteroids) in emotionally labile and fearful children than in less emotional children who were regarded as leaders by their peers (Montagner et al., 1978). Additionally, 1-year-old infants who were prone to extreme distress following maternal separation in the home also showed higher urinary cortisol levels than those who were minimally distressed (Tennes, Downey, & Vernadakis, 1977).

Physiological Activity Across the Variables

The inhibited, in contrast to the uninhibited, children in Cohort 1 were more likely to show the peripheral physiological consequences predicted from the hypothesis of lower thresholds of reactivity in limbic lobe. However, only about one-third of the inhibited children showed signs of higher activity in all three stress circuits, and most of the intercorrelations among the physiological variables described above were low and nonsignificant. With the exception of the correlation of .84 between heart period and heart period variability, the remaining 27 correlations ranged from −.26 to + .33, with a median coefficient of + .10. (See Nesse et al., 1985, for a similar finding.)

In order to assess the degree of concordance in responsivity across the indexes, we computed a mean standard score, and standard deviation, for eight physiological variables quantified on Cohort 1 at $5\frac{1}{2}$ years of age. The eight variables were: (1) cortisol level in the morning at home, (2) cortisol level obtained in the laboratory, (3) heart period during cognitive tasks, (4) heart period variability during cognitive tasks, (5) pupillary dilation during cognitive tasks, (6) variability of pitch periods of the voice under the second cognitive stress, (7) standard deviation of all the fundamental frequency values, and (8) total norepinephrine level in the laboratory urine sample. We reversed the values for variables 3, 4, 6, and 7 so that a high standard score indicated greater limbic arousal. The correlations between the mean across all eight physiological variables and each of its component scores ranged from .36 to .56, with heart period, heart period variability, cortisol in the laboratory, and variability of the pitch periods having the highest correlations with the aggregate mean (r = .56, .53, .51, and .51). The standard deviation of the eight physiological variables was unrelated to the individual measures and to the mean index ($r = -.17$).

We examined the relation between the aggregate mean of the eight physiological variables and the index of behavioral inhibition at each age for 22 inhibited and 21 uninhibited children (see Table 1). The correlation was highest with the original index of inhibition at 21 months ($r = .70, p < .001$) but statistically significant at the two later ages ($r = .66$ with the behavioral index at age 4; $r = .58$ with the aggregate behavioral index at 5½ years). Additionally both heart period and heart period variability values obtained on these children at 4 years of age were positively related to the physiological index at 5½ years ($r = -.44, -.36, p < .05$).

Two of three formerly inhibited children with the lowest physiological indexes had become increasingly less inhibited across the period from 21 months to 5½ years. Two of the three formerly uninhibited children with the highest physiological indexes had become more inhibited at 5½ years. Thus the direction of change in behavior over the 4 years of study was accompanied by an expected level of physiological reactivity at 5½ years. But none of the uninhibited children was as physiologically reactive as the top quartile of inhibited children. A combination of both behavioral and biological variables led to a more accurate diagnosis of the children who remained inhibited or uninhibited over time than either variable alone. However, a multiple regression analysis that made inhibition at 21 months and the aggregate physiological index at 5½ years the two predictors, and the aggregate index of behavioral inhibition at 5½ years the criterion, was not significantly higher than the correlation with the index of inhibited behavior at 21 months (multiple $R = .62$ for both predictors vs. a correlation of .52 between the behavioral indexes at 21 months and 5½ years).

DISCUSSION

When children are selected in the second or third years to be extremely inhibited or uninhibited in their behavioral reactions to the unfamiliar, there is preservation of these two behavioral profiles over a period of 4 years. There is also a theoretically consistent association between inhibited behavior and peripheral physiological processes that originate in activity in the limbic lobe, especially the amygdala and the hypothalamus. These facts imply that a small proportion of children, estimated to be about 10%, has a low threshold of reactivity in those parts of the limbic lobe that are responsive to unfamiliarity and challenge, while another 10% has a higher threshold in these areas.

The use of an aggregate index of responsivity across the eight physiological variables does not presume an abstract state of general arousal. A study of eight endocrine and physiological variables in adult phobic women exposed to psychological stress revealed that very few women showed increased reactivity on all of the biological indexes, and the correlations among the variables were generally low (Nesse et al., 1985). The aggregate score is useful, and often yields more robust relations than any single index, because any single variable can be the product of a factor unrelated to the hypothetical mechanisms mediating inhibited and uninhibited temperaments. Pooling several indexes dilutes the contribution of any one of these extraneous factors. For example, a child who did not have an inhibited temperament but was highly motivated to solve the cognitive problems might show a high and stable heart rate and a large pupil, but this child should show low levels of cortisol and high variability in the vocal perturbation index.

Inhibition of motor activity is the biologically prepared initial response to states of uncertainty and to discharge of one or more of the stress circuits in infants and young children, and if assimilation is not possible, crying or other signs of distress may occur. The prepared behavioral reaction in 2–3-year-olds is cessation of play and speech and seeking a target of attachment. That is why the second year, especially 20–30 months, is a sensitive time to detect the behavioral tendencies toward inhibition or lack of inhibition to the unfamiliar. In the final section of the article we turn to three general issues related to this research.

Biological Mechanisms

Explanations of individual differences in behavior that involve temperamental constructs have become more popular during the last decade. Two of the most popular are, first, the tendency either to approach or to avoid challenge and unfamiliarity and, second, the ease with which the emotional states of uncertainty, anxiety, and fear are generated. These qualities are different and, in adults, are statistically independent. Introversion-extraversion and neuroticism emerge as independent factors in the questionnaire responses of unselected samples of adults (Eysenck, 1982). However, these dimensions are moderately correlated in young children who fall at the extremes on the tendency to approach or to withdraw from unfamiliarity. Therefore, there is a potential utility, at least for young children, to a conjunctive construct for young children that we might call "variation in the ease of generation of psychological uncertainty and physiological arousal and, as a consequence, withdrawal, rather than approach, to unfamiliar or challenging situations."

There are several possible explanations of the variation among children in this complex quality or qualities. During the 40 years when behaviorism and psychoanalytic theory shared popularity, many American and European psychologists viewed the variation in fearful behavior as learned. The American behaviorists offered a logically consistent and intuitively appealing argument based on the conditioning of a state of fear and the biologically prepared response of avoidance to formerly neutral events. The popular textbook example is of the infant who acquired a fear of a white rat. In this model, a child who was consistently shy with unfamiliar adults must have had painful experiences with adults in the past. Thus many psychologists teaching during that era explained intense stranger anxiety in the infant as a consequence of unpleasant experiences with strangers. In a similar vein, an extreme degree of separation anxiety was the result of experiences of hunger or pain when the mother was away from the home; hence, the mother's absence became the conditioned stimulus for an anxiety reaction. Although this explanation seemed reasonable 30 years ago, only a small number of contemporary psychologists continue to favor a version of this argument.

Two related explanations that are gaining initial consensus do not deny the influence of learning from experience but implicate the role of inherent individual differences in central nervous system functioning. One explanation holds that children differ in ease of excitability—or threshold of response—in those parts of the central nervous system that contribute to states of psychological uncertainty and physiological arousal. Most investigators assume that limbic structures play a central part in this phenomenon (Gray, 1982). A more specific variant of this hypothesis is that some infants are born with low thresholds of reactivity in amygdala and hypothalamus when the child encounters unfamiliarity or challenge for which there is no immediate coping response. A related, complementary, explanation emphasizes the effectiveness of processes that inhibit the discharge of limbic structures. As Rothbart and Derryberry (1981) note, these two mechanisms are different, even though investigators working with humans cannot measure each separately at the present time. Pavlov chose to emphasize the inhibition function, suggesting that organisms differed in the "strength of the central nervous system," where strength meant the ability to inhibit the buildup of excitation. Pavlov implied that fearful dogs and shy children had a "weak nervous system." The Polish psychologist Jan Strelau (1985) is responsible for a modern version of Pavlov's ideas.

The environment presents children with at least three classes of events that invite some form of response. The first refers to unfamiliar events that provoke attempts at assimilation (e.g., an unfamiliar sound or sight). The second class includes events, usually the actions of people, to which the child must issue some action (e.g., an unfamiliar person approaches and offers a toy). Finally, the environment presents problem situations to which the child must generate cognitive solutions (e.g., test questions in our battery). Most of the time children and adults assimilate unfamiliar events easily, issue socially effective actions to others, and generate correct cognitive solutions with minimal delay and, therefore, minimal limbic lobe arousal. But when there is a delay in the generation of a coping response, the child is simultaneously alerted psychologically and aroused physiologically. We believe that this state should be treated as a special psychological cum physiological condition mediated in part by limbic structures. We choose to call this state *uncertainty;* others may prefer a different word.

The state of uncertainty often has peripheral physiological consequences because the amygdala and hypothalamus mutually influence each other, and the latter influences the pituitary-adrenal axis, reticular activating system, and sympathetic chain. Hence, the physiological signs that are characteristic of inhibited children could be due to tonically lower thresholds of reactivity in these brain structures. As a result, the inhibited children show increases in muscle tension, a rise and stabilization of heart rate, pupillary dilation, or increased cortisol to minimally unfamiliar or challenging events, whereas most children would not show these physiological reactions to the same relatively innocuous experiences. This speculative suggestion is in accord with results of neurobehavioral studies of the amygdala and the hypothalamus over the last 20 years. One primary function of the amygdala is to receive evaluated, meaningful information from secondary, or associative, sensory areas and the hippocampus, and through projections to the hypothalamus and the autonomic nervous system generate visceral reactions that are often accompanied by behavioral signs of fear and feelings of increased emotionality (Aggleton & Passingham, 1981; Gloor, 1978; Sarter & Markowitsch, 1985; Turner, Mishkin, & Knapp, 1980). Indeed, one team of investigators has suggested that a person's conscious awareness of internal feeling tone is generated in the amygdala (Hebben, Corkin, Eichenbaum, & Shedlack, 1985).

The idea that inhibited and uninhibited children differ in the excitability of the amygdala and the hypothalamus finds support in studies of domestic cats differing in degree of defensive, nonaggressive behavior with rats. The descriptions of the defensive, in contrast to the nondefensive, cats resemble closely our descriptions of inhibited and uninhibited children. The defensive cats are less likely to attack rats and are more inhibited in novel environments, as well as with humans. These behavioral qualities are stable over periods as long as 3 years (Adamec & Stark-Adamec, 1986). Stimulation of the basal amygdala evoked stronger multiple unit activity in the limbic structures of defensive compared with nondefensive animals. Further, when the amygdala was stimulated with single pulses of increasing intensity, the peak height of the evoked potential in the ventromedial hypothalamus was significantly greater in defensive than in nondefensive cats. Finally, while orienting to rats, the defensive cats showed both larger and more prolonged increases in multiple unit activity in the amygdala than did the nondefensive animals. The authors, who believe that the behavioral differences between defensive and nondefensive cats may be due, in part, to a lower threshold of response in the amygdala, wrote, ". . .Some form of synaptic potentiation underlies [this] behavioral disposition [or bias]. . .the behavioral outcome may be determined by the normally occurring excitatory status of limbic substrates" (p. 142), . . ."some form of potentiation of synaptic transmission" (p. 132; Adamec & Stark-Adamec, 1986). This suggestion, together with data indicating that the amygdala appears to mediate the state of conditioned fear in the rat (Hitchcock & Davis, 1986), renders a bit more credible the idea that differences in responsivity of limbic structures make an important contribution to the contrasting behaviors of inhibited and uninhibited children.

The reasons for the lower thresholds of reactivity in the amygdala and hypothalamus are unclear, but one possible contributing factor is high levels of central norepinephrine. Central norepinephrine appears to amplify the brain's reaction to novelty by suppressing background neural activity and, therefore, increasing the psychological salience of an incentive stimulus (Aston-Jones & Bloom, 1981; Charney, Heninger, & Breier, 1984; Charney & Redmond, 1983; Reiser, 1984). Further, rats who are unable to avoid shock show increased norepinephrine activity, especially in the amygdala and the hypothalamus (Tsuda & Tanaka, 1985), and assays of a large number of autonomic and hormonal variables in phobic women exposed to the sources of their fear reveal that blood levels of norepinephrine have the largest number of correlations with the other physiological indexes (Nesse et al., 1985) (see also Bandura, Taylor, Williams, Mefford, & Barchas, 1985).

The locus coeruleus is a major source of central norepinephrine and its axons synapse on many parts of the brain, including the amygdala and the hypothalamus. The fact that neurons of the locus coeruleus of rats fire to the novelty of unexpected tones and lights led Aston-Jones and Bloom (1981) to suggest that the increased state of vigilance to novelty is accompanied by increases in the concentration of central norepinephrine, as if the locus coeruleus-norepinephrine system "rendered ordinarily neutral innocuous stimuli anxiety provoking" (Reiser, 1984). Thus, one possible hypothesis, albeit speculative, is that inhibited children have tonically higher levels of norepinephrine than uninhibited children due to enhanced reactivity of the locus coeruleus. As a result, a mildly unfamiliar or challenging event is more likely to produce activity in the amygdala and hypothalamus of inhibited children and, during the early years, an accompanying disposition to become quiet, to cease playing, and to withdraw from the event.

The Role of Experience

Although there may be an inherited biological contribution to the profile of behaviors we have described, there is also an important role for learning. First, most American families regard consistent fear and withdrawal to challenge as undesirable qualities (Singer, 1984). Hence, parents reward their children for inhibition of excessive fear and may discourage consistent display of its outward manifestations. Second, by 4 years of age, most inhibited children have become aware of their behavioral reactions to novelty and the fact that they might be afraid, and want to control these responses. One 5½-year-old inhibited boy in our study told his mother, "I know I am afraid, but I'm trying to not be." Many inhibited children who are motivated to control behavioral signs of fear learn to react to the states of uncertainty and arousal with less fearful, timid behavior. These children may gradually acquire the ability to interrupt the prepared response of inhibition. As these coping behaviors become stronger, they might even mute the uncertainty and arousal that occur in unfamiliar settings. This suggestion may explain why the index of inhibition at 5½ years of age was a slightly poorer correlate of the aggregate biological index than inhibited behavior at 21 months ($r = .58$ vs. $.70$). Just as knowledge about the reversibility of a Necker cube makes it easier to see it in both perspectives, so, too, might knowledge about one's physiological and behavioral reactions to unfamiliarity make it easier to influence them. Whether this alteration is context specific or can become more general is still not clear.

Although there is no question that inhibited children can become uninhibited in surface behaviors, it is less clear if these behavioral changes are accompanied by changes in the thresholds of responsivity in the limbic system. However, we suspect these changes are also possible, for a few older children who had been very inhibited at 21 months were both behaviorally uninhibited and showed minimal signs of physiological arousal when seen at 5½ years. It is possible, of course, that if more serious stressors had been used, these children would be more likely than the average child to react with the physiological signs they displayed at a younger age.

Inhibition: A Quality or a Quantity?

Finally, these data invite consideration of a choice between continuous quantities or discrete qualities in describing these children. The traditional strategy is a return to the popular concept of general arousal as a continuum with individuals varying in magnitude of the state. Hence, the small group of children who showed reactivity in all of the target systems originating in limbic structures would be regarded as highly aroused; those who showed reactivity in only a few would be moderately aroused. However, one can also regard the children as falling into qualitatively different groups. Those who show reactivity in most of the target systems are coherently aroused; those who show reactivity in none are coherently nonaroused; those who show reactivity on only a few indexes are not coherently aroused. These groups of children are to be regarded as differing in "quality of arousal," not in "degree of arousal." When we treated heart rate, heart rate variability, and inhibited behavior at 21 and 48 months in Cohort 1 as continua and used these variables as predictors in a multiple regression equation with the index of inhibition at $5\frac{1}{2}$ years as the criterion, neither heart rate nor variability had any significant amount of unique variance over and above the variance attributable to behavioral inhibition at 21 and 48 months. However, when we created four discrete groups—inhibited with a high and stable heart rate, inhibited with a low and variable heart rate, uninhibited with a high and stable heart rate, and uninhibited with a low and variable heart rate—the 13 children who were inhibited and had a high and stable heart rate were significantly different from the other three at $5\frac{1}{2}$ years. These children stared more at the unfamiliar peer and spent significantly more time close to the mother in the peer play session and, in another room, avoided contact with novel objects that suggested risk of harm. During the first year of life these children showed at least one of the following symptoms: chronic constipation, allergy, extreme irritability, and sleeplessness. Thus, treating inhibited children with a high and stable heart rate as a qualitatively special category yielded results that did not emerge when behavior and heart rate variability were treated as continua reflecting degree of arousal.

Scientists can choose among many possible dimensions when they summarize the similarities and differences between two classes of events they believe to be related theoretically. Prior premises, the question of interest, and the sources of evidence will determine whether the dimensions selected imply a continuum or qualitatively different categories. We chose to emphasize the qualitative differences between inhibited and uninhibited children because we selected children at the behavioral extremes and, therefore, minimized behavioral overlap in the original groups. Additionally, the forms of the distributions of the behavioral data gathered subsequently (e.g., time proximal to the mother and time staring at an unfamiliar child) did not suggest a continuous trait, for very few uninhibited children spent a long time near their mother or staring at the unfamiliar child. The pattern of behavioral stabilities and the intercorrelations also favored the hypothesis of qualitatively discrete groups because inhibited children with a high and stable heart rate at 21 months were different at 5½ years from inhibited children with a low and variable heart rate. Further, the fact that some obviously uninhibited children had a high and stable heart rate led us away from the notion of a continuum of arousal. If there were such a continuum, inhibited behavior and a high and stable heart rate should have covaried better than they did, and there should have been fewer uninhibited children with a high and stable heart rate. As our work proceeded, we began to develop the hypothesis that an inhibited temperament might be influenced by biological factors. As a result, we were tempted to emphasize dimensions that were unique to inhibited children, like their later-born ordinal position, high cortisol levels, and presence of infant symptoms such as colic, allergy, and constipation. These characteristics imply qualitative differences between inhibited and uninhibited children. However, if we had believed that experience was the primary cause both of inhibited behavior and the correlated physiological signs, we would have selected dimensions implying constructs such as strength of conditioned anxiety, motivation to control fear, and ability to deal with uncertainty. These concepts can be applied to all children to differing degrees. As a result, we would have treated the differences between inhibited and uninhibited children as continuous.

Many readers may feel, with us, that pragmatic factors will decide which descriptive category—qualitative categories of children or quantity of arousal in children—is theoretically more profitable for a given corpus of data. The description that leads to the more robust predictions and the more satisfying explanations is always the one to be preferred. For those who wish to emphasize the important environmental contributions to the formation of and change in inhibited and uninhibited behavior, the major dimensions will refer to experiences and imply continua. For those who wish to emphasize the possibility of a biological contribution to these profiles, and especially genetic influences, the dimensions selected will emphasize qualities. Each perspective has validity, given the investigator's initial assumptions and intentions, and, of course, the form of the evidence.

This conclusion is the central theme in Bohr's famous essay on complementarity, which attempted to resolve the debate as to whether electromagnetic energy should be treated as a continuous wave or as discrete quanta. Bohr (1950) suggested that the frame adopted depended upon the question and mode of data analysis. Each perspective was valid in its own domain of inquiry, leading the physicist J. J. Thomson to suggest the metaphor of a tiger and a shark to represent the two perspectives; each animal was potent in its own ecological niche, but impotent in the niche of the other (Wheaton, 1983).

REFERENCES

Adamec, R. E., & Stark-Adamec, C. (1986). Limbic hyperfunction, limbic epilepsy, and interictal behavior. In B. K. Doane & K. E. Livingston (Eds.), *The limbic system* (pp. 129–145). New York: Raven.

Ainsworth, M. D. S., Blehar, M. C., Waters, E., & Wall, S. (1978). *Patterns of attachment.* Hillsdale, NJ: Erlbaum.

Aggleton, J. P., & Passingham, R. E. (1981). Syndrome produced by lesions of amygdala in monkeys *(Macaca mulatta). Journal of Comparative and Physiological Psychology, 95,* 961–977.

Akselrod, S., Gordon, D., Madwed, J. B., Snidman, N. C., Shannon, D. C., & Cohen, R. J. (1985). Hemodynamic regulation: Investigation by spectral analysis. *American Journal of Physiology: Heart and Circulatory Physiology, 249,* 867–875.

Akselrod, S., Gordon, D., Ubel, F. A., Shannon, D. C., Barger, D. C., & Cohen, R. J. (1981). Power spectrum analysis of heart rate fluctuation: A quantitative probe of beat-to-beat cardiovascular control. *Science, 213,* 220–222.

Aston-Jones, G., & Bloom, F. E. (1981). Norepinephrine-containing locus coeruleus neurons in behaving rats exhibit pronounced responses to non-noxious environmental stimuli. *Journal of Neuroscience, 1,* 887–900.

Bandura, A., Taylor, C. B., Williams, S. L., Mefford, I. N., & Barchas, J. D. (1985). Catecholamine secretion as a function of perceived coping self-efficiency. *Journal Consulting Clinical Psychology, 53,* 406–414.

Bohr, N. (1950). On the notions of causality and complementarity. *Science, 111,* 51–54.

Charney, D. S., Heninger, G. R., & Breier, A. (1984). Noradrenergic function in panic anxiety. *Archives of General Psychiatry, 41,* 751–763.

Charney, D. S., & Redmond, D. E. (1983). Neurobiological mechanisms in human anxiety. *Neuropharmacology, 22,* 1531–1536.

Chess, G. F., Tam, R. M., Calaresu, F. R. (1975). Influence of cardiac neural inputs on rhythmic variations of heart period in the cat. *American Journal of Physiology, 228,* 775–779.

Ciarenello, R. D. (1983). Neurochemical aspects of stress. In N. Garmezy & M. Rutter (Eds.), *Stress, coping, and development in children* (pp. 85–105). New York: McGraw-Hill.

Coe, C. L., Wiener, S. G., Rosenberg, L. T., & Levine, S. (1985). Endocrine and immune responses to separation and maternal loss in nonhuman primates. In M. Reite & T. Field (Eds.), *The psychobiology of attachment and separation* (pp. 163–199). New York: Academic Press.

Coster, W. (1986). *Aspects of voice and conversation in behaviorally inhibited and uninhibited children.* Unpublished doctoral dissertation, Harvard University.

Cranach, B. V., Grote-Dham, R., Huffner, U., Marte, F., Reisbeck, G., & Mittelstadt, M. (1978). Das social Gehemmte Kind im Kindergarten. *Praxis der Kinderpsychologie und Kinderpsychiatrie, 27,* 167–179.

Eysenck, H. J. (1982). *Personality, genetics, and behavior.* New York: Praeger.

Fredrikson, M., Sundin, O., & Frankenhaeuser, M. (1985). Cortisol excretion during the defense reaction in humans. *Psychosomatic Medicine, 4,* 313–319.

Garcia-Coll, C., Kagan, J., & Reznick, J. S. (1984). Behavioral inhibition in young children. *Child Development, 55,* 1005–1019.

Gersten, M. (1986). *The contribution of temperament to behavior in natural contexts.* Unpublished doctoral dissertation, Harvard Graduate School of Education.

Glick, G., & Braunwald, E. (1965). Relative roles of the sympathetic and parasympathetic nervous systems in the reflex control of heart rate. *Circulation Research, 16,* 363–375.

Gloor, P. (1978). Inputs and outputs of the amygdala: What the amygdala is trying to tell the rest of the brain. In K. E. Livingston & O. Hoznykiewicz (Eds.), *Limbic mechanisms* (pp. 189–209). New York: Plenum.

Gray, J. A. (1982). *The neuropsychology of anxiety.* Oxford: Clarendon.

Hebben, N., Corkin, S., Eichenbaum, H., & Shedlack, K. (1985). Diminished ability to interpret and report internal states after bilateral medial temporal resection: Case H.M. *Behavioral Neuroscience, 99,* 1031–1039.

Hitchcock, J., & Davis, M. (1986). Lesions of the amygdala, but not of the cerebellum or red nucleus block conditioned fear as measured with the potentiated startle paradigm. *Behavioral Neuroscience, 100,* 11–22.

Kagan, J., Reznick, J. S., Clarke, C., Snidman, N., & Garcia-Coll, C. (1984). Behavioral inhibition to the unfamiliar. *Child Development, 55,* 2212–2225.

Karoum, F. (1983). Mass fragmentography in the analysis of biogenic amines: A clinical, physiological, and pharmacological evaluation. In S. Parvez, T. Nagatsu, I. Nagatsu, and H. Parvez (Eds.), *Methods in biogenic amine research* (pp. 237–255). Amsterdam: Elsevier.

Katona, P. G., & Jih, F. (1975). Respiratory sinus arrhythmia. *Journal of Applied Physiology, 39,* 801–805.

Levine, S., Coe, C. L., Smotherman, W. P., & Kaplan, J. N. (1978). Prolonged cortisol elevation in the infant squirrel monkey after reunion with mother. *Physiology and Behavior, 20,* 7–10.

Lieberman, P. (1961). Perturbations in vocal pitch. *Journal of Acoustical Society of America, 33,* 597–603.

Montagner, H., Henry, J. C., Lombardot, M., Benedini, M., Burnod, J., & Nicolas, R. M. (1978). Behavioral profiles and corticosteroid excretion rhythms in young children, Part 2. In N. Blurton-Jones & V. Reynolds (Eds.), *Human behavior and adaptation* (Vol. 18, pp. 229–265). London: Taylor & Francis.

Nesse, R. M., Curtis, G. C., Thyer, B. A., McCann, D. S., Huber-Smith, M., & Knopf, R. F. (1985). Endocrine and cardiovascular responses during phobic anxiety. *Psychosomatic Medicine, 47,* 320–332.

Pomeranz, B., Macaulay, R. J. B., Caudill, M. A., Kutz, I., Adam, D., Gordon, D., Kilborn, K. M., Barger, A. C., Shannon, D. C., Cohen, R. J., & Benson, H. (1985). Assessment of autonomic function in humans by heart rate spectral analysis. *American Journal of Physiology, 248,* 151–153.

Porges, S. W., McCabe, P. M., & Yongue, B. G. (1982). Respiratory-heart rate interactions: Psychophysiological implications for pathophysiology and behavior. In J. Cacciopo & R. Petty (Eds.), *Perspectives in cardiovascular psychophysiology* (pp. 223–264). New York: Guilford.

Reiser, M. F. (1984). *Mind, brain, body.* New York: Basic.

Reznick, J. S., Kagan, J., Snidman, N., Gersten, M., Baak, K., & Rosenberg, A. (1986). Inhibited and uninhibited behavior: A follow-up study. *Child Development, 57,* 660–680.

Rothbart, M. K., & Derryberry, D. (1981). Development of individual differences in temperament. In M. E. Lamb & A. L. Brown (Eds.), *Advances in developmental psychology* (Vol. 1, pp. 37–86). Hillsdale, NJ: Erlbaum.

Sarter, M., & Markowitsch, H. J. (1985). Involvement of the amygdala in learning and memory. *Behavioral Neuroscience, 99,* 342–380.

Singer, J. L. (1984). *The human personality.* San Diego: Harcourt Brace Jovanovich.

Snidman, N. (1984). *Behavioral restraint and the central nervous system.* Unpublished doctoral dissertation, University of California, Los Angeles.

Snow, M. E., Jacklin, C. N., & Maccoby, E. E. (1981). Birth order differences in peer sociability at 33 months. *Child Development, 52,* 589–595.

Stevens, K. N., & Hirano, M. (Eds.). (1981). *Vocal fold physiology.* Tokyo: University of Tokyo Press.

Strelau, J. (1985). Temperament and personality: Pavlov and beyond. In J. Strelau, F. H. Farley, & A. Gale (Eds.), *The biological bases of personality* (Vol. 1, pp 25–44). Washington, DC: Hemisphere.

Tennes, K., Downey, K., & Vernadakis, A. (1977). Urinary cortisol excretion rates and anxiety in normal one-year-old infants. *Psychosomatic Medicine, 39,* 178–187.

Tsuda, A., & Tanaka, M. (1985). Differential changes in noradrenaline turnover in specific regions of rat brain produced by controllable and uncontrollable shocks. *Behavioral Neuroscience, 99,* 802–817.

Turner, B. H., Mishkin, M., & Knapp, M. (1980). Organization of the amygdalopetal projections from modality-specific cortical association areas in the monkey. *Journal of Comparative Neurology, 19,* 515–543.

Vallbo, A. B., Hagbarth, K. E., Torebjork, H. E., & Wallin, B. G. (1979). Somatosensory, proprioceptive, and sympathetic activity in human peripheral nerves. *Physiological Reviews, 59,* 919–957.

Walker, R. F. (1984). Salivary cortisol determinations in the assessment of adrenal activity. In D. B. Ferguson (Ed.), *Steroid hormones in saliva* (pp. 33–50). Basel: Karger.

Walker, R. F., Riad-Fahmy, D., & Read, G. F. (1978). Adrenal status assessed by direct radioimmunoassay of cortisol in whole saliva or parotid fluid. *Clinical Chemistry, 24,* 1460–1463.

Wheaton, B. R. (1983). *The tiger and the shark.* Cambridge: Cambridge University Press.

6

Behavioral State as a Lead Variable in Neonatal Research

John Colombo and Frances Degen Horowitz
University of Kansas, Lawrence

Research on the perceptual and cognitive capacities of the human newborn has revealed that state variables typically will interfere with or override the neonate's attentional and stimulus processing tendencies. It is proposed that this finding argues for the power of early state variables as behavioral determinants, a position that has not received sufficient attention in recent neonatal research. It is further suggested that such neonatal state measures might provide good prediction of later developmental status, especially in combination with other early behavioral components. Data relevant to this position are discussed, and recommendations for future research are made.

The most basic ideas about the human infant, and particularly the human neonate, have changed drastically in the last half century. The prevailing popular conceptualization of the human neonate in the 1930s was that it was a vegetative and reflexive organism. However, it is now clear that the newborn is a perceptually and socially competent organism. This newer conceptualization has become so pervasive that the introductions of most

Reprinted with permission from the *Merrill-Palmer Quarterly,* 1987, Vol. 33, No. 4, 423–437. Copyright 1987 by Wayne State University Press.

We are grateful to Marion O'Brien, Jeff Coldren, D. Wayne Mitchell, Diane Bythell, Diana Anderson-Goetz, Madelyn Moss, and Yvonne Caldera for their comments on various earlier versions of the manuscript. Preparation of the manuscript was supported by NIMH grant 5T32HD07173–04 awarded to the Department of Human Development at the University of Kansas, ADAMHA grant 1-R01-MH41395–01 awarded to J. Colombo, and by NICHHD grant 1-R01-HD18290–01A1 to F. D. Horowitz.

current research reports on the neonate routinely begin by calling attention to the neonate's wide behavioral repertoire.

The interest in the psychological abilities of the neonate was a natural result of the renaissance in infancy research that began in the late 1950s and which has continued unabated to the present day (see Haith & Campos, 1983). From the proliferation of research on neonatal behavior that has emerged in this time, evidence has amassed to suggest that the neonate is receptive to and interactive with its environment, even at its earliest contact. The newborn has come to be characterized as having the ability (a) to process sensory-perceptual information (e.g., Lewis & Maurer, 1980; Zelazo, Brody, & Chaika, 1984) and (b) to learn within traditional conditioning paradigms (e.g., Blass, Ganchrow, & Steiner, 1984; see, however, Sameroff & Cavanaugh, 1979). Thus the newborn has been depicted as a relatively mature and sophisticated organism, capable of not only processing external input (e.g., stimulation, contingencies) but responding systematically to such input. This conceptualization has led naturally and logically to various studies of higher order stimulus processing early in life (e.g., Antell & Keating, 1983; Slater, Morison, & Rose, 1984), as well as to examinations of the young infant's social abilities and interactions (e.g., Field, Cohen, Garcia, & Greenberg, 1984).

Another major step in the effort to understand and characterize the newborn has been the development of an instrument for assessing the newborn's behavioral repertoire and responses to various types of visual and auditory stimuli, the Neonatal Behavioral Assessment Scale (NBAS; Brazelton, 1973/1986; see also Horowitz, Sullivan, Byrne, & Mitchell, in preparation; Sameroff, 1978). Closely following the development of the NBAS have been revisions and supplemental items (Horowitz, Sullivan, & Linn, 1978) as well as a number of systems for examining specific item subsets (Als, 1978; Lester, Emory, Hoffman, & Eitzman, 1976).

One of the assumptions implicit in such neonatal research has been that early stimulus processing abilities form the basis for more complex abilities that develop later. A logical step beyond this assumption was the hope that the assessment of such basic abilities might allow some prediction of later abilities, and perhaps of the individual's eventual developmental status in childhood. That is, a linear developmental continuity might exist for cognitive ability from the newborn period through childhood. Such cognitive continuity, however, remains largely undemonstrated. What little data exist do not indicate that there are strong and direct relationships between neonatal stimulus processing abilities and later stimulus processing abilities, or developmental outcome (e.g., Sameroff, 1978; Zelazo, 1979). The purpose of the present paper is to provide an account of this relationship, and perhaps examine what other variables might be important in the "equation" that yields later developmental outcome.

The basic proposition here is that, in the neonatal period, state variables are powerful behavioral determinants, and that they are, in fact, the dominant characteristic of neonatal behavior. As such, state may be considered as a *lead* variable in the early behavioral repertoire, and may therefore carry significant weight within the developmental equation. Korner (1972) noted nearly 15 years ago that state was primarily regarded as an "obstacle" or a nuisance factor within infant and neonatal research. The position proposed here, similar to Korner's view, is that state is an important variable in its own right, and that it may be considered most fruitfully as part of the solution in understanding neonatal behavior, rather than part of the problem in studying it.

To make this case, we first review some of the literature on information processing and cognition in neonates and discuss the difficulties in the work, with an emphasis on the overriding tendencies of early state variables. We then briefly discuss the mechanisms by which state variables might provide opportunities for prediction of later development. Finally, we discuss data relevant to our proposals, and make some recommendations for future research.

DIFFICULTIES WITH NEONATAL RESEARCH

Progress in documenting the early human cognitive and perceptual repertoire has been accomplished in spite of considerable difficulty. The human newborn is not the most cooperative of organisms, and in most research on neonatal stimulus processing there is typically a high rate of subject attrition. That is, many more subjects are tested than actually provide data. Considering the reasons for such attrition is illuminating. Two major factors contribute to subject attrition: One relates to the maintenance of state, and the other involves the display of the behavior of interest.

Failure to Maintain Optimal State

It is frequently reported that a substantial proportion of subjects are excluded from the final analyses in newborn research because they failed to maintain the state constraints imposed by the experimenter. Wolff (1966) observed two decades ago that the full-term newborn has about six distinct behavioral states that may be reliably classified. Of these six, only one (Alert Inactivity, or State 4 in the current NBAS framework) is considered by most developmental psychologists to be appropriate for the direct observation of the stimulus processing capacities of the human neonate. The vast majority of reports on neonatal stimulus processing typically include only subjects who maintain this state throughout the experimental procedures. Such exclusion for failure to maintain an alert state for the experimental procedures is completely justifiable, of course, on theoretical grounds. Investigators are interested in demonstrating the upper limits of newborns' stimulus processing, and therefore must restrict their observations to periods in which the young infant is awake, alert, and available to attend to stimuli. Obviously, the behavior of interest is not likely to occur in nonalert states.

In any case, the imposition of this State 4 constraint in newborn research raises a serious issue. Of all the behavioral states exhibited by the newborn, State 4 is among the least representative (Wolff, 1966). The classic estimates of the proportion of total time spent in State 4 during the first month of life range from 11% to 21% (Thoman, 1975; Wolff, 1965; see also Prechtl, 1974). As a result of the imposition of constraining data collection to periods during which infants maintain a State 4, a large proportion of recruited subjects must be excluded from the final analyses.

We conducted a brief review* of state-dependent subject attrition in 40 published studies (49 experiments) of infants up to 2 months of age and found that it was indeed high, both in an absolute sense, as well as relative to research with older infants. The average subject loss attributed to state (i.e., fussing, crying, sleeping, too much motor activity) was 37%. This percentage is about three times as much as the average loss we have experienced in our laboratory with infants 3 months of age and older during projects here at the University of Kansas over the past 4 years (12%).

The proportion of neonatal attrition varied widely from study to study, with a standard deviation of 17% and a range of 0% (Maurer & Salapatek, 1976) to 71% (Haith, 1981; Study III). However, studies which reported subject loss lower than 20% to 30% (e.g., Maurer & Salapatek, 1976) invariably allowed procedural "breaks" to manipulate subjects' state when infants started to cry or fall asleep. Attrition did not appear to be affected by the actual dependent measure or measurement technique used.

This high attrition is accepted typically as part of the difficulty associated with doing research on very young infants. It is common to find comments

---

*The survey of information processing studies in infants up to 2 months of age was not exhaustive, but included mostly studies over the past 8 years that were published in *Child Development, Developmental Psychology, Infant Behavior and Development, Journal of Experimental Child Psychology,* and *British Journal of Developmental Psychology,* as well as some classic studies published elsewhere or earlier. The complete list of papers and subject-loss calculations is not given here, but can be obtained by contacting the authors. The calculation of the mean for state-dependent attrition stabilized somewhere after 20 studies and neither increased nor decreased substantially by doubling the sample size of reports.

within such reports that attest to this resignation (e.g., Maltzoff & Moore, 1983). Perhaps as a result, attrition data are sometimes not presented in much detail (e.g., Blass et al, 1984) or may not be documented at all (e.g., Crassini & Broerse, 1980; Field et al., 1984; Freidman & Jacobs, 1981; Salapatek, 1968). Although it might be argued that such high attrition reduces the external validity of these studies, the reliability of single occasion-to-occasion measures of neonatal irritability are too low to support the contention that a particular group of infants is being excluded, or that some kind of selection bias is being introduced due to such practices (e.g., Lancioni, Horowitz, & Sullivan, 1980; Sameroff, 1978; Steichen Asch, Gleser, & Steichen, 1986).

Failure to Exhibit the Behavior of Interest

A second class of attrition in neonatal behavior occurs when researchers exclude infants who did not exhibit the behavior(s) of interest. Usually, no specific interfering variable is called on to account for nonbehavior, although the specific reasons given for this type of exclusion are generally related to the data collection procedure involved in the specific experiments. For example, in studies using non-nutritive sucking as a dependent measure, some infants (up to 17%) are invariably excluded for failure to take a pacifier or meet certain criteria for sucking (Ashmead, Reilly, & Lipsitt, 1980; Bertonucci & Mehler, 1981; DeCasper & Carstens, 1981; Milewski & Siqueland, 1975; Nelson, Clifton, Dowd, & Field, 1978; Werner & Siqueland, 1978).

In studies using response habituation, infants are excluded for not habituating (up to 18%: e.g., Bertonucci & Mehler, 1981; Bridger, 1961; Friedman, Bruno, & Vietze, 1974; Milewski & Siqueland, 1975). In one study of newborn auditory localization, over 10% of the total sample was excluded because they failed to localize (Zelazo et al., 1984). Finally, in many studies of visual processing, infants are excluded for (a) failing to look at the provided stimulus (up to 10%: Friedman et al., 1974; Lewis & Maurer, 1980; Maurer, 1983); (b) failing to look at all the stimuli when more than one are provided (up to 20%: Slater, Morison, & Rose, 1984; Slater, Rose, & Morison, 1984); or (c) failing to look at the stimulus long enough to provide sufficient data (up to 59%: Fantz, 1963; Lewis & Maurer, 1980; Maurer, 1983; see also relevant data in Hainline & Lemerise, 1982).

It is important to note that these examples are not presented to challenge the validity of the results of any of these studies. The results reported in these studies are undoubtedly valid in their own right and make important contributions to the literature. Rather, the information on these issues is presented to emphasize the point that stimulus seeking and processing may not constitute the most prominent activity of the very young human infant.

Indeed, even under conditions that maximize the occurrence of such stimulus oriented behavior, it seems fragile and difficult to elicit.

Implications

This brief review of the difficulties with neonatal perceptual-cognitive research leads to two tentative but potentially very important conclusions. The first is that the neonate's perceptual and cognitive abilities can be observed only under fairly constrained (indeed, perhaps optimal) situations that are among those least representative of the overall behavioral character of the neonate. Further, when these abilities are observed, they appear fragile, perhaps even transient. Given the fragility of these abilities, it does not seem surprising that early cognitive variables are not very predictive of later cognitive-intellectual abilities. A second conclusion is that state variables may be the more robust and powerful determinants of the neonate's behavior. Given the pervasiveness of state in the characterization of the neonate's behavioral patterns, it seems reasonable to suggest that we stop fighting with it and instead explore state as a dominant and important variable in its own right, one which might be involved significantly in the prediction of later development.

STATE ORGANIZATION AS A LEAD VARIABLE IN NEONATAL BEHAVIOR

The idea that it might prove fruitful to focus more closely on state or state organization* as lead variables in neonatal research is by no means new. As noted earlier, Korner (1972) has previously argued this position by observing that state is more frequently considered as a nuisance variable rather than an important behavioral aspect in its own right. This point of view has characterized the programmatic research conducted by Thoman and her associates (e.g., Thoman, Acebo, & Becker, 1983; Thoman, Denenberg, Sievel, Zeidner, & Becker, 1981; Thoman, Korner, & Kraemer, 1976; Thoman & Tynan, 1979; Tynan, 1986) on neonatal sleep-wake states and the stability of individual state organization patterns.

---

*We use the term *state organization* in this paper. At present, we must use this term to refer to a very general, overall construct of behavioral state assessment which we would propose to include a number of parameters: (a) the quality or distinctiveness of states (a developmental parameter); (b) the distribution of states within assessments (e.g., lability, range) and across repeated assessments (e.g., stability-instability); and (c) the pattern of state change in response to external stimuli (e.g., reactivity, self-regulation). Our hope is that this paper will foster progress toward the refinement and specification of this construct.

Thus, state per se may be seen as a very prominent, and perhaps dominant, component of neonatal behavior. Therefore, it may prove worthwhile to consider the development of state maturation and regulation, and the use of state as a source for prediction of later behavior. More specifically, it is proposed that early state variables or factors carry more predictive weight than do stimulus processing variables or factors. There are at least two obvious mechanisms by which state may carry such predictive weight for later development.

State as a Measure of CNS Integrity

Aylward (1981) and Berg and Berg (1979) have suggested that the emergence of well-defined behavioral states distinguishes pre-term from full-term infants. Although technically the end of the newborn period is the 28th day, it could be plausibly argued that the entrainment of state into fairly regular sleep-wake and activity-rest cycles during the third month of life (Berg & Berg, 1979) may provide a true terminus of the newborn period. Thus, state variables could be seen as reflecting some postnatal refinement of the central nervous system (CNS), and changes in state organization (i.e., cyclicity, distinctiveness, regulation, control variability, etc.) could indicate the speed or status of CNS development itself. This mechanism is apparently the one that forms the rationale for Thoman's descriptive research on sleep-wake states in the newborn (e.g., Thoman, 1975; Thoman & Tynan, 1979; Thoman et al., 1976), and her research on predictive validity of state organization (Thoman et al., 1981).

Within this framework, the wide individual differences in alert inactivity that Wolff (1966) observed more than 20 years ago might provide an index that contributes to outcome prediction. Even if speed of CNS maturation per se is not wholly predictive of later development, such an index may be predictive in combination with measures of early environmental experience. This explanation fits well with our knowledge of the effects of external stimulation or input within periods of rapid developmental change (Colombo, 1982; Gottleib, 1983; Scott, Stewart, & DeGhett, 1974).

State as a Modulating Influence for Early Stimulation

The amount of alertness or state control an infant possesses also may greatly affect the newborn's opportunity for early stimulation. This is a mechanism that Korner (1972) hypothesized in her call for the direct investigation of infant state. As an infant matures, state boundaries become more distinct, and there are more sustained periods of alert, organized behavior during which the infant is truly responsive to external input. If this mature status is attained earlier, such organization may allow newborns to exploit more frequently the upper limits of their stimulus processing capacities. Again, this behavior relates to the hypothesized importance of early stimulus input to the maintenance and facilitation of early CNS development (e.g., Gottleib, 1983).

Furthermore, state variables also may influence early social interactions. That is, specific state organization patterns may influence the kind of interactions that occur between caretaker and newborn, therefore affecting the kind or amount of active stimulation the infant receives. There are several straightforward directions in which such stimulation might occur. For example, parents obviously have the opportunity to interact longer and more with an infant whose state organization contains more alert awake periods. Alternatively, given that individual neonates differ in initial tendencies toward sleep, or in the rate at which sustained alertness is attained (Wolff, 1966), some infants will have therefore more opportunities for stimulation than others because parents do not generally wake sleeping babies for purposes of social engagement.

Caregiver variables can come into play within this alternative view as well. A mother who is adept at manipulating state may provide more opportunities for her infant to be stimulated by the environment, which may be especially important in cases where the infant is unable to modulate such stimulation herself or himself. Because state, to some degree, can be externally manipulated with powerful stimuli such as particular types of vestibular movement (Byrne & Horowitz, 1981; Korner & Grobstein, 1966; Korner & Thoman, 1972), an environment which consistently encourages and/or maintains sustained periods of quality alertness within a stable alternation of sleep might predict good developmental outcome.

DATA RELEVANT TO THE POSITION

When Korner (1972) initially proposed that infant state per se may provide important insights into behavioral development, there were few longitudinal data to support a contention that early state variables were predictive of later development. In the subsequent 15 years, some data relevant to this position have become available. We briefly review them here in order to assess further the plausibility of this position.

One group of findings involve NBAS items or clusters and later developmental status scores. Unfortunately, the follow-up measures reported in these studies typically have been Bayley Scale scores (Bayley, 1970), whose long-term prognostic ability is dubious (see McCall, Eichorn, & Hogarty,

1977). At any rate, some weak but positive relationships have been reported. Vaughn, Taraldson, Crichton, and Egeland (1980) found that an NBAS cluster based on state variables predicted Bayley mental performance at 9 months of age, whereas a stimulus-based *interactional* cluster did not correlate with later development. Vaughn et al. (1980) found that a *motoric processes* cluster significantly predicted 9-month Bayley mental scores as well.

Sostek and Anders (1977) reported a weak but statistically significant relationship between a state factor and 10-week Bayley scores. Caldera, Schwartz, and Horowitz (1985) found that the pattern of change of a *regulation of state* cluster from repeated NBAS testings significantly predicted Bayley scores at 30 months of age ($R = .51$). Furthermore, Moss (1985) reported that an NBAS *range of state* cluster significantly predicted performance on a visual discrimination task at 3 months of age ($r = .49$), and Bayley performance at 12 months, whereas orientation scores did not. This finding was replicated subsequently with a comparable sample (Moss, Colombo, Mitchell, & Horowitz, 1987).

Along with these positive findings of relationships between NBAS state ratings or clusters and later developmental measures, there are several null findings as well (e.g., Sameroff, 1978; Zelazo, 1979). One reason for the finding of weak or inconsistent relationships between NBAS state measures and later developmental assessments may lie, perhaps, in the fact that researchers using the NBAS as the neonatal measure typically employ only one very brief neonatal assessment. Numerous studies have demonstrated that a single NBAS assessment has fairly low reliability (Horowitz et al., 1978; Kaye, 1978; Sameroff, 1978; Steichen Asch et al., 1986). Given an important variable that is measured with such low reliability, it is plausible that inconsistency from study to study would result.

Indirect support for this contention may be found in several studies of the reliability of various measures of visual attention and discrimination in older infants (Colombo, 1987). In these studies, multiple measures of infants' visual discrimination performance were taken. Whereas the relationship of infant performance on any one task to any other task was typically low (e.g., *rs* averaging about + .20), the reliability of infants' average recognition task performance at one point with their average recognition task performance at some later point was considerably better (*rs* ranging from about + .40 to almost + .60). These findings suggest that valid individual differences in infant behavior may not be assessed validly in single measurements.

A persuasive case also may be made for the use of extended state observations. Although Thoman et al. (1981) report the use of 7.5-hour observations, other suggested lengths have generally varied from 2 hours (Prechtl, Fargel, Weinmann, & Bakker, 1979) to 1 hour (Dittrichova, 1966;

Thoman & Tynan, 1979). All such observations are considerably longer than the NBAS examination, which typically takes 30 min, and in which data are collected on many other variables besides behavioral state.

In any case, meaningful measurements may be available only through a more intensive approach, involving both longer periods of observation and multiple assessments. Such a systematic and focused approach characterizes the work of Thoman and her colleagues, and, perhaps as a result, their findings regarding state and developmental status are somewhat more consistent and convincing.

Thoman et al. (1976) demonstrated that there is considerable consistency (test-retest $r = + .52$) in neonatal state patterns when observed intensively across a 1-hour recording period (see also Thoman, 1975; Thoman & Tynan, 1979). Thoman et al. (1981) compiled weekly profiles of normal, low-risk infants' state in extensive observation conducted over the first month of life. They found that the degree of stability across these early assessments of state organization predicted developmental outcome at 30 months of age. Furthermore, infants who exhibited extreme instability across these multiple sessions experienced developmental delays and/or severe medical problems at later observations at 6 and 30 months.

In two subsequent studies, Tynan (1986) made multiple state observations on 25 neonates from an intensive care unit. In these studies, it again was found that less stable state profiles across the multiple observations were predictive of various severe medical conditions (e.g., seizures, sensory handicaps) as well as infant mortality 10 weeks later.

CONCLUSIONS AND RECOMMENDATIONS

These preliminary indications are presented here only to support the feasibility of an alternative conceptualization of state as a dominant neonatal behavior. They support the position that state is an important variable in its own right, and deserving of direct attention in the design and analysis of future neonatal research, especially longitudinal research.

It is important to note that the dominance of state in the determination of early behavioral patterns must be characterized along a developmental continuum. For example, the establishment of stable and distinct states may be the most pressing goal for the premature or at-risk infant. In the healthy neonate, where such distinct patterns may exist, the primary function of state variables may be in the affordance of opportunities for stimulation, or in the internal modulation of stimulus processing. Finally, by the third month, truly state-independent patterns of behavior may finally emerge. This developmental framework fits well with other accounts of major behavioral reorganizations in early infancy (e.g., Emde, Gaensbauer, & Harmon, 1976).

More precise specifications of the parameters of state that are most relevant to later prediction are needed. Such specificity would eliminate a major weakness of the current proposal. The dimension of stability-instability in state organization may represent one such important parameter (e.g., Thoman et al., 1981; Tynan, 1986; see also Horowitz, 1985). In any case, serious and sustained consideration of state or state organization may prove to be a key to demonstrating the existence of developmental continuity and, indeed, may carry a significant weight in equations that predict later development.

Such a position leads to the following recommendations for future research. First, it seems that basic, detailed research on individual differences in behavioral state should be given a high priority. This research should be designed to yield important parametric data on various aspects of the infant's state patterns and organization, such as the research conducted by Thoman and her associates. Second, it is important to consider the inclusion of state variables in all longitudinal research in which infants are followed from the newborn period. Third, on the basis of the limited available research, state variables should be explored in the assessment of neonatal risk, at least in the short term (e.g., Tynan, 1986). Such an emphasis would benefit both basic research aimed at an early identification strategy by which the risk status of neonates can be discerned, as well as the applied settings in which extra medical attention may be warranted.

The emphasis on the importance of state maturation and control as a necessary condition for or (especially) in combination with the development of information processing abilities in infants incorporates an understanding of both the neonate's behavioral competence and behavioral limitations in responding to the environment. Such a strategy should yield a more accurate characterization of the earliest period of postnatal human development. In turn, this more accurate picture of the newborn could yield a more precise understanding of the mechanisms of early development.

REFERENCES

Als, H. (1978). Assessing an assessment: Conceptual considerations, methodological issues, and a perspective on the future of the Neonatal Behavioral Assessment Scale. In A. Sameroff (Ed.), Organization and stability of newborn behavior: A commentary on the Brazelton Neonatal Behavior Assessment Scale. *Monographs of the Society for Research in Child Development, 43* (5–6, Serial No. 177).

Antell, S. E., & Keating, D. P. (1983). Perception of numerical invariance in neonates. *Child Development, 54,* 695–701.

Ashmead, D., Reilly, B., & Lipsitt, L. (1980). Neonates' heart rate, sucking rhythm, and sucking amplitude as a function of the sweet taste. *Journal of Experimental Child Psychology, 29,* 264–281.

Aylward, G. (1981). The developmental course of behavioral states in preterm infants: A descriptive study. *Child Development, 52,* 564–568.

Bayley, N. (1970). *The Bayley Scales of Infant Development.* New York: The Psychological Corp.

Berg, W., & Berg, K. (1979). Psychophysiological development in infancy: State, sensory function, and attention. In J. Osofsky (Ed.) *Handbook of infant development* (pp. 283–392). New York: Wiley.

Bertonucci, J., & Mehler, J. (1981). Syllables as units in infant speech perception. *Infant Behavior and Development, 4,* 247–280.

Blass, E., Ganchrow, J., & Steiner, J. (1984). Classical conditioning in newborn humans 2–48 hours of age. *Infant Behavior and Development, 7,* 223–235.

Brazelton, T. B. (1973). *The Neonatal Behavioral Assessment Scale.* Philadelphia: Lippincott.

Bridger, W. (1961). Sensory habituation and dishabituation in the human neonate. *American Journal of Psychiatry, 117,* 991–996.

Byrne, J., & Horowitz, F. D. (1981). Rocking as a soothing intervention: The influence of direction and type of movement. *Infant Behavior and Development, 4,* 207–218.

Caldera, Y., Schwartz, S., & Horowitz, F. (1985, April). *Prediction of later developmental status from repeated neonatal assessments.* Paper presented at the meeting of the Society for Research in Child Development, Toronto.

Colombo, J. (1982). The critical period concept: Research, methodology, and theoretical issues. *Psychological Bulletin, 92,* 260–275.

Colombo, J. (1987, April). *The psychometrics of infant visual attention.* Paper presented at the meeting of the Society for Research in Child Development, Baltimore, MD.

Crassini, B., & Broerse, J. (1980). Auditory-visual integration in neonates: A signal detection analysis. *Journal of Experimental Child Psychology, 29,* 144–155.

DeCasper, A. J., & Carstens, A. A. (1981). Contingencies of stimulation: Effects on learning and emotion in the neonate. *Infant Behavior and Development, 4,* 19–35.

Dittrichova, J. (1966). Development of sleep in infancy. *Journal of Applied Physiology, 21,* 1243–1246.

Emde, R. N., Gaensbauer, T. J., & Harmon, R. J. (1976). Emotional expression in infancy: A biobehavioral study. *Psychological Issues, 10* (Monograph No. 37).

Fantz, R. (1963). Pattern vision in newborn infants, *Science, 140,* 296–297.

Field, T., Cohen, D., Garcia, R., & Greenberg, R. (1984). Mother-stranger face discrimination in the newborn. *Infant Behavior and Development, 7,* 19–25.

Friedman, S., Bruno, L., & Vietze, P. (1974). Newborn habituation to visual stimuli: A sex difference in novelty detection. *Journal of Experimental Child Psychology, 18,* 242–251.

Friedman, S., & Jacobs, B. (1981). Sex differences in neonates behavioral responsiveness to repeated auditory stimulation. *Infant Behavior and Development, 4,* 175–183.

Gottlieb, G. (1983). The psychobiological approach to developmental issues. In M. Haith & J. Campos (Eds.), *Handbook of child psychology: Vol. 2. Infancy and developmental psychobiology* (4th ed., pp. 1–26). New York: Wiley.

Hainline, L., & Lemerise, E. (1982). Infants' scanning of geometric forms varying in size. *Journal of Experimental Child Psychology, 33,* 235–256.

Haith, M. M. (1981). *Rules that babies look by.* Hillsdale, NJ: Erlbaum.

Haith, M. M., & Campos, J. J. (Eds.) (1983). *Handbook of child psychology: Vol. 2. Infancy and developmental psychobiology* (4th ed.). New York: Wiley.

Horowitz, F. (1985, April). *Stability and instability as a dimension of infant behavior.* Paper presented at the International Conference on Infant Studies, Los Angeles, CA.

Horowitz, F., Sullivan, J., Byrne, J., & Mitchell, D. W. (in preparation). *An atlas of newborn behavior.*

Horowitz, F., Sullivan, J., & Linn, P. (1978). Stability and instability in the newborn infant: The quest for elusive threads. In A. Sameroff (Ed.), Organization and stability of newborn behavior: A commentary on the Brazelton Neonatal Behavior Assessment Scale. *Monographs of the Society for Research in Child Development, 43* (5–6, Serial No. 177).

Kaye, K. (1978). Discriminating among normal infants by multivariate analysis of Brazelton scores: Lumping and smoothing. In A. Sameroff (Ed.), Organization and stability of newborn behavior: A commentary on the Brazelton Neonatal Behavior Assessment Scale. *Monographs of the Society for Research in Child Development, 43* (5–6, Serial No. 177).

Korner, A. F. (1972). State as a variable, as obstacle, and as a mediator of stimulation in infant research. *Merrill-Palmer Quarterly, 18,* 77–95.

Korner, A. F., & Grobstein, R. (1966). Visual alertness as related to soothing in neonates: Implications for maternal stimulation and early deprivation. *Child Development, 37,* 867–876.

Korner, A. F., & Thoman, E. (1972). The relative efficacy of contact and vestibular proprioceptive stimulation in soothing neonates. *Child Development, 43,* 443–453.

Lancioni, G., Horowitz, F., & Sullivan, J. (1980). The NBAS-K: 1. A study of its stability and structure over the first month of life. *Infant Behavior and Development, 3,* 341–359.

Lester, B., Emory, B., Hoffman, S., & Eitzman, D. (1976). A multivariate study of the effects of high-risk factors on the performance on the Brazelton Neonatal Assessment Scale. *Child Development, 47,* 515–517.

Lewis, T., & Maurer, D. (1980). Central vision in the newborn. *Journal of Experimental Child Psychology, 29,* 475–480.

Maurer, D. (1983). The scanning of compound figures by young infants. *Journal of Experimental Child Psychology, 35,* 437–448.

Maurer, D., & Salapatek, P. (1976). Developmental changes in the scanning of faces by young infants. *Child Development, 47,* 523–527.

McCall, R., Eichorn, D., & Hogarty, P. (1977). Transitions in early mental development. *Monographs of the Society for Research in Child Development, 42* (3, Serial No. 171).

Meltzoff, A., & Moore, M. (1983). Newborns imitate adult facial gestures. *Child Development, 54,* 702–709.

Milewski, A. E., & Siqueland, E. (1975). Discrimination of color and pattern novelty in one-month human infants. *Journal of Experimental Child Psychology, 19,* 122–136.

Moss, M. (1985). *Neonatal behavioral organization and visual processing at three months*. Unpublished master's thesis, University of Kansas Infant Study Center, Lawrence, KS.

Moss, M., Colombo, J., Mitchell, D., & Horowitz, F. (1987). *Newborn behavioral organization and visual processing at three months*. Manuscript submitted for publication.

Nelson, M. N., Clifton, R. K., Dowd, J. M., & Field, T. M. (1978). Cardiac responding to auditory stimuli in newborn infants: Why pacifiers should not be used when heart rate is the dependent measure. *Infant Behavior and Development, 1,* 277–290.

Prechtl, H. F. R. (1974). The behavioural states of the newborn (A review). *Brain Research, 76,* 185–212.

Prechtl, H. F. R., Fargel, J., Weinmann, H., & Bakker, H. (1979). Postures, motility, and respiration of low-risk preterm infants. *Developmental Medicine and Child Neurology, 21,* 3–27.

Salapatek, P. (1968). Visual scanning of geometric figures by the newborn. *Journal of Comparative and Physiological Psychology, 66,* 247–258.

Sameroff, A. (1978). Summary and conclusions: The future of newborn assessment. In A. Sameroff (Ed.), Organization and stability of newborn behavior: A commentary on the Brazelton Neonatal Behavior Assessment Scale. *Monographs of the Society for Research in Child Development, 43* (5–6, Serial No. 177).

Sameroff, A. J., & Cavanaugh, P. J. (1979). Learning in infancy: A developmental perspective. In J. D. Osofsky (Ed.), *Handbook of infant development* (pp. 344–392). New York: Wiley.

Scott, J. P., Stewart, J., & DeGhett, V. (1974). Critical periods in the organization of systems. *Developmental Psychobiology, 7,* 489–513.

Slater, A., Morison, V., & Rose, D. (1984). Habituation in the newborn. *Infant Behavior and Development, 7,* 183–200.

Slater, A., Rose, D., & Morison, V. (1984). Newborn infants' perception of similarities and differences between two- and three-dimensional stimuli. *British Journal of Developmental Psychology, 2,* 287–294.

Sostek, A., & Anders, J. (1977). Relationships among the Brazelton neonatal scale, Bayley infant scales, and early temperament. *Child Development, 48,* 320–323.

Steichen Asch, P., Gleser, G., & Steichen, J. (1986). Dependability of Brazelton neonatal behavioral assessment cluster scales. *Infant Behavior and Development, 9,* 207–320.

Thoman, E. B. (1975). Sleep and wake behaviors in neonates: Consistencies and consequences. *Merrill-Palmer Quarterly, 21,* 295–314.

Thoman, E. B., Acebo, C., & Becker, P. T. (1983). Infant crying and stability in the mother-infant relationship. *Child Development, 54,* 653–659.

Thoman, E. B., Denenberg, V. H., Sievel, J., Zeidner, L., & Becker, P. T. (1981). State organization in neonates: Developmental inconsistency indicates risk for developmental dysfunction. *Neuropediatrics, 12,* 45–54.

Thoman, E. B., Korner, A., & Kraemer, H. (1976). Individual consistency in behavioral states in neonates. *Developmental Psychobiology, 9,* 271–283.

Thoman, E. B., & Tynan, W. D. (1979). Sleep states and wakefulness in human infants: Profiles from motility monitoring. *Physiology and Behavior, 23,* 519–523.

Tynan, W. D. (1986). Behavioral stability predicts morbidity and mortality in infants from a neonatal intensive care unit. *Infant Behavior and Development, 9,* 71–79.

Vaughn, B., Taraldson, B., Crichton, L., & Egeland, B. (1980). Relationships between neonatal behavioral organization and infant behavior during the first year of life. *Infant Behavior and Development, 3,* 47–66.

Werner, J., & Siqueland, E. (1978). Visual recognition memory in the preterm infant. *Infant Behavior and Development, 1,* 79–94.

Wolff, P. H. (1965). The development of attention in young infants. *Annals of the New York Academy of Sciences, 118,* 815–830.

Wolff, P. H. (1966). The causes, controls, and organization of behavior in the neonate. *Psychological Issues, 5* (Monograph No. 17).

Zelazo, P. R. (1979). Reactivity to perceptual-cognitive events: Application for infant assessment. In R. B. Kearsley & I. E. Sigel (Eds.), *Infants at risk: Assessment of cognitive functioning* (pp. 49–82). Hillsdale, NJ: Erlbaum.

Zelazo, P. R., Brody, L., & Chaika, H. (1984). Neonatal habituation and dishabituation of head turning to rattle sounds. *Infant Behavior and Development, 7,* 253–264.

Part II

CHILD-CARE ISSUES

As Phillips, McCartney, and Scarr point out in the first paper of this section, some form of nonparental care is the norm for over half of all American children. As more and more young children spend more and more time out of the home, child care can no longer be viewed as a uniform intervention. Research into the developmental effects of child care must begin to take both differences in programmatic organization and family background into account. This carefully designed and well-controlled investigation, which specifically examines the consequences of social development of 166 children who attended nine different child-care centers that varied widely in quality, is an exemplar of this much-needed shift in research direction. The overall quality of the children's child-care environments was found to have made a significant contribution to their social development. More specifically, the director's experience and the amount of verbal interaction between caregivers and children were the most consistent predictors of the children's social development in child care, while child-staff ratios showed a more modest degree of influence. However, of great importance in view of changing national trends, age at entry and time in care were relatively poor predictors of the children's social development in child care. The investigators suggest that program features such as staff training and experience exert their influence by facilitating positive interactions among staff and children. The further clarification of the processes that underlie the influence of child-care quality on child development await further research, but on a practical level, the regulation of the readily measurable aspects of program quality identified in this investigation need not await the detailed specification of mechanisms of action.

The paper by Zigler approaches the question of out-of-home experience for young children from the perspective of a critical examination of the recent movement toward enrolling four-year-olds in academic programs. Zigler suggests that the current impetus for earlier schooling is rooted in the concern generated by the recent proliferation of negative evaluations of our public secondary schools. The success of some excellent broad-based remedial

143

programs for economically disadvantaged children has encouraged many decision makers to advocate the downward extension of public schooling to four-year-olds. However, successful intervention programs and conventional schooling are not comparable. In intervention programs, not only does the target child receive academic instruction, but assistance in the form of primary health and social services is also provided to the family as a whole. Zigler suggests that those who argue in favor of universal preschool education ignore evidence indicating that early schooling is inappropriate for many four-year-olds. The supervision of very young children must be a distinct form of care, suited to the rapid developmental changes and high dependency of these children, not a scaled-down version of a grade-school curriculum. The real question is how to provide the best experience during the day for four-year-olds, specifically for those who cannot remain at home with a consistent, competent caregiver. Zigler concludes that parents do not need children who read at age four, but they do need affordable, good quality child care, which could be provided through the development of programs that utilize community schools as local centers for all the social services required by a surrounding neighborhood.

Yet another aspect of nonparental care for young children is the subject of the paper by Galambos and Lerner. These investigators examined the relative influence of child, maternal, and demographic characteristics on the labor force participation of mothers with young children enrolled in the New York Longitudinal Study. Multiple regression analyses revealed that child characteristics such as temperamental difficulty and the presence of physical problems were as potent as demographic features in predicting the mother's labor market activities throughout the child's early years. Recognizing that it is difficult to generalize the results of this study of mothers whose children were born in the late 1950s and early 1960s to mothers of young children in the 1980s, the authors conclude that there appears to be no reason to dismiss the likelihood that child characteristics have an influence on present-day mothers' career-decision-making processes as well. However, difficult temperament in toddlerhood, together with the number of young children at year three and physical problems, accounted for less than a quarter of the variance in mothers' labor force participation during the toddler and preschool years. Thus many mothers who do work do so under conditions of increased stress, a factor which also needs to be considered in the design of quality programs of nonparental care.

7

Child-Care Quality and Children's Social Development

Deborah Phillips
Bush Center in Child Development and Social Policy,
Yale University, New Haven, Connecticut
Kathleen McCartney
Harvard University, Cambridge, Massachusetts
Sandra Scarr
University of Virginia, Charlottesville

This study examined the influence on children's social development of variation in the quality of their child-care environments. The sample consisted of 166 children attending representative child-care centers that varied widely in quality. Possible relations associated with age, child-care experience, and family background were controlled using hierarchical multiple regression. Both global estimates of child-care quality and specific program features, such as director experience, ratios, and verbal interactions, were obtained from observational measures and staff questionnaires. Measures of social development were derived from parent and caregiver ratings of the children. Of greatest importance is the finding that overall quality, caregiver-child verbal interactions, and director experience were each highly predictive of the children's social development in child care. Family background measures

Reprinted with permission from *Developmental Psychology*, 1987, Vol. 23, No. 4, 537–543. Copyright 1987 by the American Psychological Association.

The larger research effort of which this study is a part was supported by grants from the William T. Grant Foundation and the Bermuda Government.

We would like to acknowledge the valuable contribution of J. Conrad Schwarz to the larger research effort from which this report derives and Susan Grajek's helpful assistance with data collection and analysis.

were also significantly predictive of several of the social outcomes, whereas child-care experience showed few significant effects. The implications for social policies and future research in child care are discussed.

The developmental effects of child care have long held interest for psychologists, first because child care represented an intriguing exception to parental care, and now because some form of child care is the norm for over half of all American children. Parallel with these demographic trends, the research literature has shifted from questions that entail comparisons of home-reared children and those enrolled in child care to more sophisticated questions about how children in child care are affected by differences in program quality (Belsky, 1984; Clarke-Stewart & Fein, 1983). A related issue concerns the identification of specific quality indicators that affect child development. A third, relatively new, empirical focus is on the joint effects of child care and family variables (Everson, Sarnat, & Ambron, 1984; Howes & Olenick, 1986; McCartney, Scarr, Phillips, Grajek, & Schwarz, 1982).

The research reported here was designed to address these contemporary issues about child care as well as to cast them in a broader theoretical framework. The principal aims of the study were (a) to examine the consequences for social development of attending child-care centers that varied widely in quality, (b) to identify specific indicators of quality—for example, staff-child ratios and verbal interactions between caregivers and children—that may account for results obtained when quality is treated as a global construct, and (c) to determine whether associations between quality and child outcomes are affected by children's day-care experience or family background. The research also addresses general theoretical issues regarding environmental influences on social development.

Within the literature on the developmental effects of child care, it is the issue of social outcomes that has generated the most contradictory findings and thus the greatest controversy. On the one hand, children who have participated in child care appear to be more socially skilled than their home-reared peers, as demonstrated by their more advanced perspective-taking skills, cooperative behavior, task orientation, and confidence in social interactions (Clarke-Stewart, 1984; Howes & Olenick, 1986; Ramey, Mac-Phee, & Yeates, 1982; Rubenstein & Howes, 1979). On the other hand, displays of aggression, negative affect, and resistance to adult requests have been reported to be more prevalent among child-care than home-reared children (Haskins, 1985; Ramey, Dorval, & Baker-Ward, 1981; Schwarz, Krolick, & Strickland, 1973).

Several reviewers of the child-care literature have reconciled this seemingly contradictory pattern of results by attributing both the positive and negative behaviors to greater social maturity on the part of children enrolled in child care (Clarke-Stewart & Fein, 1983; Rutter, 1981), to earlier acquisition of adult social values (Belsky, Steinberg, & Walker, 1982; Schwarz, Strickland, & Krolick, 1974), or to differences in the structure of the programs (Haskins, 1985).

Other factors that may explain the diverse social outcomes ascribed to child care include variation in the quality of the child-care programs studied, the children's timing and history of child-care attendance, and family variables that affect both the choice and effects of child care. Among these factors, only the contribution of child-care quality has received systematic empirical attention.

When direct comparisons are made of programs that vary in quality, results suggest that social development is enhanced by higher quality care (Golden et al., 1978; McCartney, Scarr, Phillips, & Grajek, 1982; Roupp, Travers, Glantz, & Coelen, 1979; Vandell & Powers, 1983). Efforts to extract the specific dimensions of quality that affect social development have revealed the major contribution of caregiver-child verbal interaction (Clarke-Stewart, 1984; Golden et al., 1978; McCartney, 1984; Roupp et al., 1979), caregiver stability (Clarke-Stewart & Gruber, 1984; Cummings, 1980), small groupings of peers and low child-staff ratios (Clarke-Stewart & Gruber, 1984; Howes & Rubenstein, 1985; Roupp et al., 1979), and specialized caregiver training and experience (Howes & Olenick, 1986; Roupp et al., 1979).

Children's social development in child care may also be affected by the age of entry or the length of time that they have been enrolled. Studies of these issues that specifically address social outcomes are just now emerging (Haskins, 1985; Howes & Rubenstein, 1985); thus, no systematic conclusions can be drawn. The work on program quality, however, has included both infant and preschool samples, implying that quality may override child-care experience as a determinant of child care's influence on social development.

Family influences on the developmental effects of child care are also richly deserving of study, because of indications (Howes & Olenick, 1986) that families served by low- and high-quality care differ significantly on measures of family stress. At the least, it is essential to control for program-selection effects in studies of child-care quality. As noted by Scarr and McCartney (1983), genotype-environment confounds characterize most studies of socialization, including studies of parent-selected child-care environments. In the absence of controls for children's family backgrounds, it is impossible to discern whether social outcomes derive from the genetic makeup or from the environment that children share with their parents.

Unfortunately, much of the research on child care can provide only limited answers to questions about both quality indicators and environmental influence. Studies of child care are typically conducted in above-average child-care programs characterized by restricted variation in key indicators of program quality. For example, the staff-child ratios in the majority of centers sampled for the National Day Care Study (Roupp et al., 1979) ranged from 5 to 9 children per staff member. In addition, few studies have controlled for possible confounds associated with differences in the family backgrounds of children in child-care programs varying in quality. Thus, effects that are attributable to child care cannot be distinguished from those that are attributable to differences in the family backgrounds of children in different programs.

This study sought to rectify the methodological shortcomings of prior child-care research on social development. It is part of a larger investigation of the developmental consequences of child-care quality designed to exemplify an emerging paradigm in child-care research that incorporates individual- and family-level influences. The findings reported here extend and clarify our previous reports, which have examined global indicators of program quality (McCartney et al., 1982) and have focused on language development (McCartney, 1984). This report addresses social outcomes and examines specific dimensions of program quality.

It was hypothesized that children attending higher-quality child-care centers would demonstrate greater social competence and adjustment. The influence of quality was expected to be attributable largely to the nature of the caregiver-child interactions and to structural features, such as child-staff ratios, that facilitate constructive interaction. Neither family background nor the children's previous child-care experience were expected to significantly affect the relation between child-care quality and social development.

METHOD

Child-Care Settings

Bermuda was chosen as the site of this research for two reasons that bear directly on the methodological shortcomings of prior research. First, a pilot study conducted in the most populated province in Bermuda revealed that approximately 85% of Bermudian children spend the majority of their day in some form of substitute care by the time they are 2 years of age. This reduces potential selection biases. Second, the child-care programs in Bermuda are remarkably stable and represent a wide range of quality, thus creating the opportunity to study a representative range of child care.

When this research project began in 1980, nine child-care centers in Bermuda had been in operation for over 4 years and accepted children from infancy through the preschool years. The directors of all nine agreed to participate in the study. This assured wide variation with respect to the children's family backgrounds and experience in child care. Eight of the child-care centers were privately owned; one of the centers was government-run and served predominantly low-income families.

Subjects

All children 3 years and older who had attended one of the nine target centers for 6 months or more and their parents were asked to participate in the study. A total of 166 families participated, with only 15 refusals. The children ranged in age from 36 to 68 months; 130 were Black and 36 were White. Fathers were present in 68% of the households, and extent of maternal education ranged from 5 to 22 years. The average age of entry into child care was 19 months for the participating children, suggesting high continuity of care.

Measures

Child-care environment. The quality of the child-care environment was assessed in three ways. First, Harms and Clifford's (1980) Early Childhood Environment Rating Scale (ECERS) was used to obtain observational ratings of quality on seven dimensions: personal care, creative activities, language/reasoning, fine-gross motor, social development, furnishing/display, and adult facilities/opportunities. The first six scales, which measure dimensions of the child's environment, were used in our study. The interrater reliability obtained in this study across all items on the ECERS was high ($r =$ .82). The six subscales were highly correlated in this study (*rs* ranged from + .60 to + .92), so only the total scale score was used.

Second, specific indicators of quality were obtained from an extensive interview with each program director, based on the Day Care Environment Inventory (Prescott, Kritchevsky, & Jones, 1972). The interview focused on descriptive aspects of the child-care facility and program, such as staff experience and training, staff-child ratios, amount and variety of play equipment, and parent involvement. From this interview, the director's years of experience and the child-staff ratio were selected for analysis as specific indicators of quality.

Third, the quality of verbal interactions between adults and children was assessed using an observational coding system (see McCartney, 1984) in which eight children (randomly selected) per center were observed for six 10-min segments. The number of functional utterances directed to children by caregivers and by peers provided the verbal environment measures for this report.

Children's social development. Social development was assessed using parent and caregiver ratings on two standardized measures. The preschool form of the Classroom Behavior Inventory (Schaefer & Edgerton, 1978), which yields factors for intelligence, considerateness, sociability, task orientation, and dependence, was used to assess social competence. Schaefer and Edgerton (1978) report internal consistency reliabilities ranging from .72 to .95, and interrater reliabilities ranging from .50 to .83.

The Preschool Behavior Questionnaire (Behar & Stringfield, 1974), specifically designed to screen preschool-age children in group-care settings for aggression, anxiety, and hyperactivity, was used to assess social adjustment. Behar (1977) reports interrater reliabilities of .93 (aggression), .60 (anxiety), and .94 (hyperactivity). The scale was also found to significantly differentiate children who attended a therapeutic preschool class (Behar, 1977).

Family background and home environment. Family background measures were derived from parent interviews that included demographic questions (e.g., family income, age and education of parents) as well as items from the Parent as Educator Interview (Schaefer & Edgerton, 1977), which was designed to assess parental values about child learning and development. The child's age of entry into child care and length of child-care attendance were also obtained during the parent interview.

Procedure

Between March and June 1980, two researchers visited each of the nine centers on at least three different days to administer the director's interview, collect the verbal environment data, and rate program quality on the ECERS. During the initial visit, the social measures were distributed to two caregivers per program. The instructions required the caregivers to rate all participating children item by item in order to reduce potential halo effects. The two caregiver ratings were averaged to produce the final caregiver rating on each social measure, as recommended by Schaefer and Edgerton (1977). Two additional program visits by two researchers were required to collect observational data on the verbal environment of the centers. Following their observations, the two coders individually rated program quality. Ten Bermudian college students who were naive to the purpose of the study conducted the parent interviews, during which the information about family background and child-care history and the parent ratings on the measures of social development were obtained.

RESULTS

Descriptive Statistics

Given the importance of obtaining data on representative child-care programs, descriptive statistics for the major predictor variables of child-care quality were first examined. Wide variation characterized each of the quality measures. Scores on the ECERS ranged from 66.5 to 191.0 ($M = 123.2$), indicating ample variation given the 37 (low) to 259 (high) possible range. Similarly, directors' experience ranged from 11.3 to 24.5 years ($M = 15.7$), and staff-child ratios ranged from 1:5.7 to 1:15 ($M = 1:10.5$).

Preliminary Correlational Analyses

Intercorrelations were examined among the parent and teacher ratings of social development, and between sex of child and the social measures.

The degree of correspondence between the parent and caregiver ratings of social development was examined using Pearson correlations. Only the parent and teacher ratings of the children's intelligence correlated significantly ($r = .35, p < .001$). The independence of parent and teacher ratings may reflect differing perceptions of the children, or may be a function of differing sources of bias for these two groups of raters. It is important to note that the rating scales used in the study were designed exclusively for use by teachers.

Intercorrelations between sex of child and each of the social-development measures were examined in light of recent suggestions that sex of child may moderate the developmental effects of child care (Gamble & Zigler, 1986). Only 1 of the 16 intercorrelations attained significance: sex with teacher ratings of the children's dependence ($r = -.20, p < .05$). Boys were rated as more dependent than girls.

Controlling for Center Selection

Because parents select child-care programs for their children, and selection biases may covary with program quality, it is essential to control for center selectivity when examining the influence of child-care quality on social development. In order to examine the issue of selectivity, stepwise multiple regression was conducted to identify the specific family-background measures that showed the strongest relation to child-care quality. Specifically, the total quality score from the ECERS was regressed on the 16 measures of family demographics and home environment obtained from the family interview. This conservative approach was used to remove the maximum variance in center selection attributable to differences in the children's family backgrounds prior to examining the influence of child-care experience and program quality in the regression analyses reported below.

The two family-background measures that emerged from this analysis were *values social skills,* a positive predictor of the total ECERS score, F (2, 84) = 8.85, $p < .01$; and *values conformity,* a negative predictor, F (2, 84) = 8.61, $p < .01$. Parents who placed a high value on social skills and a low value on conformity selected higher-quality child-care centers than did other parents. In the hierarchical regression analyses that follow, these two family-background variables were entered prior to measures of the day-care environment. This provided a more rigorous control for center selectivity than that used in prior reports of this research (see McCartney et al., 1982), because empirically-derived, rather than estimated, predictors of selectivity were used as controls.

Data Analysis Strategy

The general strategy for the quality analyses involved controlling for age of the child, family background, and child-care experience prior to obtaining an estimate of the contribution of child-care quality to children's social development. Specifically, a hierarchical regression model was used in which the child's age at testing was entered in the first equation, followed by the two proxies for family background that affected center selection. Age at entry into care and total hours of attendance were added in the third equation. The total quality score was entered in the fourth and final equation. The model was computed separately for each of the parent and caregiver ratings of social development. A second set of analyses, using the same model, was then conducted to evaluate the influence of specific indicators of program quality: the director's years of experience, child-staff ratio, caregiver-child verbal interaction, and verbal interaction among peers.

Effects of Overall Quality

The overall quality of the children's child-care environments made a significant contribution to their social development. Table 1 presents the change in R^2 at each step of the regression analysis. Six of the 10 factors from the Classroom Behavior Inventory and one of the six subscales from the Child Behavior Questionnaire yielded significant effects for program quality,

Table 1. Hierarchical Regression of Children's Social Development on Age, Family Background, Child-Care Experience, and Overall Quality

Measure/Rater	Change in R^2		
	Family background: Values conformity, Values social skill	Experience: Age at entry, Time in care	Quality: ECERS
Considerateness			
Parent	.019	.004	.088**
Caregiver	.054*	.002	.329***
Dependence			
Parent	.069*	.008	.000
Caregiver	.022	.041**	.021
Sociability			
Parent	.025	.007	.050*
Caregiver	.087**	.001	.390***
Intelligence			
Parent	.010	.005	.009
Caregiver	.038	.016	.213***
Task orientation			
Parent	.008	.004	.000
Caregiver	.023	.012	.141***
Aggression			
Parent	.027	.015	.005
Caregiver	.002	.022	.018
Hyperactivity			
Parent	.002	.007	.027
Caregiver	.000	.028	.018
Anxiety			
Parent	.008	.011	.001
Caregiver	.056*	.060**	.081**

Note. ECERS = Early Childhood Environment Rating Scale. Age at entry was entered prior to the two family background measures. $N = 156$ for the parent ratings and 153 for the caregiver ratings.
* $p < .05.$ ** $p < .01.$ *** $p < .001.$

controlling for the influence of age, child-care experience, and family background.

For the parent ratings, child-care quality was predictive of greater considerateness and greater sociability. The caregiver ratings corroborated these results, with quality accounting for more than a 30% increase in their ratings of considerateness and sociability. Overall quality also contributed significantly to the caregiver ratings of the children's intelligence and task orientation, so that children in higher-quality centers were rated as higher in intelligence and more task oriented. With respect to the scales of social adjustment, quality emerged as a significant predictor of caregiver ratings of anxiety, so that caregivers in higher-quality programs rated the children as more anxious.

Prior to removing the variance accounted for by center quality, several other predictors yielded significant results. Children who were older at the time of testing were rated by their caregivers as less dependent and more intelligent and task oriented. The parents of older children rated them as more intelligent, as well, and as less aggressive and less hyperactive.

The two measures of parent values showed only a few modest relations to the social-outcome measures. For the parent ratings, the higher the value placed on conformity, the greater the child's dependence. The caregivers rated children from homes that placed a low value on conformity as more considerate, sociable, and anxious.

Age at entry and time in care were relatively poor predictors of the children's social development in child care. Only two significant relations emerged, both for the caregiver ratings. Children who spent less time in child care were rated as more dependent and more anxious, and children who entered care at an earlier age were rated as more anxious. Time in child care accounted for a 4% increment in the variance accounted for in the dependence ratings. Age of entry and time in care, combined, accounted for 6% additional variance in the anxiety ratings.

In sum, overall quality of the child-care environment exerted a consistent influence on social development. Indeed, overall child-care quality was predictive of 8 of the 16 measures of social development, in spite of the fact that measures of family background, child-care experience, and child's age were entered first. Family background typically accounted for smaller increments in the total variance than did the quality score, and child-care experience showed only two significant effects. A comparison of the amount of variance contributed by quality for the parent and caregiver ratings revealed that the caregiver ratings showed a much stronger association between quality and social development. Finally, the measures of social competence, assessed using the Classroom Behavior Inventory, were much more sensitive to differences in program quality than were the measures of social adjustment derived from the Child Behavior Questionnaire.

Effects of Specific Indicators of Child-Care Quality

The finding that overall center quality affects children's social development, although theoretically significant, is of little use to practitioners and policy makers who seek to influence specific program features that predict positive outcomes for children. The next analyses were, therefore, designed to answer the question, "What aspects of quality affect social development?"

Four variables provided the focus of these analyses: director experience, child-staff ratio, verbal interaction with caregivers, and verbal interaction with peers. They were selected on the basis of their demonstrated importance in prior child-care research and the variance they exhibited across the 9 participating child-care centers.*

The hierarchical regression model used to assess the influence of overall quality was also used for these analyses, entering each of the quality indicators in the fourth and final equation. Table 2 presents the additional proportion of variance accounted for (change in R^2) by each of the specific quality indicators for the 16 measures of social development.

For the 10 measures of social competence, the director's experience and the amount of verbal interaction between caregivers and children were the most consistent predictors of the children's social development in child care. Director experience was a negative predictor of the caregiver ratings of considerateness, dependence, and sociability. Alternatively, verbal interaction between caregivers and children emerged as a positive predictor of beneficial social development in child care. Both parents and caregivers in centers with higher amounts of adult-child verbal interaction rated the children as more considerate, and caregivers also rated them as more sociable, intelligent, and task oriented.

Child-staff ratio showed a more modest degree of influence, accounting for a 3.8% increment in the variance accounted for in the parent ratings of their child's considerateness. Higher—that is, better—ratios corresponded to greater considerateness on the part of the children. Verbal interaction among peers showed a mixed pattern of influence, corresponding to greater dependence and lower task orientation, yet greater sociability as revealed by the caregiver ratings.

For the measures of aggression, hyperactivity, and anxiety, director experience again emerged as a significant predictor, although here it presents a more consistently positive picture. Caregivers in centers directed by adults with more child-care experience rated the children as less aggressive, hyperactive, and anxious. These results were not corroborated by parents.

Child-staff ratio showed a single significant result. An additional 13% of the variance in the caregiver ratings of child anxiety was attributable to child-

---

*Caregiver training, a significant predictor of child outcomes in prior research (see Roupp et al., 1979), showed minimal variation in these Bermudian centers and was thus excluded from the regression analyses.

Table 2. Hierarchical Regression of Children's Social Development on Age, Family Background, Child-Care Experience, and Specific Quality Indicators

Measure/Rater	Change in R^2			
	Director experience	Child–Staff ratio	Caregiver: Verbal interaction	Peer: Verbal interaction
Considerateness				
Parent	.003	.038*	.047*	.026
Caregiver	.097**	.002	.355***	.008
Dependence				
Parent	.001	.003	.012	.006
Caregiver	.263***	.005	.009	.203***
Sociability				
Parent	.001	.021	.028	.020
Caregiver	.181***	.009	.222***	.125***
Intelligence				
Parent	.023	.002	.016	.004
Caregiver	.011	.016	.234***	.000
Task orientation				
Parent	.008	.001	.001	.006
Caregiver	.001	.001	.279***	.041*
Aggression				
Parent	.009	.002	.005	.003
Caregiver	.037*	.018	.000	.051*
Hyperactivity				
Parent	.000	.008	.021	.000
Caregiver	.041*	.004	.005	.021
Anxiety				
Parent	.005	.003	.029	.013
Caregiver	.056**	.130***	.002	.143***

Note. Each of the four quality variables was entered last in separate hierarchical multiple regression equations. The following variables were entered first: age at testing, values conformity and values social skills, age at entry, and time in group care.
* $p < .05$. ** $p < .01$. *** $p < .001$.

staff ratios, so that children in programs with better ratios were rated as more anxious by their caregivers. The parent ratings of anxiety did not corroborate this puzzling result. The final predictor, verbal interaction with peers, emerged as a negative indicator of quality. Children in programs with higher levels of child-to-child verbal interaction were rated by their caregivers as more aggressive and more anxious.

To summarize the results for the specific indicators of center quality, children appear to fare better in child-care centers characterized by large amounts of caregiver-child verbal interaction and, consequently, relatively low amounts of verbal interaction among peers. Director experience also emerged as an important predictor of children's social development in child care, although the direction of its influence was not consistent. Social competence appears to suffer in programs run by directors with more experience, as indicated by lower caregiver ratings of considerateness and sociability. Yet the ratings of aggression, hyperactivity, and anxiety suggested that children in programs directed by adults with more experience are better adjusted. Child-staff ratios, like overall quality, showed a perplexing positive association with anxiety. Ratios, however, also showed a positive, but modest relation to parent ratings of considerateness. In general, the caregiver ratings of social development were much more sensitive than the parent ratings to variation in the specific indicators of program quality.

DISCUSSION

The most important finding to emerge from this research is that the overall quality of the child-care environment affects many aspects of children's social competence and adjustment. The influence of quality was found in analyses that, unlike those used in other studies of child-care quality, included controls for the effects of the children's age, family background, and child-care experience.

Convergence of the findings with previous reports of the Bermuda study in which child-care quality was found to have a significant impact on children's cognitive and language development (McCartney, 1984), with analyses comparing the high-quality government-run child-care program in Bermuda with the lower-quality private centers (McCartney, Scarr, Phillips, & Grajek, 1985), and with the reports of other investigators (Howes & Rubenstein, 1985; Roupp et al., 1979; Vandell & Powers, 1983) lends additional support to the assertion that variation in child-care quality affects child development. It is particularly significant that these results have emerged from research that examines representative rather than high-quality child-care centers or expensive early intervention programs that fail to reflect the real child-care choices available to most families.

The study's major weakness is the exclusive use of questionnaire measures of social development, and the notable differences in the results obtained with the caregiver and parent ratings. Moreover, the anomalous associations found between anxiety and both overall quality and ratios are perplexing and deserve further study. It should be noted, however, that the actual range of anxiety scores in this study (1.00 to 2.67) is well within the normal range on the Preschool Behavior Questionnaire, on which the standardization sample averaged 1.96 (SD = 2.34) and a comparison sample of disturbed children averaged 6.73 (Behar, 1977).

On a theoretical level, our study provides persuasive evidence of environmental influences on development, because of the inclusion of empirically derived controls for family-based center-selection confounds. Although it is entirely possible that some remaining variance due to center selection was not eliminated, the results nonetheless lend support to the optimistic stance assumed by most intervention programs that nonfamilial early childhood environments can promote positive development. Particularly significant is the new evidence that child care not designed as early intervention can nevertheless serve in this capacity if it is of adequate quality (Scarr & Weinberg, 1986).

With respect to the question "What aspects of quality affect social development?", children appear to profit from a verbally stimulating environment in which adult caregivers and children are frequently engaged in conversation. Similar findings were reported by McCartney (1984) for children's cognitive and language development. In contrast, verbal interaction with peers, perhaps because it replaces the more important caregiver talk, appears to have deleterious effects on social development. Again, this pattern matches that found for children's language development in prior reports of the Bermuda study (McCartney, 1984).

The director's experience showed a contradictory pattern of results, with lower social competence, yet better social adjustment in programs run by more experienced directors. Perhaps director experience plays a role in preventing maladjustment in child care, but does not play sufficiently powerful or constructive a role to promote social competence. In the National Day Care Study (Roupp et al., 1979), caregivers—not directors—with more years of experience were found to engage in less social interaction and cognitive stimulation with infants and toddlers. On the other hand, Howes (1983) found that experienced caregivers were more responsive to children's bids for attention. Clearly, "experience" is a multifaceted construct requiring more sensitive measures capable of deciphering beneficial features of experience and of examining their relation to competent caregiving.

The final indicator of quality examined in this research, child-staff ratios, predicted parent ratings of considerateness and caregiver ratings of anxiety. Ratios have frequently emerged in child-care research as a significant positive indicator of quality (Howes, 1983; Howes & Rubenstein, 1985; Roupp et al., 1979). In comparison, the results of the current study are relatively modest. And the link between ratios and anxiety—like that between overall quality and anxiety—challenges one's intuitive views of child-care quality as well as the thrust of most research evidence.

Taken as a whole, these results have implications for social policies and future research on child care. This study also provides a useful model for research designed to examine general issues of environmental influence on development.

In terms of social policy, this research adds further documentation to the importance of investing in high-quality child care. Unfortunately, issues of program quality are generally overshadowed by concerns about the sheer availability and cost of child care (Phillips, 1984). Quality is monitored exclusively at the state level by regulations that establish a floor below which children's health and safety are presumed to be jeopardized, not a ceiling designed to promote positive development (Gamble & Zigler, 1986; Phillips & Zigler, in press). The research evidence reported here suggests not only that higher standards of quality are imperative if children are to thrive in child care, but that specific features of child care that are amenable to regulation can be identified.

The research implications call attention to the critical need to take into account variation in quality when child care is studied, rather than to revert to prior models of research in which child care is treated as a uniform intervention. Just as home care varies in quality, day care varies in quality. The challenge facing researchers is to advance understanding of the processes that underlie the influence of child-care quality on child development. Available evidence suggests that tangible program features, such as staff-child ratios and staff training and experience, exert their influence by facilitating positive interactions among staff and children.

This study also exemplifies an emerging research paradigm that attempts to control for family background variables when examining environmental—including child care—predictors of child development. Variation in quality must be examined in concert with family factors to obtain an accurate portrayal of how children fare in child care. Exposure effects that entail examining interactions between program quality and time in care also warrant study because of many families' extensive reliance on child care. Longitudinal research on child care, as distinct from early intervention programs, is also essential because of the political and theoretical significance of documenting the long-term consequences of child care.

REFERENCES

Behar, L. (1977). The Preschool Behavior Questionnaire. *Journal of Abnormal Child Psychology, 5,* 265–275.

Behar, L., & Stringfield, S. A. (1974). A behavior rating scale for the preschool child. *Developmental Psychology, 10,* 601–610.

Belsky, J. (1984). Two waves of day care research: Developmental effects and conditions of quality. In R. C. Ainslie (Ed.), *The child and the day care setting* (pp. 1–34). New York: Praeger.

Belsky, J. A., Steinberg, L. D., & Walker, A. (1982). The ecology of daycare. In M. Lamb (Ed.), *Childrearing in nontraditional families* (pp. 71–116). Hillsdale, NJ: Erlbaum.

Clarke-Stewart, A. (1984). Day care: A new context for research and development. In M. Perlmutter (Ed..), *The Minnesota Symposia on Child Psychology: Vol. 17. Parent-child interaction and parent-child relations in child development* (pp. 61–100). Hillsdale, NJ: Erlbaum.

Clarke-Stewart, A., & Fein, G. G. (1983). Early childhood programs. In P. H. Mussen (Series Ed.) & M. Haith and J. Campos (Vol. Eds.), *Handbook of child psychology: Vol. II. Infancy and developmental psychobiology* (pp. 917–1000). New York: Wiley.

Clarke-Stewart, A., & Gruber, C. P. (1984). Day care forms and features. In R. C. Ainslie (Ed.), *The child and the day care setting* (pp. 35–62). New York: Praeger.

Cummings, E. H. (1980). Caregiver stability and day care. *Developmental Psychology, 16,* 31–37.

Everson, M. D., Sarnat, L., & Ambron, S. R. (1984). Day care and early socialization: The role of maternal attitude. In R. C. Ainslie (Ed.), *The child and the day care setting* (pp. 63–97). New York: Praeger.

Gamble, R., & Zigler, E. (1986). Effects of infant day care: Another look at the evidence. *American Journal of Orthopsychiatry, 56* (1), 26–42.

Golden, M., Rosenbluth, L., Grossi, M. T., Policare, H. J., Freeman, H., Jr., & Brownlee, E. M. (1978). *The New York City Infant Day Care Study.* New York: Medical and Health Research Association of New York City.

Harms, R., & Clifford, R. M. (1980). *Early Childhood Environment Rating Scale.* New York: Teachers College Press.

Haskins, R. (1985). Public aggression among children with varying day care experience. *Child Development, 57,* 202–203.

Howes, C. (1983). Caregiver behavior in center and family day care. *Journal of Applied Developmental Psychology, 4,* 99–107.

Howes, C., & Olenick, M. (1986). Family and child care influences on toddlers' compliance. *Child Development, 57,* 202–216.

Howes, C., & Rubenstein, J. (1985). Determinants of toddlers' experiences in daycare: Age of entry and quality of setting. *Child Care Quarterly, 14,* 140–151.

McCartney, K. (1984). The effect of quality of day care environment upon children's language development. *Developmental Psychology, 20,* 244–260.

McCartney, K., Scarr, S., Phillips, D., & Grajek, S. (1985). Day care as intervention: Comparisons of varying quality programs. *Journal of Applied Developmental Psychology, 6,* 247–260.

McCartney, K., Scarr, S., Phillips, D., Grajek, S., & Schwarz, J. C. (1982). Environmental differences among day care centers and their effects on children's development. In E. Zigler and E. Gordon (Eds.), *Day care: Scientific and social policy issues* (pp. 126–151). Boston: Auburn.

Phillips, D. (1984). Day care: Promoting collaboration between research and policymaking. *Journal of Applied Developmental Psychology, 5,* 91–113.

Phillips, D., & Zigler, E. (in press). The checkered history of federal child care regulation. In E. Rothkopf (Ed.), *Review of Research in Education* (Vol. 14). New York: Teachers' College Press.

Prescott, E., Kritchevsky, S., & Jones, K. (1972). *The day care environment inventory.* Washington, DC: U.S. Department of Health, Education and Welfare.

Ramey, C., Dorval, B., & Baker-Ward, L. (1981). Group day care and socially disadvantaged families: Effects on the child and the family. In S. Kilmer (Ed.), *Advances in early education and day care* (pp. 69–106). Greenwich, CT: JAI Press.

Ramey, C., MacPhee, D., & Yeates, K. (1982). Preventing developmental retardation: A general systems model. In L. Bond & J. Joffee (Eds.), *Facilitating infant and early childhood development: Vol. 6. Primary prevention of psychopathology* (pp. 343–401). Hanover, NH: University Press of New England.

Roupp, R., Travers, J., Glantz, F., & Coelen, C. (1979). *Children at the center: Final results of the National Day Care Study.* Boston: Abt Associates.

Rubenstein, J. L., & Howes, C. (1979). Caregiving and infant behavior in day care and in homes. *Developmental Psychology, 15,* 1–24.

Rutter, M. (1981). Social-emotional consequences of day care for preschool children. *American Journal of Orthopsychiatry, 51,* 4–28.

Scarr, S., & McCartney, K. (1983). How people make their own environments: A theory of genotype—environment effects. *Child Development, 54,* 424–435.

Scarr, S., & Weinberg, R. A. (1986). The early childhood enterprise: Care and education of the young. *American Psychologist, 41,* 1140–1146.

Schaefer, E., & Edgerton, M. D. (1977). *Parent as educator interview.* Unpublished manuscript. University of North Carolina at Chapel Hill.

Schaefer, E., & Edgerton, M. D. (1978). *A method and a model for describing competence and adjustment: A preschool version of the classroom behavior inventory.* Paper presented at the 86th Annual Meeting of the American Psychological Association, Toronto, Ontario, Canada.

Schwarz, J. C., Krolick, G., & Strickland, R. (1973). Effects of early day care experience on adjustment to a new environment. *American Journal of Orthopsychiatry, 43,* 340–346.

Schwarz, J. C., Strickland, R., & Krolick, G. (1974). Infant day care: Behavioral effects at preschool age. *Developmental Psychology, 10,* 502–506.

Vandell, D. L., & Powers, C. P. (1983). Day care quality and children's free play activities. *American Journal of Orthopsychiatry, 53,* 493–500.

8

Formal Schooling for Four-Year-Olds? No

Edward F. Zigler
Yale University, New Haven, Connecticut

This article examines the recent movement toward enrolling four-year-olds in academic programs. The research base and political forces that guided the direction of the movement are considered: remedial intervention programs for economically disadvantaged children, the need for change in decaying school programs, and the urgent need for increased day-care services. It is determined that the research base does not demonstrate that early schooling will be beneficial to middle-class children who constitute the majority of four-year-olds. It is suggested that early schooling may be an inappropriate solution to the current crisis in child care for working parents and that children's development may suffer if limited educational funds are expended on nonfunctional programs. Developmentally appropriate care programs carried out in school buildings by specialists in early childhood development are suggested as an alternative.

A developing momentum is moving our nation toward universal preschool education (Zimiles, 1985). Many decision makers are currently advocating the downward extension of public schooling to four-year-olds. New York's Mayor Koch has not only made all-day kindergarten mandatory but has also appointed a commission charged with the creation of a public school program for all four-year-olds. A recent *New York Times* editorial entitled "School at 4: A Model for the Nation" (1985) hailed Koch's initiative as the most sensible way to "save the next generation" (p. 22). American Federation of

Teachers president Albert Shanker has also endorsed preschool education. So many positive voices have been heard that it is easy to assume that schooling for four-year-olds is a nonvalenced issue that is met only with popular support and enthusiasm. Indeed, the Commissioner for Education in New York State, Gordon Ambach (1985), stated that it was impossible to find anyone to uphold the negative side of the issue. However, there are some negative voices, and they are beginning to be heard. Herbert Zimiles (1985), a leading thinker in the field of early childhood education, recently argued that the movement toward universal preschool education is characterized more by enthusiasm than thought. The Commissioner of Education for the State of Connecticut, Gerald Tirozzi, another champion of public education for four-year-olds, established a committee to study the issue within the general context of children's services. In their recommendations, this committee concluded that "under no circumstances do we believe it appropriate for all four-year-olds to be involved in a 'kindergarten-type' program within the public schools" (Kagan, 1985, p. 3). In this article, I will add my voice to those who have argued that the issue of universal schooling for four-year-olds requires more thought than it has been accorded.

The current impetus for earlier schooling has two sources. The first is the concern generated by the recent proliferation of negative evaluations of our public secondary schools. The National Commission on Excellence in Education's (1983) report, *A Nation at Risk,* detailed the failures of secondary schooling in America. Similar studies (e.g., Boyer, 1983; Sizer, 1984) soon followed. These reports emphasized the need for higher academic standards, more attention to basics, more rigor in teaching, and longer school days and years. Few of them proposed earlier schooling as a solution to our educational problems.

An ostensible exception to this, Mortimer Adler's thoughtful *Paideia Proposal* (1982) did link school reform and early childhood education. Adler stated that "preschool deprivation is the cause of backwardness or failure in school . . . hence at least one year—or better, two or three years of preschool tutelage must be provided for those who do not get such preparation from favorable environments" (pp. 37–38). Too often, however, Adler's caveat with regard to the purely remedial nature of preschool for the disadvantaged is ignored. It was not Adler's opinion, nor is it mine, that the more advantaged children in our society require a year of preschool education at the state's expense.

A second source of the momentum toward universal preschool education is the inappropriate generalization of the effects of some excellent broad-based remedial programs for the economically disadvantaged. Several preschool intervention programs such as Head Start (Lazar & Darlington,

1982), the New York University Institute for Developmental Studies (Deutsch, Deutsch, Jordan, & Grallo, 1983), the Ypsilanti-based Perry Preschool Program (Berrueta-Clement, Schweinhart, Barnett, Epstein, & Weikart, 1984), the New York State prekindergarten program (Ambach, 1985), and the Brookline Early Education Program (Pierson, Tivnan, & Walker, 1984) have succeeded in spurring the developmental and cognitive growth of economically disadvantaged three- and four-year-old children. But extrapolation to all children from these programs is inappropriate for two reasons. First, benefits were obtained only for economically disadvantaged children. Second, these intervention programs differ from standard school fare in a number of important ways, providing primary health and social services, in addition to remedial academic programs. In addition, unlike conventional schooling, this assistance is provided to the family as a whole, not simply to a target child. These are vital differences, as many theorists believe that preschool programs are most successful when parents participate (Bronfenbrenner, 1974; Deutsch, Deutsch, Jordan, & Grallo, 1983; Radin, 1969; Slater, 1971; Sparrow, Blachman, & Chauncey, 1983; Valentine & Stark, 1979; Waksman, 1980) and that the basic needs of children and their families must be met before schooling can have any effect.

Public preschool education shares few of these services and concerns, nor can they become the primary focus of the educational establishment. It is an open question whether early school-based programs will result in the same increases in social competence found by the Cornell Consortium (Royce, Darlington, & Murray, 1983) following early intervention programs for the economically disadvantaged—benefits that may well be a consequence of services having very little to do with formal education. It was precisely the differences between Head Start and formal schooling, as I have outlined here, that led many of us to oppose President Carter's proposal to move Head Start into the new Department of Education, and that in the end prevented its inclusion.

THE PERRY PRESCHOOL PROGRAM

Additional differences must be considered when interpreting the benefits of the Perry Preschool Program. This well-known exemplary intervention effort achieved remarkable success and is deserving of the praise it has received from many quarters. It is one of the few intervention efforts that attempted to assign participants randomly to experimental and control groups. Further, it is one of the ever-smaller number of intervention efforts that have met my dictum that the assessment of early intervention efforts should include a cost-benefit analysis (Zigler & Berman, 1983). Generalization from the results of this unique effort to typical public programs is highly problematic for three reasons, however. First, it is very unlikely that a preschool program mounted in the typical public school will be of the quality represented by the Perry Preschool Project. The program's experimental character ensured that it would be exceptionally well planned, monitored, and managed. Furthermore, participating in an experiment can stimulate and motivate staff. Researchers worked extensively with direct child caregivers in analyzing and constructing the program (Barnett, personal communication, September 20, 1985), and visiting experts held weekly seminars for the entire preschool staff (Weikart, 1967). Although the consequences of these program features were not analyzed, their potential effects on the program's outcome may well have been substantial.

Second, the Perry sample was not only nonrepresentative of children in general, but there is also some question whether it was representative of even the bulk of economically disadvantaged children. The sample was limited to Black children, when in fact the majority of low-income children are White (U.S. Department of Commerce, Bureau of the Census, personal communication, March 1984). It is even problematic as to whether the sample was representative of low-income Black children. The Perry Project was limited to children with IQs between 61 and 88. Yet, the median IQ of Black children in the U.S. was 80 to 85 in the early 1960s (Kennedy, Van de Riet, & White, 1963). Another argument against generalizing from the Perry Preschool Project involves the fact that participation was fully voluntary, which introduces a self-selection phenomenon. How the families that did not choose to volunteer differed from those in the final project sample is an open question.

Finally, the Perry Project poses a number of methodological difficulties. First, to be assigned to the intervention group, children had to have a parent at home during the day, resulting in a significant difference between control and intervention groups on the variable of maternal employment. Second, primary data collectors were community people who had close and supportive ties with the families involved in the project, resulting in a confound between the effects of the intervention *per se* and the process of maintaining the sample. Third, assignment to experimental and control groups was not wholly random, producing the problems of interpretation noted by Haskins and Gallagher (1984). Finally, criticisms have been advanced that the Perry program's cost-benefit analyses overestimate the benefits attributed to the intervention (Hanke & Anwyll, 1980).

I concur with Gottfried and Gottfried (1984) and Larsen (1985) that caution should be exercised in generalizing from one population to another. I would like to see the outcome of the High/Scope model when mounted by people with less expertise than those employed in the Perry Project. Furthermore, evaluations of any intervention should be conducted by researchers not involved in the development of the model being evaluated (Zigler & Berman, 1983). Given the pervasiveness of self-fulfilling prophecies (Merton, 1948; Rosenthal & Jacobson, 1968), this caveat represents merely a common-sense concern. I should note, however, that Campbell (in press) has recently argued that it is appropriate for those who mount programs to do their own evaluations in order to retain their qualitative, subjective insights in project analyses.

APPROPRIATE CANDIDATES FOR INTERVENTION

The High/Scope data generate the intriguing hypothesis that preschool intervention is particularly effective for the most economically disadvantaged children, a view supported by the New York State evaluation of its experimental preschool program (Irvine, Flint, Hick, Horan, & Kikuk, 1982). The New York study indicated that the only cognitive gains that lasted beyond the preschool period were among children whose mothers were of the lowest educational index.

This view has apparently not escaped educational decisionmakers. Almost all the states that now provide school-sponsored programs for four-year-olds limit enrollment to low-income, handicapped and in some cases, non-English speaking youngsters (Kagan, 1985). Even the Ypsilanti group recognizes that these are the children who can most profit from intervention (Berrueta-Clement et al., 1984, p. 7). Although Pierson, Tivnan, and Walker (1984) made some claims for the effectiveness of preschool programs for middle-class children, their criterion for socioeconomic status was questionable. In any case, the gains made by children of educated parents were far fewer than those made by the children of less educated parents. What is more, such differences as were found may turn out to be shortlived, because no long-term assessment of the intervention and control groups has been carried out. (Pierson, Tivnan, & Walker, 1984).

In contrast, there is a large body of evidence indicating that there is little if anything to be gained by exposing middle-class children to early education (c.f., Adler, 1982; Caruso & Detterman, 1981; Clarke, 1984; Darlington, Royce, Snipper, Murray, & Lazar, 1980; Swift, 1964). For example, the only advantage Swift (1964) could find as a result of preschool education was a minimal degree of initial enhanced social development at school entrance, with children not involved in preschool reaching the same level of social adjustment in less than two years. Similarly, Abelson, Zigler, and DeBlasi (1974) found that although an extensive four-year intervention program benefited low-income children, it had no effect on middle-class youngsters. In his review of research on preschool intervention, English specialist on child development and education Martin Woodhead (1985) stated:

> Three main considerations affect the validity of drawing general conclusions for early education policy. First, the populations served by these projects were severely disadvantaged, mainly black children, and the evidence for wider replicability is inconclusive. Secondly, the projects all featured a carefully designed, well-supported programme with low ratios of children to teachers. Finally the effectiveness of pre-school may also be conditional on features of the educational and family context in which intervention took place. (p. 133).

American schools are already under great financial pressure and must make the most efficient use possible of limited economic resources. I have long been an advocate of cost-benefit analyses for all types of social programs (Zigler & Berman, 1983). As previously stated, our best thinking suggests we can make the most effective use of limited funds by investing them in intervention programs that target three overlapping groups: (a) the economically disadvantaged child, (b) the handicapped, and (c) the bilingual (Casto & Mastropieri, 1984; Kagan, 1985; White & Casto, 1984). Spreading education budgets to cover preschool education for all four-year-olds would spread them too thin. Such an extension would not only have little effect on the more advantaged mainstream but would also diminish our capacity to intervene with those who could benefit the most.

There is, however, one potential advantage to universal preschool education. A weakness of Head Start and programs like Head Start is their built-in economic segregation of children. Poor children go to Head Start, while more affluent children go elsewhere. Universal preschool would better integrate children across socioeconomic lines, and as Zimiles (1985) has noted, would introduce equity into early childhood programs. Although this would waste funding on children who have little to gain from early education, it would guarantee its availability to those who could not otherwise afford it.

Furthermore, Abelson, Zigler, and DeBlasi (1974) and Coleman et al. (1966) suggested there are educational advantages to mixed socioeconomic and racial groupings. Yet, although we would be well advised to promote the integration of children from diverse social and ethnic backgrounds, the cost of doing so through universal preschool education outweighs its potential benefits.

THE REAL PROBLEM

Educators in several states point to parental pressure for all-day kindergarten as evidence of the value parents place on early education, but I believe they have misread this demand. What many parents are expressing is less a burning desire for infant academics than their desperate need for quality day care. Fifty-nine percent of the mothers of three- and four-year-olds are now employed outside their homes. Many of these mothers have enrolled their children in child care programs that provide organized educational activities (Chorvinsky, 1982). Yet, ironically, not even all-day kindergarten programs are able to fill the day-care needs of families with both parents working outside the home. Schools tend to adjourn around 3:00, two hours before most working days end. Thus, the day-care problem has only been moved back for a few hours. This token improvement may actually lead parents to take fewer precautions during this relatively short period of time.

Day care can be prohibitively expensive for many families, and it is not surprising that many would prefer to shift the cost to the public school system. The Perry Preschool Project was estimated by its originators to cost approximately $1,500 per year per child in 1963. Given the number of three- and four-year-olds in the nation today, and adjusting these figures for inflation, the total cost of a universal child development program would be many billions of dollars per year. Unfortunately, advocates of universal preschool education continue to behave as though these vast sums will magically appear. Fiscal reality demands that we target populations who can most benefit from care and provide them with the more inclusive programs best suited to their particular needs.

We must also listen to those families who neither need nor want their young children to be placed in preschool. The compulsory aspect of many of the proposed early education plans has angered many parents and set them in opposition to school officials—a poor beginning to the positive home-school relationship that is vital to the educational process (Bronfenbrenner, 1974; Lazar & Darlington, 1982). Decision makers must be sensitive to the individual needs of children and parents and recognize that, when the family situation is appropriate, the best place for a preschool child may be at home.

We must be sensitive to the individual differences between young children. Some four-year-olds can handle a five- or six-hour school day. Many others cannot. Whenever it is best for the children to be at home with their parents, we should not needlessly deprive families of valuable time they could spend together. This is not to ignore the fact that home may be a place of abuse or neglect, a welfare hotel, or a confusing and insecure environment without what we have come to accept as adequate resources. For these children, day care may be the best available alternative. Yet many competent, caring parents who are at home resent school administrators' proposals to keep their preschool children in a full-day early education program. In fact, recent work by Tizard and her colleagues has demonstrated that the conversations children carry on at home may be the richest source of linguistic and cognitive enrichment for children from all but the most deprived backgrounds (Hughes, Carmichael, Pinkerton, & Tizard, 1979; Tizard, Carmichael, Hughes, & Pinkerton, 1980; Tizard & Hughes, 1984; Tizard, Hughes, Carmichael, & Pinkerton, 1982, 1983; Tizard, Mortimore, & Burchell, 1981). This body of work highlights the vast scope of the information and ideas that are transmitted at home, as opposed to the circumscribed agenda of the school. The fact that parents and child share a common life and frame of reference allows them to explore events and ideas in intimate conversations with great personal meaning. At a time when universal early education, the earlier the better, is being advocated, the Tizard work reminds us of other, equally important roots of cognitive development.

A TIME FOR CHILDHOOD

I concur with Elkind (1981) and Winn (1983) that we are driving our young children too hard and thereby depriving them of their most precious commodity—their childhood. The image of the four-year-old in designer jeans, miniature executive briefcase in hand may seem cute, but rushing children from cradle to school denies them the freedom to develop at their own pace. Children are growing up too fast today, and prematurely placing four-year-olds and five-year-olds into full-day preschool education programs will only compound this problem.

Those who argue in favor of universal preschool education ignore evidence indicating that early schooling is inappropriate for many four-year-olds and may even be harmful to their development (Ames, 1980; Collins, 1984; Elkind, 1981; Gesell, 1928; Yarrow, 1964; Zimiles, 1985). For example, Marie Winn (1983) noted in *Children Without Childhood* that premature schooling can replace valuable play time, potentially slowing or reducing the child's overall development. This is particularly dangerous given the present cognitive thrust in education, increasing the danger of an overemphasis on formal and overly structured academics (Ames, 1980; Zimiles, 1985). The supervision of very young children must be a distinct form of care, suited to the rapid developmental changes and high dependency of these children, not a scaled-down version of a grade-school curriculum.

At the same time we must remember that although early childhood is an important and sensitive period, it is not uniquely so. In the 1960s we believed early childhood was a magic period during which minimal intervention efforts would have maximal, indelible effects on the child. In the current push toward early formal education we can see the unfortunate recurrence of this idea.

Every age in a child's life is a magic age. We must be just as concerned for the 6-year-old, the 10-year-old, and the 16-year-old as we are for the 4-year-old (Clarke & Clarke, 1976). In fact, the proposed New York plan is especially troubling in that it includes a suggestion to add a year of education at the beginning of formal schooling and to drop a year at the end of high school. The work of Feuerstein (1970; Feuerstein, Rand, Hoffman, & Miller, 1980) and Hobbs and Robinson (1982), to name but a few scholars in this area, has demonstrated that adolescence is itself a sensitive and fluid period in the life of the child. We must guard against shortchanging one age group in our efforts to help another.

THE EASY WAY OUT

This is not the first time universal preschool education has been proposed. As a consultant to the California school system, I was called on when Wilson Riles, then California State Superintendent of Schools, advocated early childhood education 10 years ago, just as school superintendents in New York and Connecticut are doing today. Then as now the arguments in favor of preschool education were that it would reduce school failure, lower drop-out rates, increase test scores, and produce a generation of more competent high school graduates. My interpretation of the evidence, the same as that finally reached by the State of California, is that preschool education will achieve none of these results. I am not simply saying that universal preschool education will be a waste of time and money. There is a danger in asserting that the solution to the poor school and later life performance of the disadvantaged will be solved by a year of preschool education. The nation is on the verge of falling into the overoptimistic trap that ensnared us in the mid-1960s, when expectations were raised that an eight-week summer program could solve all the problems of the poor. If we wish to improve the lives of the economically disadvantaged we must abandon the short-term "solutions" of the 1960s and work for much deeper social reforms (Zigler & Berman, 1983). The purely symbolic function served by relying on educational innovations alone to solve the problems of poor children has been noted by historian Marvin Lazerson (1970):

> Too often discussions of education reform appear to be a means of
> avoiding more complex and politically dangerous issues . . .

education is . . . cheaper than new housing and new jobs. We are left with greater school responsibility while the social problems which have the greatest effect on schooling are largely ignored. The schools—in this case, preschool—are asked to do too much, and given too little support to accomplish what they are asked. A variety of interest groups, however, are satisfied: educators, because they get status and funds, social reformers, because they believe in education, and government officials because they pass positive legislation without upsetting traditional social patterns. (p. 84).

We simply cannot innoculate children in one year against the ravages of a life of deprivation. Even champions of early childhood education have made sobering statements warning us not to expect too much while doing too little. Fred Hechinger (1985) wrote, "Part of the problem is to overpromise and under finance. The hard fact is that there are no educational miracles for the effects of poverty" (p. C10). In an incisive analysis, Senator Daniel Patrick Moynihan (1984) agreed, warning that exaggerated reports of success in the field of early childhood education lead inevitably to near nihilism when these extravagant hopes are unfulfilled: "From finding out that not everything works, we rush to the judgement that nothing works or can be made to work" (p. 8). Moynihan noted that the Ypsilanti researchers were restrained in their claims of the benefits of early childhood education, stating that such programs are "part of the solution, not the whole solution" (quoted in Moynihan, 1984, p. 13). In editorializing these results, however, the *New York Times* unabashedly stated, "Yes, after all the years of experiment and disappointment, American society does know one sure way to lead poor children out of a life of poverty" (quoted in Moynihan, p. 13). Moynihan's point that research is threatened when results are exaggerated in this fashion is well taken. Just as the credibility of researchers can be damaged, so too can the credibility of educators if they insist on promising more than they can possibly deliver. Barbara Tizard (1974) stated:

In so far, then, as the expansion of early schooling is seen as a way of avoiding later school failure or of closing the social class gap in achievement, we already know it to be doomed to failure. It would perhaps be sensible for research workers to point this out very clearly to public authorities at an early stage. This is not, of course, to say that such an expansion has no value—no one would agree that a young child should not be fed well, because his present diet may not affect his adult weight and height. Nursery schooling, or particular forms of it, may help to develop the child's social and cognitive skills as well as add to the happiness of both child and mother. What seems certain, however, is that without continuous reinforcement in the primary school or home, pre-school education has no long-term effect on later school achievement. (p. 4).

A REALISTIC SOLUTION

Educators must realize they cannot reform the world or change the basic nature of children. The real question is how to provide the best experience during the day for four-year-olds, specifically for those who cannot remain at home with a consistent, competent caregiver. Parents do not need children who read at age four, but they do need affordable, good quality child care. The most cost-effective way to provide universally available—again, not compulsory—care would be to work from the school. I am advocating a return to the concept of the community school as a local center for all the social services required by the surrounding neighborhood. These full-service schools would, in addition to supplying other programs, provide full-day, high quality child care for four- and even three-year-old children in the school facilities already present in the community. Although such preschool programs would include a developmentally appropriate educational component, they would primarily be places for recreation and socialization—the real business of preschoolers. In-school day care could also easily accommodate older children after school is dismissed. Another investigator summarized the need in this way: "We must . . . align the goals of programs for infants, preschoolers, and early elementary school-aged pupils so that such programs become components of an integrated, consistent plan for educating young children" (Weinberg, 1979, p. 915).

Such a program, although operating on school grounds, should not be staffed solely by teachers. Instead I propose that school-based day-care programs be staffed with teachers in a supervisory capacity and with child development associates (CDAs), certified child caregivers currently being used in our nation's Head Start program. The National Day Care Study (Ruopp, Travers, Glantz, & Coelen, 1979) found that the one background characteristic of teachers that related to program quality was early childhood training. Certification of CDAs is based on both educational attainment and their proven competence in meeting children's needs.

Finally, in thinking of three- and four-year-olds, let us not neglect the needs of five-year-olds. I believe that a full-day of formal schooling is too much even for these children. Instead, I would propose a half-day kindergarten program to be followed by a half-day in school day care for those who need it. The extra cost could be borne by parents on a sliding-fee basis, with financial assistance available to needy families. Licensed qualified teachers would teach a half day in the morning and certified CDAs would care for the children in the afternoon. A half day of education is sufficient for a five-year-old. Again, let me emphasize that the day-care element should be strictly voluntary; no parent who wants his or her child at home after school ends at noon should be denied this option. Furthermore, such a program would do well to adopt a whole-child approach such as that exemplified by Biber (1984) in her Bank Street model, rather than treating kindergarten like a miniature elementary school with a heavy cognitive-academic orientation. New York University's Institute for Developmental Studies educational enrichment program is another excellent example of a program using a sound whole-child approach.

On a larger scale, many aspects of the funding issue will have to be addressed, such as tax base and licensing procedures. Federal support might be expected to subsidize costs for economically disadvantaged children. Cost containment would also be enhanced by making use of existing school facilities.

In short, we must ask ourselves, what would we be buying for our children in universal preschool education programs and at what cost? The family-oriented, multi-service community school could meet the many different needs of preschoolers and their families with a variety of programs from which families could select to suit their wants. Such services could include comprehensive intervention programs, health and nutrition components, and high quality, affordable day care, to name only a few possibilities. Our four-year-olds do have a place in school, but it is not at a school desk.

REFERENCES

Abelson, W., Zigler, E., & DeBlasi, C. (1974). Effects of a four-year Follow Through program on economically disadvantaged children. *Journal of Educational Psychology, 66,* 750–771.

Adler, M. (1982). *The paideia proposal.* New York: MacMillan.

Ambach, G. (1985, March). *Public school for four year olds, yes or no?* Paper presented at the meeting of the American Association of School Administrators. New York, NY.

Ames, L. B. (1980, March). Kindergarten—not for four-year-olds! *Instructor,* pp. 32, 37.

Berrueta-Clement, J., Schweinhart, L., Barnett, W., Epstein, A., & Weikart, D. (1984). *Changed lives.* Ypsilanti, MI: High/Scope Press.

Biber, B. (1984). *Early education and psychological development.* New Haven, CT: Yale University Press.

Bronfenbrenner, U. (1974). Is early intervention effective? In M. Guttentag & E. L. Struening (Eds.), *Handbook of evaluation research* (Vol. 2, pp. 519–605). Beverly Hills, CA: Sage.

Boyer, E. I. (1983). *High school: A report on secondary school in America.* New York: Harper & Row.

Campbell, D. (in press). The interface between evaluation and service providers. In E. Zigler & S. L. Kagan (Eds.), *Family support programs: The state of the art.* New Haven, CT: Yale University Press.

Caruso, D., & Detterman, K. (1981). Intelligence research and social policy. *Phi Delta Kappan, 63,* 183–186.

Casto, G., & Mastropieri, M. (1984). *The efficacy of early intervention programs for handicapped children: A meta-analysis.* Logan, UT: Utah State University, Early Intervention Research Institute.

Chorvinsky, M. (1982). *Preprimary enrollment 1980.* Washington, DC: National Center for Education Statistics.

Clarke, A. M. (1984). Early experience and cognitive development. In E. W. Gordon (Ed.), *Review of research in education II* (pp. 125–161). Washington, DC: American Educational Research Association.

Clarke, A. M., & Clarke, A. D. B. (Eds.). (1976). *Early experience: Myth and evidence.* New York: Free Press.

Coleman, J. S., Campbell, E. Q., Hobson, C. J., McPartland, J., Mood, A., Weinfeld, F., & York, R. (1966). *Equality of educational opportunity.* (FS5–238–38001). Washington DC: U.S. Department of Health, Education, and Welfare, U.S. Government Printing Office.

Collins, G. (1984, September 4). Experts debate impact of day care. *New York Times,* p. B11.

Darlington, R. B., Royce, V. M., Snipper, A. S., Murray, A. W., & Lazar, I. (1980). Preschool programs and later school competence of children from low-income families. *Science, 208,* 202–204.

Deutsch, M., Deutsch, C., Jordan, T., & Grallo, R. (1983). The IDS Program: An experiment in early and sustained enrichment. In Consortium for Longitudinal Studies (Ed.), *As the twig is bent* (pp. 377–411). Hillsdale, NJ: Erlbaum.

Elkind, D. (1981). *The hurried child.* Boston, MA: Addison-Wesley.

Feuerstein, R. A. (1970). A dynamic approach to the causation, prevention and alleviation of retarded performance. In H. C. Haywood (Ed.), *Social-cultural aspects of mental retardation* (pp. 341–378). New York: Appleton-Century-Crofts.

Feuerstein, R., Rand, Y., Hoffman, M. B., & Miller, R. (1980). *Instrumental enrichment: An intervention program for cognitive modifiability.* Baltimore, MD: University Park Press.

Gesell, A. (1928). *Infancy and human growth.* New York: MacMillan.

Gottfried, A., & Gottfried, A. (1984). Home environment and cognitive development in young children of middle-socioeconomic-status families. In A. Gottfried (Ed.), *Home environment and early cognitive development: Longitudinal research* (pp. 57–115). Fullerton, CA: Academic Press.

Hanke, S. H., & Anwyll, J. B. (1980). On the discount rate controversy. *Public Policy, 28,* 171–183.

Haskins, R., & Gallagher, J. (1984, August). *The voices of children project: A report to the Carnegie Foundation.* Chapel Hill: University of North Carolina at Chapel Hill, Bush Institute for Child and Family Policy.

Hechinger, F. (1985, April 23). Schools and the war on poverty. *New York Times,* p. C10.

Hobbs, N., & Robinson, S. (1982). Adolescent development and public policy. *American Psychologist, 37,* 212–223.

Hughes, M., Carmichael, H., Pinkerton, G., & Tizard, B. (1979). Recording children's conversations at home and at nursery school: A technique and some methodological considerations. *Journal of Child Psychology and Psychiatry, 20,* 225–232.

Irvine, D. J., Flint, D. L., Hick, T. L., Horan, M. D., & Kikuk, S. E. (1982). *Evaluation of the NY State experimental preschool program: Final report.* Albany, NY: State Education Department.

Kagan, S. L. (Ed.). (1958). *Four year olds—who is responsible?* Unpublished report presented to the Connecticut Board of Education by the committee on four year olds, their families and the public schools.

Kennedy, W., Van de Riet, V., & White, J. (1963). Normative sample of intelligence. *Monographs of the Society for Research in Child Development, 28* (6, Serial No. 90).

Larsen, J. (1985, April). *Family influences on competence in low-risk preschool children.* Paper presented at the bienniel meeting of the Society for Research in Child Development, Toronto, Canada.

Lazar, I., & Darlington, R. (1982). Lasting effects of early education: A report from the Consortium for Longitudinal Studies. *Monographs of the Society for Research in Child Development, 47* (2–3, Serial No. 195).

Lazerson, M. (1970). Social reform and early childhood education: Some historical perspectives. *Urban Education, 5,* 84–102.

Merton, R. (1948). The self-fulfilling prophecy. *Antioch Review, 8,* 193–210.

Moynihan, D. P. (1984). *On the present discontent.* Paper presented at the convocation for the 140th Anniversary of the School of Education. State University of New York, Albany, NY.

National Commission on Excellence in Education (1983). *A nation at risk* (A report to the nation and the Secretary of Education, United States Department of Education). Washington, DC: Author.

Pierson, D., Tivnan, D., & Walker, T. (1984). A school based program from infancy to kindergarten for children and their parents. *Personal and Guidance Journal, 4,* 448–455.

Radin, N. (1969). The impact of a kindergarten home counseling program. *Exceptional Children, 36,* 251–256.

Rosenthal, R., & Jacobson, L. (1968). *Pygmalion in the classroom.* New York: Holt, Rinehart & Winston.

Royce, J., Darlington, R., & Murray, H. (1983). Pooled analysis: Finding across studies. In Consortium for Longitudinal Studies (Ed.), *As the twig is bent* (pp. 411–461). Hillsdale, NJ: Erlbaum.

Ruopp, R., Travers, J., Glantz, F., & Coelen, C. (1979). *Children at the center* (Final report of the National Day Care Study, Vol. 1). Cambridge, MA: Abt Books.

School at 4: A model for the nation. (February 20, 1985). *New York Times,* p. 22.

Sizer, T. (1984). *Horace's compromise: The dilemma of the American high school.* Boston: Houghton Mifflin.

Slater, B. R. (1971). Perceptual integration. *Encyclopedia of Educational Research, 3,* 1213–1218.

Sparrow, S., Blachman, B., & Chauncey, S. (1983). Diagnostic and prescriptive intervention in primary school education. *American Journal of Orthopsychiatry, 53,* 721–729.

Swift, J. W. (1964). Effects of early group experience: The nursery school and day nursery. In M. L. Hoffman & L. W. Hoffman (Eds.), *Review of child development research* (Vol. 1, pp. 249–289). New York: Russell Sage.

Tizard, B. (1974). *Early childhood education: A review and discussion of current research in Britain.* Atlantic Highlands, NJ: Humanities Press.

Tizard, B., Carmichael, H., Hughes, M., & Pinkerton, G. (1980). Four year olds talking to mothers and teachers. In L. A. Hersov, M. Berger, & A. R. Nichol (Eds.), *Language and language disorders in childhood* (pp. 49–76). Oxford, England: Pergamon Press.

Tizard, B., & Hughes, M. (1984). *Young children learning.* Cambridge, MA: Harvard University Press.

Tizard, B., Hughes, M., Carmichael, H., & Pinkerton, G. (1982). Adults' cognitive demands at home and at nursery school. *Journal of Child Psychology and Psychiatry, 23,* 105–116.

Tizard, B., Hughes, M., Carmichael, H., & Pinkerton, G. (1983). Children's questions and adult's answers. *Journal of Child Psychology and Psychiatry, 24,* 269–281.

Tizard, B., Mortimore, J., & Burchell, B. (1981). *Involving parents in nursery and infant schools.* London: Grant McIntyre.

Valentine, J., & Stark, E. (1979). The social context of parent involvement in Head Start. In E. Zigler & J. Valentine (Eds.), *Project Head Start: A legacy of the war on poverty* (pp. 291–315). New York: Free Press.

Waksman, M. (1980). Mother as teacher: A home intervention program. *Interchange, 10,* (4), 40–52.

Weikart, D. (1967). *Preschool intervention: Preliminary results of the Perry Preschool Project.* Ann Arbor, MI: Campus Publishers.

Weinberg, R. (1979). Early childhood education and intervention: Establishing an American tradition. *American Psychologist, 34,* 912–916.

White, K., & Casto, G. (1984). *An integrative review of early intervention efficacy studies with at-risk children: Implications for the handicapped.* Logan, UT: Utah State University, Early Intervention Research Institute.

Winn, M. (1983). *Children without childhood.* New York: Penguin Books.

Woodhead, M. (1985). Pre-school education has long-term effects: But can they be generalised? *Oxford Review of Education, 11* (2), 133–155.

Yarrow, L. J. (1964). Separation from parents during early childhood. In M. L. Hoffman & L. W. Hoffman (Eds.), *Review of child development research* (Vol. 1, pp. 89–137). New York: Russell Sage.

Zigler, E., & Berman, W. (1983). Discerning the future of early childhood intervention. *American Psychologist, 38,* 894–906.

Zimiles, H. (1985, April). *The role of research in an era of expanding preschool education.* Paper presented at the meeting of the American Educational Association, Chicago, IL. (Revised version of an invited address entitled "Four-year-olds in the public schools: What research does and does not tell us").

PART II: CHILD-CARE ISSUES

9

Child Characteristics and the Employment of Mothers with Young Children: A Longitudinal Study

Nancy L. Galambos
Technical University of Berlin, Federal Republic of Germany
Jacqueline V. Lerner
The Pennsylvania State University, University Park

The present longitudinal study investigated the relative influence of child, maternal, and demographic characteristics on the labor force participation of 93 mothers with young children in the New York Longitudinal Study. Multiple regression analyses revealed that child characteristics such as temperamental difficulty and the presence of physical problems were as potent as demographic features in predicting the mother's labor market activities through-out the child's early years. Conclusions were that multiple aspects of the context, including child characteristics, must be addressed if a more comprehensive picture of the employment patterns of mothers is to be gained.

The phenomenon of women seeking employment outside of the home has been a focus of much scientific inquiry. Since the 1940s there has been a general trend in women joining the labor force in increasing numbers. Yet the most dramatic change in employment rates has occurred for married women

Reprinted with permission from the *Journal of Child Psychology and Psychiatry,* 1987, Vol. 28, No. 1, 87–98. Copyright 1987 Association for Child Psychology and Psychiatry, Pergamon Journals Ltd.

The authors thank Ann C. Crouter and Richard M. Lerner for their critical reading of an earlier version of this paper.

Jacqueline V. Lerner's work on this paper was supported in part by grants from the John D. and Catherine T. MacArthur Foundation and by the W. T. Grant Foundation.

177

with young children (Fox & Hesse-Biber, 1984). By mid-1983 nearly 50% of married mothers with children under the age of six were engaged in employment outside the home (Waldman, 1983). This unprecedented rate of labor force participation by mothers of preschoolers is striking because of its relationship to numerous changes within the family, for example, changes in spousal and parental roles, family structure (Hetherington, Cox & Cox, 1982), and the nature of the child's early experiences (Belsky, Steinberg & Walker, 1982; Hetherington, Cox & Cox, 1978).

A social change as dramatic as the increase in mothers' labor force participation raises a number of critical questions, a key one being, "What accounts for a mother's decision to seek employment outside the home?" Most studies which have investigated the mother's employment status as a dependent variable have looked generally at two sets of variables as predictors. First, demographic characteristics such as the mother's level of education, work history prior to marriage, number of children in the family, and the husband's income have been found to be associated with differential rates of female employment (Ewer, Crimmins & Oliver, 1979; Gordon & Kammeyer, 1980; McLaughlin, 1982). Second, attitudinal variables such as the mother's career versus family orientation, her sex role attitudes, and the attitudes of her husband regarding the desirability of women's employment have been shown also to account for variance in the mother's decision to be employed outside the house (Ferber, 1982; Gordon & Kammeyer, 1980). Features other than demographic characteristics or career and family attitudes, such as child characteristics however, have been studied less frequently.

One exception to this is a recent longitudinal investigation by Morgan & Hock (1984) in which a variety of psychosocial attributes were assessed in order to predict the mother's labor force participation when her child was one, three, and six years of age. In addition to attitudinal, personality, and demographic indices, Morgan & Hock (1984) included a measure of the mother's aversion to fussiness in her infant, an infant characteristic associated with the domain of attributes usually labeled as temperamental ones (Buss & Plomin, 1984; Thomas & Chess, 1977). The inclusion of this latter variable in this type of investigation, although it did not attain significance as a predictor, was unique because of the recognition that the mother's response to her child's behavioral (temperamental) individuality could potentially influence the mother's decision to work outside of the home.

The issue of mothers' labor force participation and the role that demographic characteristics, parental attitudes, and child attributes play in influencing this phenomenon may be cast as a sample case of the contextually-oriented life-span approach to human development. The characteristic assumptions of this approach are that: (a) development is a lifelong process; (b) bi-directional relations between the context and the individual occur such that features of the context influence as well as change in response to individual development; and (c) the individual is a producer of its own development (Baltes, Reese & Lipsitt, 1980; R. Lerner & Busch-Rossnagel, 1981). Insofar as the mother's employment is viewed as one aspect of her development, then demographic and child attributes may be conceptualized as relevant features of the context that will influence that development. Moreover, maternal attitudes and behaviors may be identified as individual characteristics that affect the mother's further development. Therefore, the issue of the mother's decision to be a wage earner is one that falls under the domain of the life-span approach. Given the bi-directional relations that are assumed to occur between the context and the mother, the child's attributes may influence the mother's development, in this case in regard to her working outside of the home.

However, while there is an abundance of research on the effects of maternal employment on the child, there is a lack of data on the effects of the child on the mother's employment (J. Lerner & Galambos, 1986). Therefore, guided by the above life-span perspective, the purpose of the present study is· to investigate the relative influence over time of three sets of variables on the young mother's labor force participation: (1) child characteristics; (2) the mother's orientation to her child; and (3) demographic variables.

Child Characteristics

Among the characteristics of the child that are believed to elicit reactions from the environment is temperament. Temperament is defined as the style with which the individual goes about daily behavior, and refers to such attributes as activity level, rhythmicity, and adaptability (J. Lerner & R. Lerner, 1983; Thomas & Chess, 1977). Children whose temperaments allow them to adapt to the demands of their contexts are thought to have "easy" temperaments while the child with a "difficult" temperament usually has a low child-context goodness-of-fit (J. Lerner & R. Lerner, 1983; Thomas & Chess, 1977). With respect to the mother's employment status, Lamb, Chase-Lansdale & Owen (1979) speculated that the difficult child's mother would be more likely to return to work while the child with an easy temperament might reinforce any employment decision. For example the "easy" baby, being adaptable to alternative care when the mother decides to work outside the home, may reinforce her decision to work and, alternatively, if the mother decides to stay home, the happy, smiling adaptable baby can reinforce her perceptions of her "mothering".

J. Lerner Galambos (1986) found, in contrast to the expectations of Lamb *et al.* (1979), that mothers with difficult children were more likely to be homemakers while mothers engaged in paid employment were likely to have children with easy temperaments. Similarly, McBride & Belsky (1985) reported that one cohort of mothers who were not employed when their infants were three months old were more likely than employed mothers to rate their infants' temperament as difficult. It may be that the mother with an easy child feels more comfortable in leaving that child in the care of others (J. Lerner & Galambos, 1986). If this is indeed the case, then we would expect that there are other prominent characteristics of the child that may likewise influence the mother's labor force participation. Children with physical problems or illnesses, for example, may be expected to elicit a range of responses from socializing others (Lamb *et al.,* 1979; J. Lerner & R. Lerner, 1983), and may make it more problematic for the mother to obtain substitute care while she is away from home. Indeed, McBride & Belsky (1985) found that mothers who had planned to work in their child's infancy but were *not* employed had infants who were less alert and responsive during observations. As a predictor of the mother's work status, then, it is expected that children who evidence physical problems or who have more difficult temperaments are more likely to have mothers who remain at home.

Maternal Attitudes

Previous research has demonstrated that the mother's attitudes toward mothering, careers, and the gender-based division of family responsibilities are significant predictors of labor force participation. Specifically, those mothers who believe that children do not need exclusive maternal care, who place the importance of a career high on their list of priorities, or who regard the duties of men and women as nearly equal, are more likely to enter the work force when they have young children than do mothers who favor more traditional sex roles (Ferber, 1982; Gordon & Kammeyer, 1980; Morgan & Hock, 1984). Moreover, it could be argued that the mother who reacts negatively toward, disapproves of, or feels little warmth for her child may be more likely to join the labor force in response to a lower desire to spend time with that child. In support of this notion, Hock, Christman & Hock (1980) reported that mothers with greater aversion to fussiness in their infants were more likely than more tolerant mothers to return to work during the first year after birth despite previous plans to stay home. Thus, in the present study, it is expected that those mothers who are family-oriented or who evidence feelings of warmth for their children will be more likely to remain at home.

Demographic Characteristics

One of the most consistent and strong predictors of mothers' labor force participation is the number of children in the family. The greater the number of young children, the less the likelihood that the mother is engaged in labor market activities (Ewer *et al.,* 1979; Gordon & Kammeyer, 1980; Hoffman, 1974; Morgan & Hock, 1984). Another important correlate of maternal employment is the mother's educational level, which is generally positively related to her working status. Mothers with more than a high school education return to work earlier after the births of their children and continue to have higher employment rates during the first year than do mothers who have lower levels of education (McLaughlin, 1982). A third predictor of mother's labor force participation is the father's level of income. As the husband's income increases, the probability of the mother being employed decreases (Ewer *et al.,* 1979; Gordon & Kammeyer, 1980). It is expected, then, that in the present sample, a small number of young children, a higher educational level attained by the mother, and the father's higher level of occupational prestige will all predict significantly the mother's greater participation in the work force.

METHOD

Sample

The subjects for this study were part of a sample of those parents and children who have participated in the New York Longitudinal Study (NYLS) from the child's early infancy. The NYLS was initiated in 1956 by Thomas & Chess (1977). The major sample is composed of 133 children, all of whom are still being followed at this writing. The characteristics of this sample and the methods used throughout the study are detailed in several previous publications (e.g. Chess & Thomas, 1984; Thomas, Chess, Birch, Hertzig & Korn, 1963; Thomas, Chess & Birch, 1968; Thomas & Chess, 1977, 1980).

The subsample used in the present investigation consists of 93 children and their mothers from families in which the parents were married throughout the child's first five years. In addition to the two-parent criterion, this subsample was selected because complete data existed on the child's temperament and the mother's work status during each of these five years, and indices of the mother's attitudes toward her child and her family orientation were available through intensive parental interviews conducted when the children were three years of age. The families in this group of 93 subjects were from white, middle- to upper-middle-class backgrounds. Over

75% of the families were Jewish with the rest divided between the Protestant and Catholic religions. The mean age of the fathers at the birth of the target children was 36.4; the mean age of the mothers was 31.6. Thirty-eight percent of the children were firstborns, 42% were secondborns, and the remaining children were either the third or fourth children in the family.

The mean occupational prestige score for the fathers when their children were age three, as indicated by the National Opinion Research Center (NORC) rankings (Davis, 1980), was 65 (range = 20–82), demonstrating their high occupational status. Most were employed in the medical, business, and academic professions. The mean NORC score for mothers who were employed when their children were three years of age was 58 (range = 29–82), reflecting their high occupational status. Many of the mothers in this sample were medical doctors and university professors. In their child's first year, 24% of the mothers were employed (17% part-time, 7% full-time), in their child's third year, 36% of the mothers were employed (25% part-time, 11% full-time), and in their child's fifth year 42% were employed (30% part-time, 12% full-time). With respect to schooling, all of these mothers had at least a high school education, 44% had college degrees, and another 36% had attained both college and postgraduate degrees by the time their children reached age three.

The women in this sample, then, were as a group unusually skilled and educated, and considering the time frame when data were collected (i.e. the late 1950s and early 1960s), they could not be considered to be representative of the larger population. It is likely that the employed mothers were employed for reasons of personal fulfillment. We are aware of the fact that the homogeneity of our sample limits the generalizability of the results to other groups of lower SES, where many mothers may be employed for reasons of economic need. However, all major, long-term longitudinal studies in the United States have non-representative samples (e.g. the Berkeley/Oakland data sets, the Fels data set), and while sampling bias may impose limitations in making generalizations about mean levels or possibly, variability, it does not necessarily constrain generalizations about structural patterns within or across time (Jessor, 1982). In this regard, Eichorn (1984) indicated that no finding derived from a major longitudinal study has been concluded to be incorrect on the basis of subsequent cross-sectional research with more representative samples. Thus, we believe that the homogeneity of our sample should not preclude our ability to discern the predictive utility of child, mother, and demographic characteristics on mother's labor force participation.

Methods

We present here an overview of those features of the NYLS methods which are relevant to the present study. Beginning in the first month of the child's life the parents were interviewed periodically (about every three months) for the first two years after which they were interviewed twice yearly, and again in adolescence and young adulthood. The interviewers routinely collected data on family characteristics such as marital status and birth of siblings; the substantive focus of the interview concerned the child's behaviors and functioning in several content areas (e.g. sleeping, eating, social behaviors, etc.). These interviews were the source for scoring the child's temperament and physical difficulty scores, and for the demographic information such as number of children in the family, the father's occupation, and the mother's work status. The techniques used to derive the temperament scores and the measurement of other variables obtained from these interviews are described in subsequent sections.

In addition to these routine interviews, an intensive interview was conducted when the target child was approximately three years of age. Mothers and fathers in the sample were interviewed separately for approximately three hours about their child care practices and attitudes, parental and spousal roles, and the effects of the child on them and the family. Each parent was interviewed and audiotaped independently by two interviewers who had no exposure to data already gathered. This semi-structured, open-ended interview obtained information pertinent to the mother's attitudes and behaviors toward her child, her family and career orientation, and her work history. It is from this interview that the maternal attitudes—rejection of the child and family orientation—were obtained. Information about the mother's work status which was collected in this interview supplemented the data collected in the routine interviews, thereby establishing a reliable five-year history of the mother's labor force participation. The variables used in the present investigation are described below.

Mother's Labor Force Participation

The mother's work status for each of the child's first five years was rated as follows: "0" = "not employed outside of the home," "1" = "employed from 5 to 29 hours a week outside of the home" (part-time), and "2" = "employed over 30 hours a week outside of the home" (full-time). Interrater reliability for this item across the five years was 100%. However, rather than studying the mother's work status within any particular one-year period it may be more relevant conceptually to investigate labor force participation during critical stages of the child's development. That is, the mother's return to the labor force depends, in part, on her perception of the child's need for intensive care (Hock, 1978, 1980), and the periods of infancy, toddlerhood, and preschool age represent stages of decreasing importance for such care and increasing independence of the child. Therefore, the mother's work status during the child's first year served as an index for labor force participation during infancy (Mean = 0.30, S.D. = 0.59), the second and third year scores were averaged to yield an index for labor force participation during toddlerhood (Mean = 0.43, S.D. = 0.65), and the fourth and fifth year work status scores were averaged to indicate the mother's labor force participation during the child's preschool years (Mean = 0.55, S.D. = 0.70).

Child Characteristics

Temperament. Each child's temperament was measured at each year during his/her first five years on each of the following dimensions: Activity Level (the amount of motor activity present in a child's functioning); Rhythmicity (the regularity of a child's functioning such as sleep-wake cycles, hunger, feeding patterns or elimination); Approach/Withdrawal (the nature of the initial response to a new stimulus); Adaptability (the ease with which the child adjusts to new or altered situations); Threshold of Responsiveness (the intensity level of stimulation needed to evoke a response); Intensity of Reaction (the energy level of a response, irrespective of its quality or direction); Quality of Mood (the amount of pleasant or unpleasant behavior); Distractibility (the effectiveness of extraneous stimuli in interfering with or altering the direction of the ongoing behavior); and Attention Span/Persistence (attention span refers to the length of time a child pursues a particular activity; persistence refers to the continuance of an activity in the face of obstacles).

As described by Thomas *et al.* (1963, 1968) scores on these nine dimensions of temperament were obtained for each subject for each year by rating the descriptions of behavior contained in the corresponding parental interviews for years one through five. Five of the nine characteristics of temperament were combined to form a "difficulty" score (a low score indicates a more difficult temperament, high score indicates an easier temperament). The signs of the Difficult Child (Thomas & Chess, 1977) are low rhythmicity, low adaptability, withdrawal responses, negative mood, and high intensity of reactions. These scores were generated by Thomas & Chess (1977), and their predictive utility has been documented in previous research using the NYLS data set (e.g. Chess & Thomas, 1984; Thomas *et al.*, 1963, 1968). Corresponding to the periods of infancy, toddlerhood, and preschool age, the difficulty score for year one (Mean = 2.00, S.D. = 0.71), the averaged difficulty scores for years two and three (Mean = 1.93, S.D. = 0.69), and the averaged difficulty scores for years four and five (Mean = 1.27, S.D. = 0.70), respectively, were calculated and used in the analyses for this study.

Our use of data collected 25 years ago precluded the possibility of obtaining measures of temperament from sources other than the mother. However, Thomas & Chess have put a strong emphasis throughout the NYLS on obtaining descriptions of behaviors rather than subjective opinions by parents. It is these descriptions that were used by objective raters to code temperament. In addition, there may be several advantages to using parental interviews. As Maccoby & Martin (1983) noted, a child's behavior varies widely across situations and some behaviors are not publicly displayed. The parent, therefore, may be the only source for this kind of information. Moreover, while Maccoby & Martin (1983) discuss the potential for unreliability of parental reports for retrospective data the temperament scores used here are based only on concurrent reports.

Physical problems in childhood. Based on the interviews with the parents, each child in the study received a rating made by the Thomas group for the severity of physical problems evidenced in childhood (from birth through age six). The ratings were: "0" = "None," "1" = "Mild," "2" = "Moderate," and "3" = "Severe," and referred to chronic problems such as asthma, infections, gastrointestinal problems, and allergies (Mean = 1.01, S.D. = 0.83).

Maternal Attitudes

Rejection and family orientation. The scores relevant to maternal attitudes were obtained from the previously described three-year maternal interviews and were established in previous research with the NYLS data set reported by Cameron (1977). Cameron selected 70 items related to parenting attitudes and practices and entered them into a cluster analysis. Eight oblique parental clusters resulted from the 70-item matrix; two are used here because they most clearly resemble constructs used in other studies investigating the role of maternal attitudes in predicting the mother's labor force participation (e.g. Morgan & Hock, 1984). These two are: (1) *rejection*—the mother's intolerance toward and disapproval of the child; and (2) *family orientation* — the mother's child-centeredness and desire for more children. Scores were standardized with a mean of 50 and a standard deviation of 10. Factor scores were computed by the "simple sum" method: the standardization of the sums of the defining terms were divided by the number of items with non-missing data.

The *family orientation* cluster was made up of three items pertaining to the mother's desire to have more children and the degree to which she indicated interest in her child. A high score indicates a more maternalistic, child-centered personality. The scores on this cluster ranged from 37 to 80 and had a mean of 49.94 (S.D. = 10.05).

The *rejection* cluster was made up of three items pertaining to the mother's tolerance and feelings for the child, her approval of the child, and the quality of the mother-child relationship. A high score on this factor indicates high bias and intolerance toward the child and a high amount of rejection. These scores ranged from 38 to 83 and had a mean of 50.32 (S.D. = 10.39).

Demographic Characteristics

Father's occupational prestige. In order to assess the father's occupational prestige when the child was three years old, we used NORC scores. The NORC ratings range from 9 to 82, with higher scores indicating higher occupational status. The reliability and validity of these ratings have been demonstrated in other research (Bose & Rossi, 1983; Hodge, Siegel & Rossi, 1965). There is a high correlation between NORC prestige ratings and level of income (Duncan, 1961). This was the only variable in the present study for which there was some missing data. Because the sample was quite homogeneous with respect to demographic characteristics, the mean value (65) for the father's occupational prestige was substituted in the five cases that were missing this variable (S.D. = 13.44).

Mother's education. The index for the level of education achieved by the mother by the child's third year was rated on the following scale: "1" = "high school graduate," "2" = "some college or technical school," "3" = "college graduate," "4" = "some graduate school," and "5" = "graduate degree." The mean level of education was 3.47 (S.D. = 1.25).

Number of children. The number of children in the family under age six when the target child was one, three and five years of age was computed from demographic information collected in interviews from the parents at regular intervals. Over 80% of the mothers in this sample had only one or two children under age six in any given year, and only a few mothers had as many as four young children.

Analyses

Analysis of the data proceeded in three steps. First, Pearson product-moment correlations were computed between the mother's labor force participation (infancy, toddlerhood, and preschool age) and the indices for child characteristics, maternal attitudes, and demographic characteristics. Second, in order to identify those groups of variables that were best able to predict the mother's labor force participation, three stepwise regressions were conducted in which the mother's labor force participation at three stages was regressed on the child, maternal, and demographic variables. In these analyses, independent variables were examined at each step for entry or removal from the regression model. In order for a variable to be included in the regression model as a significant predictor, the probability of the F-to-enter was set at 0.10. The probability of F-to-remove was also set at 0.10.

In order to arrive at a final regression model with the best predictors, the final step was to conduct another set of three stepwise regressions including only those independent variables that achieved significance in the initial set of stepwise regressions. However, a more stringent criterion was applied, that is, the probability of F-to-enter was set at 0.05.

RESULTS

Table 1 shows the correlations between the mother's labor force participation in three stages of the child's life and child, maternal, and demographic variables. Only one variable was significantly related to the mother's labor force participation during the infancy period. In this case, difficult child temperament in toddlerhood was related to his/her mother not being gainfully employed.

The child's difficult temperament as measured in infancy and toddlerhood and the presence of more severe physical problems were related to the mother's lower level of employment when the child was a toddler. Furthermore, the greater the number of children under age six when the target child was age three and five, the less the likelihood was that the mother was employed outside of the home during her child's toddlerhood. Similar results were obtained for the mother's level of employment during the child's preschool years. That is, the child's difficult temperament, as measured in infancy and toddlerhood, and the greater number of young children present when the target child was three and five years old, were related to the mother's lower level of labor force participation. The correlation between presence of physical problems in the child and maternal employment during the preschool period did not attain significance.

Table 1. Pearson Correlations Between Mothers' Labor Force Participation and Child, Maternal and Demographic Variables

Variables	Labor force participation		
	Infancy	Toddlerhood	Preschool age
Child characteristics			
Difficulty (infancy)	− 0.16	− 0.18*	− 0.26†
Difficulty (toddlerhood)	− 0.28†	− 0.34‡	− 0.36‡
Difficulty (preschool age)	− 0.04	− 0.08	− 0.02
Physical problems	− 0.12	− 0.18*	− 0.13
Maternal attitudes			
Rejection of the child	− 0.04	0.04	0.02
Family orientation	− 0.07	− 0.08	− 0.02
Demographic characteristics			
Father's prestige	0.17	0.10	0.04
Mother's education	0.09	0.12	0.15
Number of children (year 1)	− 0.09	− 0.16	− 0.08
Number of children (year 3)	− 0.16	− 0.22*	− 0.20*
Number of children (year 5)	− 0.14	− 0.18*	− 0.23*

*$p < 0.05$.
†$p < 0.01$.
‡$p < 0.001$.

Neither of the maternal attitudes—rejection of the child and family orientation—was significantly related to the mother's level of employment at any stage. The father's occupational prestige and the mother's level of education also failed to correlate significantly with the mother's work status. Furthermore, difficult temperament during the preschool years and the number of children when the child was in his/her first year were not related significantly to the mother's employment.

In order to establish the relative contribution of child characteristics, maternal attitudes, and demographic characteristics to the mother's level of employment, stepwise multiple regressions were employed. In the initial set of regressions, the same three variables met the 0.10 probability of F-to-enter for each stage of labor force participation. These three variables were child's temperamental difficulty in toddlerhood, physical problems in childhood, and number of young children when the child was three. In the final set of regressions with the probability of F-to-enter set at a more stringent 0.05 level, the same three variables achieved significance as predictors of the mother's employment during the toddlerhood and preschool stages. Only difficult temperament, however, reached significance for the mother's work status during the child's infancy.

Table 2 presents results from the final set of regressions for the dependent variables of mothers' labor force participation during the child's infancy, toddlerhood, and preschool years. Eight percent of the variance in the mother's level of employment in the infancy period was explained by the predictor of difficult temperament in toddlerhood. Difficult temperament in toddlerhood, together with the number of young children at year three and physical problems, accounted for 23% of the variance in the mother's labor force participation during the toddlerhood years. These three variables also emerged as significant predictors of the mother's level of employment during the preschool years, accounting for 22% of the variance.

DISCUSSION

In a highly educated, middle- to upper-middle-class sample, characteristics of the child such as temperamental style and physical problems contributed significantly to the mother's decision to be gainfully employed in the child's early years. Although child characteristics alone did not explain a great deal of the variance (ranging from 8 to 18%), the results suggest that features of the child may play an important role in the mother's career development and should be included in future studies of women's labor force participation patterns. A child who has a difficult temperament or who has physical problems that require more intensive care may present too many demands on the mother who under less stressful conditions would like to pursue employment. These findings are in concordance with those of McBride & Belsky (1985), who used a contemporary sample. The high association between the number of young children in the family and mothers' employment status, a finding that is also consistent with other studies, reinforces the notion that family demands may depress the mother's level of employment. Of course, the direction of causality in this study was not investigated, and it could be that the child of the mother who is employed becomes less demanding. In fact, the child's temperament during toddlerhood was related to the mother's maternal employment status during the child's first year. We believe, in accordance with the life-span perspective, that the relationship between the mother's employment and the child's characteristics are characterized by bi-directionality so future research should address the issue of causal relations.

It was somewhat surprising that neither of the maternal attitudes measured in this study, that is, maternal rejection of the child and mother's family orientation, related to the mother's employment situation. Perhaps a

Table 2. Regression of Mothers' Labor Force Participation (Infancy, Toddlerhood, Preschool) on Predictor Variables

Dependent variable	Predictor variables	Unstandardized beta	Standardized beta	Multiple R	R^2
Mother's labor force participation (infancy)	Difficulty (toddlerhood)	−0.23	−0.28	0.28	0.08
		$F(1,91) = 7.48, p < 0.01$			
Mother's labor force participation (toddlerhood)	Difficulty (toddlerhood)	−0.34	−0.36	0.34	0.12
	Number of children (year 3)	−0.26	−0.28	0.41	0.17
	Physical problems	−0.20	−0.25	0.48	0.23
		$F(3,89) = 8.90, p < 0.0001$			
Mother's labor force participation (preschool age)	Difficulty (toddlerhood)	−0.39	−0.38	0.36	0.13
	Number of children (year 3)	−0.25	−0.25	0.42	0.18
	Physical problems	−0.17	−0.19	0.47	0.22
		$F(3,89) = 8.19, p < 0.001$			

measure of career salience rather than family orientation would have been more potent, as devotion to one's children neither precludes nor is precluded by investment in one's career. Although rejection of the child was not an important predictor in this study, it seems that future studies might do well to examine the mother's attitudes toward her child since child characteristics such as a difficult temperament could be linked to maternal employment status through the mother's feelings about those characteristics.

The mother's education and the father's occupational prestige did not predict significantly the mother's employment. This is probably attributable to the homogeneity of the sample with respect to educational and occupational attainments. Furthermore, most mothers who were employed were engaged in occupations that demand a great deal of personal dedication, and given the relatively high prestige levels of their spouses we may assume that many of the mothers were employed for personal rather than economic reasons.

Although it is difficult to generalize the results from this study to mothers of young children in the 1980s, there seems to be no reason to dismiss the likelihood that child characteristics have an influence on the mother's career decision-making process. It is recognized that the mother's labor force participation is a product of the mother and her context, and relevant features of both can and should be studied in order to learn more about a dramatic change, occurring over the last 40 years, that has had effects at all levels of society.

REFERENCES

Baltes, P. B., Reese, H. W. & Lipsitt, L. P. (1980). Life-span developmental psychology. *Annual Review of Psychology, 31,* 65–110.

Belsky, J., Steinberg, L. D. & Walker, A. (1982). The ecology of day care. In M. E. Lamb (Ed.), *Nontraditional families: Parenting and child development* (pp. 71–116). Hillsdale, NJ: Lawrence Erlbaum Associates.

Bose, C. E. & Rossi, P. H. (1983). Gender and jobs: Prestige standings of occupations as affected by gender. *American Sociological Review, 48,* 316–330.

Buss, A. H. & Plomin, R. (1984). *Temperament: Early developing personality traits.* Hillsdale, NJ: Erlbaum.

Cameron, J. R. (1977). Parental treatment, children's temperament, and the risk of childhood behavioral problems: I. Relationships between parental characteristics and changes in children's temperament over time. *American Journal of Orthopsychiatry, 47,* 568–576.

Chess, S. & Thomas, A. (1984). *Origins and evolution of behavior disorders.* New York: Brunner/Mazel.

Davis, J. A. (1980). *General social surveys, 1972–1980 cumulative codebook.* Chicago: University of Chicago.

Duncan, O. D. (1961). A socioeconomic index for all occupations. In A. J. Reiss, Jr., O. D. Duncan, P. K. Hatt & C. C. North (Eds), *Occupations and social status* (pp. 109–161). Glencoe, IL: The Free Press.

Eichorn, D. (1984, October). Comments made at the Radcliffe Conference on "The use of archival data to study women's lives." Cambridge, MA.

Ewer, P. A., Crimmins, E. & Oliver, R. (1979). An analysis of the relationship between husband's income, family size, and wife's employment in the early stages of marriage. *Journal of Marriage and the Family, 41,* 727–738.

Ferber, M. A. (1982). Labor market participation of young married women: Causes and effects. *Journal of Marriage and the Family, 44,* 457–467.

Fox, M. F. & Hesse-Biber, S. (1984). *Women at work.* Palo Alto, CA: Mayfield.

Gordon, H. A. & Kammeyer, K. C. W. (1980). The gainful employment of women with small children. *Journal of Marriage and the Family, 42,* 327–336.

Hetherington, E. M., Cox, M. & Cox, R. (1978). The aftermath of divorce. In J. H. Stevens, Jr. & M. Mathews (Eds), *Mother-child, father-child relations* (pp. 149–176). Washington, DC: National Association for the Education of Young Children.

Hetherington, E. M., Cox, M. & Cox, R. (1982). Effects of divorce on parents and children. In M. E. Lamb (Ed.), *Nontraditional families: Parenting and child development* (pp. 233–288). Hillsdale, NJ: Lawrence Erlbaum Associates.

Hock, E. (1978). Working and nonworking mothers with infants: Perceptions of their careers, their infants' needs, and satisfaction with mothering. *Developmental Psychology, 14,* 37–43.

Hock, E. (1980). Working and nonworking mothers and their infants: A comparative study of maternal characteristics and infant social behavior. *Merrill-Palmer Quarterly, 26,* 79–101.

Hock, E., Christman, K. & Hock, M. (1980). Factors associated with decisions about return to work in mothers of infants. *Developmental Psychology, 16,* 535–536.

Hodge, R. W., Siegel, P. M. & Rossi, P. H. (1965). Occupational prestige in the United States, 1925–63. *American Journal of Sociology, 70,* 286–302.

Hoffman, L. W. (1974). The employment of women, education, and fertility. *Merrill-Palmer Quarterly, 20,* 99–119.

Jessor, R. (1982, Dec. 10–11). *Psychosocial development in adolescence: Continuities with young adulthood.* Paper presented at Social Science Research Council Subcommittee on "Child Development in Life-Span Perspective" Conference on "Pubertal and Psychosocial Change." Tucson, Arizona.

Lamb, M. E., Chase-Lansdale, L. & Owen, M. T. (1979). The changing American family and its implications for infant social development: The sample case of maternal employment. In M. Lewis & L. A. Rosenblum (Eds), *The child and its family* (pp. 267–291). New York: Plenum Press.

Lerner, J. V. & Galambos, N. L. (1986). The child's development and family change: The influences of maternal employment. In L. P. Lipsitt (Ed.), *Advances in infancy research* (Vol. 4, pp. 39–86). Hillsdale, NJ: Ablex.

Lerner, J. V. & Lerner, R. M. (1983). Temperament and adaptation across life: Theoretical and empirical issues. In P. B. Baltes & O. G. Brim, Jr. (Eds), *Life-span development and behavior* (Vol. 5, pp. 197–231). New York: Academic Press.

Lerner, R. M., & Busch-Rossnagel, N. A. (1981). Individuals as producers of their development: Conceptual and empirical bases. In R. M. Lerner & N. A. Busch-Rossnagel (Eds), *Individuals as producers of their development: A life-span perspective* (pp. 1–36). New York: Academic Press.

Maccoby, E. E. & Martin, J. A. (1983). Socialization in the context of the family: Parent-child interaction. In E. M. Hetherington (Ed.), *Handbook of child psychology: Vol. 4. Socialization, personality, and social development* (pp. 1–101). New York: Wiley.

McBride, S. L. & Belsky, J. (1985, April). *Maternal work plans, actual employment and infant temperament.* Paper presented at the Biennial Meeting of the Society for Research in Child Development, Toronto, Canada.

McLaughlin, S. D. (1982). Differential patterns of female labor-force participation surrounding the first birth. *Journal of Marriage and the Family, 44,* 407–420.

Morgan, K. C. & Hock, E. (1984). A longitudinal study of psychosocial variables affecting the career patterns of women with young children. *Journal of Marriage and the Family, 46,* 383–390.

Thomas, A. & Chess, S. (1977). *Temperament and development.* New York: Brunner/Mazel.

Thomas, A. & Chess, S. (1980). *The dynamics of psychological development.* New York: Brunner/Mazel.

Thomas, A., Chess, S. & Birch, H. G. (1968). *Temperament and behavior disorders in children.* New York: New York University Press.

Thomas, A., Chess, S., Birch, H. G., Hertzig, M. E. & Korn, S. (1963). *Behavioral individuality in early childhood.* New York: New York University Press.

Waldman, E. (1983, December). Labor force statistics from a family perspective. *Monthly Labor Review, 106,* 16–19.

Part III

METHODOLOGICAL ISSUES

When new statistical models—such as multiple regression analysis—are developed, they can sometimes become powerful aids in extending the boundaries of our analyses of complex bodies of behavioral data. A recent development has been the introduction of an elaborate statistical model, known as Structural Equation Modeling (SEM), whose primary purpose is the testing of causal theories using nonexperimental and even experimental data. The use of SEM by developmental psychologists and sociologists has increased dramatically in the past year. This prompted the journal *Child Development* to devote a special section to this subject in their February 1987 issue (Vol. 58).

We feel that the use of SEM is now sufficiently widespread so that some general idea of the claims for its special statistical power, as well as some of the criticisms and skepticisms regarding its usefulness, make it appropriate to include in *Annual Progress.* Most of the articles in this special section of *Child Development,* however, are highly technical. We have therefore included only two of the articles: 1) the brief introduction by Connell and Tanaka, which outlines the nature of the articles included in the special section; and 2) a paper by Martin that puts the logic of SEM in simple terms and provides readers with a set of five statements and questions to guide them in their attempts to understand research reports using SEM models.

One of Martin's statements, which applies to statistical methods in general and especially to SEM, is worth emphasizing:

> The actual value of a piece of research to the advancement of any substantive field like child development rests in large measure on the clarity of the presentation of the theoretical framework that motivates the research. When *method* (rather than theory)

becomes the major focal point of substantive research, the tail (as it has been said) wags the dog. . . .Mathematical and statistical elegance can obfuscate inherent weaknesses in statistical methods and lead substantive researchers to turn the control of their data-analytic procedures to so-called statistical experts.

Well said, and most important to say!

10

Introduction to the Special Section on Structural Equation Modeling

James P. Connell
University of Rochester, New York
J. S. Tanaka
New York University, New York City

As coeditors of this Special Section, our mission was to provide readers of *Child Development* with a clearer view of Structural Equation Modeling (SEM) as a potential tool for research. Here, we provide an overview of what the section contains and of what has been omitted.

In the first article, Biddle and Marlin provide a nontechnical statement that should be valuable to SEM novices as well as experts; they point out what SEM is, its relation to other more familiar data-analytic techniques, and some of the potentials and pitfalls of SEM in analyzing developmental data. Structural equation modeling is often referred to as "causal modeling," and users of these methods have sometimes been criticized for interpretational biases in attributing "causal" meaning to the results of SEM analyses (Baumrind, 1983; Martin, 1982). Mulaik's conceptually demanding but extremely stimulating treatise on the nature of causality addresses the often misunderstood link between causal inference and SEM. His discussion of design, data-analytic strategies, and their role in causal inference should prove extremely useful to developmental researchers who employ either experimental or nonexperimental methods. Martin's contribution provides a set of "guidelines" for evaluating SEM research; although not everyone who uses SEM methods may agree with his perspective, this article gives insight

Reprinted with permission from *Child Development,* 1987, Vol. 58, 2–3. Copyright 1987 by the Society for Research in Child Development, Inc.

into how someone familiar with SEM would judge the adequacy of a study that uses such methods.

The next three articles describe applications of SEM in developmental data sets and demonstrate a spectrum of approaches to its uses in the building, testing, and evaluation of theory. Crano and Mendoza consider what could be described as exploratory uses of SEM; Anderson compares types of model specifications using either measured variables (path analysis) or latent-variable models; and Bentler provides a prototypic "confirmatory" application of SEM that also introduces a structural equations computer program, EQS.

The following three articles focus on the specification and testing of models of change, a problem central to developmental research. Gollob and Reichardt claim that when applied to cross-sectional data, standard SEM procedures almost invariably lead to misleading findings concerning relations among variables. They then suggest how notions of "causality" can be tested when only cross-sectional data are available. Hertzog and Nesselroade challenge the typical treatment of causal effects in longitudinal data, that is, to view causal relations only in light of the stability of interindividual differences. They argue that models should be conceptualized and tested in ways that directly reflect prior assumptions as to the trait- or state-like nature of the variables, and provide examples demonstrating that meaningful longitudinal studies of state variables can be conducted without assuming their stability over time. In presenting their latent growth curve model, McArdle and Epstein take the position that studies of developmental change should deal with individual growth curves. They then compare this new approach (chronometric models) to other existing strategies for investigating change (psychometric models).

Turning to technical issues, Tanaka considers the problem that arises when researchers do not have the large sample sizes optimally desired in SEM; he discusses how small sample size affects assessment of model fit and provides a new estimator that may be beneficial for use in small-sample situations. Huba and Harlow demonstrate how violations of the assumption that the observed variables are normally distributed may affect conclusions about models and address the issue of the robustness of findings under such conditions.

In the concluding contribution, Connell lists three criteria that can codetermine whether a new methodological technique is embraced by developmental researchers, and critically evaluates the potential impact of SEM from this perspective.

The contributions included in the Special Section provide a diverse sampling of conceptual, empirical, and theoretical work in SEM; however, a number of equally important issues have not been covered. Applications of SEM in experimental settings represent one such omission; readers may refer to Blalock (1985) for a general discussion, and to Fiske, Kenny, and Taylor (1982) as well as Geiselman, Woodward, and Beatty (1982) for examples of such uses. Discussion of models applicable to data that are categorical or discrete in nature has also been omitted; those interested in this topic could refer to Clogg and Shockey (in press), Goodman (1984), or Muthén (1984).

In closing, we thank the reviewers with whom we worked on this section for their careful and useful feedback on the original versions of these contributions, the contributors for their stalwart efforts at meeting the mission of the section, and the editors of *Child Development* (particularly associate editor Wanda Bronson, with whom we were most closely involved) for their encouragement and support of this project.

REFERENCES

Baumrind, D. (1983). Specious causal attributions in the social sciences: The reformulated stepping-stone theory of heroin use as an exemplar. *Journal of Personality and Social Psychology, 45,* 1289–1298.

Blalock, H. M., Jr. (Ed.). (1985). *Causal models in panel and experimental designs.* New York: Aldine.

Clogg, C. C., & Shockey, J. W. (in press). Multivariate analysis of discrete data. In J. R. Nesselroade & R. B. Cattell (Eds.), *Handbook of multivariate experimental psychology* (2d ed.). New York: Plenum.

Fiske, S. T., Kenny, D. A., & Taylor, S. E. (1982). Structural models for the mediation of salience effects on attribution. *Journal of Experimental Social Psychology, 18,* 105–127.

Geiselman, R. E., Woodward, J. A., & Beatty, J. (1982). Individual differences in verbal memory performance: A test of alternative information-processing models. *Journal of Experimental Psychology: General, 111,* 109–134.

Goodman, L. A. (1984). *The analysis of cross-classified data having ordered categories.* Cambridge, MA: Harvard University Press.

Martin, J. A. (1982). Application of structural modeling with latent variables to adolescent drug use: A reply to Huba, Wingard, and Bentler. *Journal of Personality and Social Psychology, 43,* 598–603.

Muthén, B. (1984). A general structural equation model with dichotomous, ordered categorical, and continuous latent variable indicators. *Psychometrika, 49,* 115–132.

PART III: METHODOLOGICAL ISSUES

11

Structural Equation Modeling: A Guide for the Perplexed

John A. Martin

California School of Professional Psychology, Berkeley

Despite seemingly incomprehensible notation and statistical complexity, the basic logic behind latent-variable structural equation modeling is quite simple. These methods are essentially an extension of familiar techniques such as multiple regression and factor analysis. In this light, readers are provided with a set of 5 statements and questions to guide them in their attempts to decipher reports of research employing structural modeling methods.

The editors of this special section on structural equation modeling have asked me to write a general commentary on the three application papers that follow this article (Anderson, 1987; Bentler, 1987; and Crano & Mendoza, 1987; all in this issue). This request was partly based, I suspect, on an article I wrote some time ago (Martin, 1982). This 1982 paper was a critique of overzealous claims made by some proponents of latent-variable structural modeling techniques and the unsupported conclusions drawn from the studies. Since 1982, the popularity of these techniques has increased tremendously, and reports of their use have appeared in increasing number. Unhappily, the general problems that were the focus of my 1982 critique have, in my opinion, persisted in many papers that use these techniques.

Reprinted with permission from *Child Development,* 1987, Vol. 58, 33–37. Copyright 1987 by the Society for Research in Child Development, Inc.

The author wishes to thank Lorna Bennett for her assistance with manuscript preparation. Send requests for reprints to the author at the California School of Professional Psychology, 1900 Addison Street, Berkeley, CA 94704.

I have very little to say about the applications papers in this issue that I did not say in my 1982 paper. However, since the 1982 paper appears to have had little impact, I thought I would use this opportunity to try again. I begin with a concise and somewhat idiosyncratic guide to the logic and use of structural modeling techniques placed within the context of more traditional nonexperimental research methods. I conclude with five brief, pointed, and admittedly partisan value statements followed by questions that readers of these and future applications of structural equation modeling methods may wish to ask themselves as they read and evaluate the appropriateness of the conclusions drawn on the basis of the methods.

THE LOGIC OF STRUCTURAL EQUATION MODELING

The primary purpose of structural equation modeling is the testing of causal theories using nonexperimental data (see Blalock, 1985, for a description of how these methods can be used with experimental data as well). Let us begin by examining the logic underlying the testing of a causal theory, whether by means of structural equation modeling or some other more modest set of methods. We begin by stating unambiguously a fully developed causal theory in terms of (generally unobservable) hypothetical constructs and processes. Next comes the *operationalization* of the major constructs and then the derivation of one or more *specific, testable* hypotheses using statistical tests that accurately reflect the nature of the theoretical "links" connecting the constructs. The hypotheses are constructed so that, if one or more can be proved *not* to be true, it then becomes *logically impossible* for the causal theory from which they were derived to be true, given the data. That is, hypotheses are constructed and tested that are *necessary* (although no one argued "sufficient") for the truth of causal theory.

So, there's nothing new about testing causal theories with data, whether the data be experimental or nonexperimental. We've been doing this for quite some time, whether we called it "testing causal theories" or not. Structural equation modeling merely represents a somewhat more powerful method* for doing precisely what we've always done. Rather complex (causal) linkages among independent and dependent variables can be specified and "tested" with structural equation modeling techniques using multiple regression-type models (Duncan, 1975); in addition, *certain* structural modeling methods (generically referred to as latent variable or LV methods by Bentler, 1980)

---

*The method is more *powerful* in the sense that a researcher can get more information from the same data set than with other methods, provided certain assumptions are met. As always, there are costs associated with power. These costs are discussed below.

like LISREL (Jöreskog & Sörbom, 1978) allow researchers to include hypotheses about measurement error and its potential impact on the relationships tested by the multiple regression-type procedures. However, the basic rules of the game remain unchanged.

Specifically, the first step in structural equation modeling is *still* that an unambiguous causal theory be specified: No statistical method can relieve us of the responsibility of stating our a priori beliefs in a substantively articulate manner. Therefore, at the level of substance—not surprisingly—these "new" methods have nothing new to offer (see Connell, 1987, in this issue, for a different view). Structural modeling *does*, however, allow researchers to test more complex hypotheses (hypotheses that must necessarily be true in order that the previously articulated causal theory remain credible) than had been possible. However, the general thrust behind the "testing" has remained unchanged: The potential value of the testing procedure rests entirely on *(a)* the status of the hypothesis, however complex, relative to the theory (i.e., that it be "necessary"), *(b)* the care with which the major constructs have been operationalized, and *(c)* the "match" between the substantive statement of the hypothesis and the statistical procedure to be used for testing it.

Herein lies the potential power of structural modeling. Psychologists generally concede that single measures can rarely be used to represent most major psychological constructs. When single measures are not appropriate, researchers often choose to obtain multiple measures: That is, several independent pieces of information pertinent to some hypothetical construct are collected and in some way put together so as to more adequately represent that construct. Different methods can be employed to do this. The traditional approach has been to employ principal components or some other factor analytic method to obtain factor scores that represent the hypothetical construct(s) in question. The factor scores are then used in correlational or multiple regression methods. The problem with this general procedure is that the "cluster" of measured variables created by the principal components or factor analytic method is (necessarily) an imperfect representation of the hypothetical construct: The *error* inherent in the cluster, as well as systematic variance in the items that is unrelated to the cluster, cannot be differentiated from the cluster itself. Consequently, statistical analyses of clusters of measured variables confound measurement error and unexplained item variance with "true" variance, rendering inference about the causal theory itself—divorced of "error"—difficult.

In contrast to this approach to the use of multiple indicators, LV models like LISREL get around this problem by performing the clustering and the multiple regression-type procedure at the same time. In this way, the error and unexplained variance that are necessary parts of the cluster can be included as part of the causal theory that is being tested; substantive statements about them can be kept separate from statements about the portion of the cluster that is neither error nor item variance (presumed to be representative of the hypothetical construct). In this way, inferences about the hypothetical constructs as operationalized by the multiple measures can be distinguished from any confounding effects both of error inherent in the construction of a composite measure of the constructs and of variability in the items that is unrelated to the constructs.

Clearly, then, as has repeatedly been claimed by proponents of structural modeling methods, these new techniques represent an important new advance over more traditional approaches to causal questions. However, statistical power is not without cost. One cost of this statistical power in the case of LV models, as in the case of other relatively powerful statistical techniques (like multiple regression compared to simple correlation), is that the maximum-likelihood methods used to test LV models like LISREL are predicated on a highly restrictive set of simplifying assumptions, conditioning statements that *must* be presumed true in order for inferences based on the methods to be true (see, e.g., Mulaik, 1987, in this issue). The simplifying assumptions upon which LV models like LISREL are based are highly restrictive, and it is not known whether psychologists will ever be able to meet them or whether violating these assumptions is likely to have serious consequences (Biddle, Slavings, & Anderson, 1985; Freedman, 1984). Yet another cost, as in factor analytic studies using a large number of variables, is that LV methods like LISREL require that a large number of cases be available for analysis (Tanaka, 1987, in this issue). This may not be a realistic requirement in light of the need, common in all research, for high-quality data on the major constructs. Psychological constructs are, for the most part, ephemeral and not easily measured; generally, it takes time and costs money to get high-quality information upon which to base measures of psychological constructs. It is unlikely that the resources of most psychologists will allow for the collection of sufficiently high-quality data upon which to rest causal inference on a large enough sample to satisfy the requirements of LV structural models. In a world of limited resources, there is generally a trade-off between sample size and the quality of measures. Data quality ought not to be wantonly sacrificed in service of a statistical method that requires a large sample size.

Presuming that both sample-size and data-quality requirements are met, and provided that the major simplifying assumptions of the LV method seem plausible (or are demonstrated to be of little importance, that is, by demonstrating the robustness of the method to violations of the assumptions), what are we able to conclude? Once again, structural equation modeling methods have nothing fundamentally new to offer at the level of causal inference. Provided that everything has been done properly up to and including this point, the causal theory *can be rejected* if the random process explanation *cannot be rejected*. Or, if the null hypothesis *is* rejected at an acceptable level of statistical significance, persons who choose to believe the causal theory are permitted to continue to entertain that belief. And this is as it has always been.

On what basis might someone choose to believe in a causal theory in the first place? Its phenomenological persuasiveness will always be an important factor, and this is based in part on the force of logic used in its construction. Another major factor is its empirical context: Since establishing the truth of a causal law necessarily requires a large and possibly unspecifiable set of simplifying and conditioning assumptions, information about the results of other studies using other samples and other contexts—perhaps testing different sectors of the causal process—will be of great importance in evaluating the importance of any additional piece of evidence. No matter how powerful the statistical method, however, no single piece of research is ever likely to achieve the status of "definitive."

Despite these criticisms and the inherent similarity of these methods to simpler ones, structural equation modeling methods may be thought of as being in many respects superior to more traditional approaches to testing causal theories. When researchers use causal modeling, they are forced to be explicit about the causal theory that motivates the statistical test(s): this constitutes perhaps the strongest argument in support of these methods. In addition, LV models like LISREL have the additional advantage that the "error" of measurement involved in operationalizing the hypothetical construct(s) can be separated from the "error-free" component of the operationalization, and various hypotheses about the error can be included in the statement of the (testable) causal model. However, in arguing for the "power" of structural equation modeling, it is important to keep in mind that the *costs* of power—namely, highly restrictive assumptions that researchers who use these methods rarely acknowledge and that may never be met with psychological data, and the need for a large sample size (and, generally, a corresponding diminution of data quality)—are substantial. It is also important to keep in mind that these "new" structural modeling methods are subject to the same major logical limitations concerning causal inference as the simpler, more widely known correlational methods.

SOME VALUE STATEMENTS, AND QUESTIONS FOR READERS

As you read the applications of latent variable structural modeling methods that follow—or other published (or unpublished) applications of these methods—I propose that you keep in mind the following points, and ask yourself the following questions. These are offered as criteria to evaluate *any* research, including research that makes use of structural equation modeling.

1. Research cannot directly answer causal questions—whether the research is experimental or nonexperimental, whether the techniques are traditional or whether more sophisticated latent variable methods are employed. Have the authors of these papers demonstrated anything about their "causal models" that had previously been inaccessible to researchers? Are these authors in any better position than anyone else to make "causal inferences"? Is their manner of presentation and the force of their claims consistent with their ability to address causal issues with nonexperimental research?

2. The actual value of a piece of research to the advancement of any substantive field like child development rests in large measure on the clarity of the presentation of the theoretical framework that motivates the research. When *method* (rather than theory) becomes the major focal point of substantive research, the tail (as it has been said) wags the dog. How well have these authors articulated their theoretical positions? If some more familiar methods that did not require full understanding of structural modeling (like partial correlation) were used instead, what would be your reaction to their presentation of their substantive concerns?

3. Careful operationalization of major constructs and collection of high-quality data are the sine qua non of any substantive research enterprise. No methodologies, no matter how powerful, allow researchers to study phenomena they have not measured well. One cannot make a silk purse out of a sow's ear, no matter how powerful the sewing machine. How carefully have these authors articulated and operationalized their major constructs? How convincing are their data? A related question: Does the use of multiple indicators salvage poor-quality data? That is, does the use of several measures of a construct improve the measurement of that construct if each measure is poor—if the aim is to produce a silk purse, are 10 sows' ears better than one?

4. The power of latent-variable structural equation modeling methods rests on *(a)* highly restrictive simplifying assumptions and *(b)* the accessibility of large samples. The usefulness of these methods when the assumptions are not met or met with small samples is questionable. Are you convinced that the additional simplifying assumptions that differentiate structural equation modeling from more conventional methods are met, or can realistically be assumed to have been met? Are you satisfied that the trade-off between sample size and data quality is defensible?

5. Mathematical and statistical elegance can obfuscate inherent weaknesses in statistical methods and lead substantive researchers to turn the control of their data-analytic procedures to so-called statistical experts. For example, the editors of this special section on structural modeling, recognizing this fact, asked us to aim our presentation to the average *CD* reader. If you consider yourself an average *CD* reader, do you find the authors' presentations in these papers clear and comprehensible? Are you tempted to infer from the complexity of the presentation that the methods themselves are unintelligible to you? If these methods were explained in plain English (e.g., Biddle & Marlin, 1987, in this issue), would you believe the conclusions? In this regard, a word of warning seems appropriate: If you find that you do not understand the method by which a researcher has reached his or her conclusions, this does *not* represent an argument for accepting (or, for that matter, rejecting) those conclusions. In all scientific enterprises, it is wise to remain skeptical unless and until convincing information is presented that might lead you to be otherwise.

REFERENCES

Anderson, J. G. (1987). Structural equation models in the social and behavioral sciences: Model building. *Child Development, 58,* 49–64.

Bentler, P. M. (1980). Multivariate analysis with latent variables: Causal modeling. *Annual Review of Psychology, 31,* 419–456.

Bentler, P. M. (1987). Drug use and personality in adolescence and young adulthood: Structural models with nonnormal variables. *Child Development, 58,* 65–79.

Biddle, B. J., & Marlin, M. M. (1987). Causality, confirmation, credulity, and structural equation modeling. *Child Development, 58,* 4–17.

Biddle, B. J., Slavings, R. L., & Anderson, D. S. (1985). Panel studies and causal inference. *Journal of Applied Behavioral Sciences, 21,* 79–93.

Blalock, H. M. (Ed.). (1985). *Causal models in panel and experimental designs.* New York: Aldine.

Connell, J. P. (1987). Structural equation modeling and the study of child development: A question of goodness of fit. *Child Development, 58,* 167–175.

Crano, W. D., & Mendoza, J. L. (1987). Maternal factors that influence children's positive behavior: Demonstration of a structural equation analysis of selected data from the Berkeley Growth Study. *Child Development, 58,* 38–48.

Duncan, O. D. (1975). *Introduction to structural equation models.* New York: Academic Press.

Freedman, D. A. (1984). Discussion of the Jöreskog-Sörbom paper. In H. Winsborough, O. D. Duncan, & P. B. Reads (Eds.), *Cohort analysis in social research.* New York: Academic Press.

Jöreskog, K. G., & Sörbom, D. (1978). *LISREL IV: Analysis of linear structural relationships by the method of maximum likelihood.* Chicago: National Educational Resources.

Martin, J. A. (1982). Application of structural modeling with latent variables to adolescent drug use: A reply to Huba, Wingard, and Bentler. *Journal of Personality and Social Psychology, 43,* 598–603.

Mulaik, S. A. (1987). Toward a conception of causality applicable to experimentation and causal modeling. *Child Development, 58,* 18–32.

Tanaka, J.J. (1987). How big is big enough? Sample size and goodness of fit in structural equation models with latent variables. *Child Development, 58,* 134–146.

Part IV

SPECIAL STRESS
AND COPING

A central characteristic of human development involves coping with physical, psychological, and social stress. Mastery of stress promotes healthy development; the inability to cope successfully has the opposite effect. Overprotective parents who attempt to shield their children from stress are not helpful and may even prevent their children from acquiring the basic sense of self-confidence and self-esteem that comes from successive mastery of the stresses and challenges that life poses at successive age-periods. On the other hand, excessive stress which the youngster may not be able to master with his own resources alone, may also have serious developmental consequences. In such situations, it is the responsibility of the caregivers and community institutions and agencies to recognize the problem and give the child the necessary support and additional resources he may need to cope successfully with such excessive stress.

These generalizations set a framework—but only a framework—for identifying the specific types of stress to which children may be exposed, as well as the different coping resources, styles, and specific strategies that children and adolescents develop in coping with stress. Compas reviews the literature on these issues, and identifies seven different lines of research. He concludes by emphasizing the need for further research that will focus on systematic comparisons of coping across different types of stress and also over time in response to a single stress.

Wertlieb and his colleagues present a carefully done investigation, statistically sophisticated, with a large population, which explores the relationships between stress, temperament, and behavior. Of interest is their differentiation between undesirable life events and "daily hassles," namely the relatively minor experiences or events encountered in the course of daily living.

The paper by Marcus and co-workers reports two longitudinal studies of the offspring of schizophrenic parents: the NIMH Israeli Kibbutz-City Study, begun in Israel in 1965, and the Jerusalem Infant Development Study, begun in 1973. Results from both studies supported the hypothesis that schizophrenic illness involves constitutional factors whose expression can be observed as early as infancy. The study also utilized an innovative data-analysis strategy involving a decision-free approach, which could differentiate subgroups within high-risk groups, rather than only group differences between high- and low-risk groups. Such a data-analytic model may make it possible to differentiate kinds and severity of stress and coping mechanisms in high-risk subgroups.

West and Prinz provide a comprehensive review of studies examining the relationship of the high stress factor of parental alcoholism and the outcome in childhood psychopathology. The paper first addresses methodological issues and then summarizes findings around eight areas of dysfunction outcome in the family and the children. The finding that not even a major portion of children from alcoholic homes are inevitably doomed to develop a psychological disorder leads the authors to point briefly and appropriately to the literature that emphasizes the resiliency and positive coping abilities of many children faced with severe stress. Their conclusion is apt: More research needs to be focused on the question "Which children of alcoholic families fare well and which do not, and why?"

Without doubt, American Indians are the most severely disadvantaged of any population within the United States. Yates documents the many severe stresses to which American Indian children are subjected and the tragic consequences in the rates of serious mental disorder and academic underachievement among the children and adolescents. The author details the methods of prevention and intervention that can easily be implemented if mainstream America faces its responsibility for the tragic lives of these seriously deprived and highly stressed youngsters.

12

Coping with Stress During Childhood and Adolescence

Bruce E. Compas

University of Vermont, Burlington

In this article, research on how children and adolescents cope with stress and coping's role in reducing the adverse psychological states associated with stress is reviewed. Child and adolescent coping is reflected in seven different lines of research—infants' responses to maternal separation, social support, interpersonal cognitive problem-solving, coping in achievement contexts, Type A behavior pattern in children, repression-sensitization, and resilience to stress. A variety of different coping resources, styles, and specific strategies are important in successfully adapting to stress, including efforts that focus directly on the problem, as well as attempts to deal with adverse emotions associated with stress. Directions for future research are identified, emphasizing the need for more systematic comparisons of coping across different types of stress and over time in response to a single stressful episode.

A central feature of human development involves coping with psychosocial stress. Beginning in infancy, individuals are confronted with a stream of potentially threatening and challenging situations that require action and adaptation. The modest to moderate correlations typically found between stressful life events and disorder during childhood and adolescence suggest that individual difference factors related to coping may moderate the stress-

Reprinted with permission from *Psychological Bulletin,* 1987, Vol. 101, No. 3, 393–403. Copyright 1987 by the American Psychological Association, Inc.

This work was supported in part by W. T. Grant Foundation Grant 85–1016–85.

The author is grateful to Lynne Bond and Harold Leitenberg for their comments on an earlier version of this article.

disorder relation (see Compas, in press, for a review). The resources available to cope with stress and the manner in which individuals actually cope may be important factors influencing patterns of positive growth and development as opposed to the onset of a host of psychological and somatic problems.

Although the study of coping with stress during adulthood has been characterized by increasing convergence in conceptualization and measurement (e.g., Lazarus & Folkman, 1984; Meneghan, 1983; Moos & Billings, 1982), this is not true for coping during childhood and adolescence. Instead, coping in younger age groups has been represented by different definitions and methods of measurement, as well as several divergent lines of research. The purpose of this review is to integrate these somewhat disparate areas of research and to identify future directions for study. First, various definitions and conceptualizations of coping are discussed. Second, empirical studies of coping during childhood and adolescence are reviewed. Finally, conclusions drawn from this research, the major issues facing the field, and directions for future research are outlined.

CONCEPTUALIZATION OF COPING

As no systematic effort has been made to conceptualize coping during childhood and adolescence, the adult literature must be drawn on for this purpose (cf. Rutter, 1981). At the most general level, coping has been considered to include all responses to stressful events or episodes. This feature is characteristic of both animal (e.g., N. E. Miller, 1980) and human (e.g., Silver & Wortman, 1980) models of coping. For example, Silver and Wortman (1980) defined coping as "any and all responses made by an individual who encounters a potentially harmful outcome" (p. 281). At this level, coping includes instinctive or reflexive reactions to threat as well as an array of learned responses to aversive stimuli. However, theorists from a variety of perspectives have argued that this definition is too broad. Coping has been further differentiated on the basis of (a) effortful versus noneffortful responses, (b) coping's function, and (c) a focus on resources, styles, or specific responses.

Coping as Effortful Responses to Stress

Several authors have argued for the importance of distinguishing coping as including effortful or purposeful reactions to stress but excluding reflexive or automatic responses (e.g., Lazarus & Folkman, 1984; Murphy, 1974). By focusing only on adaptational responses involving effort, coping is distinguished from instinctual mechanisms that are beyond the individual's volitional control. With regard to coping responses of children, Murphy and associates (Murphy, 1974; Murphy & Moriarity, 1976) have placed coping at the middle of a continuum ranging from reflexes that are present from birth to automatized mastery responses that have been learned to the extent that they no longer require conscious control. Purposeful responses may become automatic after being repeated many times. Lazarus and Folkman (1984) pointed out that focusing on effortful responses avoids the pitfall of defining coping so broadly that it includes everything that individuals do in relating to the environment.

This perspective on coping is best reflected by Lazarus and Folkman's (1984) definition: "We define coping as constantly changing cognitive and behavioral efforts to manage specific external and/or internal demands that are appraised as taxing or exceeding the resources of the person" (p. 141). They pointed out that managing stress includes accepting, tolerating, avoiding, or minimizing the stressor as well as the more traditional view of coping as mastery over the environment. Coping is not limited to successful efforts but includes all purposeful attempts to manage stress regardless of their effectiveness.

Functions of Coping

Coping efforts have been delineated into those intended to act on the stressor (problem-focused coping) and those intended to regulate emotional states associated with or resulting from the stressor (emotion-focused coping; Folkman & Lazarus, 1980). Efforts to act on the stressor include strategies for problem solving or altering the stressful relation between the individual and the environment. Alternatively, adjustment or adaptation can be facilitated by emotional regulation achieved through avoiding the stressor, cognitively reframing the stressor, or selectively attending to positive aspects of the self or situation. Problem- and emotion-focused coping can be carried out through either cognitive or behavioral channels.

Resources, Styles, and Specific Coping Efforts

It is also useful to distinguish among the resources available to the individual in coping with stress, the styles of coping that characterize an individual's responses, and the specific coping efforts displayed in a particular stressful episode (e.g., Menaghan, 1983). Coping resources include those aspects of the self (e.g., problem-solving skills, interpersonal skills, positive self-esteem) and the social environment (e.g., the availability of a supportive social network) that facilitate or make possible successful adaptation to life stress. Coping styles are methods of coping that characterize individuals' reactions to stress either across different situations or over time within a given situation. These may partly reflect the ways of coping preferred by individuals because they are consistent with personal values, beliefs, and goals. Coping styles do not necessarily imply the presence of underlying personality traits that predispose the person to respond in a particular way (Lazarus & Folkman, 1984). Instead, coping styles may reflect the tendency to respond in a particular way when confronted with a specific set of circumstances (e.g., an individual may display different coping styles in controllable vs. uncontrollable situations). Finally, specific coping efforts or strategies refer to the cognitive or behavioral actions taken in the course of a particular stressful episode. These may vary across time and context depending on the nature of the stressful encounter.

Child and Adolescent Coping

Applying these general notions of coping to the actions of children and adolescents requires some alterations and additions. First, the nature of the infant or young child's dependence on adults for survival emphasizes the need to include the child's social context in understanding his or her coping resources, styles, and efforts (Leiderman, 1983). Thus, adaptive coping cannot be characterized by a description of the individual's skills or resources alone but instead lies in the relation between the child and the environment. Whereas this relational definition of coping may apply throughout life, it should be especially important early in development. Second, the child's coping efforts will be constrained by his or her psychological and biological preparedness to respond to stress. For example, temperament is frequently cited as playing a central role in influencing the child's coping responses (e.g., Kagan, 1983; Lerner, Baker, & Lerner, 1985; Rutter, 1981). The child's temperament may define a range of responsivity to stress and influence the style that characterizes the child's coping. Children differ in their sensitivity to the environment, with some showing signs of arousal and distress to a much wider array of stimuli than others. More responsive children may need to cope with a greater number of situations than less responsive youngsters. Further, individual differences are apparent in the ways children react once they are aroused or threatened, for example, in the degree of inhibition of behavior and expressions of fear they display in response to a stressful stimulus (e.g., Garcia Coll, Kagan, & Reznick, 1984). Third, basic features of cognitive and social development are likely to affect what children experience as stressful and how they cope (e.g., Maccoby, 1983). Important aspects of development include self-perceptions (Harter, 1983) and self-efficacy beliefs

(Bandura, 1981), self-control or inhibitory mechanisms (Harter, 1983), attributions of cause (Ruble & Rholes, 1981), friendships (Hartup, 1983), and parental relationships (Maccoby & Martin, 1983), among others. Although it is beyond the scope of this discussion to review each of these areas, it is important to recognize the ways in which the study of coping during childhood and adolescence can contribute to as well as benefit from research on these fundamental aspects of human development.

Not surprisingly, it appears that coping during childhood is affected by both personal and environmental factors. The degree to which coping is effective may depend on the goodness of fit between the child and the environment (e.g., Lerner et al., 1985; Lerner & Lerner, 1983). For example, if a child's temperamental style does not effectively elicit caretaking responses from the parents, then a poor fit exists and the child's coping efforts will not facilitate successful adaptation to stressful encounters with the environment. Thus, research investigating coping during childhood must account for the environmental context in which the stressful episode occurs (including both the nature of the stressor and the availability of resources for coping), the individual's developmental level, the personal resources the individual brings to the situation, the prior history of and preferred ways of coping, and the actual coping responses.

EMPIRICAL INVESTIGATIONS

Aspects of coping as just conceptualized have been central themes in seven areas of research, all concerned with adaptation to stress during childhood and adolescence—(a) attachment and separation during infancy (e.g., Ainsworth, 1979), (b) social support (e.g., Barrera, 1981), (c) interpersonal cognitive problem solving (e.g., Spivack & Shure, 1982, 1985), (d) coping in achievement contexts (e.g., Dweck & Wortman, 1982), (e) Type A and B behavior patterns (e.g., Matthews, 1981), (f) coping styles of repression and sensitization (e.g., Krohne & Rogner, 1982) or monitoring and blunting (e.g., S. M. Miller & Green, 1984), and (g) resilience or invulnerability to stress (e.g., Garmezy, 1983). The common theme among these lines of research is that they all concern the responses of children and adolescents to stressful stimuli.

Attachment and Separation

The attachment of the infant to the mother or caretaker and evidence of distress in reaction to separation from the mother are fundamental aspects of human social development. More specifically, the infant's reactions to separation from the mother may be the infant's first experiences in coping with stress. Although there is considerable variability in infants' responses to maternal separation, indications of behavioral inhibition, fear, and distress are common (e.g., Garcia Coll et al., 1984). This distress is typically relieved by renewed contact with the mother. Thus, behaviors displayed by the infant in response to separation that promote the mother's return can be seen as the earliest forms of coping an individual displays.

The "strange situation" paradigm developed by Ainsworth and colleagues (e.g., Ainsworth, 1979) is the context used most often for the study of infants' reactions to maternal separation. Infants are observed for brief periods in an unfamiliar laboratory setting in the presence of their mother, with a stranger, with the mother and the stranger, and alone. Whereas the primary purpose of this research is to classify the quality of the attachment between the infant and mother, and the representativeness of infant behavior in this context has been called into question (e.g., Kagan, 1984; Lamb, Thompson, Gardner, Charnov, & Estes, 1984), the behavior observed with the strange situation can be seen as an interesting example of infant coping (cf. Hock & Clinger, 1981). The pattern labeled as representing a secure attachment (i.e., mildly protesting after the mother leaves, seeking proximity to the mother when she returns, and being easily placated by her) might reflect a pattern of coping with an event that is experienced by the infant as mildly stressful. Alternatively, less effective coping may be reflected in the behavior of insecurely attached children, who become seriously distressed when the mother leaves and are not easily soothed by their mothers' attempts to calm them. Finally, a third group of avoidant children, who do not protest the mother's departure and do not seek her out when she returns, may reflect a group not experiencing the event as stressful and, thus, not being mobilized to cope.

The study of responses to maternal separation highlights two intriguing problems that confront coping researchers, particularly in studying young children. First, if it is accepted that coping involves effortful but not reflexive responses, it is unclear whether infants' reactions to maternal separation actually represent coping, as opposed to predisposed patterns of responding. Although there is substantial variability among infants in their patterns of response, there is considerable stability in individuals' reactions across time. Thus, infants' reactions to separation may reflect stable temperamental factors to a great extent (Kagan, 1983). However, temperament may affect the likelihood or degree to which separation is experienced as stressful but not necessarily infants' attempts to cope with the event. Kagan (1984) and Hock and Clinger (1981) have argued that some infants who fail to display distress when the mother departs may be better able to cope with uncertainty rather than being poorly attached to mother. Their behavior may imply that "babies who do not become upset in the Strange Situation have acquired adaptive coping strategies to deal with stress" (Kagan, 1984, p. 61). These adaptive strategies are probably influenced by parenting patterns that value self-reliance and the capacity to control fear. Thus, infant responses are likely to reflect the effects of both temperamental patterns and learned effortful behavior.

The second dilemma of coping research illustrated by studies of separation distress involves the overlapping nature of stress and coping. The constellation of behaviors that indicates that separation is stressful (inhibition of exploratory behavior, fretting, and crying) is simultaneously defined as the infant's effort to cope with the separation by promoting the mother's return. Further, the absence of distress may indicate that the separation is not stressful, and it may also represent more adaptive coping. The interdependent and reciprocal nature of the relation between stress and coping is evident in other literature on coping during childhood and adolescence.

Social Support

The continued importance of social bonds and relationships throughout childhood and adolescence is evident in studies of social support. This concept has been approached by numerous researchers and has involved several different conceptualizations. Most of these investigators have applied definitions of social support developed in work with adult populations to the use of the construct with children and adolescents (e.g., Cauce, Felner, & Primavera, 1982; Kaplan, Robbins, & Martin, 1983). Barrera (1981) developed the most comprehensive definition of social support during childhood and adolescence. He argued that the concept must include explication of the providers of support, the individual's subjective appraisal of support, and the activities involved in the provision of support. Whereas social support is typically viewed as a form of coping or a factor that facilitates coping, Barrera's (1981) conceptualization goes the furthest in this regard by outlining examples of socially supportive behaviors. These are likely to include attempts to assist the individual in mastering emotional distress, sharing responsibilities, providing advice, teaching skills, and providing material aid.

In studies of social support as a resource for coping among children and adolescents, researchers have examined both the direct relation between social support and adjustment and the interaction of life events and social support in relation to well-being. Evidence for a direct relation between social support and levels of psychological or physical symptomatology or both has been strong; Barrera (1981), Cauce et al. (1982), Compas, Slavin, Wagner, and Vannatta (1986), Compas, Wagner, Slavin, and Vannatta (1986), Felner, Ginter, and Primavera (1982), Sandler (1980), and Sandler and Barrera (1984) reported significant relations. Although it is clear that the quality of one's social support is related to symptom levels, this relation varies as a function of a number of subject characteristics (e.g., gender, age, and socioeconomic status) and the aspect or dimension of social support under investigation (e.g., number of supportive relationships, satisfaction with social support, and others' socially supportive behaviors). Differences in subjects, measures, and research designs make it difficult to draw conclusions in this literature at present.

Studies of interactive effects of social support have been more mixed in their findings. Compas, Slavin, et al. (1986) and Gad and Johnson (1980) failed to find any interaction between life events and social support in predicting symptom level. The Life Event × Social Support interactions that have been reported are limited to certain types of subjects, particular aspects of social support, specific symptoms, or all three. For example, in a study of stressful events and social support in pregnant adolescents, Barrera (1981) found that negative life events interacted with total size of the social network and unconflicted network size in predicting depression. No interactions occurred, however, in regression equations predicting anxiety or total symptom level. The socially supportive behaviors of others and satisfaction with social support did not interact with negative life events in predicting any symptomatology. The inconsistent nature of the findings of this and other studies (Hotaling, Atwell, & Linsky, 1978; Sandler, 1980; Sandler & Barrera, 1984; Sandler & Lakey, 1982) prohibit making any conclusions regarding the differential effects of life events among individuals with high and low social support.

Interpersonal Cognitive Problem Solving (ICPS)

Spivack, Shure, and their colleagues' work has provided extensive evidence on the ways in which children and adolescents respond to problems encountered in interpersonal relationships (see reviews by Spivack, Platt, & Shure, 1976; Spivack & Shure, 1982, 1985). Specifically, they have addressed the way an individual recognizes a problem and thinks during an interpersonal situation. The cognitive steps one goes through in response to a social problem are viewed as mediators of the quality of social and personal adjustment. Their research has contained a strong developmental flavor, centered around the proposition that interpersonal cognitive problem-solving skills may differ in their significance as a function of age. Interpersonal cognitive problem-solving skills contain the following components: genera-tion of alternative solutions, consideration of consequences of social acts, development of means-ends thinking, development of social causal thinking, sensitivity to problems, and a dynamic orientation (see Spivack & Shure, 1982). Spivack and Shure have acknowledged that their research deals with one mode of coping (cognitive problem solving) in reference to one type of stressful situation (interpersonal). Although they have speculated on other cognitive responses to interpersonal problems (e.g., not thinking and defensive thinking), they have not attempted to conceptualize these or other coping strategies or to address tactics to deal with nonsocial problems (e.g., a school examination or a physical illness).

Empirical investigations by the Spivack and Shure group have had three focuses—(a) delineation of the component skills that constitute ICPS, (b) examination of the relation of these skills to adaptive functioning, and (c) examination of the effects of programs to increase ICPS skills on children's and adolescents' well-being. Their findings have generally been positive in each of these areas (Spivack & Shure, 1982). First, they have shown that six separate skills compose ICPS (see previous paragraph), and that these skills emerge at different points in development. For example, the ability to generate alternative solutions to a problem emerges as important as early as age 4 or 5 and remains a valuable skill throughout life (e.g., Shure & Spivack, 1978, 1980). In contrast, the development of means-ends thinking, defined as mentally articulating the sequence or step-by-step means necessary to carry out a particular solution to an interpersonal problem, does not become significant for adjustment until approximately ages 8 to 10 (Spivack et al., 1976). The investigators raised the plausible hypothesis that means-ends thinking requires complex cognitive processes that are not sufficiently developed in younger children.

Studies of the relation between ICPS skills and levels of adjustment have consistently shown a strong association between the two. The typical design used in these studies has been to identify a sample of well-adjusted children or adolescents and a matched sample of youngsters displaying emotional or behavioral problems (see Spivack & Shure, 1982). The level of ICPS skills of the two groups has then been compared. Each of the six ICPS skills has been shown to discriminate problem from nonproblem samples, but their effects have varied as a function of age. The generation of alternative solutions, consideration of consequences of social acts, and development of means-ends thinking have been studied most extensively (Spivack & Shure, 1982). It is not clear, however, whether ICPS skills are important in modifying the impact of stress, are directly related to adjustment independent of stress, or both.

Finally, data from intervention studies have been somewhat more mixed regarding the importance of ICPS skills for coping with interpersonal problems. Intervention programs have been designed for preschool and school-age children (Spivack & Shure, 1982) and adolescents (Spivack et al., 1976). Increased ICPS skills were found to be related to enhanced adjustment in three studies, but improved adjustment was not associated with problem-solving training in seven studies (Durlak, 1983, 1985). Specifically, only the Hahnemann group (Spivack & Shure, 1982) was able to show that increased ICPS skills are associated with improved behavioral adjustment. These varied results may suggest that certain elements are essential for ICPS interventions to affect children's functioning (e.g., the use of dialoguing on an ongoing basis is a central part of Spivak and Shure's work). Alternatively, these programs may be more effective for children experiencing high levels of stress than for those under relatively less stress. This possibility has not been investigated.

Coping in Achievement Contexts

The coping of children in achievement contexts has been studied extensively in both laboratory and field investigations. This work is best exemplified by Dweck and her colleagues' investigations of "helpless" and "mastery-oriented" children (see reviews by Dweck & Licht, 1980; Dweck & Wortman, 1982). This conceptualization of coping parallels Spivack and Shure's work in that the primary emphasis is on the cognitive strategies used by children to adapt to aversive experiences. Coping strategies are viewed as individuals' efforts to minimize distress and to maximize performance (Dweck & Wortman, 1982). Implicit in this work is a distinction between effective and ineffective coping with failure on academic achievement tasks. Mastery-oriented children are examples of effective copers in that they sustain high levels of motivation, persist in attempts at problem solving, increase their concentration, and display enhanced performance. Alternatively, helpless children display ineffective coping, as reflected by their reduced levels of effort, high levels of discouragement, and deteriorated performance. Observations of these children indicate that the behavior of the two groups is quite similar prior to experiencing failure but differs dramatically following failure. The cognitive coping strategies used in response to failure distinguish the two groups (Dweck & Licht, 1980).

In early studies of causal attributions for achievement tasks, researchers found that mastery-oriented youngsters attribute success to their abilities and failure to changeable factors such as effort, whereas helpless children blame their failure on a lack of personal ability and see success as caused by variable factors (e.g., Dweck & Reppucci, 1973). When helpless children were taught to attribute failure to a lack of personal effort, improvements occurred in their persistence and level of performance (Dweck, 1975). Further, the attribution pattern of helpless children was found to occur more often in girls and to be linked to socialization practices observed in school classrooms (e.g., Dweck & Bush, 1976; Dweck, Davidson, Nelson, & Enna, 1978; Dweck, Goetz, & Strauss, 1980).

The role of causal attributions in these coping patterns was subsequently explored more extensively by using an alternative research design. In the early studies, an experimenter instructed the children to provide explanations for the cause of their performance. In a later series of studies, Diener and Dweck (1978, 1980) allowed children to freely report their thoughts while working on a similar achievement task. They found that the key difference between mastery-oriented and helpless children may not be in the types of attributions they make but in whether they generate attributions for the cause of their behavior at all. Few of the mastery-oriented children made any attributions of causality. Instead, they focused their thinking on problem-solving strategies, generating alternative solutions, and task-relevant information. Helpless children continued to focus their attention on an explanation for the cause of their failure and made attributions of cause to uncontrollable factors with high frequency. Dweck and Wortman (1982) hypothesized that the reactions of these children to success and failure in an achievement situation depend on the meaning of the outcome for the individual. They suggested that failure has self-evaluative meaning for helpless children and task-relevant information value for mastery-oriented children. The attribution search for an explanation of the cause of failure is short-circuited in the adaptive responders. This may have a dual benefit. First, they avoid focusing attention on the fact that they have failed and thereby avoid the aversive emotions associated with it. Second, they are free to invest more of their cognitive activity in trying to generate more adaptive coping strategies and, therefore, increase their likelihood of doing so.

Type A Behavior Pattern

The importance of more generalized coping styles is seen in studies of Type A behavior in children and adolescents. Descriptions of the antecedents of the Type A coronary-prone behavior pattern have been focused on personality styles or traits as determinants of coping behavior (e.g., Matthews, 1981, 1982). This style of responding has been observed in children and adolescents in contexts similar to those used in studying adults (e.g., Matthews, 1979; Matthews & Volkin, 1981). Based on laboratory and field research. Matthews (1981) conceptualized children's Type A behaviors as "a distinctive style of coping with potentially uncontrollable events" (p. 243). Emphasis is placed on the three major behavioral components of Pattern A—competitive achievement striving, a sense of time urgency and impatience, and aggressiveness-hostility. Viewed from a developmental perspective, these patterns in childhood and adolescence are seen as precursors of coronary heart disease in adulthood and are influenced by certain child-rearing practices (Matthews, 1977).

Empirical work concerning Type A behavior in children has entailed measurement development, generation of a base of descriptive information about the characteristics of Pattern A in children, and examination of factors that contribute to the development of Type A behavior. Of the four measures for assessment of Type A behavior in children, the Matthews Youth Test for Health (MYTH; Matthews & Angulo, 1980) is the most psychometrically sound (see Matthews, 1981, for a comparison of the different measures). Studies with the MYTH and other assessment instruments have provided a picture of the characteristics of Type A behavior in children. The Type A behavior pattern observed in children closely parallels the style observed in adults, especially in situations in which individuals feel threatened by a loss of control (Matthews, 1979). That is, Type A children make more efforts to control than do Type Bs when initially threatened by a loss of control. High levels of Type A behavior are inversely related to empathy level in children, suggesting that the competitive, impatient, and hostile feelings associated with Type A behavior distract the individual from concern about another's welfare (Matthews, Barnett, & Howard, 1979). Available developmental data have failed to reveal any effects of age on level of Type A behavior, but a consistent gender effect, with boys higher in Type A behavior than girls, has been reported at all ages (Matthews & Angulo, 1980).

Research on the antecedents of Type A behavior has been concentrated on familial influences, which include genetic factors, modeling of Type A behavior by parents, and child-rearing practices. Twin studies designed to assess genetic contributions to Type A behavior have produced conflicting findings, with no effects reported on structured interviews assessing Type A behavior but support for a genetic contribution when self-report measures have been used (Rahe, Hervig, & Rosenman, 1978). Matthews (1981) argued that any conclusions regarding genetic contributions to the Type A behavior pattern would be premature and must await further research that addresses methodological problems in prior studies. Similarly, data on the effects of parental modeling on children's Type A behavior are only at a preliminary level (e.g., Bortner, Rosenman, & Friedman, 1970; Matthews & Krantz, 1976). Data indicating the effects of child-rearing practices on Type A behavior are somewhat stronger. Glass (1977) reported that when observed in an experimental setting, Type A boys were treated differently than Type B boys by their mothers. Type A boys were given fewer positive evaluations of task performance than were Type B boys. Further, Type A boys were pushed to try harder than Type B boys, particularly by Type B mothers. Matthews (1977) found that this pattern of feedback was not elicited from female strangers, indicating that it is unlikely that Type A boys elicit these behaviors from their mothers.

More recently, attention has been focused on early temperament factors in the development of Type A behavior patterns in adulthood (Steinberg, 1985). In a follow-up of data from the New York Longitudinal Study, Steinberg found that temperament ratings obtained at ages 3 and 4 were significant predictors of Type A behavior 20 years later. Although the role of socialization and constitutional factors in the development of Type A patterns is not clear, this behavioral style appears to have roots very early in development and to be stable over time in at least some individuals.

Repression–Sensitization

The sixth conceptualization of coping during childhood and adolescence is similar to the notion of the Type A pattern in that it focuses on personality styles or traits. A number of investigators have argued that coping behavior can be assigned to a point on the unidimensional, bipolar personality characteristic of repression-sensitization (e.g., Bryne, 1964; Krohne & Rogner, 1982). Whereas individuals in the middle range of the continuum are considered to be coping adaptively, those at either end are viewed as responding maladaptively. Specifically, repressors neglect or avoid information in threatening situations, and sensitizers focus their attention on cues that indicate danger in such situations. Krohne (1979) suggested that these coping patterns depend on an individual's learning history, especially certain characteristics of family socialization. These characteristics include inconsistency in patterns of punishment and reward administered by parents, parental restriction of certain coping responses by the child, or failure to provide an adequate model of adaptive coping. Similarly, S. M. Miller (S. M. Miller, 1981; S. M. Miller & Green, 1984) has distinguished between two styles of coping that she has labeled "monitoring" and "blunting." Monitoring, similar to the strategies used by sensitizers, involves being alert for and sensitized to the negative or potentially negative aspects of an experience. Alternatively, blunting parallels repressing in that it involves distraction from and cognitively protecting oneself from sources of danger. S. M. Miller and her associates have not yet examined factors influencing the development of monitoring or blunting coping styles.

Empirical examinations of the repressor-sensitizer or monitor-blunter dimension in the coping styles of children and adolescents have been rare. Krohne (1979) reported two studies in which parental child-rearing practices were examined in relation to children's coping styles. Parental inconsistency, restrictiveness, and use of punishment were all related to repression-sensitization in children, providing preliminary support for Krohne's (1979) conceptualization. These associations were more pronounced for boys than for girls. Krohne cautioned that these studies were based on questionnaire data and should be viewed only as preliminary. No data are available on the psychological or behavioral outcomes of repression or sensitization in children.

Direct evidence on monitoring and blunting in children is also sparse. An extensive literature has developed, however, on the use of information-seeking and information-avoidant coping styles in children during uncontrollable aversive events (see S. M. Miller & Green, 1984). These studies have been focused on interventions designed to prepare children for dental or medical procedures (e.g., Burstein & Meichenbaum, 1979; Melamed, 1982; Melamed & Siegel, 1975; Siegel & Peterson, 1980). These procedures are characterized as highly aversive and beyond the personal control of children who undergo them. Interventions that facilitate selective attention to nonaversive aspects of the procedure, filtering of information about the event, distraction from salient aversive cures, and focusing attention on less threatening cures are associated with reduced arousal and anxiety (S. M. Miller & Green, 1984). Although the coping styles of monitoring and blunting have not been assessed in these studies, these findings indicate that increasing children's use of strategies similar to blunting in these situations is efficacious.

Resilience or Invulnerability to Stress

Finally, coping of children and adolescents has been described in studies of resilience or invulnerability to stress. This line of research grew from investigations of factors that predispose individuals or place them at risk for developing psychopathology. Findings from several studies have indicated that a portion of youngsters who have been exposed to grossly deprived or disadvantaged environments during development do not suffer emotional or psychological problems (e.g., Rutter, 1979). This has led to an interest in so-called *protective factors,* defined by Garmezy (1983) as "those attributes of persons, environments, situations, and events that appear to temper predictions of psychopathology based upon an individual's at-risk status" (p. 73). Interest has centered around stable characteristics of the child or the environment that reduce the potentially deleterious effects of chronic stressors.

Garmezy (1983) summarized five approaches to the study of invulnerability—(a) the epidemiological studies conducted by Rutter and his colleagues (Rutter, 1979; Rutter, Cox, Tupling, Berger, & Yule, 1975; Rutter, Yule, et al., 1975) on the Isle of Wight and in an inner-city area of London, (b) studies of competent black children in urban ghettos who have been exposed to the stressors of poverty and prejudice (see Garmezy, 1981), (c) a longitudinal-developmental study from birth to adulthood of a cohort of children born on the island of Kauai in the Hawaiian islands (Werner & Smith, 1982), (d) a longitudinal-developmental examination of ego resilience in children (Block & Block, 1980), and (e) studies of children growing up in war (e.g., Fields, 1977; Zuckerman-Bareli, 1982). Garmezy (1983) found that these diverse lines of investigation shared the following characteristics:

> (1) an emphasis on prospective developmental studies of children who (2) have been exposed to stressors of marked gravity (3) which can be accentuated by specific biological predispositions, familial and/or environmental deprivations (4) typically associated with a heightened probability of present or future maladaptive outcomes but (5) which are not actualized in some children whose behavior instead is marked by patterns of behavioral adaptation and manifest competence. (p.73)

These studies differ from most of the other literature concerned with coping during childhood and adolescence in that they have not emphasized what youngsters do to cope with stress. Instead, they have focused on the identification of stable, enduring characteristics of resilient children and their environments that distinguish them from others who respond maladaptively to stress. The following three broad factors have been consistently found to characterize invulnerable children across various studies (see Garmezy, 1983): (a) dispositional and constitutional characteristics of the child, including temperament, high self-esteem, internal locus of control, and autonomy; (b) the presence of a supportive family environment, including parental warmth, cohesiveness, closeness, and order and organization; and (c) a supportive individual or agency in the environment that provides the child with a support system to aid in coping and positive models for identification. Although the methodological rigor of these studies varies greatly, the consistency with which these themes have appeared is encouraging.

SUMMARY AND EVALUATION

Empirical investigations of coping during childhood and adolescence have generated a rich and interesting picture of the diverse nature of coping in these age groups. Psychometrically adequate measures of certain aspects of coping have been developed, research designs used in both laboratory and field settings have been sound, and many of the findings have been quite consistent and dramatic. Clearly, children and adolescents' efforts at coping can have a powerful effect in moderating the impact of stress. This research will now be discussed in terms of the three themes outlined in the introduction to this article.

Coping as Effortful Responses to Stress

In prior research concerned with child and adolescent coping, both reflexive and purposeful behavior has been addressed. Regarding the former, childhood temperament has been examined in studies of attachment and separation, Type A behavior patterns, and invulnerability to stress. Children's responses to stress appear to be influenced by dispositional factors, and these effects may carry into coping patterns during adulthood (e.g., Steinberg, 1985). On the other hand, effortful or purposeful responses to stress have been addressed extensively in the literature concerning child and adolescent coping. In particular, such behaviors are the central feature of interpersonal problem solving, coping in achievement contexts, and monitoring-blunting. However, similar to the study of coping during adulthood (Lazarus & Folkman, 1984), the concept of coping becomes meaningless when it is applied to both the broad domains of effortful and automatic behavior of children and adolescents. Coping needs to be distinguished from the whole of human development and adaptation. Thus, it seems necessary to limit the use of the term to a subset of adaptational actions involving effort (cf. Lazarus & Folkman, 1984; Murphy, 1974).

A central task facing researchers is to examine the relation between coping and reflexive or automatized adaptive behaviors. Initial work in this regard might focus on the relation between temperament and coping. Temperament factors may influence coping by restricting the range of coping responses of an individual or by affecting the types of situations perceived as stressful. Prospective longitudinal research is needed for examining whether the use of various problem- and emotion-focused coping strategies is affected by a child's temperamental style. For example, "difficult" infants who display low adaptability to change and intense negative emotional responses (Chess & Thomas, 1984) may have greater difficulty in developing a diverse set of coping strategies than more adaptable, less emotional infants. In a sense, a youngster may need to learn to cope with his or her own temperamental style, in addition to coping with stress in the environment. This would be more likely if the child's style is a poor match for the caretaking environment.

Functions of Coping

Studies of child and adolescent coping suggest that both problem- and emotion-focused coping are important in successful adaptation to stress. For example, Spivack and Shure have shown the importance of one type of problem-focused coping, cognitive problem solving. However, they indicated that other coping strategies aimed at emotional regulation may also be important to positive adjustment (Spivack & Shure, 1985). This is evident in studies showing the effectiveness of distraction and reframing (emotion-focused coping) in dealing with stressful medical procedures (S. M. Miller & Green, 1984). The importance of problem- and emotion-focused coping may vary in response to different types of stress or different points in time (see Suls & Fletcher, 1985, for a discussion of this issue regarding adults coping with health-related problems). Further, studies with adults indicate that both problem- and emotion-focused coping are used during almost all stressful episodes (Folkman & Lazarus, 1980, 1985) and that the use of relatively more problem- or emotion-focused coping varies in effectiveness across different types of stressors (Forsythe & Compas, in press).

Because both problem- and emotion-focused strategies are important in coping with stress, effective coping is likely to be characterized by flexibility and change. New demands require new ways of coping, and thus, no single coping strategy is effective for all types of stress. A closer examination of studies of child and adolescent coping indicates that a strategy that may be adaptive for dealing with one stressor may be maladaptive when used in a different context or at a different point in time in response to the same stressor. Several examples are offered to clarify this point. First, generating attributions for the cause of a stressful event has received mixed praise from researchers. An analysis of the cause of a problem is seen as a component of effective ICPS. Spivack and Shure (1982) stated, "The better adjusted individual not only weighs alternatives but sees a problem in the light of prior causes and later effects" (p. 329). In contrast, Dweck and her colleagues' findings, which indicate that effective copers (mastery-oriented children) did not attempt to generate attributions for the cause of failure, whereas helpless children did make causal attributions, have been cited. The situations in which attributions have been found to be beneficial, as opposed to harmful, differ in a number of ways. For example, it may be useful to analyze causes for personal or interpersonal problems but not for impersonal problems like the tasks in Dweck's studies. Alternatively, it may be useful to generate attributions at some points in time during a given stressful encounter but not at others. Spivack and Shure's (1982) subjects were analyzing the causes of an event that had already occurred. In contrast, Dweck studied children during a stressful encounter. Analyzing causes may facilitate coping after an event by helping prepare for similar stressful encounters in the future but impede coping during an event by distracting attention from more important features of the situation.

Similar disagreement exists about the effectiveness of cognitively "reframing" or avoiding certain features of a stressor. Attempts to enhance children's preparation for medical or dental procedures indicate that information about the event is most beneficial when it is presented in an attenuated form (S. M. Miller & Green, 1984). Selectively attending to less threatening aspects of the event, transforming how the event is cognitively processed, and even being distracted from the event itself have all been found to benefit children's coping. In contrast, Spivack and Shure (1982) argued that dysfunctional coping with interpersonal problems is characterized by daydreaming, fantasizing, and attempting to avoid or escape the problem. The stressful situations discussed by these authors may differ in the amount of personal control that children have or perceive that they have. Cognitive strategies to reframe a stressor may be beneficial when it appears beyond the personal control of an individual, as in the case of surgery. These strategies may not be useful, however, when dealing with an interpersonal problem over which one might have considerable control (cf. Forsythe & Compas, in press).

A related theme in the child and adolescent coping literature involves the costs and benefits that may result from particular coping strategies and resources. While researchers have focused almost exclusively on the positive consequences of various types of coping (i.e., reduction of psychological distress or somatic problems), it is apparent that coping has negative side effects as well. This is most apparent regarding social relationships and social support. Negative consequences of social support in adults have been identified in several lines of research (e.g., Kessler & McLeod, 1984; Rook, 1984). Adverse effects of social support include greater vulnerability to stress because of the loss of supportive others, experiencing the effects of stressful events in the lives of members of one's social network, and negative interpersonal exchanges with others. With regard to children and adolescents, the possible costs of social ties in early development are reflected in the attachment and separation literature. Infants classified as having formed an attachment to the mother, whether secure or insecure, experience maternal separation as stressful, whereas the avoidant group, infants considered not to have formed the attachment, does not display signs of distress. Thus, infants who have formed an attachment with the mother may be experiencing, for the first time, the costs and benefits of a close social bond. These processes are less clearly understood in later childhood and adolescence and should be a focus of future research.

Resources, Styles, and Specific Coping Efforts

The availability of personal and social resources for coping, cross-situational or temporally stable coping styles or both, and coping strategies used in specific situations have all been shown to be important in the efforts of children and adolescents to manage or overcome psychosocial stress. Although each of these factors appears to be important in coping, the distinction between them is somewhat blurred in the literature already described. Their importance as well as sources of confusion among them are briefly summarized.

With regard to resources, the importance of social resources to assist children in coping with stress is the focus of studies concerned with early social bonds and attachment, social support, and invulnerable children. Supportive relationships with parents or adults outside the family or both (Garmezy, 1983), peers (Cauce et al., 1982), and siblings (Sandler, 1980) have all been found to be resources for coping with stress. Personal resources that facilitate coping appear to include high self-esteem (Garmezy, 1983) and the requisite skills to solve interpersonal (Spivack & Shure, 1982) and impersonal problems (Dweck & Wortman, 1982).

To a certain extent, all of the literature reviewed here is concerned with coping styles. The invulnerability literature has examined broad dispositional factors related to positive adaptation under adverse circumstances, that is, the coping styles of those youngsters who adapt successfully. The social support literature is concerned with the use of support in coping across a variety of stressors in an individual's life. The other literature has been somewhat more limited in scope, focusing on the ways individuals cope with a specified type of stress. For example, interpersonal problems, achievement tasks, medical procedures, and uncontrollable situations have each been addressed separately. Children and adolescents are typically classified into groups based on their style of responding in a given type of stressful situation, and differences between the groups in symptoms and well-being are examined. For example, children characterized as mastery-oriented (i.e., those who generate alternative solutions to a problem, focus on task-relevant information, and use problem-solving strategies) functioned better than helpless children on achievement-related tasks. Thus, coping styles have been conceptualized at two levels. At the first, coping is assumed to be consistent across a wide variety of stressful situations, similar to a broad personality trait. At the second, coping is assumed to be consistent under similar circumstances but possibly vary as features of the environment or cognitive appraisals of the environment change (Compas, Forsythe, & Wagner, 1987). Among those coping styles whose adaptive consequences have been studied, it is apparent that no single style of coping is adaptive in all situations.

Finally, specific coping strategies have been examined in some detail in studies of interpersonal cognitive problem solving, coping on achievement tasks, monitoring-blunting, and social support. As already indicated, both problem- and emotion-focused strategies have been shown to be important in coping with stress. It has not been determined, however, which strategies are most effective in coping with which types of stress at what points in time.

Although the distinctions among coping resources, styles, and strategies have been important in conceptualizations of the coping process (e.g., Lazarus & Folkman, 1984; Menaghan, 1983), the differences among these concepts are not completely clear in the study of child and adolescent coping. In particular, researchers have failed to adequately distinguish between coping styles and specific strategies. That is, coping styles have typically been assessed through self-report measures that ask youngsters how they usually respond in a given type of situation or how they would respond in a hypothetical situation (e.g., Krohne & Rogner, 1982; Matthews & Angulo, 1980; Spivack & Shure, 1982). This method may, however, disguise variability in the coping strategies used by children and adolescents because they are not reporting on the ways they actually coped in different stressful episodes (see Lazarus & Folkman, 1984, pp. 128–130, for a discussion of this problem in studies of adult coping). Those investigators who have studied samples of children's coping in specific stressful situations (e.g., Dweck & Wortman, 1982; Hock & Clinger, 1981) have inferred that these samples of behavior represent styles of coping, at least in similar situations. This may be an accurate inference, but it remains to be tested by observing multiple samples of the coping behavior of the same children over time in similar situations.

Directions for Future Research

The first task confronting researchers interested in further clarifying the nature of coping during childhood and adolescence involves the development of comprehensive measures of coping that will allow for systematic comparisons of responses to different stressors and over time in response to the same stressful episode. Questionnaires for the assessment of coping styles or strategies used in a specific stressful encounter have been developed for adults (e.g., Billings & Moos, 1981; Folkman & Lazarus, 1985; Pearlin & Schooler, 1978). This has facilitated investigations of consistency and change in the ways adults cope with stress. Development of such a measure of child and adolescent coping will, in all probability, require different versions for various age groups to reflect changes in cognitive development and response capabilities. Whereas adult measures have typically relied on structured checklists, recent work with more open-ended formats (Stone & Neale, 1984) indicates that this may be a promising method to pursue with children and adolescents.

The second area for future research involves the relation between effortful coping responses and more stable, nonvolitional factors, such as temperament. This would serve to clarify further the distinction between coping and other adaptational responses to stress. In addition, research in this area might clarify the ways in which stable features of individuals limit or constrain the type of coping responses they are willing or able to use.

Third, the relation between various social contexts or ecologies and the coping behavior of children and adolescents needs to be examined in greater detail. Foremost among these is the role of the family. For example, it is unclear whether children learn some or much of their coping behavior through observations of their parents' efforts to manage stress in their own lives. Although several investigators have noted the potential importance of parental modeling of coping (e.g., Krohne, 1979; Matthews, 1981), these processes have received little attention in empirical studies. More broadly, socialization practices as a whole may influence the development and use of different coping strategies. Gender identity and sex-role socialization may affect the types of coping displayed by boys and girls, as suggested by the work of Dweck and her colleagues (e.g., Dweck & Bush, 1976; Dweck et al., 1978, 1980). Parents, teachers, and peers all influence children's values and beliefs, which may in turn either facilitate or impede the use of different coping strategies.

Finally, prospective longitudinal studies are needed for clarifying the ways in which coping resources, styles, and behaviors change or remain constant with development. Spivack and Shure's (1982, 1985) work indicates that cognitive problem-solving skills change with age, probably as a result of cognitive development. Similar changes probably occur in emotion-focused coping strategies, but this has not been investigated. Similar changes associated with social development may affect coping. For example, the changing nature of children's friendships (e.g., Hartup, 1983) indicates that the nature of social support may change with development.

In sum, research concerned with coping during childhood and adolescence has been conducted in several independent lines of investigation and has yielded numerous important findings. However, it now seems necessary to look for factors and processes that may be common to effective coping across a wide variety of stressful experiences. The important features of effective coping with failing an exam at school and with an argument with one's parents may ultimately differ substantially, but both may be characteristics of an individual who is capable of dealing purposefully and effectively with the wide-ranging demands that are part of human development.

REFERENCES

Ainsworth, M. D. S. (1979). Infant-mother attachment. *American Psychologist, 34,* 932–937.

Bandura, A. (1981). Self-referent thought: A developmental analysis of self-efficacy. In J. H. Flavell & L. Ross (Eds.), *Social cognitive development: Frontiers and possible futures* (pp. 200–239). Cambridge, England: Cambridge University Press.

Barrera, M. (1981). Social support in the adjustment of pregnant adolescents: Assessment issues. In B. H. Gottlieb (Ed.), *Social networks and social support* (pp. 69–96). Beverly Hills, CA: Sage.

Billings, A. G., & Moos, R. H. (1981). The role of coping responses in attenuating the impact of stressful life events. *Journal of Behavioral Medicine, 4,* 139–157.

Block, J. H., & Block, J. (1980). The role of ego-control and ego-resiliency in the organization of behavior. In W. A. Collins (Ed.), *Development of cognition, affect and social relations* (pp. 39–101). Hillsdale, NJ: Erlbaum.

Bortner, R. W., Rosenman, R. M., & Friedman, M. (1970). Familial similarity in Pattern A behavior. *Journal of Chronic Disease, 23,* 39–43.

Burstein, S., & Meichenbaum, D. (1979). The work of worrying in children undergoing surgery. *Journal of Abnormal Child Psychology, 7,* 121–132.

Byrne, D. (1964). Repression-sensitization as a dimension of personality. In B. A. Maher (Ed.), *Progress in experimental personality research* (Vol. 1, pp. 169–220). New York: Academic Press.

Cauce, A. M., Felner, R. D., & Primavera, J. (1982). Social support in high-risk adolescents: Structural components and adaptive impact. *American Journal of Community Psychology, 10,* 417–428.

Chess, S., & Thomas A. (1984). *Origins and evolution of behavior disorders: From infancy to early adult life.* New York: Brunner/Mazel.

Compas, B. E. (in press). Stress and life events during childhood and adolescence. *Clinical Psychology Review.*

Compas, B. E., Forsythe, C. J., & Wagner, B. M. (1987). *Consistency and variability in cognitive appraisals and coping with stress.* Manuscript submitted for publication.

Compas, B. E., Slavin, L. A., Wagner, B. M., & Vannatta, K. (1986). Relationship of life events and social support with psychological dysfunction among adolescents. *Journal of Youth and Adolescence, 15,* 205–221.

Compas, B. E., Wagner, B. M., Slavin, L. A., & Vannatta, K. (1986). A prosective study of life events, social support, and psychological symptomatology during the transition from high school to college. *American Journal of Community Psychology, 14,* 241–257.

Diener, C. I., & Dweck, C. S. (1978). An analysis of learned helplessness: Continuous changes in performance, strategy, and achievement cognitions following failure. *Journal of Personality and Social Psychology. 36,* 451–462.

Diener, C. I., & Dweck, C. S. (1980). An analysis of learned helplessness: II. The processing of success. *Journal of Personality and Social Psychology, 39,* 940–952.

Durlak, J. A. (1983). Social problem-solving as a primary prevention strategy. In R. D. Felner, L. A. Jason, J. N. Moritsugu, & S. S. Farber (Eds.), *Preventive psychology: Theory, research and practice* (pp. 31–48). New York: Pergamon Press.

Durlak, J. A. (1985). Primary prevention of school maladjustment. *Journal of Consulting and Clinical Psychology, 53,* 623–630.

Dweck, C. S. (1975). The role of expectations and attributions in the alleviation of learned helplessness. *Journal of Personality and Social Psychology, 31,* 674–685.

Dweck, C. S., & Bush, E. S. (1976). Sex differences in learned helplessness: I. Differential debilitation with peer and adult evaluators. *Developmental Psychology, 12,* 147–156.

Dweck, C. S., Davidson, W., Nelson, S., & Enna, B. (1978). Sex differences in learned helplessness: II. The contingencies of evaluative feedback and III: An experimental analysis. *Developmental Psychology, 14,* 268–276.

Dweck, C. S., Goetz, T. E., & Strauss, N. L. (1980). Sex differences in learned helplessness: IV. An experimental and naturalistic study of failure generalization and its mediators. *Journal of Personality and Social Psychology, 38,* 441–452.

Dweck, C. S., & Licht, B. G. (1980). Learned helplessness and intellectual achievement. In J. Garber & M. E. P. Seligman (Eds.), *Human helplessness: Theory and applications* (pp. 197–221). New York: Academic Press.

Dweck, C. S., & Reppucci, N. D. (1973). Learned helplessness and reinforcement responsibility in children. *Journal of Personality and Social Psychology, 25,* 109–116.

Dweck, C. S., & Wortman, C. B. (1982). Learned helplessness, anxiety, and achievement motivation: Neglected parallels in cognitive, affective, and coping responses. In H. W. Krohne & L. Laux (Eds.), *Achievement, stress, and anxiety* (pp. 93–125). Washington, DC: Hemisphere.

Felner, R. D., Ginter, M., & Primavera, J. (1982). Primary prevention during school transitions: Social support and environmental structure. *American Journal of Community Psychology, 10,* 277–290.

Fields, R. M. (1977). *Society under siege: Studies in childhood bereavement.* Philadelphia, PA: Temple University Press.

Folkman, S., & Lazarus, R. S. (1980). An analysis of coping in a middle-aged community sample. *Journal of Health and Social Behavior, 21,* 219–239.

Folkman, S., & Lazarus, R. S. (1985). If it changes it must be a process: A study of emotion and coping during three stages of a college examination. *Journal of Personality and Social Psychology, 48,* 150–170.

Forsythe, C. J., & Compas, B. E. (in press). Interaction of cognitive appraisals of stressful events and coping: Testing the goodness of fit hypothesis. *Cognitive Therapy and Research.*

Gad, M. T., & Johnson, J. H. (1980). Correlates of adolescent life stress as related to race, sex, and levels of perceived social support. *Journal of Clinical Child Psychology, 9,* 13–16.

Garcia Coll, C., Kagan, J., & Reznick, J. S. (1984). Behavioral inhibition in young children. *Child Development, 55,* 1005–1019.

Garmezy, N. (1981). Children under stress: Perspectives on antecedents and correlates of vulnerability and resistance to psychopathology. In A. I. Rabin, J. Aronoff, A. M. Barclay, & R. A. Zucker (Eds.), *Further explorations in personality* (pp. 196–269). New York: Wiley Interscience.

Garmezy, N. (1983). Stressors of childhood. In N. Garmezy & M. Rutter (Eds.), *Stress, coping and development in children* (pp. 43–84). New York: McGraw-Hill.

Glass, D. C., (1977). *Behavior patterns, stress, and coronary disease.* Hillsdale, NJ: Erlbaum.

Harter, S. (1983). Developmental perspectives on the self-system. In P. H. Mussen & E. M. Hetherington (Eds.), *Handbook of child psychology: Vol. 4. Socialization, personality, and social development* (pp. 275–385). New York: Wiley.

Hartup, W. W. (1983). Peer relations. In P. H. Mussen & E. M. Hetherington (Eds.), *Handbook of child psychology: Vol. 4. Socialization, personality, and social development* (pp. 103–196). New York: Wiley.

Hock, E. & Clinger, J. B. (1981). Infant coping behaviors, *Journal of Genetic Psychology, 138,* 231–243.

Hotaling, G. T., Atwell, S. G., & Linskey, A. A. (1978). Adolescent life changes and illness: A comparison of three models. *Journal of Youth and Adolescence, 7,* 393–403.

Kagan, J. (1983). Stress and coping in early development. In N. Garmezy & M. Rutter (Eds.), *Stress, coping, and development in children* (pp. 191–216). New York: McGraw-Hill.

Kagan, J. (1984). *The nature of the child.* New York: Basic Books.

Kaplan, H. B., Robbins, C., & Martin, S. S. (1983). Antecedents of psychological distress in young adults: Self-rejection, deprivation of social support, and life events. *Journal of Health and Social Behavior, 24,* 230–244.

Kessler, R. C., & McLeod, J. D. (1984). Sex differences in vulnerability to undesirable life events. *American Sociological Review, 49,* 620–631.

Krohne, H. W. (1979). Parental child-rearing behavior and the development of anxiety and coping strategies in children. In I. G. Sarason & C. D. Speilberger (Eds.), *Stress and anxiety* (Vol. 7, pp. 233–245). Washington, DC: Hemisphere.

Krohne, H. W., & Rogner, J. (1982). Repression-sensitization as a central construct in coping research. In H. W. Krohne & L. Laux (Eds.), *Achievement, stress, and anxiety* (pp. 167–193). Washington, DC: Hemisphere.

Lamb, M. E., Thompson, R. A., Gardner, W. P., Charnov, E. L., & Estes, D. (1984). Security of infantile attachment as assessed in the "strange situation": Its study and biological interpretation. *Behavioral and Brain Sciences, 7,* 127–171.

Lazarus, R. S., & Folkman, S. (1984). *Stress, appraisal and coping.* New York: Springer.

Leiderman, P. H. (1983). Social ecology and childbirth: The newborn nursery as environmental stressor. In N. Garmezy & M. Rutter (Eds.), *Stress, coping, and development in children* (pp. 133–159). New York: McGraw-Hill.

Lerner, J. V., Baker, N., & Lerner, R. M. (1985). A person-context goodness of fit model of adjustment. In P. C. Kendall (Ed.), *Advances in cognitive-behavioral research and therapy* (Vol. 4, pp. 111–136). New York: Academic Press.

Lerner, J. V., & Lerner, R. M. (1983). Temperament and adaptation across life: Theoretical and empirical issues. In P. B. Baltes & O. G. Brim, Jr. (Eds.), *Life-span development and behavior* (Vol. 5, pp. 197–231). New York: Academic Press.

Maccoby, E. E. (1983). Social-emotional development and response to stressors. In N. Garmezy & M. Rutter (Eds.), *Stress, coping and development in children* (pp. 217–234). New York: McGraw-Hill.

Maccoby, E. E., & Martin, J. A. (1983). Socialization in the context of the family: Parent-child interaction. In P. H. Mussen & E. M. Hetherington (Eds.), *Handbook of child psychology: Vol. 4. Socialization, personality and social development* (pp. 1–101). New York: Wiley.

Matthews, K. A. (1977). Caregiver-child interactions and the Type A coronary-prone behavior pattern. *Child Development, 48,* 1752–1756.

Matthews, K. A. (1979). Efforts to control by children and adults with the Type A coronary-prone behavior pattern. *Child Development, 50,* 842–847.

Matthews, K. A. (1981). "At a relatively early age . . . the habit of working the machine to its maximum capacity": Antecedents of the Type A coronary-prone behavior pattern. In S. S. Brehm, S. M. Kassin, & F. X. Gibbons (Eds.), *Developmental social psychology* (pp. 235–248). New York: Oxford University Press.

Matthews, K. A. (1982). Psychological perspectives on the Type A behavior pattern. *Psychological Bulletin, 91,* 293–323.

Matthews, K. A., & Angulo, J. (1980). Measurement of the Type A behavior pattern in children: Assessment of children's competitiveness, impatience-anger, and aggression. *Child Development, 51,* 466–475.

Matthews, K. A., Barnett, M. A., & Howard, J. A. (1979). *Children's empathic responses and the Type A behavior pattern.* Unpublished manuscript, University of Pittsburgh.

Matthews, K. A., & Krantz, D. S. (1976). Resemblances of twins and their parents in pattern A behavior. *Psychosomatic Medicine, 28,* 140–144.

Matthews, K. A., & Volkin, J. I. (1981). Efforts to excel and the Type A behavior pattern in children. *Child Development, 52,* 1283–1289.

Melamed, B. G. (1982). Reduction of medical fears: An information processing analysis. In J. Boulougouris (Ed.), *International symposium on practical applications of learning theories in psychiatry.* New York: Wiley.

Melamed, B. G., & Siegel, L. J. (1975). Reduction of anxiety in children facing hospitalization and surgery by use of filmed modeling. *Journal of Consulting and Clinical Psychology, 43,* 511–521.

Menaghan, E. G. (1983). Individual coping efforts: Moderators of the relationship between life stress and mental health outcomes. In H. B. Kaplan (Ed.), *Psychosocial stress: Trends in theory and research* (pp. 157–191). New York: Academic Press.

Miller, N. E. (1980). A perspective on the effects of stress and coping on disease and health. In S. Levine & H. Ursin (Eds.), *Coping and health* (NATO Conference Series III: Human Factors, pp. 323–353). New York: Plenum Press.

Miller, S. M. (1981). Predictability and human stress: Toward clarification of evidence and theory. In L. Berkowitz (Ed.), *Advances in experimental social psychology* (Vol. 14, pp. 203–255). New York: Academic Press.

Miller, S. M., & Green, M. L. (1984). Coping with stress and frustration: Origins, nature, and development. In M. Lewis & C. Saarni (Eds.), *The socialization of emotions.* New York: Plenum Press.

Moos, R. H., & Billings, A. G. (1982). Conceptualizing and measuring coping resources and processes. In L. Goldberger & S. Breznitz (Eds.), *Handbook of stress: Theoretical and clinical aspects* (pp. 212–230). New York: Free Press.

Murphy, L. B. (1974) Coping, vulnerability, and resilience in childhood. In G. V. Coelho, D. A. Hamburg, & J. E. Adams (Eds.), *Coping and adaptation* (pp. 101–124). New York: Basic Books.

Murphy, L. B., & Moriarity, A. E. (1976). *Vulnerability, coping, and growth.* New Haven, CT: Yale University Press.

Pearlin, L. I., & Schooler, C. (1978). The structure of coping. *Journal of Health and Social Behavior, 22,* 337–356.

Rahe, R. H., Hervig, L., & Rosenman, R. H. (1978). The heritability of Type A behavior. *Psychosomatic Medicine, 40,* 478–486.

Rook, K. S. (1984). The negative side of social interaction: Impact on psychological well-being. *Journal of Personality and Social Psychology, 46,* 1097–1108.

Ruble, D. N., & Rholes, W. S. (1981). The development of children's perceptions and attributions about their social world. In J. H. Harvey, W. Ickes, & R. F. Kidd (Eds.), *New directions in attribution research* (Vol. 3, pp. 1–36). Hillsdale, NJ: Erlbaum.

Rutter, M. (1979). Protective factors in children's responses to stress and disadvantage. In M. W. Kent & J. E. Rolf (Eds.), *Social competence in children* (pp. 49–74). Hanover, NH: University Press of New England.

Rutter, M. (1981). Stress, coping, and development: Some issues and some questions. *Journal of Child Psychology and Psychiatry, 22,* 323–356.

Rutter, M., Cox, A., Tupling, C., Berger, M., & Yule, W. (1975). Attainment and adjustment in two geographical areas: I. The prevalence of psychiatric disorder. *British Journal of Psychiatry, 126,* 493–509.

Rutter, M., Yule, B., Quinton, D., Rowlands, O., Yule, W., & Berger, M. (1975). Attainment and adjustment in two geographical areas: III. Some factors accounting for area differences. *British Journal of Psychiatry, 126,* 520–533.

Sandler, I. N. (1980). Social support resources, stress, and maladjustment of poor children. *American Journal of Community Psychology, 8,* 41–51.

Sandler, I. N., & Barrera, M. (1984). Toward a multimethod approach to assessing the effects of social support. *American Journal of Community Psychology, 12,* 37–52.

Sandler, I. N., & Lakey, B. (1982). Locus of control as a stress moderator: The role of control perceptions and social support. *American Journal of Community Psychology, 10,* 65–78.

Shure, M. B., & Spivack, G. (1978). *Problem-solving techniques in childrearing.* San Francisco, CA: Jossey-Bass.

Shure, M. B., & Spivack, G. (1980). Interpersonal problem-solving as a mediator of behavior adjustment in preschool and kindergarten children. *Journal of Applied Developmental Psychology, 1,* 29–43.

Siegel, L. J., & Peterson, L. (1980). Stress reduction in young dental patients through coping skills and sensory information. *Journal of Consulting and Clinical Psychology, 48,* 785–787.

Silver, R. L., & Wortman, C. B. (1980). Coping with undersirable life events. In J. Garber & M. E. P. Seligman (Eds.), *Human helplessness: Theory and applications* (pp. 279–340). New York: Academic Press.

Spivack, G., Platt, J. J., & Shure, M. B. (1976). *The problem solving approach to adjustment.* San Francisco, CA: Jossey-Bass.

Spivack, G., & Shure, M. B. (1982). The cognition of social adjustment: Interpersonal cognitive problem-solving thinking. In B. B. Lahey & A. E. Kazdin (Eds.), *Advances in clinical child psychology* (Vol. 5, pp. 323–372). New York: Plenum Press.

Spivack, G., & Shure, M. B. (1985). ICPS and beyond: Centripetal and centrifugal forces. *American Journal of Community Psychology, 13,* 226–243.

Steinberg, L. (1985). Early temperamental antecedents of adult Type A behaviors. *Developmental Psychology, 21,* 1171–1180.

Stone, A. A., & Neal, J. M. (1984). New measure of daily coping: Development and preliminary results. *Journal of Personality and Social Psychology, 46,* 892–906.

Suls, J., & Fletcher, B. (1985). The relative efficacy of avoidant and nonavoidant coping stategies: A meta-analysis. *Health Psychology, 4,* 249–288.

Werner, E. E., & Smith, R. S. (1982). *Vulnerable but invincible: A study of resilient children.* New York: McGraw-Hill.

Zuckerman-Bareli, C. (1982). The effect of border tension on the adjustment of kibbutzim and moshavim on the northern border of Israel. In C. D. Spielberger, I. G. Sarason, & N. A. Milgram (Eds.), *Stress and anxiety* (Vol. 8, pp. 81–91). Washington, DC: Hemisphere.

13

Temperament as a Moderator of Children's Stressful Experiences

Donald Wertlieb
Tufts University, Medford, Massachusetts
Carol Weigel and Tamar Springer
Institute for Health Research, Harvard Community Health Plan
Michael Feldstein
Department of Biostatistics, Harvard School of Public Health

Data on 158 children, six and nine years old, are analyzed for the relationship between stress and behavior. Undesirable life events and intense "hassles" were particularly correlated with behavioral symptoms. Statistically, temperament appears to moderate this influence but, lacking appreciable variance of symptoms in the models including these interaction effects, the more parsimonious main-effects concept may be more useful.

Clear and consistent relationships between stressful life experiences and problems in children's psychosocial adjustment and adaptation have been demonstrated during several decades of research.[13,14,19,35] Over the course of childhood, children and their families cope with numerous challenges and tasks which tax their resources. Some of these experiences can be regarded as major life events; for example, serious illness of a family member, divorce, death of a loved one, or relocation in a new school or neighborhood. Stress also emanates at the level of more ongoing or pervasive experiences which can be irritating or annoying. The daily functioning of children and their

Reprinted with permission from the *American Journal of Orthopsychiatry*, 1987, Vol. 57, No. 2, 234–245. Copyright 1987 by the American Orthopsychiatric Association, Inc.

Research was supported in part by the Institute for Health Research (a joint program of Harvard Community Health Plan and Harvard University), W. T. Grant Foundation grant 82083500, and National Institute of Mental Health grant MH 37970.

families involves such "hassles" as time pressures, inefficiency, or disruptions in routines. In his major critical review of the extant literature, Rutter[34] accentuated important individual differences in the organization and effect of these various stressors. Of particular concern is variation in relationships entailing a range of indices of health, developmental status, and behavioral symptomatology.

A focus on these relationships for the developing child in the context of the family is relatively recent, in contrast to a longer tradition of research and clinical interest in adults.[16,22] Shifting focus to children and families confronts the researcher with significant conceptual and methodological challenges, given the saliency of quantitative and qualitative developmental distinctions.[30,34,38] One popular strategy employs checklists of life-events, modeled after classical measures of life change and stress used with adults.[8,19,31] Through self-report or parent-report, stress is operationalized as a count of events or sum of distress weightings marked off on a comprehensive checklist of major events in the life of a child, such as illness of a parent, birth of a sibling, or marital separation of parents. Such stress scores are generally found to correlate moderately but significantly with behavioral symptomatology scores. Though important, these relationships are quite limited in meaning.

> Correlations of this magnitude (.20 to .30) indicate that life stress usually accounts for less than 10% of the variance in the dependent measures employed. Such findings suggest that life stress measures considered alone are not likely to be especially useful in predicting health and adjustment problems.[19]

Another strategy in adult stress research shows promise for inclusion in studies of child and family stress. Rather than rely only on the major life events noted above as indices of stress, Kanner *et al.*[20] included a measure of "daily hassles," relatively minor annoyances which may or may not be associated with the readjustment to experiences included on the more traditional major life events checklists. In a community sample of adults they found the stress index for daily hassles to be a significant predictor of psychological distress, with significantly increased amounts of the variance accounted for above and beyond variance accounted for by the major life events index. The extent to which this distinction may be evident in children is of concern in this and other reports of our work.[40] Technology for measuring hassles for children is only in its earliest stages.[21] The present report uses a maternal report of her daily hassles as one index of family stress.

The level of stress experienced by the major caretaker has been shown to be an important predictor of children's behavior problems.[4,5,9]

As noted above, researchers have been able to account consistently for about 10% of the variance in behavioral and adjustment problems with a range of measures of life stress. Recently, the necessity of considering moderator variables to account for some of the individual differences observed in the relationship has been emphasized. Moderator variables would include psychological or environmental elements which might buffer or mediate the impact of stress as it is manifest in behavioral symptoms. For instance, it has been demonstrated that stress effects can be reduced or buffered in a context of high levels of social support.[40] Another such moderator, temperament, a cluster of variables characterizing the style of an individual's behavior, figures centrally in several important conceptual frameworks for child development and mental health[36,37] as well as more specific formulations on the mediation of the effects of stress.[7,24,34]

> Temperament-environment interactions appear to play a contributing role in behavioral problems, the physiological disturbances of colic and night waking, the incidence of accidents and illness visits, minor developmental delay, and school performance. They seem likely to be involved also in child abuse, failure-to-thrive, obesity and other psychosomatic problems.[7]

The definition and measurement of temperament remain elusive and controversial.[11,25,27-29,32] The present study adopts the constructs and definitions of the New York Longitudinal Study[36,37] as operationalized in a parent-report measure, the Middle Childhood Temperament Questionnaire.[17] Nine dimensions of temperament are assessed, each involving individual differences that are constitutionally based and relatively stable, though not fixed, from infancy into adulthood. Each of the dimensions is defined in Table 1.

Considerable empirical evidence exists for individual differences in temperament in association with a range of developmental and health correlates and outcomes. However,

> . . . there is very little direct evidence on either the extent or nature of the contribution of temperament in modifying children's reactions to stress events. What are largely lacking are studies of the role of temperament in reactions to stress events.[34]

The few extant data are very supportive of the importance of such endeavors. In the landmark Kauai Longitudinal Study of vulnerability in a

Table 1. Dimensions of Temperament[2] (with Sample Items from the Middle Childhood Temperament Questionnaire[17])

ACTIVITY: The motor component of child's functioning. ("Jumps about or wiggles when talking to parents")	MOOD: The amount of pleasant, joyful and friendly behavior, as contrasted with unpleasant, crying and unfriendly behavior ("Cheerful or agreeable on waking up in the morning")
ADAPTABILITY: The ease with which initial responses are modified in the desired direction. ("Bothered by changing activities—play, reading, etc.—at parent's request")	PERSISTENCE: The continuation of an activity direction in the face of obstacles; related to attention span or the length of time the child pursues an activity. ("Loses interest as soon as difficulty arises when working on a project of his/her own choice")
APPROACH: The nature of the initial response to something new, a toy, food, person, etc. Displayed through mood expression or activity as approach or withdrawal. ("Approaches new visitors in the home")	PREDICTABILITY: The regularity or rhythmicity in timing and organization of biological functioning and other behavior. ("Remembers to do homework without being reminded")
DISTRACTIBILITY: The effectiveness of extraneous environmental stimuli in interfering or altering the direction of ongoing behavior. ("Looks up right away when telephone or doorbell rings")	THRESHOLD: The intensity level of stimulation that is necessary to evoke a discernible response regardless of the specific form that the response might take or the sensory modality affected. ("Notices differences in taste or consistency of food—brand, recipe, etc.")
INTENSITY: The energy level of behavior and responses, regardless of quality or direction. ("Laughs hard, shouts, squeals, etc. when happy")	

ᵃAdapted from Thomas and Chess.[37]

1955 birth cohort of 633 high-risk children, temperamental differences in activity level and social responsiveness or approach were key discriminators of resilient versus problem-plagued children. Active, approach-oriented styles were associated with positive outcomes.[39]

In examining the specific stressful situation of integrating a newly born child into the family, Dunn and Kendrick[12] reported significant correlations between temperament and changes in children's behavior after the birth of the sibling. Further, these individual differences interacted with the mother's emotional state and with the quality of mother-child interaction.

> The implication is that the child's temperamental features increased the liability to behavioral changes after the birth of a sibling, but that this increased liability was due in part to the effect of temperamental features in modifying children's responses to altered parental behavior.[34]

Whether these relationships are evident in the context of other major stressors or cumulative stress is among the foci of this report.

These studies, along with the theoretical and conceptual frameworks cited earlier, emphasized the importance of considering individual differences in temperament as a possible buffer or moderator of the relationship between stress and behavioral symptoms. This paper presents initial findings from an ongoing longitudinal study of stress and coping processes in childhood. The specific questions addressed are:

1. What are the relationships among stress, temperament and behavioral symptoms in school-age children?
2. How do alternative measurements of stress alter our view of these relationships?
3. To what extent is temperament a moderator of the relationship between stress and behavioral symptoms?

METHOD

Participants

Participants in this study were 158 children and their mothers, volunteers from a large health maintenance organization (HMO), enrolled in a longitudinal study of stress and health. Each family with a six- or nine-year-old child was contacted by mail and telephone follow-up. One hundred and twenty five of the families, our "normative" group, were selected on a stratified random basis from a pool of volunteers with two-parent homes, two years' membership in the HMO, and no record of use of mental health services. The sample was enriched with 33 volunteers from a pool of families who had experienced a marital separation or divorce within the four year period prior to study entry, thus having a greater likelihood of experiencing a series of stressful events associated with marital disruption. These families were identified in the initial mail and telephone follow-up mentioned above. They, too, had at least two years membership in the HMO but there was no exclusion on the basis of mental health utilization. These families constituted a relatively "high stress" group though, as will be noted below, they differed from our "normative" group on very few of the variables under study. Stratification aimed at an even distribution by gender and geographical representation of the HMO population. Table 2 describes the sample in sociodemographic terms.

MEASURES

As part of an extensive battery of measures administered in home visits during the first year of the study, the following instruments generated data on stress level, temperament, and behavioral symptomatology.

The Life Events Scale (LES)[8] is a 35-item checklist of major events experienced by children. Ten events comprise a subscale of undesirable events

Table 2. Sample Sociodemographics

FACTOR	TOTAL (N = 158)	NORMA- TIVE (n = 125)	HIGH STRESS (n = 33)
Age Cohort			
6 yr. old	93	76	17
9 yr. old	65	49	16
Age in months			
Mean	96.47	95.86	98.76
SD	19.2	19.2	19.4
Gender			
boys	79	64	15
girls	79	61	18
Socioeconomic Status[a]			
Mean	55.26	55.76	53.39
SD	9.0	9.5	6.9

[a]Hollingshead[18] Four Factor Index reflecting an upper middle and upper class sample of professional, business and technical occupations.

such as death of a parent, hospitalization of a sibling, or failure to achieve something a child really wanted. A set of eight events comprises a subscale of desirable events, such as recognition for excelling in a sport. An additional set of 17 items is considered as family events, such as birth of a sibling. In completing the LES, the mother indicated which events and how many times each event had happened to the target child during the previous twelve-month period. Scoring takes these frequencies into account as well as universalized weightings of stressfulness derived from professional judgments. Data on reliability and validity are presented by Coddington.[8]

The Hassles Scale[20] is a 116-item check-list of "daily hassles," relatively minor experiences or events commonly encountered in the course of daily living (*e.g.*, inconsiderate smokers, too many interruptions, misplacing or losing things). Mothers indicated which hassles they had experienced in the previous thirty days and rated each on a three-point scale of mildly, moderately, or extremely severe. Thus, the family's level of stress is indexed by the mean severity of the mother's hassles ratings. Reliability and validity data were reported by Kanner *et al.*[20] and Delongis *et al.*[10]

The Middle Childhood Temperament Questionnaire (MCTQ)[17] is a 99-item parent-report form using six-point frequency scales. The temperament categories assessed, along with sample items, are defined in Table 1. Reliability and validity data were reported by Hegvik *et al.*[17] and Maziade *et al.*[29]

The Child Behavior Checklist (CBC)[2] provides parent reports of symptomatic behavior frequency and severity over the past year. A total score based on the 113 items, as well as Internalizing and Externalizing scale scores are generated. Norms, reliability, and validity data were reported by Achenbach and Edelbrock.[1,2] Analyses reported here use the standardized scores (*T*-scores) provided by Achenbach and Edelbrock.[2]

Data analyses mapped relationships among stress, temperament, and behavioral symptoms, guided by the research questions noted above. In correlational and multiple regression analyses, indices of stress and temperament were investigated as predictors of behavioral symptom outcomes.

RESULTS

Data were examined for group differences in terms of age, gender, and stress group. In testing for such differences, no effect of gender was evident, therefore data from boys and girls were pooled. Only one variable showed a statistically significant age difference, with older children scoring higher on undesirable life events ($t = 2.02, p < .05$). Data from both age groups were pooled and the influence of this single group difference was tested in subsequent analyses where appropriate. When differences between the normative and high stress group were examined, two of the four indices of stress differentiated the groups in the expected direction. The high stress group experienced more family events ($t = 3.93, p = .0001$) and higher intensity of hassles ($t = 2:56, p = .01$). Table 3 presents means and standard deviations for each study variable.

Relationships among the variables were then examined, in response to the research questions noted above. They were first examined with Pearson product-moment correlations. This analysis addresses some aspects of the research questions as well as identifying data reduction possibilities. Within the stress indices, Coddington Life Events subscales correlated strongly with the Total Scale Score (each $p < .0001$) but only minimally to moderately with one another. Desirable and undesirable events related most strongly to each other ($r = .44, p < .0001$). Family events did not relate significantly to either desirable or undesirable events subscale scores. The Hassles score correlated moderately and significantly with undesirable events ($r = .34, p < .001$) and family events ($r = .18, p < .03$). Hassles and desirable events were unrelated ($r = .12$, NS). Given this set of relationships, all four stress variables—three life events subscales and the hassles intensity score—were retained for subsequent analyses.

A considerable degree of overlap is evident in the temperament scale scores. The matrix of correlations is presented in Table 4. The correlations are generally consistent with some of the theoretical and clinical clustering proposed in the literature;[17,37] however, a sound psychometric basis for

Table 3. Means (and Standard Deviations) of Stress, Temperament, and Behavioral Symptomatology for Normative and High Stress Children

FACTOR	TOTAL (*N* = 158)	NORMATIVE (*n* = 125)	HIGH STRESS (*n* = 33)	GROUP DIFFERENCES*
Stress				
Life Events				
Desirable	105.69(97.9)	107.28(99.4)	99.67(93.1)	NS
Undesirable	55.04(74.8)	50.26(76.8)	73.18(64.4)	*p* = .09
Family	68.15(81.1)	54.62(74.2)	119.39(86.7)	*p* = .0001
Hassles	0.28 (.21)	0.26 (.19)	0.38 (.26)	*p* = .01
Temperament				
Activity	3.38 (.89)	3.43 (.91)	3.18 (.78)	NS
Adaptability	2.86 (.74)	2.85 (.74)	2.89 (.78)	NS
Approach	2.63 (.97)	2.63 (.98)	2.64 (.97)	NS
Distractibility	3.94 (.97)	3.97 (1.0)	3.82 (.76)	NS
Intensity	3.76 (.86)	3.78 (.90)	3.67 (.71)	NS
Mood	3.00 (.69)	2.96 (.69)	3.14 (.71)	NS
Persistence	2.67 (.75)	2.65 (.71)	2.74 (.87)	NS
Predictability	2.88 (.72)	2.86 (.69)	2.94 (.82)	NS
Threshold	3.67 (.72)	3.70 (.72)	3.55 (.71)	NS
Behavioral Symptoms				
Total Severity	54.10(10.7)	53.98(10.8)	54.55(10.5)	NS
Internalizing	55.17(10.3)	54.73(10.0)	56.85(11.2)	NS
Externalizing	53.06(10.2)	53.06(10.5)	53.09 (9.4)	NS

*t-test.

Table 4. Pearson Correlations Between Temperament Subscales (N = 158)

CHARACTERISTIC	1	2	3	4	5	6	7	8
1. Activity								
2. Adaptability	.36***							
3. Approach	.07	.29**						
4. Distractibility	.35***	.24**	−.01					
5. Intensity	.62***	.39***	−.06	.17*				
6. Mood	.34***	.64***	.24**	.18*	.41***			
7. Persistence	.47***	.49**	.19*	.27**	.25**	.45**		
8. Predictability	.44***	.49**	.11	.17*	.33***	.43***	.65***	
9. Threshold	.16*	.13	.08	.44***	.19**	.19**	−.03	.07

*p<.05; **p<.01; ***p<.0001.

demarcating these clusters in a valid and reliable manner in not yet available, so each scale score was retained in the analyses that follow.

In terms of behavioral symptomatology, the externalizing and internalizing scores were highly correlated with on another (r = .77, p < .0001) and each with the total score (r = .93, p < .0001). Because of the important clinical and conceptual distinctions between the scales, they were retained for analysis despite the covariation.

The bivariate relationships between stress indices and behavioral symptoms were strong. There were statistically significant relationships between stress indices and behavioral symptoms and between all but one of the nine temperament dimensions and behavioral symptoms. The magnitude and statistical significance of these bivariate relationships is documented in Table 5.

The analyses thus far document statistically significant relationships between stress and behavioral symptoms and between temperament and behavioral symptoms. A more refined mapping of these relationships requires simultaneous consideration of both sets of variables as well as explicit examination of possible mediating or buffering influences. A series of stepwise multiple regression models was generated to articulate these issues.

To evaluate the main effects of life events, hassles, and temperament, each LES subscale score, hassles intensity score, and the nine temperament scale scores were entered into a step-wise multiple regression procedure along with background or classifying variables, including the child's age group, gender, socioeconomic status,[18] and stress group (normative *vs* high stress). Table 6 depicts the resulting model which accounts for 55% of the variance in total behavioral symptom scores ($p < .0001$). Both undesirable life events and daily hassles exerted significant main effects, as did five of the nine temperament scales. That the two stress indices each contributed independently and significantly to the model suggests the importance of considering both conceptualizations of stress in articulating the relationship between stress and behavioral symptoms. In none of the multiple regression analyses did the group classification of normative *vs* high stress emerge as significant.

Table 5. Percent of Variance Shared Among Stress, Temperament, and Behavioral Symptoms ($N = 158$)

CATEGORY	TOTAL BEHAVIORAL SYMPTOMS	EXTERNALIZING SYMPTOMS	INTERNALIZING SYMPTOMS
Stress			
Desirable Events	01	02	00
Undesirable Events	08*	08*	06*
Family Events	01	00	01
Hassles	16**	11**	18**
Temperament			
Activity	22**	29**	10**
Adaptability	32**	36**	23**
Approach	06*	02	10**
Distractibility	11**	12	09*
Intensity	20**	27**	11**
Mood	24**	23**	20**
Persistence	23**	24**	16**
Predictability	20**	23**	14**
Threshold	01	01	01

*p<.01; **p<.0001.

Table 6. Multiple Regression Model—Main Effects of Life Events, Hassles, and Temperament in Predicting Total Behavioral Symptoms

VARIABLE[a]	REGRESSION COEFFICIENT	F-STATISTIC[c]	p-VALUE
Adaptability	3.55	12.30	.0006
Approach	1.79	7.42	.0072
Intensity	3.46	20.03	.0001
Distractibility	2.19	9.27	.0028
Threshold	−1.96	4.13	.0439
Persistence	1.63	2.74	.0998
Undesirable Events	.02	5.24	.0234
Desirable Events	−.01	2.65	.1056
Hassles	10.62	12.07	.0007
Intercept	17.45		
Total Model[b]			
$R^2 = .55$		20.37	.0001

[a]Also allowed to compete in the stepwise procedure, but not entering into the model as significant were: age group, gender, SES, family events score, mood, activity, predictability.
[b]$N = 158$.
[c]F-statistic based on the Type III Sum of squares.

Separate regression analyses predicting total behavioral symptoms were performed, first using only the life events subscales and then only the hassles score as stress indices. Highly significant models emerged in each instance, along with significant independent contributions by temperament scales. With life events variables as the stress indices, a model with $R^2 = .50$ ($p < .001$) included undesirable events ($p < .01$) and five temperament scales. In another model, hassles was the only stress index ($p < .001$), $R^2 = .47$ ($p < .0001$), along with Activity and Adaptability as significant temperament predictors ($p < .0001$).

These analyses provide strong evidence for important "main effects" of stress and temperament on behavioral symptoms. Our third research question examines the notion of temperament as a moderator or buffer of the relationship between stress and symptoms. Empirical substantiation of such an influence would require demonstration of "stress × temperament" interaction effects in regression models such as those presented above. Table 7 presents the model which emerges when such interaction terms are included in a multiple regression analysis. Each significant main effect from the preceding model (Table 6), along with a stress × temperament cross-product for each was allowed to compete in a stepwise procedure predicting total behavioral symptom scores. The model accounted for 56% of the variance ($p < .0001$). Stress indices were retained only as parts of interaction terms. Two temperament scales exhibited significant main effects, Adaptability ($p < .0001$) and Intensity ($p < .0001$), while three additional scales entered as elements of interaction terms. The findings are similar when each stress index

Table 7. Multiple Regression Model—Interaction Effects, Stressful Life Events, Hassles, and Temperament Predicting Total Behavioral Symptoms

VARIABLE[a]	REGRESSION COEFFICIENT	F-STATISTIC[c]	p-VALUE
Adaptability	4.28	22.12	.0001
Intensity	3.58	23.04	.0001
Distractibility × Undesirable Events	.004	4.36	.0384
Distractibility × Hassles	7.36	21.05	.0001
Threshold × Hassles	−8.72	19.51	.0001
Approach × Hassles	6.46	13.84	.0003
Intercept	23.36		
Total Model[b] $R^2 = .56$		31.67	.0001

[a]Also allowed to compete in the stepwise procedure but not entering the model as significant were: age group, gender, SES, approach, distractibility, threshold, undesirable events, hassles, and all other hassles × temperament, and undesirable events × temperament interaction terms derived from statistically significant main effects reported above in TABLE 6.
[b]$N = 158$.
[c]F-statistic based on the Type III sum of squares.

is considered separately, with those models accounting for slightly less variance, though each is highly significant.

Each model was also run substituting the Internalizing or Externalizing Behavioral Symptom score as the outcome. As would be expected, given the relationship between these and with the Behavioral Symptom Total, each model was highly significant ($p < .0001$). There was some important variation in which specific temperament dimensions were represented in the different models, as depicted in Table 8. Six of the nine temperament scales are included either through main or interaction effect in one or another of the three models. All three models include adaptability, intensity and distractability as elements of the predictive model. Predictability, persistence, or mood are not represented in any of the three models. All three models are highly significant. The relationship among stress, temperament, and symptomatology accounts for more variance in externalizing symptoms ($R^2 = .61$) than in internalizing symptoms ($R^2 = .46$).

DISCUSSION

The findings presented here address each of the research questions raised above. So far as the relationships among stress, temperament, and behavioral symptoms are concerned, the data reveal that there are several highly significant relationships to be considered. Higher levels of stress, whether measured in terms of undesirable life events or daily hassles, are associated with higher levels of behavioral symptoms. Eight of the nine temperament dimensions assessed showed highly significant associations with behavioral symptomatology, all in the expected direction (Table 5). When considered simultaneously in multiple regression analyses, six of the nine dimensions are included as significant. The following temperament orientations are associated with behavioral symptoms: high activity level, low adaptability, withdrawal from new stimuli, distractability, high intensity, unpleasant or unhappy mood, a lack of persistence, and an irregular or unpredictable behavioral style. The similarity between what might be called behavioral problems and "difficult" temperament, and the possible circularity of this conceptualization will be further considered below.

Temperament appears to be differentially related to internalizing and externalizing behavioral symptomatology. Dimensions of high activity, high distractability, and a low threshold of stimulation are more relevant to externalizing problems than to internalizing problems. Withdrawal is more relevant to internalizing problems, as would be expected. Interestingly, mood, which might be supposed to be most strongly related to internalizing problems, is excluded from the multiple regression models (Tables 6–8), though the bivariate relationships are significant (Table 5).

The second question concerned the effect of alternative measurements of stress on our view of these relationships. Recent conceptualizations and empirical data from adults[10,20] as well as our recent report on stress and social support in children[40] distinguished stress associated with major life events from stress associated with daily hassles. Findings reported above indicate that this distinction should also be applied in relating temperament to behavioral symptoms. The stress associated with undesirable life events and the stress associated with higher intensity of daily hassles make independent,

Table 8. Temperament Characteristics and Temperament/Stress Interactions Included in Models Predicting Behavioral Symptomatology

statistically significant contributions to the variation in behavioral symptomatology (Table 6). In addition, there are differences in how these stressors interact with temperament as factors in behavioral symptoms (Table 7). A current controversy in the measurement of stress in childhood centers on the distinction between chronic stressful conditions (*e.g.,* poverty) and major life events.[15] Our data indicate that the relatively more immediate or microscopic sources of stress operationalized as daily hassles must also be included in the debate.

The third research question asked to what extent temperament is a moderator of the relationship between stress and behavioral symptoms. The identification of a statistically significant interaction is often put forth as evidence of a buffering or moderating effect in the stress and illness relationship.[23] A number of such highly significant effects are included in the models presented above (Tables 7 and 8). However, when a model using only main effects (Table 6) is compared to the model with interaction terms (Table 7), the increase in the magnitude of R^2 is relatively small, a difference between 55% and 56%. Though statistical evidence for stress buffering is obtained, the failure of these effects to enhance the predictive power of the model suggests that the simpler, more parsimonious, independent main-effects model is as useful, if not more so.

These findings lend further empirical support to the notion that temperament is relevant to socioemotional functioning and the outcome of stress reactions in school-age children.[24] These cross-sectional data do not directly address the more complex theoretical questions facing researchers as to whether personal explanations or "goodness-of-fit" explanations capture better the nature of temperament context interactions.[41] Rutter[33] criticized Cameron's[6]

> geological metaphor of temperament reflecting "fault lines" in the emerging personality so that behavioral "earthquakes" arise in those children with "fault lines" who experience environmental strain. (p.14)

How particular temperamental patterns may be "faulty" or may put a child at risk remains unclear. The data do support an association between certain temperamental characteristics and behavioral symptoms, as well as relationships with a range of stressors. Greater specification of these developmental or psychopathological processes depends upon results of longitudinal analyses.

An important set of limitations on the findings reported here involves the considerable conceptual and methodological controversy that surrounds each of the stress and temperament predictor variables. Some of this debate is the direct focus of the research questions, *i.e.,* the relative contributions of "major life events" and "daily hassles" measures of stress. Other debates are sidestepped through assumptions and commitments to particular applications of the construct. For example, considerable problems are inherent in a reliance upon parent report for assessment of temperament.[3,27] The longitudinal study from which these findings emerge will include a child self-report of temperament[26] which will be included in forthcoming reports and thus address some of these problems.

Another limitation inherent in the simultaneous use of a parental assessment of temperament and a parental assessment of behavioral problems is the overlap, even confusion, in terms of vocabulary or description. Though conceptually quite distinct, operationally there is a sufficient degree of item similarity to warrant caution in interpreting the large R^2 values reported above. Some items are really identical on the behavioral problem and temperament scales. For instance, "Fidgets when he has to stay still" is an item on the Activity Scale of the MCTQ; "Can't sit still, restless or hyperactive" is an item on the Externalizing Behavior Scale of the CBCL. Some of the shared variance is obviously related to this circularity. Yet, independent and conceptually-relevant distinctions are apparent in the results reported above. The activity scale and externalizing behavioral symptom score are significantly but moderately correlated ($r = .52, p < .0001$). It will be important for future research to refine the search for correlations with item and subscale analyses, controlling for this circularity and correcting for biases emerging from a single source for both assessments.

The data reported here represent a pioneering effort to examine the relationships among stress, temperament, and behavioral symptoms in middle childhood. We have recently reported a related set of analyses examining the role of social support as a moderator of stress.[40] The present study provides evidence for Lerner and East's[24] hypothesis that "temperament may be a quite salient moderator of a person's reactions to stressors" (p. 158). As our study progresses, we will test their assertion that,

> not only does temperament moderate other intraindividual moderators of stress reactions, but it interacts . . . with key contextual moderators such as social support. (p. 158)

The documentation of these relationships in concurrent predictive models is of major interest to research and application in childhood stress and coping and developmental psychopathology. Even more important will be the construction of the longitudinal prospective models which will be presented as our efforts continue.

REFERENCES

1. Achenbach, T. and Edelbrock, C. 1981. Behavioral problems and competencies reported by parents of normal and disturbed children aged four through sixteen. Monger. Soc. Res. Child Devlpm. 46:1–82.
2. Achenbach, T. and Edelbrock, C. 1983. Manual for the child behavior checklist and revised child behavior profile. Privately published, Burlington, Vt.
3. Bates J.E. 1980. The concept of difficult temperament. Merrill-Palmer Quart. 26(4):299–319.
4. Belle D., ed. 1982. Lives in Stress: Women and Depression. Sage, Beverly Hills.
5. Bond, C.R. and McMahon, R.J. 1984. Relationships between marital distress and child behavior problems, maternal personal adjustment, maternal personality, and maternal parenting behavior. J. Abnorm. Psychol. 93(4):348–351.
6. Cameron, J.R. 1978. Parental treatment, children's temperament, and the risk of childhood behavioral problems. 2: initial temperament, parental attitudes, and the incidence and form of behavioral problems. Amer. J. Orthopsychiat. 48:141–147.
7. Carey, W.B. 1981. The importance of temperament-environment interaction for child health and development. *In* The Uncommon Child, M. Lewis and L. Rosenblum, eds. Plenum Press, New York.
8. Coddington, R.D. 1984. Measuring the stressfulness of a child's environment. *In* Stress in Childhood, J.H. Humphrey, ed. AMS Press, New York.
9. Conger R.D. et al. 1984. Perception of child, child-rearing values, and emotional distress as mediating links between environmental stressors and observed maternal behavior. Child Devlpm. 55:2234–2247.
10. Delongis, A. et al. 1982. Relationship of daily hassles, uplifts and major life events to health status. Hlth Psychol. 1:119–136.
11. Derryberry, D. and Rothbart, M.K. 1984. Emotion, attention, and temperament. *In* Emotions, Cognition, and Behavior, C.E. Izard, J. Kagan, R.B. Zajonc, eds. Cambridge University Press, Cambridge.
12. Dunn, J. and Kendrick, C. 1980. Studying temperament and parent-child interaction: comparison of interview and direct observation. Devlpm. Med. Child Neurol. 22:494–496.
13. Felner, R. 1984. Vulnerability in childhood: a preventive framework for understanding children's efforts to cope with life stress and transitions. *In* Prevention of Problems in Childhood, M. Roberts and L. Peterson, eds. John Wiley, New York.
14. Garmezy, N. and Rutter, M., eds. 1983. Stress, Coping and Development in Children. McGraw-Hill, New York.
15. Gersten, J.C. et al, 1977. An evaluation of the etiologic role of stressful life-change events in psychological distress. J. Hlth Soc. Behav. 18:228–244.
16. Goldberger, L. and Breznitz, S., eds. 1982. Handbook of Stress: Theoretical and Clinical Aspects. Free Press, New York.
17. Hegvik, R.L., McDevitt, S.C. and Carey, W.B. 1982. The middle childhood temperament questionnaire, J. Devlpm. Behav. Pediat. 3(4): 197–200.

18. Hollingshead, A.B. 1975. Four factor index of social status. Unpublished manuscript.
19. Johnson, J.H. 1982. Life events as stressors in childhood and adolescence. *In* Advances in Clinical Child Psychology, Vol. 5, B. Lahey and A. Kazdin, eds. Plenum Press, New York.
20. Kanner, A.D. et al. 1981. Comparison of two modes of stress measurement: daily hassles and uplifts versus major life events. J. Behav. Med. 4:1–39.
21. Kanner, A.D., Harrison, A., and Wertlieb, D. 1985. The development of the children's hassles and uplifts scales: a preliminary report. Presented to the American Psychological Association, Los Angeles.
22. Kaplan, H.B., ed. 1983. Psychosocial Stress: Trends in Theory and Research. Academic Press, New York.
23. Kessler, R.C. 1983. Methodological issues in the study of psychosocial stress. *In* Psychosocial Stress: Trends in Theory and Research, H.B. Kaplan, ed. Academic Press, New York.
24. Lerner, R.M. and East, P.L. 1984. The role of temperament in stress, coping and socioemotional functioning in early development. Infant Ment. Hlth J. 5(3):148–159.
25. Lerner, J.V. and Lerner, R.M. eds. 1986. New Directions for Child Development, Vol. 31: Temperament and Social Interaction in Infants and Children. Jossey-Bass, San Francisco.
26. Lerner, R.M. et al. 1982. Assessing the dimensions of temperamental individuality across the life span: the dimensions of temperament survey (DOTS). Child Devlpm. 53:149–159.
27. Lyon, M.E. and Plomin, R. 1981. The measurement of temperament using parental ratings. J. Child Psychol. Psychiat. 22:47–53.
28. Martin, R.P. and Holbrook, J. 1985. Relationship of temperament characteristics to the academic achievement of first-grade children. J. Psychoed. Assess. 3:131–140.
29. Maziade, M. et al. 1986. Family correlates of temperament continuity and change across middle childhood. Amer. J. Orthopsychiat. 56(2):195–203.
30. Menaghan, E. 1983. Individual coping efforts and family studies: conceptual and methodological issues. Marr. Fam. Rev. [Special issue] 6(½):113–135.
31. Monaghan, J.H., Robinson, J.O., and Dodge, J.A. 1979. Children's life events inventory. J. Psychosomat. Res. 23:63–68.
32. Porter, R. and Collins, G., eds. 1982. Ciba Foundation Symposium 89: Temperamental Differences in Infants and Young Children. Pitman Books, London.
33. Rutter, M. 1982. Temperament: concepts, issues and problems. *In* Ciba Foundation Symposium 89: Temperamental Differences in Infants and Young Children, R. Porter & G. Collins, eds. Pitman Books, London.
34. Rutter, M. 1983. Stress, coping, and development: some issues and some questions. *In* Stress, Coping, and Development in Children, N. Garmezy & M. Ruttter, eds. McGraw-Hill, New York.
35. Sterling, S. et al. 1985. Recent stressful life events and young children's school adjustment. Amer. J. Comm. Psychol. 13(1):87–98.
36. Thomas, A. and Chess, S. 1981. The role of temperament in the contributions of individuals to their development. *In* Individuals as Producers of Their Development, R.M. Lerner and N.A. Busch-Rossnagel, eds. Academic Press, New York.

37. Thomas A., and Chess, S. 1984. Genesis and evolution of behavioral disorders: from infancy to early adult life. Amer. J. Psychiat. 14(1):1–9.
38. Walker, A.J. 1985. Reconceptualizing family stress. J. Marr. Fam. 47(4): 827–837.
39. Werner, E.E. and Smith, R.S. 1982. Vulnerable but Invincible: A Study of Resilient Children. McGraw-Hill, New York.
40. Wertlieb, D., Weigel, C., and Feldstein, M. 1987. Stress, social support and behavior symptoms in middle childhood. J. Clin. Child Psychol. (in press)
41. Windle, M. and Lerner, R.M. 1986. The "goodness of fit" model of temperament-context relations: interaction or correlation? *In* New Directions for Child Development, Vol. 31: Temperament and Social Interaction in Infants and Children, J.V. Lerner and R.M. Lerner, eds. Jossey-Bass, San Francisco.

14

Review of the NIMH Israeli Kibbutz-City Study and the Jerusalem Infant Development Study

Joseph Marcus and Sydney L. Hans
University of Chicago, Illinois
Shmuel Nagler*
University of Haifa, Israel and Oranim Teacher's College, Tivon, Israel
Judith G. Auerbach
Hebrew University, Jerusalem, Israel
Allan F. Mirsky
National Institute of Mental Health, Bethesda, Maryland
Annie Aubrey
University of Chicago, Illinois

The National Institute of Mental Health (NIMH) Israeli Kibbutz-City Study has followed the development of offspring of schizophrenic parents from middle childhood through early adulthood. During childhood, a subgroup of offspring of schizophrenic patients showed clear neurobehavioral deficits often accompanied by poor social competence. Early followup data suggest that this subgroup of high-risk children is at greatest risk for adult schizophrenia spectrum illness. The Jerusalem Infant Development Study has followed a similar population of children at risk for schizophrenia from before birth through middle childhood. A subgroup of high-risk children showed sensorimotor dysfunctioning in the first year

From *The Schizophrenia Bulletin*, 1987, Vol. 13, No. 3, 425–438. (Articles from *The Schizophrenia Bulletin* are in the public domain, unless otherwise specified.)
Editor's Note. Acknowledgments for this NIMH study are found on p. 277.
*See In Memoriam on p. 277.

of life, which was followed by perceptual, motor, and attentional dysfunctioning in childhood—identical to that found in the NIMH cohort. Results from both studies support the hypothesis that schizophrenic illness involves constitutional factors whose expression can be observed as early as infancy. Results also illustrate the importance of using data-analytic approaches that (1) look for subgroups within high-risk groups rather than only group differences between high- and low-risk groups, and (2) examine profiles of behavior rather than only single variables.

This article discusses two studies of the offspring of schizophrenics: the National Institute of Mental Health (NIMH) Israeli Kibbutz-City Study, begun in Israel in 1965, and the Jerusalem Infant Development Study (JIDS), begun in Israel in 1973. The JIDS, an outgrowth of the earlier study, which lacked data on the early development and experience of high-risk children, recruited a high-risk sample before the birth of the children. Since data are now being collected on the JIDS subjects at school age, the two studies will soon converge, providing a more complete picture of schizophrenic development from birth to breakdown.

NIMH KIBBUTZ-CITY HIGH-RISK STUDY

The sample consisted of 100 subjects, 46 boys and 54 girls, who ranged in age from 8.1 to 14.8 years when they were first studied in 1967. The mean age of the boys was 11.3; of the girls, 11.4.

Characteristics of the Sample

Definition of risk status. The high-risk group were offspring of a schizophrenic parent, either mother or father; the control group were offspring of parents who had no mental illness. The sample was divided into four subgroups: 25 high-risk children reared from birth in a kibbutz; 25 high-risk children reared in a traditional family setting in town; 25 control children reared from birth in a kibbutz; and 25 control children reared in a traditional family setting in town (Nagler 1985).

Diagnostic criteria for parents. Because *DSM-III* (American Psychiatric Association 1980) and Research Diagnostic Criteria (RDC) (Spitzer et al. 1975) were not available, patients were selected whose records showed: (1) diagnosis of schizophrenia or any subgroup of schizophrenia; (2) several hospitalizations for this disease; and (3) at least three symptoms from a checklist of classical signs (see *Schizophrenia Bulletin,* Vol. 11, No. 1, 1985).

We believe that virtually all of the parents' illnesses would have been classified as some subtype of schizophrenia or as schizoaffective psychosis by *DSM-III* criteria. A review, with *DSM-III* criteria in mind, of the original clinical records and subsequent medical histories is now underway.

Comparison groups. The kibbutz index cases were chosen first because of the small pool available. The sample contains almost all school-age kibbutz children with schizophrenic parents who resided in Israel at the time of the study. Matched control subjects were selected from classmates of each index child. Identical educational setting was the most important matching criterion, followed by age, ethnic origin, family size, parental educational level, and parental cultural level. On the basis of the same criteria, city pairs were chosen to match each kibbutz pair, so that the 100 subjects were divided into 25 "quadrons." It was assumed that middle-class city children provided the best match in socioeconomic status (SES) for kibbutz-reared children.

Because some kibbutz school classes were small and nonhomogeneous with respect to age, a few compromises were made in matching. Age differences of up to 1.5 years were unavoidable for a few pairs, although for the majority they were not more than 5 months. More emphasis was given to original educational level than to present occupation because parents' education was often superior to occupation in the kibbutz (*Schizophrenia Bulletin,* Vol. 11, No. 1, 1985; see table 1).

Sample biases. Several biases were introduced by the method of sample selection. "Soft" cases of schizophrenia such as those receiving diagnoses popular at the time (e.g., pseudoneurotic and borderline) were excluded, creating a bias toward a chronic type of schizophrenia.

The average IQ and SES of the sample children are high. The range of Wechsler Intelligence Scale for Children IQs was 72–144 (Sohlberg 1985). The means IQs for each group were as follows: index kibbutz, 112.96; index town, 111.40; control kibbutz, 110.58; and control town, 117.75. The sample is predominantly middle class. There is a bias toward intact family structures with two parents (for details, see *Schizophrenia Bulletin,* Vol. 11, No. 1, 1985).

Table 1. Index offspring by sex and ill parent ($n = 50$)

	Mother schizophrenic	Father schizophrenic
Boys	17	6
Girls	21	6
Total	38	12

Attrition. Attrition was low and almost exclusively due to families emigrating. At the 5-year followup, only one child refused examination; six others were out of the country and could not be tested. At the 13-year followup, one child had died; nine who were out of the country could not be tested because of limited financial resources (Mirsky et al. 1985). The low attrition resulted from an effort to establish strong personal relationships, to keep in touch, and from Israel's practice of requiring registration on moving.

Procedures for Index Offspring Assessment

Initial assessment. On entry into the study, index and control offspring were given two series of examinations on different days a week apart. The first series consisted of a two-part clinical interview; a set of psychomotor tasks measuring individual rhythm, mirror drawing, distractibility, learning, digit span, and decision making; a psychometric test battery including figure drawing, the Bender-Gestalt Test (Koppitz 1964), the Wechsler Intelligence Scale for Children (WISC) (Wechsler 1949), four verbal subtests, and the Taylor Closure Test (Snyder et al. 1961). The second part included a specially designed sentence completion test; the Sarason General Anxiety Scale for Children (Sarason 1960); and the Rorschach and Thematic Apperception Tests coded for communication deviance (Singer and Wynne 1966). Electrophysiological (galvanic skin response; GSR) and developmental neurological examinations were conducted on the second test day.

All examiners assessed behavior using a uniform observation score sheet. Children were observed during school using a time-sample method, with special attention given to automatic movements. The entire class was given a sociometric test to assess the social standing of subjects. Parents and teachers were interviewed about children's behavior (for further information on assessments, see *Schizophrenia Bulletin,* Vol. 11, No. 1, 1985).

At this writing, analyses have been done on the neuropsychological testing, some behavioral observations, and attentional, perceptual, psychophysiological, and sensorimotor measures. The information analyzed has proved valuable with the exception of parents' retrospective reports. Parents' reports on present behavior, however, were validated by other sources (interviews with child and teacher, and examiner ratings).

Subsequent assessments. Two subsequent assessments have been carried out: The first was done after 5 years on 93 of the subjects, most of them in their late teens. The second was done in 1981, 13 years after the initial examination, on 90 of the subjects, then in their mid-twenties—well into the age of greatest risk for onset of schizophrenia. A third assessment is now underway.

Developmental problems in assessment. We encountered few problems of assessment at any age. Examiners observed few signs of anxiety during the examinations. To attain an appropriate sample size, it was necessary to enroll a wide age range. Some instruments were not appropriate for such a broad range. The developmental neurological tests, for example, were designed for children under 11 and generally revealed fewer problems in older children. The adolescent assessment instruments were similar to those used 5 years earlier. The parent interview was omitted, and the neurological test was modified to make it more age appropriate.

Psychiatric assessments. At the third examination (1981), a test battery was administered to subjects consisting of the Schedule for Affective Disorders and Schizophrenia-Lifetime Version (SADS-L) (Endicott and Spitzer 1978), the Social Adjustment Scale (SAS) (Weissman and Bothwell 1976), and six subtests of the Wechsler Adult Intelligence Scale (WAIS) (Wechsler 1955; Mirsky et al. 1985). A *DSM-III* diagnosis was established from the SADS-L interview by consensus of two team members in the United States.

Use of the SADS-L and *DSM-III* systems creates some problems. To get a schizoid personality diagnosis, it was necessary to supplement the SADS-L with the SAS. Because the SADS-L has skip rules limiting the use of questions on schizotypal features to cases in which there is another diagnosis, strict adherence to these rules might miss cases in the schizophrenia spectrum. Moreover, the SADS-L does not have questions that would permit a borderline personality diagnosis. We are also concerned that compared to other classification systems, *DSM-III* may be overdiagnosing affective disorders relative to schizophrenia spectrum disorders (20 percent of our index cases did receive affective disorder diagnoses at this third assessment, and 18 percent received schizophrenia spectrum diagnoses). Finally, the *DSM-III* is an evolving classification system. Thus, longitudinal studies must define their risk populations not by diagnosis alone but by a profile of parameters such as pedigree, symptoms, biological indicators, and assessment of neurobehavioral, cognitive, or social functioning that will remain standard no matter how classificatory systems change.

Other outcome criteria. At both childhood and adolescent ages, assessment was not limited to achieving a diagnosis but included a large battery of measures of many types and from many sources. Analyses of parts of the data by members of the research team appear in the *Schizophrenia Bulletin* (Vol. 11, No. 1, 1985).

Multidimensional Scalogram Analysis found a subgroup of offspring of schizophrenics with a neurointegrative defect (Marcus et al. 1985*a*). A replication analysis on data from Mednick's obstetric study in Copenhagen (Marcus et al. 1985*b*) found that a similar-sized subgroup of offspring had profiles of "neurological" dysfunctioning. These analyses demonstrate the efficacy of multidimensional analyses of individual profiles and provide a model that could be used in other replication analyses on existing data of other consortium members.

Current Psychiatric Status of Index Offspring

Age groups. The sample was between the ages of 26 and 32 as of April 1985. Seventy-four percent were between the ages of 26 and 29, and 26 percent were over 30.

Breakdowns and dysfunction to date. At the 13-year (young adult) followup, 26 subjects received *DSM-III* diagnoses—22 in the index group and 4 in the control group (table 2; Mirsky et al. 1985). Sixteen subjects with diagnoses (three schizophrenia, three other schizophrenia spectrum disorders, five major affective disorders, and five minor affective disorders) were in the kibbutz index group. *DSM-III* diagnoses in the town index cases were two schizophrenia, one schizophrenia spectrum, and three "other" (mostly phobias). Of the four diagnoses in the control group, three (one minor affective and two "other") were from the kibbutz group, and one "other" was from the town group. None of the control cases developed schizophrenia. Thus, there was a disproportionately greater number of affective and "other" diagnoses, but not schizophrenia-spectrum diagnoses, in the kibbutz high-risk group. Mirsky et al. (1985) speculated that the small, closed nature of the kibbutz community would make it difficult, if not impossible, to escape one's family history and proved stressful to the high-risk children. However, they left open the question of which environmental influences on kibbutz-reared youths interact with a schizophrenic family history to produce so many cases of psychopathology. Because the risk period for schizophrenia may extend to age 50, they view the reported result as interim and are now carrying out further assessments of these subjects and their families to clarify the finding.

Several yet unexplored factors may have influenced the greater psychopathology in the kibbutz-reared high-risk group. For example, we have no knowledge of the psychopathology or the pedigree of the index parents' spouses. Some of these may have had affective disorders, and it is possible that more such spouses were present in the kibbutzim. Moreover, we lack extensive information about recent life stressors that could be related to affective disorders. One major stressor affecting Israeli youth, military service, is not a likely contributor to this finding since 11 of the individuals with affective disorders were females (Mirsky et al. 1985), and the military experience of women in Israel is less dangerous and presumably less stressful than that of males. Some of the reasons for the excess of psychopathology in

Table 2. *DSM-III* diagnoses of offspring

		Diagnostic category						
Group	n	Schizophrenia	Other schizophrenia spectrum	Major affective	Minor affective	Other diagnosis	No diagnosis	Total *DSM-III*
Kibbutz-index	23	3	3	5	4	1	7	16
Town-index	23	2	1	1	0	3	16	7
Kibbutz-control	23	0	0	0	1	2	20	3
Town-control	21	0	0	0	0	1	20	1
Totals	90	5	4	6	5	7	63	27

Note. — *DSM-III* diagnoses were based on information gained in the Schedule for Affective Disorders and Schizophrenia-Lifetime Version (SADS-L) interview. A χ^2 test performed on the cell frequencies in the 6 columns of diagnostic categories yielded a value of 47.6. For 15 *df*, $p < .0001$. Further comparisons yielded the following, all with 5 *df*: kibbutz-index vs. town-index, $\chi^2 = 18.4$, $p < .005$; kibbutz-index vs. kibbutz-control, $\chi^2 = 21.9$, $p < .0005$; kibbutz-index vs. town-control, $\chi^2 = 23.2$, $p < .0003$; town-index vs. kibbutz-control, NS; town-index vs. town-control, NS. Another parallel series of χ^2 tests was performed on the frequencies yielded by pooling all (or total) *DSM-III* diagnoses and comparing this with no diagnosis (i.e., comparing the last 2 columns in table 1). In every case, the parallel χ^2 on the pooled data yielded statistically significant values where they had been found in the unpooled data.

the kibbutz index group will be clarified by further study of the probands, their health records, and their parents. Another possible explanation for the excess of psychopathology in the kibbutz-reared individuals has to do with administration of the interview used for arriving at diagnoses. The version of the SADS-L used in the Israeli study included a lengthy list of questions related to affective disorders. However, a skip rule prescribed that these questions not be asked if the subject reported never having sought treatment for depression or never having been told by others that he had a problem with depression. It is arguable that city-reared individuals have poorer access to mental health services and have a smaller pool of individuals from whom they might receive feedback than do kibbutz-reared individuals. These factors would make it more likely that city-reared subjects would not be asked the full series of affective questions, and would thus have their incidence of affective disorders underestimated.

Social adequacy. Mirsky et al. (1985) found that control subjects were significantly more involved in social and leisure activity, had more relations with their extended family, and had a better overall score on the SAS ($p <$ .05).

Predictors of Vulnerability

Modern theories of the etiology of schizophrenia are multifactorial. They assume that some combination of constitutional diathesis (specific or nonspecific, genetic or induced), when coupled with environmental stress (either general or in some specific aspect of the family interaction), will produce schizophrenic illness. To identify the true predictors of subsequent schizophrenic illness from research data, we believe it is necessary to analyze multifactorial profiles of individuals over the process of development. Thus far, we have carried out three principal multifactorial studies: (1) an analysis of profiles of neurological and neuropsychological signs and behaviors; (2) a multidimensional analysis of social behavior; and (3) an analysis of a decision-tree model, which includes the previous sets of behavior as well as intervening parental behaviors. Our approach enables us to combine multidimensional statistical analyses with clinical case studies to increase our understanding of the multiple causes of adult disorder.

If schizophrenia requires a genetically transmitted central nervous system (CNS) diathesis, there should be at least three types of individuals in a sample with schizophrenic parents: (1) vulnerable individuals who have a constitutional CNS deficiency and later become schizophrenic; (2) vulnerable individuals who have a constitutional CNS deficiency but avoid eventual schizophrenic breakdown because of compensatory personal abilities or a protective environment; and (3) invulnerable individuals who have no inherited CNS deficiency and cope adequately with life's stress.

Neurobehavioral markers. Several studies have now shown that a subgroup of offspring of schizophrenics have childhood signs of nonfocal neurobehavioral dysfunctioning (Fish and Hagin 1973; Marcus 1974; Erlenmeyer-Kimling 1975; Ragins et al. 1975; Hanson et al. 1976; Orvaschel et al. 1979; Rieder and Nichols 1979; Marcus et al. 1981, 1985a, 1985b; Erlenmeyer-Kimling et al. 1982; Marcuse and Cornblatt, in press), including attentional problems (Rutschmann et al. 1977; Asarnow et al. 1978; Erlenmeyer-Kimling and Cornblatt 1978; Neuchterlein et al. 1981; Erlenmeyer-Kimling et al. 1982; Cornblatt and Erlenmeyer-Kimling 1984; Weintraub and Neale 1984). Some investigators have also noted the similarity between the type of functioning seen in this subgroup and the pattern seen in children with attentional deficit disorder (ADD) (Bellak 1979). As of this writing, however, there are few reports of whether attentional and neurological signs co-occur as a constellation of symptoms in some subgroup of offspring of schizophrenics, and whether such signs, individually or in combination, mark those children who eventually become schizophrenic.

Because we were interested in studying "ADD-like" neurointegrative deficits in children at risk for schizophrenia, two psychologists not involved in the original assessment examined the available items from the assessment battery to select those that were relevant to the diagnosis of ADD and ADD-like behavior (Marcus and Hans 1984; Marcus et al., in preparation). Since ADD and similar diagnostic categories such as minimal brain dysfunction (MBD) are rather vaguely defined in the literature, we formalized our own concept of ADD-like behavior to provide a clear rationale for selection of the items. We chose to define the syndrome by a brief mapping sentence taken from our facet design of child development (Marcus and Aubrey 1982; Marcus and Hans 1982; Hans et al. 1984; Marcus et al. 1984).

There are two facets especially relevant to the diagnosis of ADD and ADD-like conditions: behavior modality (cognitive or motor), and behavior function (control or coordination). The Cartesian cross-product of these two facets yields five categories of behavior, here identified also by familiar terminology: lack of motor control (hyperkinesis), lack of cognitive control (poor concentration), lack of motor coordination (motor dyscoordination), lack of cognitive coordination (perceptual signs), and poor verbal abilities. Items measuring these five concepts were found in several parts of the assessment battery, including interviews with child, teacher ratings, neurological examination, cognitive and psychomotor testing, and observations made by the examiners.

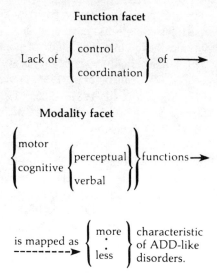

For analysis, each score from the various scoring schemes used was converted into one of three categories: worrisome sign, mild sign, and no sign. Then each child received a score for each of the five ADD variables that was equal to the most extreme score seen by any examiner. Final scoring was: 2 = at least one of the five sources reported a worrisome sign; 1 = at least one of the five sources reported a mild sign; and 0 = none of the five sources reported signs. This method of scoring was used instead of averages because of the possibility of certain ADD-like behaviors (especially those related to the function of control) appearing only sporadically or only in specific contexts.

To examine the patterns of the five variables simultaneously, a Partial Order Scalogram Analysis by Coordinates (POSAC) (Shye 1980; Marcus et al. 1984) was computed. The results of this POSAC analysis yielded a variable structure with motor control as one axis, cognitive control as an orthogonal axis, and the three coordination variables as intermediate (joint) axes (figure 1). POSAC is a multidimensional data-analytic technique that both reveals the structure of the set of variables and produces plots of individual subjects within this structure.

A line is drawn on the POSAC plot separating the children with ADD-like poor neurobehavioral scores (a sum ≥ 8 of the five variables). Twenty-four of the index cases (48 percent) were in the region of poor neurobehavioral

Figure 1. POSAC of childhood neurobehavioral profiles.

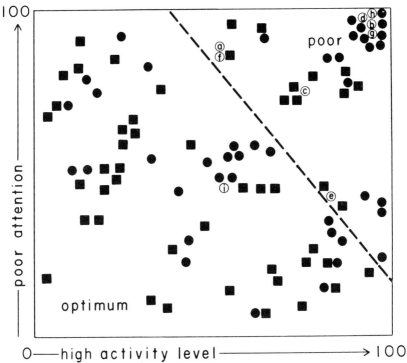

Squares = control cases; circles = index cases. Index cases with young-adult schizophrenia spectrum diagnoses are marked by letters a–i. POSAC = Partial Order Scalogram Analysis by Coordinates.

scores; only 13 of the control cases (26 percent) were in this region. Eight of the nine individuals who later received diagnoses of schizophrenia spectrum disorders were in the region of poor neurobehavioral scores. The one exception (case i) was atypical in that she was an older female (and thus at low risk for such signs) and, as an adult, had only a schizoid personality disorder diagnosis combined with an affective diagnosis. Even so, she exhibited mild neurobehavioral signs. Without exception, all the psychotic schizophrenic breakdowns were in cases exhibiting poor neurobehavioral signs. We do not consider these children identical to children diagnosed as ADD; some aspects of their behavior are, however, similar (Marcus 1986).

Interpersonal markers. A second set of analyses (Hans and Marcus 1985) examined data on interpersonal behavior from parent, child, and teacher interviews. As a group, index children showed more pathology: their behavior was less desirable, less active, less sociable (more withdrawn), and less compliant (more antisocial). There was a mix of types of poor social adjustment, but the strongest discrimination of index from control children lay in withdrawn behavior.

Eight of the nine adults receiving schizophrenia spectrum diagnoses had shown undesirable interpersonal behavior at school age. None had shown excellent interpersonal adjustment in childhood. Males had shown extremely undesirable behavior (antisocial behavior, social withdrawal, or both) that was clearly observable by the child, teachers, and parents. Females had shown less overt dysfunctioning. Although parents and teachers observed adequate interpersonal adjustment, the girls themselves had reported acute feelings of rejection and not belonging.

Multiple etiological factors. Finally, to broaden the view of the multiple developmental factors that might relate to later psychopathology, Hans and Marcus (in press) made a third report, which included neurobehavioral and interpersonal factors as well as parental factors. Using a decision-tree data analytic model and a diathesis-stressor theoretical model, they identified several variables that seem to predict schizophrenic breakdown.

Differential diagnosis can be understood as a problem of deriving a categorical decision (in this case, schizophrenia) from a set of multiple cues. Some models for differential diagnosis, such as those using linear discriminant analysis, have relied on statistics for selecting cues that are the most powerful discriminators in a particular sample. A process model, in contrast, uses a set of sequential cues dictated by a logical model derived before the beginning of analysis, here from theory about the etiology of schizophrenia. A decision tree is an especially simple and flexible structure for representing this process. The developmentally ordered decision cues and their operationalization in the NIMH sample were:

1. *Is there a family history of schizophrenia?* Was the child in the index or control group?
2. *Does the child show early neurobehavioral signs that might reflect a constitutional deficit?* Did the child's neurobehavioral profile place him in the region of poor functioning in figure 1?
3. *Is the childhood environment, particularly the family environment, stressful?* Does the child have at least one parent whose parenting style shows at least two of the following: overinvolvement, inconsistency, hostility?

4. *Are there premorbid childhood signs of poor social adjustment?* Did the child show moderate to severe signs of social withdrawal or antisocial behavior in the analyses?
5. *Does schizophrenia spectrum illness emerge in adulthood?* Does the young adult receive a *DSM-III* diagnosis in the schizophrenia spectrum?

Figure 2 shows the application of this decision model to the data of the NIMH study. Of the nine cases who received *DSM-III* diagnoses within the schizophrenia spectrum, seven followed the "worst" developmental course: they had a schizophrenic parent, showed signs of neurobehavioral dysfunctioning, had stressful family environments, and showed premorbid signs of social maladjustment. Only four cases following the worst pathway have not received a *DSM-III* diagnosis, but because the group is relatively young, these "false positives" might no longer be "false" at a later followup. Also, we have not yet systematically examined protective factors that might be operating in the lives of these four individuals.

The decision cues selected do seem to be specific to the etiology of schizophrenia. Individuals with other diagnoses appeared scattered across the branches of the tree. We believe that such a decision tree model is an exceptionally straightforward and flexible way of looking at the process of development. The decision cues can be whatever univariate or multivariate cues the scientist believes, for theoretical reasons, should be important to the discrimination. A decision cue allows for changes in the significance of cues over time as well as the interaction of cues within time periods. When parsimoniously constructed, such a model, because it does not force an essentially dynamic system into a static model, can offer insight into underlying developmental processes.

Possible Protective Factors

We have not looked systematically at protective factors. For the whole group, a well-integrated CNS seems to protect against the development of schizophrenia, but this may just be a way of identifying those who are not at "real risk." In E. James Anthony's model (Anthony 1974), these are the children made from metal rather than wood or clay. To identify protective factors, one must first identify those children who seem to be at risk biologically.

A structured, nondemanding environment may be a protective factor for those who would appear to be at real risk as in the case of one of our subjects, who showed numerous signs of early neurobiological and physiological

Figure 2. Decision-tree model for development of schizophrenia: Application to Israeli high-risk study data.

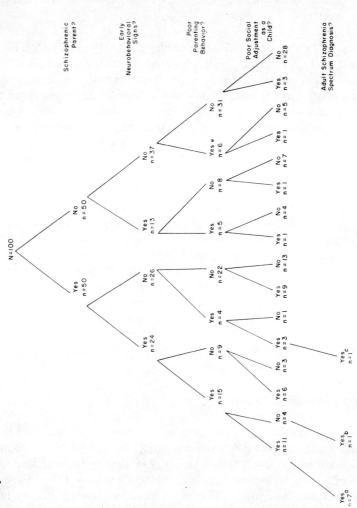

Breakdown cases marked "a" = 1 residual-type schizophrenia, 3 paranoid schizophrenia, 2 schizoid personality disorders, and 1 mixed spectrum disorder.
Breakdown case marked "b" = 1 residual-type schizophrenia. Breakdown case marked "c" = 1 schizoid personality disorder with dysthymic disorder.

dysfunctioning, but as an adult functions adaptively within the structured and nondemanding lifestyle of the religious setting. This environment may, therefore, be assumed to be a "protective factor."

Recommendations

Even though the NIMH study collected a wide range of data, some useful information on this sample remains to be analyzed or collected. There was no organized or complete information on perinatal history or early development other than mothers' retrospective reports. Also, information about the parents should be more complete. In particular, a more complete assessment of CNS functioning in the parents and direct observations of family interaction would be valuable. Since young adult diagnoses change, a second round of diagnoses of both parents and offspring is needed. Because of assortative mating, we see absence of a diagnosis of the second parent as one of the serious holes in the NIMH study. Brain imagery, biochemical measures, and pedigrees should be included in future studies. Some of these are now being carried out. New, more comprehensive studies could be designed, but we recommend making fuller use of existing studies before initiating expensive new ones.

JERUSALEM INFANT DEVELOPMENT STUDY

An important issue that could not be addressed by the NIMH study was the role of perinatal history in the causation of CNS defects. To determine this, it was necessary to start with a cohort of schizophrenic women who were pregnant and obtain detailed data on the perinatal period and the development of the infant offspring. Other methodological improvements were use of multiple control groups, use of the Current and Past Psychopathology Scale (CAPPS) (Endicott and Spitzer 1972) to obtain diagnostic information on the parents, and use of *DSM-II* (American Psychiatric Association 1968) and RDC to establish diagnoses. These offspring were studied during the first year of life (Marcus et al. 1981), and we have been following the families since then with visits and questionnaires. We recently completed a round of followup examinations of these children, as well as some of their siblings.

Characteristics of the Sample

Fifty-four couples and their infants participated. Data from 58 of 67 infants born into the study were used. Nine infants were excluded because of lack of consensus on parental diagnosis, parental diagnosis of primarily organic disorder, twin birth, loss of contact with the mother, and death of the infant.

Definition of risk status. Based on parental diagnosis, four diagnostic categories were formed: schizophrenic (19 cases), affective disorders (six cases), personality disorders and neuroses (14 cases), and no mental illness (19 cases).

Diagnostic criteria for parents. DSM-II was used to make the initial diagnoses from a clinical interview based on the CAPPS, psychiatric case histories, and the CAPPS computer diagnosis. Diagnoses were later refined using updated information and RDC. All reported analyses are based on the RDC diagnoses. When there were differences of opinion, a consensus diagnosis was made by two psychiatrists, two psychiatric social workers, and a psychologist.

Families were recently reinterviewed to obtain a current parent diagnosis. The SADS-L (based on *DSM-III*) and RDC are being used. Final diagnosis will be according to RDC. On initial perusal of the data, there seems to be an increase in pathology among the no-mental-illness group (e.g., major depression, usually situational, and Briquet's disorder), and an increase in severity of pathology among groups with pathology. When *DSM-III* guidelines for diagnosis are used, some cross-cultural difficulties arise. For instance, antisocial personality in Israel is of a different order than the *DSM-III* antisocial personality. In Israel, most antisocial types have close emotional attachments to their families. Therefore, the criterion of shallow affective relationships should not be included for the Israeli sample.

Dimensionalized assessments. All parents were categorized according to severity and chronicity of disorder. There was a relationship between chronicity of maternal mental illness and motor development during the infant's first year. High chronicity was associated with maternal perception of low infant activity level at 4 and 8 months, and with delayed acquisition of motor milestones.

Comparison groups. The control groups were also defined by RDC based on CAPPS interviews and other available materials. Normality was defined as "no mental illness."

Sample biases. The sample was citywide, recruited from maternal and child care centers of Jerusalem between 1973 and 1978. About 90 percent of the population, mostly middle and lower classes, use these centers. Because the well-to-do and ultra-Orthodox do not, they were excluded. The schizophrenia group contains mixed subtypes. Some schizophrenic-group children have ill mothers; others, ill fathers. Middle and lower classes, Ashkenazi and Sephardic Jews, Israeli-born, and immigrant Jews are represented. Only family structure is homogeneous; all families were intact.

Attrition. From the original 54 families, five have dropped out. We included as many age-appropriate siblings of the project child in the followup study as we could find.

Procedures for Index Offspring Assessment

Infants were assessed at 3 and 14 days of age with the Neonatal Behavioral Assessment Scale (NBAS) (Brazelton 1973), and at 4, 8, and 12 months of age with the Bayley (1969) Scales of Infant Development. Information about prenatal, perinatal, and postnatal difficulties was obtained from obstetrical records and rated on the Rochester Obstetrical Scale (Zax et al. 1977). When the offspring were 4 and 8 months of age, mothers were interviewed about the temperament of their babies with the Carey Temperament Interview (Carey 1970). Few problems were encountered in carrying out the study and administering the instruments. If performance of the infant seemed to be affected by illness, the test was redone within a week. A just completed school-age followup study has assessed social competence, school performance, cognitive behavior, neurological status, attentional behavior, and motor behavior. Most instruments are identical to those used in the NIMH study, so we can eventually pool the data from these studies to create a convergence-like model.

Current Psychiatric Status of Index Offspring

All the children are now between the ages of 7 and 12. Followup data have just been collected and have not been analyzed. In addition to repeating many of the analyses done in the NIMH study (and in the process constructing the multidimensional, multifactorial profiles described earlier), we intend to pool individual profiles from the two cohorts and identify "pairs" or small subgroups of children with identical or similar profiles. Using this variation of a convergence model, we will be able to make inferences about the perinatal history and early development of the children from the NIMH study who eventually had breakdowns or who proved to be "invulnerable."

Predictors of Vulnerability

Among the measures used to test infants, the motor and sensorimotor items were valuable (Marcus et al. 1981). Analyses of temperament were not helpful, partly because of the questionable validity of the Carey Temperament Interview and partly because our data were incomplete. It was hypothesized that infants' motor and sensorimotor functioning would be related to parental diagnosis. For each of the five points at which testing was done (3 days, 14 days, 4 months, 8 months, and 12 months), a Multidimensional Scalogram Analysis was done of the motor and sensorimotor items on either the NBAS or Bayley scales. Two main subgroups emerged. A subgroup of 13 infants born to schizophrenics showed repeatedly poor motor and sensorimotor performance during the first year of life, although their overall developmental functioning was often in the normal range. The low birth weights of most of these children may be a result of genetically determined intrauterine growth retardation and not, as some have suggested, a cause of their poor sensorimotor functioning. Their performance could not be accounted for by the existence of prenatal, perinatal, and postnatal complications. Thus, it seems most likely that the etiology of this subgroup's poor performance is a genetic-neurointegrative deficit (Marcus et al. 1981). Other infants who performed poorly were scattered among the other three diagnostic groups. We were also able to identify a subgroup of possibly "invulnerable" infants who had a schizophrenic parent, good motor and sensorimotor functioning, and no signs of a neurointegrative deficit. The followup study will attempt to determine whether the subgroups identified as vulnerable and invulnerable in infancy remain so at school age. Although not all children have been reexamined, we do have many interesting cases that illustrate a continuity of functioning from the first year of life to school age, and whose functioning is identical to that of the children in the NIMH cohort.

RECOMMENDATIONS

The major findings of the two studies described here provide evidence for the roles of both constitutional and environmental factors. Our data on the offspring of schizophrenics point to the existence of a subgroup of children who clearly have constitutional (possibly genetic) CNS deficits combined with social deficits—principally withdrawn behavior—or a combination of withdrawn and antisocial behavior. The CNS deficits express themselves in early signs of motor, perceptual, and attentional difficulties. This combination of deficits seen in individuals who eventually had psychotic schizophrenic breakdowns resembles the syndrome of behavioral patterns that is currently defined in *DSM-III* as ADD. We feel, however, that there are probably subtle differences in the patterns of attentional deficits between ADD children and children with schizophrenic parents, and in their underlying biological dysfunctions as well (Marcus 1986). More research directly comparing these two groups, such as that of Neuchterlein (1984), could yield interesting results.

Our data also clearly point to the existence of a second, nonvulnerable subgroup who exhibit behavior indicative of an intact, normally maturing CNS. We consider them to be physiologically protected from schizophrenia, but not other psychopathology and, most likely, they do not carry any genetic vulnerability. They are not at "real risk" for schizophrenia.

In contrast, the finding of different rates of mental disorder in high-risk children reared in different environments (kibbutz vs. city) suggests that environmental factors—their specific nature as yet undetermined—influence the development of psychopathology, although not necessarily of schizophrenia. It is especially notable that a number of cases were diagnosed with affective disorders. We are trying to reinvestigate these cases to learn more about the existence of affective disease in the family (especially in the nonschizophrenic parent) that could be related to the major affective disorder breakdowns, and of later life stressors that could account for minor affective disorders.

We have learned a number of methodological lessons. It is necessary to study a wide range of background variables, including socioeconomic factors, biological and psychopathological status of both parents and other family members, cognitive functioning of both parents, and various environmental issues. Using type of parent illness as the only "independent" variable in a risk study can lead to fallacious conclusions. Group differences between at-risk and control groups may often be confounded by other factors.

We have also found the study of individual profiles more revealing than group trends and more consonant with clinical approaches. Indispensable to this approach have been Facet Theory (Shye 1978; Marcus and Aubrey 1982; Marcus and Hans 1982; Marcus et al. 1984) and programs for the multidimensional analysis and geometrical presentation of item structure and individual profiles (Guttman 1968; Shye 1980). Facet design provides an a priori scheme for conceptualizing variables and a framework for replication studies. We know that any high-risk group has to be heterogeneous; not all of its members will break down. Analysis of the profiles of those who do break down, especially over time, provides insight into the combination of factors affecting development. Facet design and multidimensional analysis of individual profiles have much to contribute to the high-risk field.

Finally, there are good ongoing studies and data bases that can still be improved upon or used for replication. These steps should precede the complicated and expensive course of initiating new studies while existing ones remain unfunded, underused, and unfinished.

REFERENCES

American Psychiatric Association. *DSM-II: Diagnostic and Statistical Manual of Mental Disorders.* 2nd ed. Washington, DC: The Association, 1968.

American Psychiatric Association. *DSM-III: Diagnostic and Statistical Manual of Mental Disorders.* 3rd ed. Washington, DC: The Association, 1980.

Anthony, E.J. A risk-vulnerability intervention model for children of schizophrenic parents. In: Anthony, E.J., and Koupernik, C. *The Child in His Family: Children at Psychiatric Risk.* New York: John Wiley & Sons, 1974. pp. 99–121.

Asarnow, R.F.; MacCrimmon, D.J.; Cleghorn, J.M.; and Steffy, R.A. The McMaster-Waterloo Project: An attentional and clinical assessment of foster children at risk for schizophrenia. In: Wynne, L.C.; Cromwell, R.L.; and Matthysse, S., eds. *The Nature of Schizophrenia: New Approaches to Research and Treatment.* New York: John Wiley & Sons, 1978. pp. 339–358.

Bayley, N. *Bayley Scales of Infant Development.* New York: Psychological Corp., 1969.

Bellak, L. Psychiatric aspects of minimal brain dysfunction in adults: Their ego function assessment. In: Bellak, L., ed. *Psychiatric Aspects of Minimal Brain Dysfunction in Adults.* New York: Grune & Stratton, 1979. pp. 73–102.

Brazelton, T.B. *Neonatal Behavioral Assessment Scale.* No. 50. Philadelphia: J.B. Lippincott Co., 1973.

Carey, W.B. A simplified method for measuring infant temperament. *Journal of Pediatrics,* 117:188–194, 1970.

Cornblatt, B., and Erlenmeyer-Kimling, L. Early attentional predictors of adolescent behavioral disturbances in children at risk for schizophrenia. In: Watt, N.F.; Anthony, E.J.; Wynne, L.C.; and Rolf, J.E., eds. *Children at Risk for Schizophrenia: A Longitudinal Perspective.* New York: Cambridge University Press, 1984. pp. 198–211.

Endicott, J., and Spitzer, R.L. Current and Past Psychopathology Scales (CAPPS): Rationale, reliability, and validity. *Archives of General Psychiatry,* 27:678–687, 1972.

Endicott, J., and Spitzer, R.L. A diagnostic interview: The Schedule for Affective Disorders and Schizophrenia. *Archives of General Psychiatry,* 27:678–687, 1978.

Erlenmeyer-Kimling, L. A prospective study of children at risk for schizophrenia: Methodological considerations and some preliminary findings. In: Wirt, R.; Winokur, G.; and Ross, M., eds. *Life History Research in Psychopathology.* Minneapolis: University of Minnesota Press, 1975. pp. 22–46.

Erlenmeyer-Kimling, L., and Cornblatt, B. Attentional measures in a study of children at high risk for schizophrenia. In: Wynne, L.C.; Cromwell, R.L.; and Matthysse, S., eds. *The Nature of Schizophrenia: New Approaches to Research and Treatment.* New York: John Wiley & Sons, 1978. pp. 359–365.

Erlenmeyer-Kimling, L.; Cornblatt, B.; Friedman, D.; Marcuse, Y.; Rutschmann, J.; and Simmens, S. Neurological, electrophysiological and attentional deviations in children at risk for schizophrenia. In: Nasrallah, H.A., and Henn, F., eds. *Schizophrenia as a Brain Disease.* New York: Oxford University Press, 1982. pp. 61–98.

Fish, B., and Hagin, R. Visual-motor disorders in infants at risk for schizophrenia. *Archives of General Psychiatry,* 28:900–904, 1973.

Guttman, L. A general nonmetric technique for finding the smallest coordinate space for a configuration of points. *Psychometrika,* 33:469–506, 1968.

Hans, S.L.; Bernstein, V.J.; and Marcus, J. Some uses of the facet approach in child development. In: Canater, D., ed. *The Facet Approach to Social Research.* New York: Springer, 1984. pp. 151–172.

Hans, S.L., and Marcus, J. "Interpersonal Behavior of Children at Risk for Schizophrenia." Presented at the meeting of the Society for Research in Child Development, Toronto, Canada, April 1985.

Hans, S.L., and Marcus, J. A process model for the development of schizophrenia. *Psychiatry: Interpersonal and Biological Processes,* in press.

Hanson, D.R.; Gottesman, I.I.; and Heston, L.L. Some possible childhood indicators of adult schizophrenia inferred from children of schizophrenics. *British Journal of Psychiatry,* 129:142–154, 1976.

Henson, L.; and Mirsky, A.F. "Offspring of Schizophrenic Parents: Vulnerable and Invulnerable Children Thirteen Years Later: A Multidimensional Analysis." In preparation.

Koppitz, E.M. *The Bender Gestalt Test for Young Children.* New York: Grune & Stratton, 1964.

Marcus, J. Cerebral functioning in offspring of schizophrenics. *International Journal of Mental Health,* 3:57–73, 1974.

Marcus, J. Schizophrenia and attention deficit disorder (ADD): An answer to Dr. Kaffman. *Schizophrenia Bulletin,* 12(3):337–339, 1986.

Marcus, J., and Aubrey, A. Multidimensional statistical analysis: A partner for clinical insight. *Zero to Three,* 3:1–7, 1982.

Marcus, J.; Auerbach, J.; Wilkinson, L.; and Burack, C.M. Infants at risk for schizophrenia: The Jerusalem Infant Development Study. *Archives of General Psychiatry,* 38:703–713, 1981.

Marcus, J., and Hans, S.L. A methodological model to study the effects of toxins on child development. *Neurobehavioral Toxicology and Teratology,* 4:483–487, 1982.

Marcus, J., and Hans, S.L. "Offspring of Schizophrenic Parents: Vulnerable and Invulnerable Children 13 Years Later." Presented at the meeting of the American Academy of Child Psychiatry, Toronto, Ont., Canada, October 12, 1984.

Marcus, J.; Hans, S.L.; Lewow, E.; Wilkinson, L.; and Burack, C.M. Neurological findings in high-risk children: Childhood assessment and five-year followup. *Schizophrenia Bulletin,* 11:85–100, 1985a.

Marcus, J.; Hans, S.L.; Mednick, S.A.; Schulsinger, F.; and Michelsen, N. Neurological dysfunctioning in offspring of schizophrenics in Israel and Denmark: A replication analysis. *Archives of General Psychiatry,* 42:753–761, 1985b.

Marcus, J.; Hans, S.L.; Patterson, C.B.; and Morris, A.J. A longitudinal study of offspring born to methadone-maintained women: I. Design, methodology and description of women's resources for functioning. *American Journal of Drug and Alcohol Abuse,* 10:135–160, 1984.

Marcuse, Y., and Cornblatt, B. Children at high risk for schizophrenia: Predictions from infancy to childhood functioning. In: Erlenmeyer-Kimling, L.; Dohrenwend, B.S.; and Miller, N., eds. *Life Span Research on the Prediction of Psychopathology.* Hillsdale, NJ: Lawrence Erlbaum, in press.

Mirsky, A.F.; Silberman, E.K.; Latz, A.; and Nagler, S. Adult outcomes of high-risk children: Differential effects of town and kibbutz rearing. *Schizophrenia Bulletin,* 11:150–154, 1985.

Nagler, S. Overall design and methodology of the Israeli high-risk study. *Schizophrenia Bulletin,* 11:31–37, 1985.

Nuechterlein, K.H. Sustained attention among children vulnerable to adult schizophrenia and among hyperactive children. In: Watt, N.F.; Anthony, E.J.; Wynne, L.C.; and Rolf, J.E., eds. *Children at Risk for Schizophrenia: A Longitudinal Perspective.* New York: Cambridge University Press, 1984. pp. 304–311.

Nuechterlein, K.H.; Phipps-Yonas, S.; Driscoll, R.M.; and Garmezy, N. The role of different components of attention in children vulnerable to schizophrenia. In: Goldstein, M.J., ed. *Preventive Intervention in Schizophrenia: Are We Ready?* DHHS Publication (ADM 81–1111). Washington, DC: Superintendent of Documents, U.S. Government Printing Office, 1981. pp. 54–77.

Orvaschel, H.; Mednick, S.; Schulsinger, F.; and Rock, D. The children of psychiatrically disturbed parents: Differences as a function of the sick parent. *Archives of General Psychiatry,* 36:691–695, 1979.

Ragins, N.; Schachter, J.; Elmer, E.; Preisman, R.; Bowes, A.E.; and Harway, V. Infants and children at risk for schizophrenia. *Journal of the American Academy of Child Psychiatry,* 14:150–177, 1975.

Rieder, R.O., and Nichols, P.L. Offspring of schizophrenics: III. Hyperactivity and neurological soft signs. *Archives of General Psychiatry,* 36:665–674, 1979.

Rutschmann, J.; Cornblatt, B.; and Erlenmeyer-Kimling, L. Sustained attention in children at risk for schizophrenia: Report on a continuous performance test. *Archives of General Psychiatry,* 34:571–575, 1977.

Sarason, S.P. *Anxiety in Elementary School Children.* New York: John Wiley & Sons, 1960.

Shye, S., ed. *Theory Construction and Data Analysis in the Behavioral Sciences.* San Francisco: Jossey-Bass, 1978.

Shye, S. "Partial Order Scalogram Analysis of Profiles and a Related Lattice Analysis of the Items by Their Scalogram Generic Roles." Unpublished manuscript, Israel Institute of Applied Social Research, June 1980.

Singer, M.T., and Wynne, L.C. Principles for scoring communication defects and deviances in parents of schizophrenics: Rorschach and TAT scoring manuals. *Psychiatry,* 29:260–288, 1966.

Snyder, S.; Rosenthal, D.; and Taylor, I.A. Perceptual closure in schizophrenia. *Journal of Abnormal and Social Psychology,* 63:131–136, 1961.

Sohlberg, S. Personality and neuropsychological performance of high-risk and control children. *Schizophrenia Bulletin,* 11:48–60, 1985.

Spitzer, R.L.; Endicott, J.E.; and Robins, E. Research Diagnostic Criteria for a Selected Group of Functional Disorders. 2nd ed. New York: N.Y. State Psychiatric Institute, 1975.

Wechsler, D. *Wechsler Intelligence Scale for Children.* New York: Psychological Corporation, 1949.

Wechsler, D. *Wechsler Adult Intelligence Scale.* New York: Psychological Corporation, 1955.

Weintraub, S., and Neale, J.M. Social behavior of children at risk for schizophrenia. In: Watt, N.F.; Anthony, E.J.; Wynne, L.C.; and Rolf, J.E., eds. *Children at Risk for Schizophrenia: A Longitudinal Perspective.* New York: Cambridge University Press, 1984, pp. 279–285.

Weissman, M.M., and Bothwell, S. Assessment of social adjustment by patient self-report. *Archives of General Psychiatry,* 33:111–115, 1976.

Zax, M.; Sameroff, A.J.; and Babigian, H.M. Birth outcomes in the offspring of mentally disordered women. *American Journal of Orthopsychiatry*, 47:218–230, 1977.

IN MEMORIAM

Shmuel Nagler passed away in March 1987, and all of us are still numb from our feelings of loss. Shmuel's central role in the National Institute of Mental Health Israeli Kibbutz-City Study was both intellectual and emotional, and all of us gained much from him in our personal and academic lives. We were enriched by our association with him, just as the knowledge base regarding the etiology of schizophrenia was enriched by the research that he spearheaded. This article is one of Shmuel's last gifts to us and to those suffering from the particularly painful disorder he researched.—J.M.

ACKNOWLEDGMENTS

The NIMH study was conceived and initiated by David Rosenthal and conducted by a large research team headed by Shmuel Nagler, clinical psychologist. The other members of the team were: Moshe Ayalon, Loni Bonvit, Zeev Glueck, Judith Heller Shottan, Shlomo Kugelmass, Michaela Lifshitz, Eitan Lewow, Joseph Marcus, Hanna Merom, Joseph Shmueli, Shaul Sohlberg, and Shoshana Yaniv. The 13-year followup was conducted by Allan Mirsky. This study has been supported by the continued funding of NIMH, and grants from NIDA (PHS 5 R18 DA-01884), the Irving B. Harris Foundation, and the University of Chicago.

The Jerusalem Infant Development Study was conducted by Joseph Marcus and Judith Auerbach. Amalia Mark and Vera Peles recruited and interviewed the parents, and Sheila Maeir examined many of the infants. Aaron Auerbach, Haim Cohen, Shoshana Sivan, and Nadina Raush are assessing children in the followup study. Sydney Hans has participated in designing the followup, and he plays an important role in the data analysis. It was supported by grants from the U.S.-Israel Binational Science Foundation (grant 598); the Chief Scientist's Office of the Israel Ministry of Health; the Olivetti Foundation; the Center for the Study of Human Sciences of the Hebrew University; the Department of Psychiatry, University of Chicago; Forest Hospital Foundation; and Mrs. Harry Jacobs. It was also supported in part by National Institute of Mental Health Psychiatry Education Branch grant MN06300–22, by National Institute of Drug Abuse grant PHS 5 R18 DA-01884, and the Grant Foundation.

15

Parental Alcoholism and Childhood Psychopathology

Melissa Owings West and Ronald J. Prinz
University of South Carolina, Columbia

Parental alcoholism can be a major source of stress for children. It is unclear, however, to what extent and in what way parental alcoholism produces psychopathology in children and adolescents. We reviewed studies about children of alcoholic parents published between 1975 and 1985 to clarify the relation between parental alcoholism and child psychopathology. We identified methodological problems in this body of literature and organized substantive findings around eight areas of outcome: (a) hyperactivity and conduct disorder; (b) substance abuse, delinquency, and truancy; (c) cognitive functioning; (d) social inadequacy; (e) somatic problems; (f) anxiety and depressive symptoms; (g) physical abuse; and (h) dysfunctional family interactions. The literature as a whole supported the contention that parental alcoholism is associated with a heightened incidence of child symptoms of psychopathology, in comparison with no increased incidence in offspring of nondisturbed parents. However, neither all nor a major portion of the population of children from alcoholic homes are inevitably doomed to childhood psychological disorder. We discuss the pattern of findings in the light of issues of causality, child resiliency, and potential qualifying factors, such as variations in family disruption, and we offer recommendations regarding methodological improvements, possible mediating variables, and a multiple-risk conceptualization.

Reprinted with permission from the *Psychological Bulletin*, 1987, Vol. 102, No. 2, 204–218. Copyright 1987 by the American Psychological Association, Inc.
We thank John Richards for his helpful comments on an earlier draft.

The most common estimate of the number of alcoholics in the United States is 10 million (Woodside, 1982). Estimates of the number of children under the age of 20 years who are living with an alcoholic parent range from 7 million (Woodside, 1983) to over 28 million (Booz-Allen & Hamilton, 1974). If parental alcoholism is a demonstrable risk factor for child psychopathology, then a large segment of the child population is at risk. The study of parental alcoholic effects on child psychological functioning offers a major opportunity to further the understanding of both the ontogeny and prevention of child psychopathology.

Others have conducted reviews of the research on children of alcoholics; el-Guebaly and Offord (1977, 1979) and Jacob, Favorini, Meisel, and Anderson (1978) have conducted the most comprehensive ones. The great majority of studies reviewed by these authors was published prior to 1975. Other recent reviews (Adler & Raphael, 1983; Watters & Theimer, 1978; Woititz, 1978) have been less extensive than the aforementioned with regard to the number of studies reviewed and, again, have described few works published since 1975. One exception is Woodside's (1983) review, which described some recent empirical work on children of alcoholics but relied on nonempirical position papers. To sample a variety of positions on this topic, the reader should refer to Arentzen (1978), Black (1979), Morehouse and Richards (1982), Nardi (1981), Richards (1980), Seixas (1982), and Straussner, Weinstein, and Hernandez (1979).

In this review, we concentrate on empirical investigations published between 1975 and 1985 on children of alcoholics. Studies of children included preschoolers through adolescents; research on fetal alcohol syndrome (FAS) was excluded. Methodological characteristics and issues are first considered for the identified body of studies. Substantive findings are considered for eight content areas: hyperactivity and conduct disorder; substance abuse, delinquency, and truancy; cognitive functioning; social inadequacy; somatic problems; anxiety and depressive symptoms; physical abuse; and dysfunctional family interactions.

RESEARCH ISSUES AND METHODS

Designs

Three types of designs were used in the empirical literature on children of alcoholics: retrospective, passive observational, and longitudinal. As reflected in Table 1, most of the reviewed studies used the passive-observational design with either of two variants: (a) identification of alcoholic parents, followed by assessment of child psychopathology, or (b) identification of children

Table 1. Research Designs for Studies (1975–1985) of Children
From Alcoholic Families

Type of design	No. studies ($N = 46$)
Passive observation, children of identified alcoholic parent	28
Passive observation, parents of psychologically disordered child	9
Longitudinal	6
Retrospective	3

experiencing difficulties, followed by assessment for parental alcoholism. Without evaluation of changes over time, however, antecedent-consequent and causal relations cannot be established (Campbell & Stanley, 1963). With the passive-observational design, child problems may have been present prior to the onset of parental alcoholism, the problems may have been precipitated by some factor unrelated to parental drinking, or parental alcoholism and a co-occurring factor may have jointly caused the child problems.

Longitudinal studies, which are important for progress in this area of inquiry, were conducted less frequently (Aronson, Kyllerman, Sabel, Sandin, & Olegard, 1985; Knop, Teasdale, Schulsinger, & Goodwin, 1985; Miller & Jang, 1977; Robins, West, Ratcliff, & Herjanic, 1978; Rydelius, 1984; Streissguth, 1976). This design is more appropriate for establishing antecedent-consequent relations, even though Achenbach (1978) cautioned against overinterpretation of findings because initial selection and subsequent attrition limit generalizability and because age, cohort, and cultural-historical effects are confounded. Longitudinal designs are advantageous, however, in tracking child and familial changes over time, which facilitates detection of functional relations between specific alcohol-related events and child behavior. Additionally, if a prospective longitudinal study is initiated early enough in the life cycle of the offspring (even including the prenatal period), then it is possible to examine the onset of child psychopathology in the context of environmental conditions.

The least used approach was the retrospective design, in which respondents recalled events that occurred when they were children. The retrospective design is the least adequate because recall of child and family functioning is affected by forgetting, defensiveness, and social desirability.

Several methodological problems were encountered across the three types of studies. Many samples varied widely in age of offspring without analyzing children and adolescents separately. Investigators who matched children of alcoholics and comparison children for age mitigated this problem. Most investigators reported after the fact that there was no significant group difference in age of children, a less precise approach.

Possible sex differences for offspring generally have not been examined. Similarly, the differential impact of sex of alcoholic parent on same-sex and opposite-sex children has also been ignored.

Assessment and Selection of Alcoholic Subjects

Varying definitions for alcoholism reduced comparability across studies. Of 46 reviewed studies, only 19 sufficiently described the diagnostic criteria. Of these, 8 applied the Feighner et al. (1972) criteria, which were adopted in the *Diagnostic and Statistical Manual of Mental Disorders* (American Psychiatric Association, 1980). The other 11 used similar diagnostic schemes in that they required particular kinds of evidence in three major areas: physical dependence (e.g., tolerance, withdrawal, blackouts, and cirrhosis); loss of control, morning drinking, or another pattern of pathological use; and adverse social and occupational consequences from drinking. Many of the remaining 27 studies noted only that one parent was in treatment for alcoholism.

Whereas variability in alcoholism criteria and assessment methods leads to difficulty in making meaningful comparisons across studies, sampling bias makes it difficult to generalize findings to the alcoholic population at large. For example, nearly all the studies reviewed used alcoholics in treatment as subjects, even though a very small proportion of all alcoholics are ever seen in treatment facilities. Treatment status, by definition, means that these cases are more severe, that they are representative of a particular segment, and that offspring status is likely to be more severe (Bacon, 1984; Heller, Sher, & Benson, 1982). Another bias in sampling lies in the fact that nearly all the samples in studies reviewed contained more male than female alcoholics, and many consisted entirely of men. Consequently, less is known about the impact of maternal alcoholism on children's risk for psychopathology.

In selecting and describing subjects, researchers ignored prenatal maternal drinking for the most part in the reviewed investigations. Designs that did not control for prenatal alcohol consumption ran the risk of confounding prenatal physiological effects with postnatal environmental effects. The prenatal issue is pertinent to the study of not only maternal alcoholics' offspring but also paternal alcoholics' offspring. Studies of assortative mating among alcoholics (Hall, Hesselbrock, & Stabenau, 1983a, 1983b; Jacob et al., 1978) indicate that male alcoholics and female alcoholics are more likely than nonalcoholics to marry heavy drinkers. Consequently, alcoholic fathers may have offspring who were exposed to prenatal maternal drinking and were, thus, candidates for FAS and sub-clinical-FAS outcomes. To offset this confounding factor, investigators can (a) at least describe the prenatal exposure of each child in the sample, (b) split the sample into subjects whose mothers did and subjects whose mothers did not drink during pregnancy and analyze accordingly, and (c) take into account both prenatally and postnatally the drinking habits of the spouse of the identified alcoholic, even when the drinking behaviors do not reach alcoholic proportions.

Assessment of Child Psychopathology

Researchers have obtained assessment information on children of alcoholics from a variety of sources. As reflected in Table 2, half of the studies tapped only one source of behavioral information, and less than 9% of the studies obtained data from more than two sources. Investigators relied heavily on information from children (61% of studies) or parents (56% of studies) and to a lesser extent on official records from schools, hospitals, or the legal system (33% of studies). Despite the acknowledged importance of teachers' observations in assessing child psychopathology, less than 9% of the studies obtained teacher data. By not assessing with multiple sources, most studies did not pursue convergence and verification of findings.

Methods of child assessment also varied considerably across studies. As reflected in Table 3, interviews (structured and semistructured) and rating

Table 2. Data Sources for Child Assessment in Studies (1975–1985) of Alcoholics' Offspring

Source	No. studies ($N = 46$)
One source ($n = 23$)	
Child	11
Parent(s)	6
Official records (school, hospital, or police)	5
Teacher	1
Two sources ($n = 19$)	
Child and parent(s)	11
Official records and parent(s)	4
Official records and child	1
Official records and residential staff	1
Teacher and child	1
Teacher and parent(s)	1
Three or four sources ($n = 4$)	
Official records, parent(s), and child	3
Official records, parent(s), teacher, and child	1

scales were the most common methods of assessing child psychopathology. Researchers used standardized tests, such as IQ or achievement tests, and tabulation of records to a moderate extent. They rarely used behavioral observation. Over half of the studies used only one method of child assessment and, consequently, were not able to establish convergence. Lack of uniformity, both in terms of method of assessment and choice of measures within a method, characterized this literature and hampered comparisons between studies.

Multiple Risk Factors and Multiple Outcomes

Parental alcoholism does not occur in a vacuum. Other adverse familial and environmental factors can influence child outcomes to varying degrees. In the reviewed studies, investigators by and large overlooked such possible contributing or mediating variables as child's age at onset of parental alcoholism, severity of alcoholism, psychopathology of alcoholic parent and spouse, extent of family disorganization (e.g., discord, separation, divorce, and multiple marriages), socioeconomic status (SES), family size, child's relationship with the nonalcoholic parent, parental criminality, and the availability of alternative sources of support. Designs that ignore the role of other risk factors could yield group differences that are due to non-alcohol-related factors; conversely, variation due to these other influences could obscure group differences. Within the population of children with alcoholic parents, the ignored dimensions could be responsible for exacerbation or mitigation of the effects of parental alcoholism.

A second multiplicity problem concerns child outcome. Most of the reviewed studies examined one child dimension at a time without considering

Table 3. Methods of Child Assessment in Studies (1975–1985) of Alcoholics' Offspring

Method	No. studies ($N = 46$)
Interview	24
Questionnaires or rating scales	24
Parent	10
Child	9
Teacher or staff	5
Tabulating official records (school, hospital, or legal system)	16
Standardized test[a]	10
Behavioral observation	3

[a] IQ, neuropsychological, or achievement tests.

the possibility of multiple outcomes across children. If parental alcoholism leads to a variety of child psychopathological outcomes, then a univariate focus would obscure this finding. An alternative approach would be to identify the diagnoses of each child and then profile the sample in terms of the incidence of each diagnostic category.

SUBSTANTIVE FINDINGS

Hyperactivity and Conduct Disorder

It is suspected that hyperactive children are more likely to have an alcoholic parent. Cantwell's (1975) review of prior research indicated that families of hyperactive children have increased prevalence of alcoholic and sociopathic fathers and of alcoholic and hysterical mothers. Because increased prevalence rates were true for biological but not adoptive parents, Cantwell (1975) concluded that parental disturbance, including alcoholism, could be genetically related to childhood hyperactivity. Little progress has been made since Cantwell's (1975) review to sharpen our understanding of the apparent link.

Recent studies have found only a weak relation. Seven of the studies began with alcoholic and nonalcoholic parents and then evaluated the children (Aronson et al., 1985; Bell & Cohen, 1981; Fine, Yudin, Holmes, & Heinemann, 1976; Knop et al., 1985; Lund & Landesman-Dwyer, 1979; Steinhausen, Nestler, & Huth, 1982; Tartar, Hegedus, Goldstein, Shelly, & Alterman, 1984). Four other studies examined parental alcoholism in children diagnosed as hyperactive (Morrison, 1980; Shaywitz, Cohen, & Shaywitz, 1980; Stewart, deBlois, & Cummings, 1980; Stewart, deBlois, & Singer, 1979).

Six of the seven studies of parent alcoholics found some association with child hyperactivity. In a study of 1,013 adolescents in residential treatment, Lund and Landesman-Dwyer (1979) found that sons (but not daughters) of alcoholics were rated significantly higher by staff than sons of nonalcoholics for hyperactivity-expansiveness, poor emotional control, and inability to delay on the Devereux Adolescent Behavior Rating Scale. Fine et al. (1976) compared 39 children and adolescents with a parent in treatment for alcoholism with two comparison groups, offspring of nonalcoholic disturbed parents and offspring of parents without alcoholic or psychological disturbance. (They did not describe the method of verification for the latter group.) Offspring of alcoholics were significantly higher than the offspring of normal parents but not the offspring of disturbed parents for maternal ratings of hyperactivity on the Devereux scale.

Bell and Cohen (1981) compared 25 children of alcoholic mothers in treatment with 25 children of nonalcoholic mothers. Teachers rated the children of alcoholic mothers as significantly more overactive on the Bristol Social Adjustment Scale. Aronson et al. (1985) also found a significantly greater incidence of hyperactivity among children of alcoholic mothers, compared with children of nonalcoholic mothers, although half of the target sample also showed signs of FAS. Steinhausen et al. (1982) compared children (4–6 years old) of alcoholic, epileptic, or healthy mothers matched on SES, age, and sex. They found, on the basis of nonblind structured interviews of the mothers, that the children of alcoholic mothers showed higher rates of hyperactivity, poor attention span, management problems, and temper tantrums than both comparison groups. The children of alcoholic mothers were, however, additionally exposed prenatally to maternal alcohol consumption, and over half had alcoholic fathers. Consequently, it was not possible to discern whether the children's behavioral outcome was attributable to living with an alcoholic mother, living with an alcoholic father, prenatal exposure to alcohol, or the combination of these factors. In the one cross-sectional study of offspring of alcoholics failing to find an association, Tarter et al. (1984) compared antisocial adolescents with and without an alcoholic parent for self-reported history and found no difference with respect to characteristics of hyperactivity and minimal brain dysfunction.

In a longitudinal study of sons of alcoholic fathers, Knop et al. (1985) reported that the teachers of this Danish cohort rated the boys as significantly higher on impulsive-restless behaviors, compared with sons of nonalcoholic fathers. This study is noteworthy for a large, carefully drawn sample and a matched comparison.

When the index sample was children with a hyperactivity diagnosis, an association with parental alcoholism did not emerge. Morrison (1980), Stewart et al. (1980), and Stewart et al. (1979) failed to find a significantly higher incidence of parental alcoholism for hyperactive children, compared with nonhyperactive children, with one minor exception: Stewart et al. (1980) found a moderate association when they excluded antisocial fathers who were also alcoholic from the analysis. Shaywitz et al. (1980) selected 15 children whose mothers were alcoholic during pregnancy from a larger sample of children referred to a clinic for learning disorders. All but one of the children showed symptoms of hyperactivity. Given the high incidence of hyperactivity for learning-disabled children and the lack of a learning-disabled comparison group, the Shaywitz et al. study cannot be interpreted as evidence for a strong association between maternal alcoholism and childhood hyperactivity.

The lack of differentiation between hyperactive children with and without concomitant problems of aggression has clouded the interpretation of results.

Because as much as a third of the population of hyperactive children also exhibits a high rate of aggressive behavior (Prinz, Connor, & Wilson, 1981), a weak but detectable association between parental alcoholism and childhood hyperactivity actually may be due to an association with conduct problems. A stronger association of parental alcoholism with conduct problems (over hyperactivity) emerged in identified studies (Fine et al., 1976; Knop et al., 1985; Merikangas, Weissman, Prusoff, Pauls, & Leckman, 1985; Steinhausen, Gobel, & Nestler, 1984; Stewart et al., 1980; Stewart et al., 1979).

Five of six studies supported an association between parental alcoholism and childhood conduct problems. Stewart et al. (1979) and Stewart et al. (1980) reported a higher incidence of alcoholism in fathers of children characterized by unsocialized-aggressive conduct disorder (with and without concomitant hyperactivity), compared with fathers of children having other psychological disorders (including hyperactivity without conduct disorder). Steinhausen et al. (1984) found that 36% of children of alcoholic fathers and 26% of children with two alcoholic parents qualified for a diagnosis of conduct disorder, compared with 0% for children of alcoholic mothers. In a larger and more adequately controlled study, Merikangas et al. (1958) found a significantly greater incidence of conduct disorder in the offspring of depressed alcoholic parents than in the offspring of normal parents and the offspring of nonalcoholic depressed parents. Fine et al. (1976) supported the general trend in finding that maternal ratings of social aggression distinguished preadolescents of alcoholic parents from offspring of normal parents and offspring of nonalcoholic but disturbed parents.

A nonconfirmatory result was noted in a longitudinal study by Knop et al. (1985), who found that teacher ratings of aggressive behavior failed to differentiate sons of alcoholic and nonalcoholic parents.

Generally, studies supported an association between parental alcoholism and childhood conduct disorder, although the role of child gender was not clarified. Results for childhood hyperactivity conflicted, in part because aggression and hyperactivity were not consistently separated. There need to be more attempts to determine whether the increased rate of attention deficit disorder with hyperactivity (ADDH) reported for children of alcoholics is in fact elevated beyond that found in offspring of disturbed but nonalcoholic parents.

It would be difficult to conclude with certainty that parental alcoholism is a major cause of childhood ADDH. The two biggest confounding factors are prenatal exposure to maternal drinking and a potential genetic link for ADDH. The studies in this section did not control for maternal alcohol consumption during pregnancy. ADDH and related symptomatology are possible outcomes from fetal exposure to alcohol even when the full-blown

FAS does not occur (Streissguth, 1978; Streissguth, Landesman-Dwyer, Martin, & Smith, 1980; Warner & Rosett, 1975).

Genetic considerations are also a threat to validity. Support for at least a partial genetic transmission of attentional and hyperactive problems has been established (Cantwell, 1975, 1976). The propensity for alcoholism and hyperactivity may be genetically linked, as suggested by findings on minor physical anomalies (Gualtieri, Adams, Shen, & Loiselle, 1982; Steinhausen et al., 1982; Waldrop, 1978). Unless specific functional-environmental relations can be identified, the roles of genetic transmission for alcoholism and ADDH cannot be readily distinguished.

Substance Abuse, Delinquency, and Truancy

Although not consistent across studies, there is a documentable relation between parental alcoholism and adolescent alcohol abuse. There was a greater incidence of parental alcoholism for alcoholic adolescents and young adults (Lund & Landesman-Dwyer, 1979; Rydelius, 1983). A group of 26 severely alcohol-abusive adolescents was identified in Lund and Landesman-Dwyer's large sample of predelinquent and disturbed adolescents in a residential treatment setting. The alcoholic adolescents reflected a 46% rate of parental alcoholism, compared with a 29% base rate for the entire residential sample. In a normative sample of 1,004 men (17–26 years old), Rydelius (1983) found that the 4% exhibiting very high levels of alcohol consumption (four or more full bottles of hard liquor during the 1-month period preceding interviews) were significantly more likely than a group of abstaining men (23% of the total sample) to have an alcoholic father (19% vs. 4%) or mother (7% vs. 1%).

Of four investigations evaluating alcohol abuse among adolescent offspring of alcoholics (Herjanic, Herjanic, Penick, Tomelleri, & Armbruster, 1977; Knop et al, 1985; Merikangas et al., 1985; Schuckit & Chiles, 1978), three found a significant relation with adolescent alcohol abuse. Herjanic et al. (1977) examined 48 adolescent offspring of male alcoholics who met the Feighner et al. (1972) diagnostic criteria and who may have been representative of the alcoholic population at large because they were not in treatment. The comparison group consisted of 26 adolescents of similar SES from a pediatric clinic. The comparison group contained adolescents whose fathers were heavy drinkers, whose mothers had been hospitalized for mental illness, whose parents took tranquilizers, or whose parents were divorced; nonetheless, the offspring of alcoholics were significantly more likely to engage in alcohol or drug use. In a supportive study, Merikangas et al. (1985) found that offspring of depressed alcoholic parents were significantly more likely to exhibit deviant drinking behavior than were offspring of depressed-only and normal parents. Schuckit and Chiles also found a higher incidence of alcohol and drug abuse among offspring of alcoholic or antisocial parents. Finally, a longitudinal investigation by Knop et al. revealed no significant differences for any aspect of current drinking pattern, drinking history, or drug use for sons of alcoholic fathers, compared with sons of nonalcoholic fathers.

Several studies supported an association between parental alcoholism and delinquent and truant outcomes for the children (Fine et al., 1976; Hughes, 1977; Miller & Jang, 1977; Offord, Allen, & Abrams, 1978; Rimmer, 1982; Robins et al., 1978; Schuckit & Chiles, 1978). Fine et al. (1976) found that child and adolescent offspring of alcoholics were rated higher than children of normal parents and children of psychologically disturbed parents with respect to the Unethical Behavior subscale of the parental Devereux Behavior Rating Scale. Whereas Lund and Landesman-Dwyer (1979) failed to replicate Fine et al.'s findings by using staff ratings of residential adolescents, Rimmer reported supportive findings. In comparing children of hospitalized alcoholics with children of hospitalized depressive parents and children of mothers hospitalized for obstetrical-gynecological reasons, Rimmer controlled for the impact of parental hospitalization, a factor that confounded other studies. On the basis of structured interviews with parents, teachers, and children, Rimmer reported elevated rates of lying, stealing, playing with matches, fighting, truancy, and discipline problems at school among the children of alcoholic parents. Although diagnostic criteria were clearly specified and assessment information was obtained from multiple sources, nonstandardized quantification prevented statistical analysis.

Hughes (1977) reported that 25 adolescent children from alcoholic families reported significantly more contacts with police during recent years than did children of nonalcoholics who were matched on age, sex, grade level, and father's occupational level. Offord et al. (1978) compared 73 families with sons known to juvenile courts with 73 families who had nondelinquent sons matched for age, school performance, IQ, and social class: The delinquent sons were significantly more likely to have an alcoholic parent. They were also more likely to live in a family with only one parent, with a mentally disturbed parent or a criminal father, and with welfare assistance. When Offord et al. compared single-parent families from both groups, these differences disappeared. In other words, parental alcoholism did not seem to increase the risk for delinquency beyond that attributable to divorce.

Robins et al.'s (1978) classic follow-up of school and police records of children of 157 black men from inner-city ghettos revealed that the children of alcoholic fathers were significantly more truant during elementary school and likely to have dropped out before high school graduation. There was no significant relation between parental alcoholism and the offspring's criminal record. When the total number of disadvantaged circumstances was held constant, there was no increased risk for truancy or dropping out as a result of having an alcoholic father. Children with alcoholic fathers but otherwise positive circumstances were no more likely to be truants or dropouts than were children of nonalcoholic fathers from similar backgrounds. Although father's alcoholism did increase the risk of the child's experiencing a disadvantaged setting, within this setting, the father's alcoholism no further increased the risk of truancy or dropping out for the child. These findings are consistent with the finding of Offord et al. (1978) that once the risk factor of parental divorce is present, parental alcoholism does not appear to place the child at further risk for delinquency. In both studies, however, parental alcoholism was associated with experiencing other disadvantaged circumstances.

Schuckit and Chiles (1978) also examined the interplay between parental alcoholism and divorced family status. They compared adolescent offspring of alcoholic and antisocial parents with offspring of affective-disordered parents, offspring of nondivorced parents without psychological disorder, and offspring of divorced parents without psychological disorder. Of all the groups, the children of alcoholic and antisocial parents had the highest percentage of suspensions and expulsions from school and the highest level of arrests before age 16. Within the group with alcoholic or antisocial parents children from divorced families had a slightly higher rate of antisocial behavior than did those from intact families.

An impressive 20-year longitudinal study by Miller and Jang (1977) followed children from lower class families with multiple problems (e.g., parental mental illness, criminality, and reliance on welfare assistance). Children of alcoholics were significantly less likely to have graduated from high school (although they were not significantly different in intellectual or cognitive skills) and more likely to have received counseling in school for psychological or discipline problems (an average of twice as many visits to school psychologists and counselors). They were more than three times as likely to have been expelled from school and significantly more likely to have received the attention of social and legal services. In addition to experiencing the stressor of parental alcoholism, these children were more likely to have experienced a variety of other family problems, that is, more than one and one half times as likely for the family to receive welfare assistance; twice as likely to have divorced parents, and almost twice as likely as children of nonalcoholics to experience such family crises as a parent's arrest, incarceration, absence, or hospitalization for alcoholism, mental illness, or criminal behavior. Thus, parental alcoholism was not the only factor differentiating the groups.

There does appear to be a relation between parental alcoholism and offspring risk for substance abuse, delinquency, and school truancy and dropping out. The greater incidence of delinquency (and associated substance abuse, school truancy, and dropping out) could be attributable to any of a number of causal pathways. For example, a greater occurrence of psychopathy and related personality disturbance in the alcoholic parent could influence the adolescent's behavior independent of any direct effects of the alcoholism. Alternatively, the family disruption associated with alcoholism may drive the child or adolescent out of the home to seek other sources of support. The estranged child may then gravitate toward and be vulnerable to the influence of delinquent youth, who often are available for greater periods of time than are other peers.

Several of the studies described in this section suggest that although parental alcoholism may not lead directly to offspring delinquency, it may increase the child's risk of experiencing other family stressors, which in turn leads to negative outcomes. Children with only one risk factor may be no more likely to experience psychological disorder than children with no risk factor at all, but a combination of several stressors may potentiate each other, resulting in much more risk of impairment than would be seen with a simple summation of the effects of separate stressors considered singly (Rutter, 1979). Those studies that looked not only at parental alcoholism but also at the child's experience of other family stressors support this model.

Evidence for a possible genetic role in drug and alcohol abuse, though controversial, cannot be ignored in this discussion (Cotton, 1979; Goodwin, 1979; Saunders & Williams, 1983; Vaillant, 1983). Separation of family environmental from purely genetic effects is an ongoing problem in this literature. Some of the adoption studies point to a definite genetic component above and beyond family environment, particularly for boys and men (Bohman, 1978; Cadoret & Gath, 1978; Goodwin, 1979; Goodwin, Schulsinger, Hermansen, Guze, & Winokur, 1973; Goodwin, Schulsinger, Moller, Hermansen, Winokur, & Guze, 1974). Peele (1986), however, in critically evaluating the alcoholism and genetics literature, argued that the role of inheritance has been assumed to be stronger than the evidence justifies. He pointed to definitional problems in the genetic transmission studies (Murray, Clifford, & Gurling, 1983), unanswered questions regarding differential alcoholism rates for gender and social class groups, and the absence of established mechanisms. Although there is undoubtedly some genetic contribution to the development of alcoholism, Peele (1986) made a strong case for a "complex interactive view of the influence of inheritance on alcoholism" (p. 71). In other words, other factors, such as family behavior and environment, must not be ignored. For example, Wolin, Bennett, and Noonan (1979) and Wolin, Bennett, Noonan, and Teitelbaum (1980) found that family environment mediated outcome for children at risk for alcoholism. In their studies, they classified alcoholic families as transmitters or nontransmitters on the basis of whether at least one of the grown children had become an alcoholic or a problem drinker. They found that the greater the change or disruption in family rituals during the episodes of parental drinking, the more likely alcoholism was to develop in the offspring. Transmitter and nontransmitter families did not differ in mean number of years of heavy drinking by the alcoholic parent or severity of parental alcoholism. Thus, despite a presumed genetic predisposition for alcoholism in all these offspring, family environment was critical in determining subsequent drinking behavior.

Cognitive Functioning

Nine investigations explored the relation between parental alcoholism and childrens' IQ. Three of these also examined childrens' neuropsychological status and found significant areas of impairment among children of alcoholics, in comparison with other groups (Aronson et al., 1985; Steinhausen et al., 1982; Tarter et al., 1984). Of the nine IQ studies, two found no significant differences (Herjanic, Herjanic, Wetzel, & Tomelleri, 1978; Tarter et al., 1984); six found significantly lower IQ scores for children of alcoholics (Aronson et al., 1985; Ervin, Little, Streissguth, & Beck, 1984; Gabrielli & Mednick, 1983; Steinhausen et al., 1982; Streissguth, 1976; Streissguth, Little, Herman, & Woodell, 1979); and one found no differences for boys and girls combined, although male children of alcoholics had significantly lower IQ scores than did male children of nonalcoholics (Kern et al., 1981). These studies varied considerably in terms of IQ measures, comparison groups, and control for prenatal exposure to alcohol and other family stressors.

To identify the impact of parental alcoholism on children's intellectual functioning, moving away from the relatively static variable of IQ toward the measurement of actual school performance, a variable more likely to be affected by the child's experience of living with an alcoholic parent, may be more productive. Of six studies that examined academic performance, five reported significantly lower performance among children of alcoholics, and one failed to find group differences. Rimmer (1982) found no significant differences in "learning problems" (defined as having to repeat a year of school or being sent to special-education classes) among children of alcoholic, depressive, and "normal" parents. The only other study in this area that used multiple comparison groups was conducted by Schuckit and Chiles (1978), who compared children of alcoholic and antisocial parents (combined in one group) with three other groups: children of affective-disordered parents, children of nondivorced parents without psychological diagnosis, and children of divorced parents without psychological diagnosis. Of all the groups, the children of alcoholic and antisocial parents had the lowest grade average in school and the highest percentage repeating a grade in school. Hughes (1977) reported that adolescent children of alcoholics reported significantly more often than did a comparison group of children of nonalcoholics (matched on age, sex, grade level, and father's occupational level) that they had been told by teachers or school guidance counselors that they were "capable of better schoolwork" (p. 947). As described earlier, in a longitudinal study of multi-problem families with and without parental alcoholism, Miller and Jang (1977) found that children from alcoholic families were significantly less likely to have graduated from high school, even though there were "no statistically significant differences between these two groups of children in terms of their intellectual or cognitive skills in school" (p. 27). Miller and Jang did not state how these skills were assessed, but it is known that the authors had access to subjects' educational records. Knop et al.'s (1985) longitudinal study revealed that sons of alcoholics were significantly more likely than sons of nonalcoholics to repeat a grade in school and to be referred to a school psychologist. There was also a nonsignificant trend for them to more often attend special classes.

Using a somewhat different approach, Shaywitz et al. (1980) examined the impact of maternal heavy drinking during pregnancy but at a level that did not result in classic FAS. Of 87 children referred to a learning disorders unit of a hospital, 15 had a history of prenatal exposure to alcohol. All 15 were within the normal range of intelligence (mean IQ = 98.2, range = 82–113); early school failure, however, was a common experience for these children. All had been recommended for special-education services by the third grade, and all but 4 had been held back because of academic failure for at least 1 year prior to their referral for special services. A major shortcoming in this study is the lack of comparison with the other learning-disabled children, who were not exposed to maternal drinking. It may be that the remainder of the sample of 87 children had similar rates of the same types of school difficulties.

To summarize, we found that investigations of the relation between parental alcoholism and children's school performance suggest moderate adverse effects. The investigations reviewed varied considerably in how they obtained school performance data, the number and nature of comparison groups used, control for prenatal exposure to alcohol, and identification of stressors in addition to parental alcoholism that may adversely affect children's school performance. As we have discussed in previous sections, evidence indicates that children of alcoholics as a group may display increased rates of hyperactivity, conduct disorder, delinquency, and truancy and may be at increased risk for suffering from abuse and neglect, parental discord, divorce, and criminality. All these factors may contribute to poor school performance, making it difficult to detect the relative impact of parental alcoholism independent of these other influences. What needs to be better documented is the ontogeny of poor school performance. Short-term longitudinal studies of elementary-school-age children of alcoholics might better detect the deterioration of academic functioning as well as the mediating factors that allow some of these children to perform adequately.

Social Inadequacy

Children of alcoholic parents are thought to have difficulties in interpersonal relationships. Arentzen (1978) and Seixas (1982) maintained that these children are ashamed to bring friends into the home. Black (1979) argued that for many of these children, the "need to be in control" leads to difficulty in having meaningful relationships. Morehouse and Richards (1982) observed how "less than ideal parenting patterns in alcoholic caretakers affect a developing child's ability to relate with others in mutually enhancing ways" (p. 22). Despite numerous assertions in the literature that children of alcoholics experience interpersonal difficulties, few investigators have examined this issue empirically. Lund and Landesman-Dwyer (1979) analyzed data obtained on the Devereux Adolescent Behavior Rating Scale for 1,013 adolescents (two-thirds male) in residential treatment facilities. The 29% with an alcoholic parent were somewhat distinguishable from those without alcoholic parents. Sons but not daughters of alcoholics were lower on the Physical Inferiority/Social Reticence scale and higher on the Approval/Dependency scale when compared with offspring of nonalcoholics. Lund and Landesman-Dwyer (1979) summarized these findings: "These males appeared to have a greater need for adult support, approval, or some type of dependent relationship, while at the same time showing an increased tendency to assert themselves physically and socially" (p. 347). In the same sample, the children of alcoholics were also significantly more likely to have experienced physical abuse, neglect, and inadequate supervision, as well as parental conflict, divorce, imprisonment, or financial problems. Thus, the observed outcomes could be the result of secondary factors caused by the alcoholism or the result of major family problems not caused by the alcoholism.

Fine et al. (1976) also used the Devereux Behavior Rating scales in their comparison of 39 children who had a parent in treatment for alcoholism with 39 children who had a parent in treatment for some other (unspecified) psychological disorder and with 523 children in a normative group (although it was not clear how the normative group was selected). For the adolescents (13–18 years old), children of alcoholics were significantly more impaired than children of other psychologically disturbed parents on the scale for Paranoid Thinking. Whereas they did not differ significantly from the normal comparison group of adolescents on Paranoid Thinking, they were higher than the normal subjects on scales for Schizoid Withdrawal and Domineering/Sadistic Behavior (indicative of aggression and causing trouble in the peer group). Neither of the scales that discriminated the adolescent children of alcoholics from those of nonalcoholics in Lund and Landesman-Dwyer's (1979) study discriminated the groups in the Fine et al. investigation. For the younger children (8–12 years old) in the Fine et al. study, children of alcoholics were significantly more impaired than were children of other psychologically disturbed parents on the scales for Emotional Detachment, Social Aggression, Pathologic Use of Senses (indicative of behavior seen in schizophrenic children), and Inadequate Need for Independence. When compared with children in the normal group, children of alcoholics differed significantly on these last four scales, as well as on the Social Isolation and Unresponsiveness scales.

Steinhausen et al. (1982) compared frequencies of various symptoms (obtained through structured interviews) seen in children of alcoholic, epileptic, and normal mothers and concluded that children of alcoholics were significantly more impaired than was either comparison group in the areas of dependency and difficulties with peers. The symptoms were ranked for severity, however, as none, slight, or marked, and neither difficulties with peers nor dependency reached a level above slight for children of alcoholics.

In summary, the paucity of empirical data in this area makes it impossible to state unequivocally what impact parental alcoholism has on children's interpersonal functioning. There was considerable variability in the makeup of samples across the three studies that were available, and there were no consistent findings across the two investigations that used the Devereux scales. None of the studies in this area used direct observation of children or peer sociometrics, either of which would have provided a more valid assessment of peer relations (Wanlass & Prinz, 1982). Because Fine et al. (1976) found evidence of impairment in interpersonal functioning of younger children that was not seen among adolescents, one may speculate that the social skills of some children of alcoholics improve as they grow older. This cannot be clearly demonstrated, however, without longitudinal data.

Somatic Problems

Of five studies examining child physical health status, three reported a significant relation with parental alcoholism (Biek, 1981; Roberts & Brent, 1982; Steinhausen et al., 1982), and two reported nonsignificant results (Moos & Billings, 1982; Rimmer, 1982). Rimmer explored the rates of health problems among children of parents who were hospitalized for alcoholism, depression, or obstetrical-gynecological problems. On the basis of information obtained from structured interviews, he found no differences among the groups in rates of children's health problems. This study differed from those that reported increased rates of health problems in that Rimmer's definition of health problems was more stringent. The second investigation based on structured interviews, which reported essentially nonconfirmatory findings, was conducted by Moos and Billings, who compared the health status of children in families of recovered versus relapsed alcoholics to those in families without an alcoholic member. Analysis of rates of five physical problems revealed no significant differences between children in any of the three groups; there was a tendency ($p < .10$), however, for the children of relapsed alcoholics to be higher than children in nonalcoholic families on a composite measure of physical problems, that is, the percentage having two or more of the five physical problems.

Roberts and Brent (1982) examined the health status of individuals in alcoholic families (excluding the alcoholics themselves), who were matched by using computerized records of a family-medicine clinic with individuals in nonalcoholic families on age, sex, race, and insurance status. Findings for children were not separated from those for adults. Roberts and Brent found that female members of alcoholic families had significantly higher physician utilization rates and higher numbers of distinct diagnoses than did their matched controls, but differences for male members were not significant on these two indexes. Steinhausen et al. (1982) conducted structured interviews to obtain frequencies (none, slight, or marked) for various symptoms in children born to epileptic, alcoholic, or healthy mothers and found that children of alcoholics were significantly more impaired than both comparison groups in rates of outpatient therapy, eating problems, headaches, and sleeping problems. However, none of the health problems of children of alcoholics reached a level above the "slight" ranking, with the exception of rates of outpatient therapy (nature of treatment unspecified).

The third investigation, which reported positive findings, was conducted by Biek (1981), who found that medical clinic outpatients who reported a problem-drinking parent had nearly twice as many somatic complaints and health concerns as those without a problem-drinking parent. Of the group reporting a problem-drinking parent, 78% were female.

In summary, three of five studies reviewed in this section suggest a tendency for alcoholic-family members, particularly girls and women, to report health problems at a higher rate than various comparison families; only one investigation (Roberts & Brent, 1982), however, used actual clinic records to explore this phenomenon. With the exception of Moos and Billings's (1982) study, which is described in more detail in the section on anxiety and depressive symptoms, these studies failed to assess family stressors other than parental alcoholism that may have accounted for some of the variance in children's health status. Variability across studies in definitions of health problems further impedes conclusive statements in this area.

Future studies relating parental alcoholism to child health status might profitably examine the onset and continued presence of child somatic symptoms as they covary (or fail to covary) with alcohol-related and familial events. Functional analyses can replace static group comparisons and lead to a better understanding of the dynamics.

Anxiety and Depressive Symptoms

Eleven investigations examined the impact of parental alcoholism on children's emotional functioning, including anxiety and depression, lowered self-esteem, and perceived lack of control over environment (Anderson & Quast, 1983; Fine et al., 1976; Herjanic et al., 1977; Herjanic et al., 1978; Hughes, 1977; Kern et al., 1981; Moos & Billings, 1982; Prewett, Spence, & Chaknis, 1981; Schuckit & Chiles, 1978; Steinhausen et al., 1984; Tarter et al., 1984). With the exception of Herjanic et al. (1978), all reported a positive association between parental alcoholism and impaired emotional functioning of offspring.

Moos and Billings (1982) assessed rates of emotional problems in children of nonalcoholics and children of relapsed and recovered alcoholics. Among children of relapsed alcoholics, there was more than twice as much reported emotional disturbance as in normal families, and they were particularly high in reported anxiety and depression. Children of recovered alcoholics functioned as well emotionally as normal children and even showed significantly less depression than the normal children. Additional variables emerged in a multiple regression analysis as predictive of children's emotional functioning. Anxiety and depression in either parent, a parent's reliance on avoidance coping, the occurrence of undesirable life-change events, and a family environment characterized by conflict and lack of cohesion and organization added significantly beyond that predicted by presence or absence of parental alcoholism.

In their 1978 study, Schuckit and Chiles took additional risk factors into account; however, they combined children of alcoholic and antisocial parents into one group. These investigators examined adolescents with a biological parent demonstrating alcoholism or antisocial personality and explored the incremental impact of broken or intact home status and having a second parent with affective disorder. They found a nonsignificant trend for offspring of alcoholic or antisocial parents from broken versus intact homes to more frequently report depressive symptoms and to have a history of psychiatric hospitalization. Subjects with a second parent with affective disorder had significantly higher rates of diagnoses of affective disorder themselves when compared with children of alcoholic or antisocial parents only (33% vs. 0%, $p < .003$).

Steinhausen et al. (1984) compared children of alcoholic mothers with children of alcoholic fathers and children of two parents with alcoholism on the basis of ICD-9 (International Classification of Diseases) diagnoses received at a child psychiatric clinic. Sixty-seven percent of children with alcoholic mothers had an emotional disorder diagnosis, 59% of children with two alcoholic parents had this diagnosis, and only 31% of children with alcoholic fathers had this diagnosis. There was no comparison with rates of emotional disorder diagnoses in children of nonalcoholic parents.

In an uncontrolled investigation, Anderson and Quast (1983) administered the Personality Inventory for Children to the nonalcoholic parent of children whose other parent was in treatment for alcoholism. As a group, these children scored significantly higher than test norms on the Anxiety and Adjustment scales, and their scores on the Depression scale approached significance.

Tarter et al. (1984) administered the Minnesota Multiphasic Personality Inventory to male antisocial adolescents, 39% of whom had an alcoholic father, and found that sons of alcoholics scored significantly higher than other boys on the Depression scale. It is unclear whether this effect can be attributed solely to parental alcoholism because the children who experienced parental alcoholism were also more likely to have experienced perinatal complications, physical abuse, maternal psychological disorder, and parental divorce.

Hughes (1977) found that alcoholics' offspring who were not members of Alateen showed significantly higher negative and lower positive mood states and significantly lower self-esteem, in comparison with children of alcoholics who were Alateen members and children of nonalcoholics.

Fine et al. (1976) found that adolescent offspring of alcoholics were significantly more impaired than normal adolescents but not adolescent offspring of other psychologically disturbed parents on the Anxious Self-Blame scale from mother-completed Devereux Behavior Rating scales. The 8- to 12-year-old children of alcoholics were significantly higher than normal children in Proneness to Emotional Upset and in Anxious-Fearful Ideation but did not differ in these areas from children of other psychologically disturbed parents.

Two studies explored the impact of parental alcoholism on children's locus of control. Kern et al. (1981) compared children of alcoholics in treatment with children of nonalcoholics from the same community on the basis of the Nowicki-Strickland Locus of Control Scale for Children and found that children of alcoholics were significantly higher in external locus of control. Although comparison children were drawn from the same community, subjects were not matched specifically on SES; thus, high externality scores may have been related to conditions associated with low SES rather than parental alcoholism. Prewett et al. (1981) overcame this problem by administering the Nowicki-Strickland locus of Control Scale to children of alcoholics in treatment and children of nonalcoholics who were matched on SES. They also found that the children with alcoholic parents had significantly more external attributions than did the comparison-group children.

Herjanic et al. (1978) administered the Piers-Harris Children's Self-Concept Scale to children of alcoholics and drug addicts from the lower one-third SES who lived in an inner-city area. Children in both groups showed normal to higher than normal self-esteem scores (compared with national test norms), which Herjanic et al. (1978) attributed to either overcompensation or impaired perception of reality. Herjanic et al. (1977) compared the same group of children of alcoholics with children of similar SES attending a pediatric clinic. The comparison group was contaminated, however, because some of the children had heavy-drinking fathers, mothers with a history of psychiatric hospitalization, or parents who took tranquilizers. A psychiatrist who interviewed the children and their mothers made all diagnoses of the children. There were no significant differences between the groups for the preadolescent children. However, the incidence of psychological disorder for the adolescent offspring of alcoholics was 54% (mostly neurotic disorder and adaptation reaction), whereas none of the adolescents seen in a pediatric clinic were characterized by psychological disorder.

The foregoing investigations suggest that children of alcoholic parents may be at risk for developing a variety of anxiety-depressive symptoms, including low self-esteem and perceived lack of control over events in their environment. This body of research is plagued, however, by many of the problems encountered in previously cited work, including the lack of accepted standards for assessment of child adjustment (Heller et al., 1982), uncorroborated self-report measures in the majority of investigations, and designs for which effects cannot be attributed directly to parental alcoholism. The single study (Fine et al., 1976) that used both normal and disturbed comparison groups found greater incidences of anxiety-related symptoms in children of alcoholic versus normal parents that were not detected in comparison with children of other psychologically disturbed parents. The two studies (Moos & Billings, 1982; Schuckit & Chiles, 1978) that explored the impact of other risk factors found that children's emotional functioning was further adversely affected by divorce, avoidance coping, anxiety, affective disorder in either parent, and undesirable changes in the family environment and life situation.

Physical Abuse

Researchers investigated an association between parental alcoholism and child abuse in three ways. First, the coincidence of parental alcoholism and child abuse was evaluated for deviant adolescents who were in residential treatment (Lund & Landesman-Dwyer, 1979) or were referred by juvenile court (Tarter et al., 1984). Second, incidence of child abuse was examined for alcoholic parents (Ellwood, 1980; Mayer, Black, & MacDonall, 1978). Third, the occurrence of alcoholism was reported for identified child-abuse cases (American Humane Association, AHA, 1980; Behling, 1979; Oliver, Cox, & Buchanan, 1978).

Lund and Landesman-Dwyer (1979) examined records on 1,013 adolescents (692 male and 321 female) 13 to 18 years old and in residential treatment facilities and found that 29% had an alcoholic parent. In this sample, child abuse was evident in 33% of the cases with an alcoholic parent, compared with 16% of the cases with no parental alcoholism. In a much smaller sample ($N = 41$), Tarter et al. (1984) found a similar pattern. For court-referred adolescents, 69% of those with an alcoholic father experienced paternal physical abuse, whereas only 12% of those with nonalcoholic fathers were abused. A strength of both studies was that offspring of alcoholics were compared with offspring of nonalcoholics who also had deviant social histories. Further analysis of group differences in both studies revealed, however, that the offspring of alcoholics also had a higher incidence of maternal psychiatric illness, parental discord and divorce, financial problems, and imprisonment of a parent. The relative impact of these factors on child abuse cannot be separated from that of parental alcoholism.

Examining child abuse in alcoholic parents, Ellwood (1980) and Mayer et al. (1978) reported an indirect association. Ellwood compared alcoholic parents (U.S. Navy families) in treatment with nonalcoholic parents and found more abusive upbringing and marital discord for the alcoholic parents, suggesting a higher potential for abuse. The alcoholic parents did not, however, report higher rates of abuse toward their own children. Mayer et al. found, on the basis of a parental questionnaire of child-rearing habits, that 75% of alcoholic parents in treatment had a high potential for abusing their children, but they made no comparison with nonalcoholic parents. Both studies were limited by sole reliance on parental report, selection of alcoholics who were in treatment, and absence of evidence that alcoholic parents were committing more abuse.

Alternatively, alcoholism was examined in families with reported child abuse. In small samples without a comparison group of families without child abuse, Behling (1979) and Oliver et al. (1978) reported 69% and 23% parental alcoholism, respectively. In a national survey of over 32,000 substantiated cases of child abuse or neglect, the AHA (1980) reported that 14.6% of the cases evidenced alcohol dependency. Orme and Rimmer (1981) criticized this survey because substantiated child-abuse cases were the only ones included and because determination of alcohol dependency was based on caseworkers' opinions. The AHA also was not able to report the incidence of alcoholism in a matched sample of nonabusive parents. The AHA finding is higher, however, than the apparent base rate of 7% for U.S. adults reported by the National Institute on Alcohol Abuse and Alcoholism (1978).

In their review of earlier work, Orme and Rimmer (1981) found no conclusive association between alcoholism and child abuse. The prevalence of alcoholism among child abusers was similar to that found in the general population. Of the seven studies reviewed above, only Lund and Landesman-Dwyer (1979) had an appropriate comparison group and an adequate sample size. They found twice as much abuse in delinquents with an alcoholic parent as in delinquents with nonalcoholic parents. The AHA (1980) also found twice as much alcoholism in families with child abuse than has been reported in the general population. It should, however, have included in its survey a comparison sample matched on socioeconomic and other relevant characteristics to permit a stronger conclusion. Mayer and Black's (1977) contention that children of alcoholics are at higher risk for abuse is still viable but has not yet been demonstrated in a manner that rules out third variables, such as SES and reporting bias.

Dysfunctional Family Interactions

Some investigators have moved beyond the simple comparison of families with and without an alcoholic member and have chosen to assess the impact of the alcoholic family's home environment and interaction style on the children (Davis, Stern, & Vandeusen, 1978; Filstead, McElfresh, & Anderson, 1981; Moos & Billings, 1982; Moos & Moos, 1984; Steinglass, 1979, 1981). Three studies used family members' responses on the Family Environment Scale (FES; Filstead et al., 1981; Moos & Billings, 1982; Moos & Moos, 1984), and three relied on direct observation (Davis et al., 1978; Steinglass, 1979, 1981).

In Moos and Billings's (1982) comparison of nonalcoholic, recovered, and relapsed alcoholic families' profiles on the FES, recovered alcoholic and nonalcoholic families did not differ significantly. Relapsed alcoholic families differed from nonalcoholic families on 6 of the 10 FES subscales, including lower cohesion and expressiveness, and displayed significantly greater husband-wife incongruence on perceived family environment. In a more recent investigation of nonalcoholic, relapsed, and recovered alcoholic families, Moos and Moos (1984) replicated the finding that families of relapsed alcoholics were significantly lower than both comparison groups for cohesion, expressiveness, and husband-wife congruence. Increased family arguments, low cohesion and expressiveness, and low levels of agreement about family environment were predicted through multiple regression by the alcoholic member's reports of high alcohol consumption and drinking problems, anxiety, depression, and physical symptoms. In addition, the nonalcoholic parent's reports of anxiety, depression, and use of avoidance-coping strategies added unique variance to the prediction of low family cohesion and expressiveness and more family arguments.

Filstead et al. (1981) administered the FES to 42 families with an alcoholic member and compared them with reference samples of normal families from Moos and Billings (1982) and Moos and Moos's (1984) work. The FES profiles for alcoholic families reflected less cohesion, expressiveness, independence, intellectual-cultural orientation, and active recreational orientation and greater conflict. The Filstead et al. study did not control for SES or for the presence of a psychologically disturbed family member.

Regarding direct observational studies, Davis et al. (1978) tested Minuchin's (1974) position that dysfunctional families fall at either extreme of an enmeshment-disengagement continuum. Alcoholic and nonalcoholic families completed a menu-planning task; this was videotaped and later observed. There were some differences in the way the two types of families completed the task, but the investigators were unable to place alcoholic families at either end of the continuum on the basis of these differences. Alcoholic families took significantly longer to complete the task, possibly indicating that they were less efficient, and parents in these families communicated less actively with each other. Whereas both types of families used enmeshed statements (characterized by "mind-reading," "mediated," and "personal control" responses), only the alcoholic families used significant numbers of controlling statements.

Steinglass (1979) classified alcoholic families into wet (active drinker) and dry (abstaining alcoholic) categories on the basis of the alcoholic member's drinking status. Steinglass (1979) observed each family performing an interactional problem-solving task, the Reiss Pattern Recognition Card Sort, which yields scores on two major dimensions. The configuration score connotes the quality of the family's solution to the problem, and the coordination score indicates how well the family works together as a group. Steinglass (1979) also assessed family perception of the impact of alcoholism on their lives by self-report. Surprisingly, the families with the highest configuration scores, that is, the best problem solutions, were those who perceived alcoholism as having the greatest impact on their lives, whereas dry families were significantly higher in coordination than wet families. In attempting to explain these apparently contradictory findings, Steinglass (1979) postulated that the wet families' lower coordination scores reflected freedom to behave independently, thereby arriving at more effective problem resolution, and that the dry families' high coordination scores reflected rigidity of interactional behavior, which impeded effective problem solving. Steinglass (1979) also found that the overall group of alcoholic families (wet and dry) displayed more variance in problem-solving approaches than did families previously observed performing this task (i.e., schizophrenic, delinquent, and normal), suggesting that alcoholic families are a heterogeneous group.

In a second investigation, Steinglass (1981) classified alcoholic families as wet, dry, or transitional (the alcoholic either began the study abstinent and resumed drinking by the end of the study or began the study drinking but was abstinent by the end of the study). During the 6-month period, two observers, using the Home Observation Assessment Method (HOAM), observed each family at home on nine occasions. Behavioral styles varied greatly across the alcoholic families, supporting Steinglass's (1979) view that alcoholic families are a heterogeneous group without a single characteristic behavior pattern based merely on the presence of an alcoholic member. The results of this study suggest that there are family-level patterns of behavior associated with the current phase of alcoholism. The three alcoholic groups were significantly different on two of the five major factors of the HOAM: distance regulation—which indicates the family members' propensity to share physical space as well as verbal contact with each other—and content variability—the extent to which decision-making conversations are held, the affective level associated with these, and the variability displayed on these two factors. Overall, families in the same phase of alcoholism did share similar patterns of interactional behavior, and a discriminant function analysis revealed that dimensions high in dry families generally were low in wet families and vice versa.

The family-interaction approach appears to be useful for assessing the impact of parental alcoholism on children's outcomes, particularly when applied to subgroups of the alcoholic family. The population of alcoholic families can be characterized as a heterogeneous one reflecting considerable variability in interactional processes, which could account for observed variability in child outcome. The assessment methodology found in the reviewed studies could, however, be significantly improved. Investigators have not conducted in-depth microanalyses of observed interactions of families with an alcoholic parent. Observational microanalyses have been accomplished with other populations, such as families with a schizophrenic member (Fontana, 1966; Jacob, 1975) and, more notably, families with an aggressive child (Patterson, 1982; Reid, 1978). Patterson and Reid have provided a prototype for intensive observation and analysis of family interaction based on multiple home observations, a complex coding system, and analyses that take into account sequential patterns and conditional behavioral relationships between family members.

Practical and ethical limitations are inherent in direct observation in naturalistic settings with the alcoholic population. Alcoholics by their nature would be resistant to observers coming into the home and might not give consent or might leave the home when the observers arrive. The families that would give their consent to home observation might not be representative of alcoholic families in general. Steinglass (1981) overcame these problems and completed nine home observations per family in a sample that included active alcoholics. The timing of observation in relation to periods of inebriation could also influence the observed interactions. Researchers also have to contend with the problem of measurement reactivity, which can undermine the validity of observational data (Johnson & Bolstad, 1973). Despite the inherent problems of naturalistic observation, Patterson (1982) was able to repeatedly observe difficult families and ferret out subtle patterns of interaction (e.g., coercive processes). Similar prospects are possible for alcoholic families. Using molecular coding systems, either in the home or in an analogue/clinic setting, alcoholism researchers can seek to determine (a) how alcoholic families differ (and do not differ) from normal families and from families with a nonalcoholic but psychologically disturbed parent; (b) the subtle interactive processes occurring in alcoholic families that are not yet in treatment, that are in treatment, and that have successfully completed treatment; (c) longitudinal changes in alcoholic families; and (d) individual differences in family-interaction patterns within the heterogeneous population of alcoholic families.

CONCLUSION

Parental alcoholism is undoubtedly disruptive to family life, but the link between parental alcoholism and specific child outcomes is more tenuous. In the reviewed body of literature on children of alcoholics, investigators focused primarily on features of child psychopathology, rather than on confirmed diagnoses of specific childhood disorders. Despite this limitation, the findings taken as a whole support the contention that parental alcoholism is associated with a heightened incidence of child symptomatology. Some general observations, however, regarding trends and qualifying considerations are warranted.

Neither all nor a major portion of the population of children from alcoholic homes are inevitably doomed to psychological disorder. This limiting conclusion derives from the relatively low magnitude of effects typically reported by investigators in this area. That is, they found significant group differences, but considerable overlap still existed in the distributions for children of alcoholic and nonalcoholic parents. Furthermore, the observed pattern of association may have been inflated by a heavy reliance on single measures of child outcome (particularly parental rating scales) and by the lack of confirmation of actual diagnoses of child psychological disorders. That childhood psychological disorder was not pervasive underscores the need to study individual differences in this population of children and to uncover specific factors that lead to positive outcome.

When psychopathological symptomatology was identified in children of alcoholics, the most prominent form was the category of externalizing problems. Conduct problems, restlessness and inattention, and poor academic performance, for example, were more strongly associated with children of alcoholics than were the internalizing problems of social inadequacy and somaticization. If degree of family disruption is a causal or mediating factor, it is not surprising that externalizing problems were more prominently associated with parental alcoholism. Hetherington and Martin (1979) noted similar trends (i.e., conduct problems) for family disruption associated with divorce, parental psychopathology, or other adverse factors. There were, however, some exceptions to this trend. Child anxiety and depressive symptoms, both considered internalizing problems, were consistently associated with parental alcoholism. Because of the chosen methods of analyses, however, it was not possible to detect whether anxiety and depressive problems occurred in the children who exhibited externalizing problems or in a different subset of children. This covariance issue, as well as a related issue of potential gender differences, needs to be resolved in subsequent work.

There was a noticeable absence of consensus about which specific stressors and features associated with alcoholic families lead to particular outcomes. It is probably unreasonable, however, to expect a direct or consistent relation between one specific environmental or biological factor and a single outcome. As Bell and Pearl (1982) noted, individuals are likely to move in and out of risk status across developmental phases. It may be more productive, as Chiland (1974) suggested, to focus not on "the risk itself but rather the relationship between the risk and the person in terms of his psychobiological make-up, his past history, his individual characteristics, and so forth" (p. 30). In using this approach, it is critically important to explore the interaction between risk factor and developmental level. Unfortunately, most of the reviewed studies collapsed across developmental levels in a search for broader patterns or as a means of generating a sufficiently large sample.

The biggest problem with this entire body of literature is the difficulty in inferring causal pathways. One viable pathway that received some support in the reviewed literature was the following: The presence of an alcoholic parent severely disrupts family interaction and equilibrium, which in turn causes child psychopathology. The critical aspect of disrupted family functioning, however, has yet to be isolated. For example, heightened marital discord could be the influential factor; we know that marital discord can result in child psychopathology (Emery, 1982). If marital conflict is the critical factor in producing child psychopathology, then the fact that not all alcoholic families have marked marital discord might explain why some of the offspring of alcoholic parents do not develop problems. Other possible specific factors include disrupted family routine, inadequate parental guidance and nurturance, and modeling of maladaptive coping style. Future studies might try to relate specific child problems (e.g., conduct problem, anxiety problem, and poor academic performance) with family features (e.g., marital conflict, disrupted routine, and low nurturance level).

Two potential mediating factors, severity of parental alcoholism and sex of alcoholic parent, received relatively little attention. Severity of alcoholism has an equivocal impact on child outcome (Herjanic et al., 1977; Rydelius, 1984; Wolin et al., 1979; Wolin et al., 1980). The limited data on maternal versus paternal alcoholism, coming primarily from Miller and Jang's (1977) longitudinal study, indicate that children of alcoholic mothers showed greater maladjustment. Severity and gender need to be examined more systematically in future studies.

It is difficult to attribute child outcomes solely to parental alcoholism when other risk factors are present in varying degrees and combinations. Several types of stressors occur at elevated rates in alcoholic families, including divorce, family conflict, parental psychopathology, substance abuse, parental criminality, poverty, physical abuse and neglect, and perinatal birth complications (Lund & Landesman-Dwyer, 1979; Miller & Jang, 1977; Moos & Billings, 1982; Moos & Moos, 1984; Offord et al., 1978; Robins et al., 1978; Tarter et al., 1984). Most of the studies of offspring of alcoholics failed to evaluate potential group differences for these other risk variables. Other methods of addressing the multiple-risk problem included (a) noting group differences on specific factors but not correcting for the problem, (b) matching groups with respect to one or more risk factors (e.g., divorce), (c) forming a separate group to systematically covary a risk factor (e.g., parental psychopathology), and (d) examining within-group differences as a function of additional risk factors. The second, third, and fourth alternatives enhance internal validity, whereas the first alternative simply acknowledges a confounded design.

Developmental level needs to be taken into account to a greater extent in research with children of alcoholics. Longitudinal designs would, of course, help address the pertinent developmental issues, such as the ontogeny of child psychopathology, the interaction between age of child and type of child psychopathology, and the differential impact of an alcoholic parent at varying ages. Cross-sectional studies can also be improved by taking into account how long and at what ages the children were exposed to the adversity of an alcoholic parent.

Future investigations of the children of alcoholic parents can be improved methodologically in the following ways:

1. Investigators can describe samples in greater detail, including the child's age at onset of parental alcoholism, presence or absence of exposure to prenatal maternal drinking, severity of parental alcoholism, extent of psychopathology and criminality of each parent, extent of marital discord, and alcoholic parent's recent treatment history.

2. Samples can be subdivided and analyzed in terms of children with and without prenatal exposure to maternal drinking for ferreting out postnatal environmental effects from prenatal factors.
3. Gender of offspring and alcoholic parent needs to be taken into account. At this stage in the research, it is not clear whether boys are more adversely affected by an alcoholic mother or an alcoholic father and whether a finding in this regard would hold for female offspring as well. Although fewer alcoholic mothers are available to study, sex differences should be analyzed whenever possible.
4. Inclusion of two comparison groups, one of children with normal-functioning parents and one of children with a nonalcoholic but psychologically disturbed parent, permits identification of outcomes associated specifically with alcoholism. Studies by Fine et al. (1976), Merikangas et al. (1985), and Steinhausen et al. (1982) exemplify this multicomparison approach.
5. Assessment of child psychopathology can be confirmed by seeking convergence across independent sources of data (e.g., teachers, parents, observers, and children). Too often, parental ratings were taken as the sole judgment of child adjustment. Furthermore, it takes more than a rating scale to make the diagnosis of a child's psychological disorder.
6. Short-term prospective designs would probably lead to stronger conclusions than cross-sectional designs have yielded. Longitudinal follow-up, if conducted sufficiently early in the child's life, may uncover the ontogeny of child problems.
7. Detailed observational analyses of family interaction, similar to the methodology used by Patterson (1982) and Reid (1978), may lead to the identification of interactional processes unique to alcoholic families.

The effects of parental alcoholism need to be viewed within a theoretical framework that considers multiple sources of stress on children. Although the role of multiple risk factors is clearly relevant to the study of children of alcoholic parents, the effects of additional risk factors may not be linear. Rutter (1979) illustrated that the combination of several stressors potentiate each other, resulting in greater impairment than expected from summation of simple effects for each stressor. Psychopathy in an alcoholic father, co-occurrence of other psychopathology in either parent, socioeconomic deprivation, child abuse, and intense marital discord (and spouse abuse) are some of the stressors that could potentiate the adverse effects of parental alcoholism.

When the occurrence of multiple stressors is taken into account, these additional factors may explain why some children of alcoholics fare worse than others. An alternative view, however, is that some children develop resiliency despite the adverse features of the parents' alcoholism and associated pathologies. Garmezy (1983), Werner (1984), and Werner and Smith (1982) have referred to these children and to others who have weathered such severe stresses as parental schizophrenia and war as "invulnerables." Research strategies based on the notion of invulnerability emphasize the identification (and, ultimately, the promotion) of protective factors that account for a child's development of coping competence. For example, Werner identified in her own longitudinal study several potentially protective factors, including nurturance from substitute care givers within the family, active use of an informal network outside the family for advice and assistance, positive classroom experiences, and an acquired sense of meaning and faith about life. Rutter (1979) maintained that factors such as positive influences at school, a stable relationship with the nondisturbed parent or another adult, parental provision of structure and control, and the child's coping skills and maintenance of self-esteem may serve a protective function. Similarly, Sameroff and Seifer (1983) pointed to parental beliefs, attitudes, and coping abilities as important mediators between environmental stress and child competence. Similar protective factors and the variables critical to their development need to be pinpointed within the population of children from alcoholic families. This type of approach would focus on competence and the absence of psychopathology and would necessitate a different set of measures. Coping styles and social support networks would invariably come into play as well. Ultimately, it will be possible to obtain more refined answers to the questions, Which children of alcoholic families fare well and which do not, and why?

REFERENCES

Achenbach, T. (1978). Psychopathology of childhood: Research problems and issues. *Journal of Consulting and Clinical Psychology, 46,* 759–776.

Adler, R., & Raphael, B. (1983). Children of alcoholics. *Australian and New Zealand Journal of Psychiatry, 17,* 3–8.

American Humane Association. (1980). *National analysis of official child neglect and abuse reporting, 1978.* Englewood, CO: Author.

American Psychiatric Association. (1980). *Diagnostic and statistical manual of mental disorders* (3rd ed.). Washington, DC: Author.

Anderson, E., & Quast, W. (1983). Young children in alcoholic families: A mental health needs-assessment and an intervention/prevention strategy. *Journal of Primary Prevention, 3,* 174–187.

Arentzen, W. (1978). Impact of alcohol misuse on family life. *Alcoholism: Clinical and Experimental Research, 2,* 349–351.

Aronson, M., Kyllerman, M., Sabel, K. G., Sandin, B., & Olegard, R. (1985). Children of alcoholic mothers: Developmental, perceptual and behavioral characteristics as compared to matched controls. *Acta Paediatrica Scandinavia, 74,* 27–35.

Bacon, S. (1984). Alcohol issues and social science. *Journal of Drug Issues, 14,* 7–29.

Behling, D. (1979). Alcohol abuse as encountered in 51 instances of reported child abuse. *Clinical Pediatrics, 18,* 87–91.

Bell, B., & Cohen, R. (1981). The Bristol Social Adjustment Guide: Comparison between the offspring of alcoholic and non-alcoholic mothers. *British Journal of Clinical Psychology, 20,* 93–95.

Bell, R., & Pearl, D. (1982). Psychosocial change in risk groups: Implications for early identification. *Prevention in Human Services, 1,* 45–59.

Biek, J. (1981). Screening test for identifying adolescents adversely affected by a parental drinking problem. *Journal of Adolescent Health Care, 2,* 107–113.

Black, C. (1979). Children of alcoholics. *Alcohol, Health, and Research World, 4,* 23–27.

Bohman, M. (1978). Some genetic aspects of alcoholism and criminality. *Archives of General Psychiatry, 35,* 269–276.

Booz-Allen & Hamilton, (1974). *An assessment of the needs of and resources for children of alcoholic parents* (Report No. PB-241-119). Springfield, VA: National Technical Information Service.

Cadoret, R. J., & Gath, A. (1978). Inheritance of alcoholism in adoptees. *British Journal of Psychiatry, 132,* 252–258.

Campbell, D., & Stanley, J. (1963). *Experimental and quasi-experimental designs for research.* Boston: Houghton Mifflin.

Cantwell, D. (1975). Familial-genetic research with hyperactive children. In D. Cantwell (Ed.), *The hyperactive child: Diagnosis, management, and current research* (pp. 93–105). New York: Spectrum.

Cantwell, D. (1976). Genetic factors in the hyperkinetic syndrome. *Journal of the American Academy of Child Psychiatry, 15,* 214–223.

Chiland, C. (1974). Some paradoxes connected with risk and vulnerability. In E. J. Anthony & C. Koupernik (Eds.), *The child in his family: Children at psychiatric risk* (pp. 23–31). New York: Wiley.

Cotton, N. (1979). The familial incidence of alcoholism. *Journal of Studies on Alcohol, 40,* 89–116.

Davis, P., Stern, D., & Vandeusen, J. (1978). Enmeshment-disengagement in the alcoholic family. In F. A. Seixas (Ed.), *Currents in alcoholism* (Vol. 4, pp. 15–27). New York: Grune & Stratton.

el-Guebaly, N., & Offord, D. (1977). The offspring of alcoholics: A critical review. *American Journal of Psychiatry, 134,* 357–365.

el-Guebaly, N., & Offord, D. (1979). On being the offspring of an alcoholic: An update. *Alcoholism: Clinical and Experimental Research, 3,* 148–157.

Ellwood, L. (1980). Effects of alcoholism as a family illness on child behavior and development. *Military Medicine, 145,* 188–192.

Emery, R. E. (1982). Interparental conflict and the children of discord and divorce. *Psychological Bulletin, 92,* 310–330.

Ervin, C., Little, R., Streissguth, A., & Beck, D. (1984). Alcoholic fathering and its relation to child's intellectual development: A pilot investigation. *Alcoholism: Clinical and Experimental Research, 8,* 362–365.

Feighner, J., Robins, E., Guze, S., Woodruff, R., Winokur, G., & Munoz, R. (1972). Diagnostic criteria for use in psychiatric research. *Archives of General Psychiatry, 26,* 57–63.

Filstead, W., McElfresh, O., & Anderson, C. (1981). Comparing the family environments of alcoholic and "normal" families. *Journal of Alcohol and Drug Education, 26,* 24–31.

Fine, E., Yudin, L., Holmes, J., & Heinemann, S. (1976). Behavioral disorders in children with parental alcoholism. *Annals of the New York Academy of Sciences, 273,* 507–517.

Fontana, A. (1966). Familial etiology of schizophrenia: Is a scientific methodology possible? *Psychological Bulletin, 66,* 214–227.

Gabrielli, W., & Mednick, S. (1983). Intellectual performance in children of alcoholics. *Journal of Nervous and Mental Disease, 171,* , 444–447.

Garmezy, N. (1983). Stressors of childhood. In N. Garmezy & M. Rutter (Eds.), *Stress, coping, and development in children* (pp. 43–84). New York: McGraw-Hill.

Goodwin, D. (1979). Alcoholism and heredity: A review and hypothesis. *Archives of General Psychiatry, 36,* 57–61.

Goodwin, D., Schulsinger, F., Hermansen, L., Guze, S., & Winokur, G. (1973). Alcohol problems in adoptees raised apart from alcoholic biological parents. *Archives of General Psychiatry, 28,* 238–243.

Goodwin, D., Schulsinger, F., Moller, N., Hermansen, L., Winokur, G., & Guze, S. (1974). Drinking problems in adopted and nonadopted sons of alcoholics. *Archives of General Psychiatry, 31,* 164–169.

Gualtieri, C. T., Adams, A., Shen, C.D., & Loiselle, D. (1982). Minor physical anomalies in alcoholic and schizophrenic adults and hyperactive and autistic children. *American Journal of Psychiatry, 139,* 640–643.

Hall, R. L., Hesselbrock, V. M., & Stabenau, J. R. (1983a). Familial distribution of alcohol use: I. Assortative mating in the parents of alcoholics. *Behavior Genetics, 13,* 361–373.

Hall, R. L., Hesselbrock, V. M., & Stabenau, J. R. (1983b). Familial distribution of alcohol use: II. Assortative mating of alcoholic probands. *Behavior Genetics, 13,* 373–382.

Heller, K., Sher, K., & Benson, C. (1982). Problems associated with risk overprediction in studies of offspring of alcoholics: Implications for prevention. *Clinical Psychology Review, 2,* 183–200.

Herjanic, B., Herjanic, M., Penick, E., Tomelleri, C., & Armbruster, R. (1977). Children of alcoholics. In F. A. Seixas (Ed.), *Currents in alcoholism* (Vol. 2, pp. 445–455). New York: Grune & Stratton.

Herjanic, B., Herjanic, M., Wetzel, R., & Tomelleri, C. (1978). Substance abuse: Its effect on offspring. *Research Communications in Psychology, Psychiatry and Behavior, 3,* 65–75.

Hetherington, E. M., & Martin, B. (1979). Family interaction. In H. C. Quay & J. S. Werry (Eds.), *Psychopathological disorders of childhood* (pp. 247–302). New York: Wiley.

Hughes, J. M. (1977). Adolescent children of alcoholic parents and the relationship of Alateen to these children. *Journal of Consulting and Clinical Psychology, 45,* 946–947.

Jacob, T. (1975). Family interaction in disturbed and normal families: A methodological and substantive review. *Psychological Bulletin, 82,* 33–65.

Jacob, T., Favorini, A., Meisel, S., & Anderson, C. (1978). The alcoholic's spouse, children and family interactions: Substantive findings and methodological issues. *Journal of Studies on Alcohol, 39,* 1231–1251.

Johnson, S. M., & Bolstad, O. D. (1973). Methodological issues in naturalistic observations: Some problems and solutions for field research. In L. A. Hammerlynck, L. C. Handy, & E. J. Mash (Eds.), *Behavior change: Methodology concepts and practice* (pp. 7–68). Champaign, IL: Research Press.

Kern, J., Hassett, C., Collipp, P., Bridges, C., Solomon, M., & Condren, R. (1981). Children of alcoholics: Locus of control, mental age, and zinc level. *Journal of Psychiatric Treatment and Evaluation, 3,* 169–173.

Knop, J., Teasdale, T., Schulsinger, F., & Goodwin, D. (1985). A prospective study of young men at high risk for alcoholism: School behavior and achievement. *Journal of Studies on Alcohol, 46,* 273–278.

Lund, C., & Landesman-Dwyer, S. (1979). Pre-delinquent and disturbed adolescents: The role of parental alcoholism. In M. Galanter (Ed.), *Currents in alcoholism* (Vol. 5, pp. 339–348). New York: Grune & Stratton.

Mayer, J., & Black, R. (1977). The relationship between alcoholism and child abuse and neglect. In F. A. Seixas (Ed.), *Currents in alcoholism* (Vol. 2, pp. 429–444). New York: Grune & Stratton.

Mayer, J., Black, R., & MacDonall, J. (1978). Child care in families with an alcohol addicted parent. In F. A. Seixas (Ed.), *Currents in alcoholism* (Vol. 4, pp. 329–338). New York: Grune & Stratton.

Merikangas, K., Weissman, M., Prusoff, B., Pauls, D., & Leckman, J. (1985). Depressives with secondary alcoholism: Psychiatric disorders in offspring. *Journal of Studies on Alcohol, 46,* 199–204.

Miller, D., & Jang, M. (1977). Children of alcoholics: a 20-year longitudinal study. *Social Work Research and Abstracts, 13,* 23–29.

Minuchin, S. (1974). *Families and family therapy.* Cambridge, MA: Harvard University Press.

Moos, R., & Billings, A. (1982). Children of alcoholics during the recovery process: Alcoholic and matched control families. *Addictive Behaviors, 7,* 155–163.

Moos, R., & Moos, B. (1984). The process of recovery from alcoholism: Comparing functioning in families of alcoholics and matched control families. *Journal of Studies on Alcohol, 45,* 111–118.

Morehouse, E., & Richards, T. (1982). An examination of dysfunctional latency age children of alcoholic parents and problems in intervention. *Journal of Children in Contemporary Society, 15,* 21–33.

Morrison, J. (1980). Adult psychiatric disorders in parents of hyperactive children. *American Journal of Psychiatry, 137,* 825–827.

Murray, R. M., Clifford, C. A., & Gurling, H. M. D. (1983). Twin and adoption studies: How good is the evidence for a genetic role? In M. Galanter (Ed.), *Recent developments in alcoholism, Vol. 1, Genetics, behavioral treatment, social mediators and prevention, current concepts in diagnosis* (pp. 25–48). New York: Plenum Press.

Nardi, P. (1981). Children of alcoholics: A role-theoretical perspective. *Journal of Social Psychology, 115,* 237–245.

National Institute on Alcohol Abuse and Alcoholism. (1978). *Alcohol and health: Third special report to the U.S. Congress* (DHEW Publication No. ADM-78-569). Washington, DC: U.S. Government Printing Office.

Offord, D., Allen, N., & Abrams, N. (1978). Parental psychiatric illness, broken homes, and delinquency. *Journal of the American Academy of Child Psychiatry, 17,* 224–238.

Oliver, J., Cox, J., & Buchanan, A. (1978). The extent of child abuse. In S. M. Smith (Ed.), *The maltreatment of children* (pp. 121–174). Baltimore, MD: University Park Press.

Orme, T., & Rimmer, J. (1981). Alcoholism and child abuse: A review. *Journal of Studies on Alcohol, 42,* 273–287.

Patterson, G. R. (1982). *Coercive family process.* Eugene, OR: Castalia.

Peele, S. (1986). The implications and limitations of genetic models of alcoholism and other addictions. *Journal of Studies on Alcohol, 47,* 63–73.

Prewett, M., Spence, R., & Chaknis, M. (1981). Attribution of causality by children with alcoholic parents. *International Journal of the Addictions, 16,* 367–370.

Prinz, R. J., Connor, P. A., & Wilson, C. C. (1981). Hyperactive and aggressive behaviors in childhood: Intertwined dimensions. *Journal of Abnormal Child Psychology, 9,* 191–202.

Reid, J. (Ed.) (1978). *A social learning approach to family intervention: Volume 2: Observation in home settings.* Eugene, OR: Castalia.

Richards, T. (1980). Splitting as a defense mechanism in children of alcoholic parents. In F. A. Seixas (Ed.), *Currents in alcoholism* (Vol. 7, pp. 239–244). New York: Grune & Stratton.

Rimmer, J. (1982). The children of alcoholics: An exploratory study. *Children and Youth Services Review, 4,* 365–373.

Roberts, K., & Brent, E. (1982). Physician utilization and illness patterns in families of alcoholics. *Journal of Studies on Alcohol, 43,* 119–128.

Robins, L., West, P., Ratcliff, K., & Herjanic, B. (1978). Father's alcoholism and children's outcomes. In F. A. Seixas (Ed.), *Currents in alcoholism* (Vol. 4, pp. 313–327). New York: Grune & Stratton.

Rutter, M. (1979). Protective factors in children's responses to stress and disadvantage. In M. W. Kent & J. E. Rolf (Eds.), *Social competence in children* (pp. 49–74). Hanover, NH: University Press of New England.

Rydelius, P. (1983). Alcohol-abusing teenage boys. *Acta Psychiatrica Scandinavica, 68,* 368–380.

Rydelius, P. (1984). Children of alcoholic fathers: A longitudinal prospective study. In D. W. Goodwin, K. T. Van Dusen, & S. A. Mednick (Eds.), *Longitudinal research in alcoholism* (pp. 27–37). Boston: Kluwer-Nijhoff.

Sameroff, A., & Seifer, R. (1983). Familial risk and child competence. *Child Development, 54,* 1254–1268.

Saunders, J., & Williams, R. (1983). The genetics of alcoholism: Is there an inherited susceptibility to alcohol-related problems? *Alcohol and Alcoholism, 18,* 189–217.

Schuckit, M., & Chiles, J. (1978). Family history as a diagnostic aid in two samples of adolescents. *Journal of Nervous and Mental Disease, 166,* 165–176.

Seixas, J. (1982). Children from alcoholic homes. In N. Estes & E. Heinemann (Eds.), *Alcoholism: Development, consequences and interventions* (pp. 193–201). St. Louis, MO: Mosby.

Shaywitz, S., Cohen, D., & Shaywitz, B. (1980). Behavior and learning difficulties in children of normal intelligence born to alcoholic mothers. *Journal of Pediatrics, 96,* 978–982.

Steinglass, P. (1979). The alcoholic family in the interaction laboratory. *Journal of Nervous and Mental Disease, 167,* 428–436.

Steinglass, P. (1981). The alcoholic family at home: Patterns of interaction in dry, wet, and transitional stages of alcoholism. *Archives of General Psychiatry, 38,* 578–584.

Steinhausen, H., Gobel, D., & Nestler, V. (1984). Psychopathology in the offspring of alcoholic parents. *Journal of the American Academy of Child Psychiatry, 23,* 465–471.

Steinhausen, H., Nestler, V., & Huth, H. (1982). Psychopathology and mental functions in the offspring of alcoholic and epileptic mothers. *Journal of the American Academy of Child Psychiatry, 21,* 268–273.

Stewart, M., deBlois, S., & Cummings, C. (1980). Psychiatric disorder in the parents of hyperactive boys and those with conduct disorder. *Journal of Child Psychology, Psychiatry, and Allied Disciplines, 21,* 283–292.

Stewart, M., deBlois, S., & Singer, S. (1979). Alcoholism and hyperactivity revisited: A preliminary report. In M. Galanter (Ed.), *Currents in alcoholism* (Vol. 5, pp. 349–357). New York: Grune & Stratton.

Straussner, S., Weinstein, D., & Hernandez, R. (1979). Effects of alcoholism on the family system. *Health and Social Work, 4,* 111–127.

Streissguth, A. P. (1976). Psychologic handicaps in children with the fetal alcohol syndrome. *Annals of the New York Academy of Sciences, 273,* 140–145.

Streissguth, A. P. (1978). Fetal alcohol syndrome, an epidemiologic perspective. *American Journal of Epidemiology, 107,* 467–478.

Streissguth, A. P., Landesman-Dwyer, S., Martin, J. C., & Smith, D. W. (1980). Teratogenic effects of alcohol in humans and laboratory animals. *Science, 209,* 353–361.

Streissguth, A. P., Little, R. E., Herman, C., & Woodell, S. (1979). IQ in children of recovered alcoholic mothers compared to matched controls. *Alcoholism: Clinical and Experimental Research, 3,* 197.

Tarter, R., Hegedus, A., Goldstein, G., Shelly, C., & Alterman, A. (1984). Adolescent sons of alcoholics: Neuropsychological and personality characteristics. *Alcoholism: Clinical and Experimental Research, 8,* 216–222.

Vaillant, G. E. (1983). *The natural history of alcoholism.* Cambridge, MA: Harvard University Press.

Waldrop, M. F. (1978). Newborn minor physical anomalies predict short attention span, peer aggression, and impulsivity at age 3. *Science, 199,* 563–564.

Wanlass, R. L., & Prinz, R. J. (1982). Methodological issues in conceptualizing and treating childhood social isolation. *Psychological Bulletin, 92,* 39–55.

Warner, R. H., & Rosett, H. L. (1975). The effects of drinking on offspring. *Journal of Studies on Alcohol, 36,* 1395–1420.

Watters, T., & Theimer, W. (1978). Children of alcoholics: A critical review of some literature. *Contemporary Drug Problems, 7,* 195–201.

Werner, E. E. (1984). Resilient children. *Young Children, 40,* 68–72.

Werner, E. E., & Smith, R. S. (1982). *Vulnerable but invincible: A study of resilient children.* New York: McGraw-Hill.

Woititz, J. (1978). Alcoholism and the family: A survey of the literature. *Journal of Alcohol and Drug Education, 23,* 18–23.

Wolin, S., Bennett, L., & Noonan, D. (1979). Family rituals and the recurrence of alcoholism over generations. *American Journal of Psychiatry, 136,* 589–593.

Wolin, S., Bennett, L., Noonan, D., & Teitelbaum, M. (1980). Disrupted family rituals: A factor in the intergenerational transmission of alcoholism. *Journal of Studies on Alcohol, 41,* 199–214.

Woodside, M. (1982). *Children of alcoholics.* New York: State Division of Alcoholism and Alcohol Abuse.

Woodside, M. (1983). Children of alcoholic parents: Inherited and psychosocial influences. *Journal of Psychiatric Treatment and Evaluation, 5,* 531–537.

PART IV: SPECIAL STRESS AND COPING

16

Current Status and Future Directions of Research on the American Indian Child

Alayne Yates

Arizona Health Sciences Center, Tucson

American Indians are the most severely disadvantaged of any population within the United States. By adolescence, Indian children show higher rates of suicide, alcoholism, drug abuse, delinquency, and out-of-home placement. School achievement is severely compromised, and many youths drop out before graduation from high school. The Indian child understands the environment through intuitive, visual, and pictorial means, but success in the Anglo school is largely dependent on auditory processing, abstract conceptualization, and language skills. This difference compounds existing problems of poverty, dislocation, alienation, depression and intergenerational conflict and can partially account for the higher rate of emotional and behavioral problems among Indian adolescents.

On the whole, American Indian tribes are remarkable in that they have withstood attempts at extermination, removal from their traditional lands, extreme poverty, deployment of their youth to boarding schools, relocation policies, and, last but not least, the white man's poison—alcohol. In spite of this, the tribes remain ethnically distinct in cognitive style, language forms, art and culture. Although there are many similarities among tribes and, in this article, Indians will frequently be referred to as a homogeneous people, the tribes are actually quite heterogeneous.

Reprinted with permission from the *American Journal of Psychiatry,* 1987, Vol. 144, No. 9, 1135–1142. Copyright 1987 by the American Psychiatric Association.

For centuries, American Indians have existed as hunters and gatherers, living off the none-too-fertile land. They became uniquely adapted to that style, developing skills which enabled them to survive. Now, American Indians are expected to "acculturate," which may mean abandoning all that is sacred and unique in their traditional life style. This expectation entails considerable stress and the risk of identity diffusion. The plight of the partially acculturated American Indian is epitomized by the Iroquois saying, "One cannot long have one's feet placed in two canoes." This quotation, in itself, is a succinct graphic metaphor, creating in our minds a rich visual picture of a concept that would entail many words. The graphic metaphor is also the cognitive language of the American Indian.

In 1900 there were 220,000 Indians in the United States; today there are somewhere between 1 and 2 million Indians in approximately 400 recognized tribes, 180 of which have a land base such as a reservation. One-third of the Indian population live on reservations, one-third are urban, and one-third move back and forth between town and reservation (1). The median age of the Indian population is 17.3 years; in the United States as a whole the median age is 29.5 years (2). This discrepancy is primarily accounted for by the birth rate among Indians, which is twice as high as that of the country at large. The death rate in certain age groups is also extraordinarily high: among 5–24-year-old Indians the death rate is two to three times higher than it is in the United States as a whole (3), and the infant mortality is the highest of any ethnic group in the United States. Twenty percent of all deaths among American Indians occur in infants and young children (2).

The disability rate among American Indians is four to six times the national average. Diabetes and the complications of alcoholism are the sources of the greatest disability among adults, and hepatitis B infection and otitis media contribute to children's disabilities (2, 4). The average income of Indian families is $2,000/year, far below the poverty level. On the reservation, the mean average income is only $900/year, well below a bare level of subsistence. Of necessity, many Indians continue to supplement this meager allotment through hunting and gathering. The overall unemployment rate is 40%, but it is as high as 75%–90% on some reservations (1). Thus, the American Indian is the most severely disadvantaged population within the United States.

MENTAL HEALTH PROBLEMS AMONG INDIAN CHILDREN

The overall rate of emotional disorders in childhood among American Indians is 20%–25% (2), compared with 5%–15% among children in the Anglo population. However, these figures must be held suspect because national statistical comparisons are usually based on small-scale tribal studies and rates of emotional disorder vary dramatically among tribes and among regions. However, there does seem to be a fascinating pattern of variance— among Indian children 5–9 years old, the rate of emotional disturbance is approximately the same as it is in the majority culture; problems consist of both learning and behavioral difficulties (5). Between ages 10 and 14 the emotional disorder rate in Indian children begins to escalate and includes delinquency and drug use as well as learning and behavioral problems. Whereas only 9% of youths in the majority culture have abused inhalants, 22% of Indian youths have abused them (6). By far the greatest number of emotional problems occur between ages 15 and 19: problems of drug and alcohol abuse and delinquency in males and unwanted pregnancy, alcohol abuse, and suicide attempts in females (5). Many authors (2, 7, 8) have described profound alienation and depression in Indian adolescents, al- though, once again, there is marked variation between tribes.

Alcohol abuse is an extensive and pervasive problem for the Indian. The overall rate of alcoholism is two to three times the national average (9, 10), although the rate varies widely among tribes. The rate of recent alcohol use is 50% among Indian adolescents and 20% in the majority culture (6). It is not uncommon to find children as young as 6 years old already drinking alcohol (11). Among adolescents, alcohol abuse is a normative pattern that facilitates interaction (5) and reduces psychological distress (8). To refuse a drink when it is offered is to insult the one who offers; the person who refuses is thought to be acting superior, like a white man (12). Solitary drinking is infrequent, but rapid drinking to become intoxicated is common. In some areas, being drunk becomes equivalent to being possessed by a spirit, which relieves the intoxicated person from responsibility for antisocial acts (13). Because of the cultural policy of noninterference, adults seldom intervene in the drinking behaviors of their children.

Associated with alcohol abuse is an inordinate number of accidents: 75 % of accidents are alcohol related, 80% of suicides are alcohol related, and 90% of homicides are alcohol related (14). In addition, alcohol-abusing adoles- cents often become alcoholic parents who tend to neglect their children and become involved in domestic violence (11). They are also three to four times as likely as members of the majority culture to succumb to cirrhosis of the liver and other complications of alcohol abuse (14). The suicide rate among Indians peaks in the adolescent and young adult years (15, 16) and is the second major cause of death in adolescence. There is substantial variation among tribes (15, 17); rates are higher in dislocated tribes where members are unable to practice the traditional life style. The suicide rate has remained low on a few reservations where traditional practices are maintained and where adolescents can attend school and work within the tribal community (18).

During adolescence, 12 of every 100 Indian youths and 2.5 of every 100 adolescents in the majority culture appear in court. The Indian youths are more likely to appear because of misdemeanors or petty offenses that are alcohol related (19). When the court appearances are controlled for alcohol intoxication, the rates are approximately the same in both cultures (9).

In spite of a common assumption to the contrary, very few Indian children are abused: 6.5/1,000 Indian boys and 2.7/1,000 Indian girls suffer maltreatment, compared with 13/1,000 black children and 15/1,000 white children (20, 21). Physical punishment is frowned upon in most Indian communities, and children are protected through informal placement within the extended family, a major resource for Indian youngsters. Most maltreated Indian children are neglected rather than physically abused (20), which is not surprising given the level of poverty on Indian reservations. In addition, Indian parents may be interpreted as neglectful by Anglo agency workers because of cultural differences (22). In some instances, the maltreatment is directly related to the alcohol abuse of one or both parents.

In spite of the lower rate of child maltreatment, five to 20 times as many Indian children as children in the culture as a whole are in out-of-home placements (23, 24). In 1976, almost 50,000 Indian children resided in boarding schools, foster homes, and adoptive homes (25). As many as 85% of these placements were in non-Indian residences (23), thus occasioning a profound rupture of cultural ties (26). "Poverty" was the most frequent rationale for out-of-home placement (27). Placement in boarding schools has been related to the unavailability of day schools in isolated areas of reservations, especially among the Navajo, 10,000 of whose elementary schoolchildren are now boarded (4). Other students are at boarding school because of the lack of adoptive or foster home placements for older, often psychiatrically disturbed, youths. The rate of psychiatric disorders is higher among children placed outside their homes (28; unpublished 1978 paper by M.D. Topper), but this may be either a cause or an effect of the placement. To date there has been no controlled outcome study of out-of-tribe versus in-tribe placement and how this variable might influence the quality of attachment and incidence of emotional disorder.

Many Indian children who live in isolated villages are never registered in public school but are taught by using whatever resources are available. A number of other children are enrolled in school but do not attend due to lack of transportation or insufficient motivation. It is likely that children who do attend school will drop out before finishing the program. The dropout rate in boarding school is 60% (29), in high school it is almost 50%, and in college it is 70% (30). There have been fewer Indian youths enrolled in government-funded boarding schools in the past decade, and there has been an effort to improve the quality of life of the Indian child who boards (31). However, as many as 75% of the boarders are said to suffer from emotional problems, alienation, and feelings of defeat and helplessness (32), perhaps related to the austere environment and to the children's attempts to match traditional values with those expected within the boarding school. When this is not possible, the result is a pattern of superficial responsiveness (33, 34). School dropouts often return to the reservation. These individuals may be reintegrated and lead productive lives, or they may continue to "drop out" on the reservation because of alcoholism, depression, and vocational failure.

To grow up as an Indian child is to grow up as a member of an extraordinarily disadvantaged minority. The pervasive emotional, physical, and social disabilities create a legacy of hopelessness and helplessness from which Indian youths must struggle to emerge. These disabilities stand as the penultimate predictors of a problematic future.

ACCULTURATION STRESS

Acculturation is a critical process that involves multiple variables at the cultural, ethnic, interpersonal, and intrapersonal levels. Adaptive acculturation can be achieved by two means: by assimilation into the dominant culture, which means that one's original cultural identity is relinquished, or by integration, which means that the original cultural identity is retained. Assimilation and integration are considered adaptive approaches. The most maladaptive approach is the rejection of either the original or the dominant culture. Some individuals and groups become marginal, existing apart from either society. Although stress is not an inevitable concomitant of acculturation, it is accentuated when the cultural distance between the two groups is great and the insistence on change is strong (35). Greater stress is found in groups who resemble the majority culture the least, who do not have a great deal of contact with the majority culture, and who have been uprooted so that their traditional and social supports are disrupted. By these measures, Indians suffer considerable stress if they remain on the reservation with little cultural interchange and if they migrate to cities or are relocated away from their traditional lands.

Stress experienced by the family affects the children. Boggs (36), in a study of the Ojibwa, found that the children of "somewhat acculturated" families were more passive and less responsive than children of either traditional or acculturated families. The parents of somewhat acculturated children interacted less in the home and appeared less involved with the children. This may be an early symptom of an important component of acculturative stress: intergenerational conflict. Young people acculturate more rapidly as they attend school and have greater contact with the majority culture. Because of their age, young people may be more open to change than are their parents. Parents feel abandoned and devalued in response to their children's greater acculturation. Studies of acculturating Hispanic families (37) demonstrated that the families with the greatest intergenerational conflict evidenced the most serious symptomatic behavior.

TRADITIONAL VALUES

If Indians, in the process of acculturation, espouse Anglo ways, they find themselves in conflict with the tribe. If they remain traditional, they may find themselves in conflict with the dominant culture, especially in the areas of sharing, allegiance, respect for elders, noninterference, orientation to present time, and harmony with nature.

Sharing

Indian children are taught to share; competitive striving is inhibited and generosity is encouraged (38). Children are unwilling to compete because they do not wish to shame the person who loses. Children playing baseball on the Papago reservation hit the ball as many times as necessary. The score is not kept and team members are not selected on the basis of skill. Because of their reluctance to compete, Indian children in Anglo schools are often labeled as unmotivated or alienated. The reluctance to compete is situation specific; Indian children can be as fiercely competitive as anyone else when circumstances are conducive.

Allegiance

Allegiance is to the family and the community rather than to the self. The youth who excels in terms of personal achievement may be ridiculed and rejected within the tribe. The following example was provided by G. Krutz.

> *Case 1.* At 17 years of age, Charlie was about to graduate from high school. He was an excellent boxer and had become the state boxing champion. During a school assembly, the principal gave Charlie a special award accompanied by a long, impassioned congratulatory address. On the way out of the auditorium, a group of other Indian boys jumped on Charlie and pummeled him

soundly. Charlie dropped out of school even though there was but 1 month to graduation.

Respect for Elders

Children are taught not to question or to look directly at adults because this would be disrespectful. As this principle also applies to teachers within the school system, Indian children have been described as withdrawn, shy, or uninterested because they avoid eye contact and do not speak up (39).

Noninterference

Indian children are not perceived as the property of their parents but as autonomous, equal individuals (40) who progress in life at their own inimitable pace and who are responsible for their own choices. Thus, toddlers choose when to eat or to sleep and grade-school children may choose not to attend school. Older children may travel to the medical clinic by themselves (26) and may decide whether to have elective surgery (41). Since there is no "right" way to raise children, parents do not interfere with the expectable course of development (42, 43). Training in developmental tasks is encouraged and rewarded but not consciously taught or forced (unpublished 1967 report by J. Ablon et al.). Thus, many Indian parents have been described as neglectful or uninvolved when, in fact, they are concerned with their children's wellbeing (22).

Orientation to Present Time

Indian children may not arrive at school on time, and Indian youth may not complete assignments or report for work as scheduled. These children, especially the girls, tend to live in and to value present time; deadlines are markers of future time (33; unpublished 1967 report by J. Ablon et al.). The following case vignette was supplied by G. Krutz.

> *Case 2.* An Indian Health Service official received authorization for a mental health services contract, to be offered to the Papago Tribal Council. He presented the document to a Tribal Council member who was also an old friend. After perusing the document, the Indian representative indicated that he would "see about it." Six months passed. Because there was a deadline on the contract the Health Service official received many memos, but he refused to pressure or even to recontact his friend. In the meantime, the

Tribal Council member was sitting with various families to discuss the pros and cons of mental health services in general. Finally, several months after the original deadline, he presented the signed contract to the Indian Health Service official.

Because of this disregard for deadlines, Indians have often been thought to be lazy or irresponsible. However, an Indian's disregard for deadlines is also context dependent, and the context often does not favor the Indian.

Harmony with Nature

To the Indian, life should be an unhurried, natural progression (unpublished 1967 report by J. Ablon et al.). White men are viewed as tampering with and distorting nature. Disease, death, and disability are accepted as milestones in the course of life's progress.

Case 3. A new, rather officious medical social worker on an Indian reservation attempted to convince the women that their children should receive polio vaccine. In spite of her well-prepared presentation, which included statements like "You don't want them to get polio, do you?" the women did not bring their children to the clinic. They listened politely and sometimes giggled among themselves. Two years later, the social worker learned through another professional that the women had named her "Woman Who Can't Stop Talking."

Because of Indians' apparent disregard for the principles of the majority culture, they can be perceived as disconnected or as uncaring and irresponsible.

THE VISUAL MODE

An important and hitherto poorly understood source of acculturation stress is the differing cognitive style of American Indians. For centuries, the Indian peoples depended on the visual pathway. They followed animals by sign and track and memorized facets of the territory. Blending with the landscape, they moved silently through the forest to avoid their enemies. The women were able to single out edible plants from a mass of vegetation. Indians predicted changes in the weather and the migration of animals by studying the sky and the earth. The principle of observation was central in the culture.

The virtue of silence has been taught to Indian children from earliest infancy. Among the Plains Indians, when a newborn baby cried the parent would place a hand over the infant's nose so that the mouth would be needed for breathing (44). Chinese and Navajo infants will accept a cloth over the nose without protest, whereas Anglo and black infants will fight the cloth; they struggle and turn away. Certain Indian tribes use cradle boards, which inhibit the infant's movement toward objects (44) and may enhance the practice of looking at objects rather than grasping them. In some tribes, such as the Papago and the Yaqui, there is little conversation in the home. When children begin to speak, baby talk is discouraged and the child is expected to enunciate properly (40). Naughty children are shamed or ignored rather than talked to or yelled at as they would be in Anglo homes. Siblings and peers often teach younger children by nonverbal encouragement and example (unpublished 1978 paper by M.D. Topper). Societal norms may be presented through fables that are memorized and handed down from generation to generation. When a fable is related, children are encouraged to listen, to be sensitive to what others think, and to obey rather than to ask questions (45). Traditional ceremonies are passed down the generations through participation and example (unpublished 1978 paper by M.D. Topper). Learning is by trial and error. An Anglocized adolescent's questioning an elder becomes a source of frustration and bewilderment, and the youth may be sharply criticized.

The construction of the Indian language is unlike that of the English language. Indian children's facility in English is among the poorest of any group in the United States; this is so even when they are reared in homes where English is spoken (40). The emphasis on observation and form is reflected in the language. For instance, in the Navajo native tongue the verb form may depend on the shape of the object of reference (46). Languages that stress form do not lend themselves readily to verbal abstractions, but they do augment the development of strategies involving the visual (graphic) metaphor, which can be viewed as a visual abstraction. Thus, it is extraordinarily difficult to translate abstractions between the Navajo and the English languages. Indian children may excel at the visual mode. For instance, Navajo children begin to sort by form rather than by color at an early age, attaining these norms in advance of other children. The most pronounced tendency to sort by form is found among the children who speak only Navajo (47).

There is evidence that the basic cognitive development of Indian children approximates that of the children of the majority culture; Piagetian tasks are attained at the expectable ages (48). Paiute children under age 2 meet expectable norms on the Gesell Developmental Profile, but their performance begins to decline as the verbal content of the scales becomes more prominent with increasing age (49). Choctaw Indian infants perform well above average on the Bayley Scale of Infant Development, a nonverbal measure, but fall below the average when they are tested later on by the McCarthy Index, a verbal measure (unpublished 1975 report by P. Quigley).

Indian children produce consistently low scores on the verbal scales of intelligence tests, but their scores on the performance scales approximate the norms of the majority culture. Boys tend to score approximately 5 points lower on the verbal scales. Children enrolled in certain Head Start programs have demonstrated marked gains (unpublished 1966 paper by H.L. Saslow), but these are not maintained when they enter the regular school system (50, 51). However, in regular schools, Indian children most often are taught by teachers who cannot speak their native tongue and who, in a subtle fashion, may be prejudiced against them.

That Indian children score within the average range on performance scales suggests that the Indian child's intelligence is intact but that our assessment instruments are biased toward verbal rather than performance skills. The tests are not culture free but depend on the language skills, competitive stance, and motivation of the children who are tested. However, in the dominant culture of the United States, academic and vocational success is largely dependent on language skills. Not only do Indian children not acquire language skills easily, but they become enmeshed in a cycle of depression, discouragement, and alienation that further impairs their test-taking ability. On the other hand, it has been shown that the performance of Indian children on some subtests of the Wechsler test can be enhanced when the examiner communicates warmth nonverbally (52).

On entering school, Indian children experience problems with language, auditory association and memory, grammatic closure and auditory processing, reading, and verbal discrimination (53–55). Not only have a great many of the children not been exposed to English before entering school (56), but they may be totally unprepared to acquire English because of the different structure of the two languages. Problems in acquiring English are augmented by the fact that the Indian child has been trained to respect adults by not asking questions and by not looking directly at them. Thus, Indian children remain largely dependent on nonverbal clues to understand their environment, and they may appear passive and uninvolved in the learning process. The impairment in acquisition of language, auditory processing, and conceptualization has profound and persistent consequences, including the recently demonstrated strong association between language disorders and psychiatric problems (57).

In spite of difficulties with the auditory pathway and language, Indian children demonstrate an unusual ability to memorize visual patterns, visualize spatial concepts, and produce descriptions that are rich in visual detail and the use of graphic metaphors (58). Unfortunately, these skills count for little in the Anglo school system if the child is unable to remember or process verbal content. Indian children are hard put to recall content that is presented verbally and not portrayed visually (59). These deficits seem fundamental to what has been called the "crossover phenomenon" by which Indian children appear to do well in school until the third grade only to begin a progressive downhill course (9, 34). The higher the grade level that Indian children achieve, the greater is their lag in performance (30).

Indian children's representational function seems to be mediated visually rather than linguistically (59), and Indian children do not spontaneously analyze their experience in verbal terms (60) but, rather, absorb the experience as a whole, using intuitive, "right brain" mechanisms (61). They do not formulate or use logical constructs as their Anglo age-mates do but, on the other hand, are more aware of their environment (40, 62). The cards seem to be stacked against Indian children from the time they enter school, and their achievement deficits become increasingly apparent as they move through the school system. Achievement and emotional problems are interrelated—it is the children with low achievement scores who exhibit anomie and low self-esteem (34), and preschoolers with signs of emotional disturbance are more likely to see themselves as poor learners (63). The dissonance in cognitive style between the Indian child and the Anglo school must be a precipitating factor in the emergence of emotional problems, depression, hopelessness, alienation, and behavioral difficulties found among older Indian children and adolescents.

INFECTIOUS AND NUTRITIONAL PROBLEMS

According to earlier estimates (64), 75% of all the Indian children were said to fall in the retarded range. Currently, 33% of Indian children are thought to have learning disabilities and 19% fall into the mentally retarded range (65), although even this figure is thought to be substantially influenced by cultural deprivation and test bias. The rate of learning problems and retardation is related to the fact that otitis media and nutritional problems are endemic on many reservations. A direct and significant relationship exists between the number of episodes of otitis media and the degree of hearing deficit and lower verbal scale scores on the WISC (66, 67). Most Indians living on a reservation are dependent on government surplus foods, which are high in carbohydrates and fats and low in protein and certain essential vitamins. Fruits, meats, and vegetables may be in short supply, too expensive, or unattractive to the Indian; this contributes to the incidence of malnutrition. Studies relating nutritional status with IQ and school performance certainly are in order.

FUTURE RESEARCH DIRECTIONS

Certain ethical considerations must be resolved before one considers directions for research. Historically, we have expected American Indian children to renounce the traditional way in order to acclimate to the majority culture. Children as young as 6 years old have been removed from their families and placed in government boarding schools so they might learn the "right" way; other children have been adopted by Mormon families interested in saving the "poor Indian" (unpublished 1978 paper by M.D. Topper). Should we continue our pressure cooker methods to coerce Indians to acculturate or should we promote the freedom of movement between cultures that would foster mutual enrichment? Clearly needed is a social policy that enhances constructive interchange, provides social supports, and militates against dislocation. Fortunately, individuals from among traditional and acculturated groups of Indians have emerged to become social and political activists. Organizations such as the Association on American Indian Affairs are lobbying to facilitate change, to increase funding, and to bring the control of social and political affairs back within the tribal community.

The complexity of the needs of various Indian groups indicates that we must place our feet squarely in three canoes: prevention, prediction, and intervention.

Prevention

Mental retardation and learning disability can be prevented to some extent. Otitis media and inadequate nutrition are likely culprits that need to be better defined and remedied. The Indian child's problem in acquiring language skills may stem from adaptive, genetic, or early environmental factors. Early environmental bases such as diminished use of language in the home may be ameliorated through early stimulation programs in which parents are encouraged to use language in interacting and playing with preschool children. It goes without saying that such programs will fail without substantial parent education and involvement as well as tribal endorsement. This cannot be achieved solely through the provision of government funding but needs to be implemented by Indian developmental specialists committed to the growth and wellbeing of the Indian people (68,

69). Indians themselves must determine their own priorities with respect to life style, occupational and social roles, the educational process, and the kinds of personal and social problems to be addressed by mental health professionals. No one other than the Indian people should determine how the individual, the tribe, and the nation should integrate with the majority culture and, at the same time, resist engulfment.

Prediction

If predictors of later social, emotional, and behavioral problems can be established for Indian children, appropriate interventions are more likely to evolve. Areas of investigation must include adaptive, genetic, and early environmental factors. This would necessitate a longitudinal study to compare the development of children reared on the reservation in the natural home with children adopted early in life and reared off the reservation in non-Indian families. Such a study would need to control for family disruption, number of child placements, socioeconomic status, adequacy of schooling, etc.

Intervention

Programs need to be developed to provide specialized aids to enhance the acquisition of language through developing diverse instructional approaches that combine visual, observational, and exploratory methods (59). These programs would also build an active, problem-solving approach to the acquisition of English (70) during early preschool and grade-school years. Teachers from the Indian culture or teachers knowledgeable about the Indian culture would be needed to offer interpersonal support, identification, and inspiration.

Programs to maximize the inherent potential of the Indian child should emphasize strengths rather than weaknesses, building on the exceptional abilities of the Indian child by individualized programs to develop fine motor, classification, visual-spatial, and visual-memory skills. Occupational training and fifth-pathway programs that begin in grade school might prepare Indian children for eventual success in such areas as forestry, art and design, interior decoration, crafts, curatorship, ethnology, agriculture, and transportation.

CONCLUSIONS

A visually based cognitive style is an additional liability for the Indian child in the Anglo system. This problem, coupled with extreme physical, economic, and acculturation stressors, must contribute to the immense emotional and behavioral difficulties found among Indian children and adolescents.

REFERENCES

1. American Indians, Subject Report, 1970 Census of the Population: PC(2)-IF. Washington, DC, US Department of Commerce, Census Bureau, 1973
2. Wallace HM: The health of American Indian children. Health Serv Rep 1972; 87:867–876
3. Kemberling SR: The Indian Health Service: commentary on a commentary. Pediatrics 1973; 51:6–9
4. Association on American Indian Affairs: Program of Activities. New York, AAIA, 1986
5. Beiser M, Attneave CL: Mental disorders among Native American children: rates and risk periods for entering treatment. Am J Psychiatry 1982; 139:193–198
6. Goldstein GS, Oetting ER, Edwards R, et al: Drug use among Native American young adults. Int J Addict 1974; 14:855–860
7. Bryde JF: Indian Students and Guidance. Boston, Houghton Mifflin, 1971
8. Holmgren C., Fitzgerald BJ, Carman RS: Alienation and alcohol use by American Indian and Caucasian high school students. J Soc Psychol 1983; 120:139–140
9. Jensen GF, Strauss JH, Harris VH: Crime, delinquency and the American Indian. Human Organization 1977; 36:252–257
10. Cockerham WC: Drinking attitudes and practices among Wind River Reservation Indian youth. J Stud Alcohol 1975; 36:321–326
11. Kahn MW: Cultural clash and psychopathology in three aboriginal cultures. Academic Psychol Bull 1982; 4:553–561
12. Westermeyer J, Neider J: Cultural affiliation among American Indian alcoholics: correlations and change over a ten year period. J Operational Psychiatry 1985; 16:17–23
13. Levy JE, Kunitz SJ: Indian Drinking: Navajo Practices and Anglo-American Theories. New York, John Wiley & Sons, 1974
14. Cohen S: Alcohol and the Indian. Drug Abuse & Alcoholism Newsletter, May 1982
15. McIntosh JL, Santos JF: Suicide among Native Americans: a compilation of findings. Omega 1981; 11:303–316
16. May PA, Dizmang LH: Suicide in the American Indian. Psychiatr Annals 1974; 4:22–27
17. Dizmang LH, Watson J, May PA, et al: Adolescent suicide at an Indian reservation. Am J Orthopsychiatry 1974; 44:43–49
18. Berlin IN: Suicide among American Indian adolescents, in Linkages for Indian Child Welfare Programs. Washington, DC. National American Indian Court Judges Association, 1984
19. Forslund MA, Meyers RE: Delinquency among Wind River Indian Reservation youth. Criminology 1974; 12:97–106
20. Nagi SZ: Child Maltreatment in the United States. New York, Columbia University Press, 1977

21. Oakland L, Kane RL: The working mother and child neglect on the Navajo Reservation. Pediatrics 1973; 51:849–853
22. Ishiasaka H: American Indians in foster care: cultural factors and separation. Child Welfare 1978; 57:299–308
23. Mindell CE, Gurwitt A: The Placement of American Indian Children—the Need for Change. Washington, DC, American Academy of Child Psychiatry, 1977
24. Byler W: The destruction of American Indian families, in The Destruction of the American Indian Family. Edited by Unger S. New York, Association on American Indian Affairs, 1977
25. Association on American Indian Affairs: Indian Child Welfare Statistical Report Submitted to the American Indian Policy Review Commission, US Congress. New York, AAIA, 1976
26. Green HJ: Risks and attitudes associated with extra-cultural placement of American Indian children: a critical review. J Am Acad Child Psychiatry 1983; 22:63–67
27. Westermeyer J: Cross-racial foster home placement among native American psychiatric patients. J Natl Med Assoc 1977; 69:231–236
28. Simon NM, Senturia AG: Adoption and psychiatric illness. Am J Psychiatry 1966; 122:858–868
29. Beiser M: Etiology of mental disorders: socio-cultural aspects, in Manual of Child Psychopathology. Edited by Wolman B. New York, McGraw-Hill, 1972
30. Zintz MV: The Indian Research Study, Final Report. Albuquerque, University of New Mexico College of Education, 1960
31. Goldstein GS: The model dormitory. Psychiatr Annals 1974; 4:85–92
32. Kleinfeld J, Bloom J: Boarding schools: effects on the mental health of Eskimo adolescents. Am J Psychiatry 1977; 134:411–417
33. Krush TP, Bjork JW, Sindell PS, et al: Some thoughts on the formation of personality disorder: study of an Indian boarding school population. Am J Psychiatry 1966; 122:868–876
34. Saslow HL, Harrover MJ: Research on psychosocial adjustment of Indian youth. Am J Psychiatry 1968; 125:224–231
35. Berry JW: Acculturation as varieties of adaptation, in Acculturation: Theory, Models, and Some New Findings. Edited by Padilla AM. Boulder, Colo, Westview Press, 1979
36. Boggs ST: An interactional study of Ojibwa socialization. Am Sociol Rev 1965; 21:191–198
37. Szapocznik J, Truss C: Intergenerational sources of role conflict in Cuban mothers, in Hispanic Families: Critical issues for Policy and Programs in Human Service. Edited by Montiel M. Washington, DC, National Coalition of Hispanic Mental Health and Human Services Organizations, 1978
38. Erikson EH: Childhood and Society, 2nd ed. New York, WW Norton, 1963
39. Philips SU: Participating structures and communicative competence: Warm Springs children in community and classroom, in Functions of Language in the Classroom. Edited by Cazden CB, John VP, Hymes D. New York, Teachers College Press, 1972
40. Blanchard EL: The growth and development of American Indian and Alaskan Native children, in The Psychosocial Development of Minority Group Children. Edited by Powell GJ. New York, Brunner/Mazel, 1983

41. Clevenger J: Cultural aspects of mental health care for American Indians, in Cross-Cultural Psychiatry. Edited by Gaw A. Littleton, Mass, John Wright-PSG, 1981
42. Hallowell A: Culture and Experience. Philadelphia, University of Pennsylvania Press, 1955
43. Wax R, Thomas R: American Indians and white people, in Native Americans Today: Sociological Perspectives. Edited by Bahr H, Chadwick B, Day R. New York, Harper & Row, 1972
44. Neithhammer C: Daughters of the Earth: The Lives and Legends of American Indian Women. New York, Macmillan, 1977
45. Garcia V: An Examination of Early Childhood Education of the American Indian: A Relationship of Culture and Cognition. Albuquerque, University of New Mexico, 1974
46. Carroll JB, Casa Grande JB: The function of language classifications in behavior, in Readings in Social Psychology, 3rd ed. Edited by Maccoby EE, Hartley EO. New York, Holt, Reinhart and Winston, 1958
47. Spellman CM: The Shift From Color to Form Preference in Young Children of Different Ethnic Backgrounds. Austin, University of Texas Child Development Evaluation and Research Center, 1968
48. Silk S, Voyet G: Cross Cultural Study of Cognitive Development on the Pine Ridge Indian Reservation: Pine Ridge Research Bulletin Number 11, DHEW Publication HSM 80–69–430. Washington, DC, Indian Health Service, 1970
49. Cazden CB, John VP: Learning in American Indian children, in Anthropological Perspective on Education. Edited by Wax NL, Diamond S, Gearing FO. New York, Basic Books, 1971
50. Wolff M., Stein A: Six Months Later: A Comparison of Children Who Had Head Start, Summer, 1965, With Their Classmates in Kindergarten. New York, Yeshiva University Ferkauf Graduate School, 1966
51. Homme LE: A System for Teaching English Literacy to Preschool Indian Children. Pittsburgh, Westinghouse Research Laboratories, Oct 11, 1965
52. Kleinfeld J: Effects of nonverbally communicated personal warmth on the intelligence test performance of Indian and Eskimo adolescents. J Soc Psychol 1973; 91:149–150
53. Lombardi T: Psycholinguistic abilities of Papago Indian school children. Except Child 1970; 36:485–493
54. Trimble JE, Goddard A, Dinges NG: Review of the Literature on Educational Needs and Problems of American Indians, 1971 to 1976: DHEW Contract 300–76–0436. Seattle, Battelle Memorial Institute, Social Change Study Center, 1977
55. McShane D: A review of scores of American Indian children on the Wechsler Intelligence Scales. White Cloud J 1980; 1:3–10
56. Gold MJ: In Praise of Diversity: A Resource Book for Multicultural Education. Washington, DC, Association of Teacher Education, 1977
57. Beitchman JH, Nair R, Clegg M, et al: Prevalence of psychiatric disorders in children with speech and language disorders. J Am Acad Child Psychiatry 1986; 25:528–535
58. Kleinfeld JS: Characteristics of Alaskan Native students, in Alaskan Native Needs Assessment in Education: Project ANNA. Juneau, Juneau Area Office, Bureau of Indian Affairs, 1974

59. John-Steiner V, Osterreich H: Learning Styles Among Pueblo Children: Final Report, DHEW-NIE Grant HEW:NE-G-00-3-0074. Albuquerque, University of New Mexico, Aug 1975

60. Shuberg J, Cropley AJ: Verbal regulation of behavior and IQ in Canadian Indian and white children. Developmental Psychol 1972; 7:295–301

61. Witelson SF: Developmental dyslexia: two right hemispheres and none left. Science 1971; 195:309–311

62. Berry JW: Ecology and socialization as factors in figural assimilation and the resolution of binocular rivalry. Int J Psychol 1969; 4:270–280

63. Bruneau OJ: Comparison of behavioral characteristics and self concepts of American Indian and Caucasian preschoolers. Psychol Rep 1984; 54:571–574

64. Anderson FN: A mental hygiene survey of problem Indian children in Oklahoma. Ment Hygiene 1936; 20:472–476

65. Report of the Council on Exceptional Children to the Bureau of Indian Affairs and the Office of Special Education and Rehabilitation. Washington, DC, Bureau of Indian Affairs, 1978

66. Roach RE, Rosecrans CJ: Verbal deficit in children with hearing loss. Except Child 1972; 1:395–399

67. Kaplan GJ, Flasman JK, Bender TR, et al: Long term effects of otitis media: a ten year cohort study of Alaskan Eskimo children. Pediatrics 1973; 52:577–585

68. Berlin R, Berlin IN: Parents' advocate role in education as primary prevention, in Advocacy for Child Mental Health. Edited by Berlin IN. New York, Brunner/Mazel, 1986

69. Caldwell BM: What does research tell us about day care? Child Today 1972; 1:1–4

70. Berlin IN: Prevention of emotional problems among Native-American children: overview of developmental issues, in Annual Progress in Child Psychiatry and Child Development. Edited by Chess S, Thomas A. New York, Brunner/Mazel, 1983

Part V

TEMPERAMENT STUDIES

Studies of temperament continue to be reported in the literature at an active and even expanded rate from year to year. These studies cover a wide range of orientations: the debate over the precision of the definition and identification of temperament and the validity and usefulness of the different categories proposed by various workers; the methodological issues involved in gathering data on temperament; the role of temperament in the child's psychological development; and the significance of temperament in the occurrence, severity, treatment, and prevention of a number of clinical conditions.

In selecting articles on temperament for the *Annual Progress* series, we have always tried to keep in mind that our own special research and clinical interest might bias us to favor papers on this subject over others in areas that might be more deserving of publication. We hope that we have been able to maintain our objectivity in this regard. At times, we have even felt that we have leaned over backwards to insure that we do not favor temperament articles inappropriately.

We have used this particular section to present papers in which the prime focus of the report is on temperament. Articles that have a different emphasis, but in which temperament appears to be one of a number of variables considered, have been grouped more appropriately in other sections of the volume (e.g., the one by Westlieb and co-workers on special stress and the two clinical articles on accidents in children).

The present section includes three papers, all by major investigators in this field. Maziade and his co-workers present another careful analysis of their extensive body of prospective data from a large population in Québec City, this one on the relationship of temperament and intellectual development. The findings of this pioneering effort are clear-cut and rather unexpected.

Matheny and his co-workers report a number of data-gathering procedures and their systematic statistical analyses bearing on the question of the validity of maternal reports of their children's behavior and on the possible sources of maternal bias when this occurs. We note with sadness the recent, untimely death of Ronald Wilson, the director of this highly productive research unit in Louisville for many years, whose informal discussions with us of temperament and related issues over many years were always stimulating, thoughtful, and challenging.

Finally, the paper by Earls and Jung confirms the significance of certain temperamental characteristics for later behavior disorder development. Marital discord was also important, and their conclusion is worth emphasizing: "Although certain temperamental characteristics are important as a first step in the development of psychopathology, environmental characteristics may become more important in determining the persistence and course of a disorder once it is set in motion."

17

Temperament and Intellectual Development: A Longitudinal Study from Infancy to Four Years

Michel Maziade, Robert Côté, Pierrette Boutin, Hugues Bernier, and Jacques Thivierge
Laval University, Sainte-Foy, Québec

Using three temperamentally different subgroups from a large birth cohort, the authors undertook a longitudinal study of the association between temperament measured in children at 4 and 8 months and IQ assessed at 4.7 years. The data suggested a strong effect of extreme temperament traits on IQ development in middle and upper socioeconomic classes and in families with superior functioning in terms of communication. The temperamentally difficult group unexpectedly displayed higher IQs, and the well-replicated effect of socioeconomic status on IQ development was observed mainly in this group. These data support the hypothesis that difficult infants activate special family resources, which stimulates intellectual development over the years.

Temperament and intelligence are concepts that have profoundly marked the evolution of developmental and clinical child psychiatry and psychology. What IQ has been to our understanding of cognition, temperament is

Reprinted with permission from the *American Journal of Psychiatry*, 1987, Vol. 144, No. 2, 144–150. Copyright 1987 by the American Psychiatric Association.

Presented at the 139th annual meeting of the American Psychiatric Association, Washington, D.C., May 10–16, 1986.

Supported by a grant from Le Fonds de Recherche en Santé du Québec.

The authors thank the families who participated in this study, Chantal Mérette and Gaétan Daigle, graduate students who participated in the data analysis, and John R. Gallup, Ph.D., for reviewing the English translation.

becoming to our comprehension of personality development. This profound influence probably stems from the fact that, unlike many concepts widely used in the behavioral field, the concepts of temperament and IQ have been and still are based on results of methodical investigations, thus keeping behind, instead of ahead of, the facts.

In addition to the child temperament model derived from the New York Longitudinal Studies (NYLS) (1), different operational definitions of temperament have been developed to which many conclusions may be empirically attached (2–4). Evidence exists that temperament is influenced by genes (5, 6) and that this influence increases with age (3). Temperament has not been associated with socioeconomic status in cross-sectional studies (7, 8) or with the type of delivery procedures or perinatal events (9). Patterns of continuity and change of temperament seem genetically modulated (10) and associated with family variables (11). An aggregation of traits resembling the NYLS "easy-difficult" typology has been replicated transculturally and at diverse age levels in our population (7, 8) and elsewhere, Moreover, the predictive value of this typology in interaction with family variables has been evidenced in our French-speaking population (12). We have previously discussed the pros and cons of temperament perceived through parental questionnaires versus temperament observed in an unusual laboratory environment (13). Although many conceptual and measurement issues remain to be clarified, child temperament is now regarded as an important variable in human development (14, 15).

Although Vernon (16) wrote in 1965 that intelligence is not a definite entity but "depends upon personality and motivational factors, organic and social drives, curiosity and interests," little is still known about the developmental interplay between personality variables and intellectual abilities (17). Marked individual changes in mental test performance during infancy and preschool years are observable but still unexplained. While intelligence can assuredly not be determined by IQ measurement alone, IQ is so far a well-documented and practical way to apprehend intellectual abilities (18).

Many well-replicated characteristics apply to children's IQs. First, IQ, like temperament, displays some genetic as well as environmental influences (19, 20). Second, in terms of predictive validity, very low IQ predicts future low achievement; however, smaller although noticeable variations around the mean (15–20 points) display inconsistent relationships with future scholastic or social achievement, indicating that other intrinsic or environmental factors interact with IQ and influence such achievement. Third, socioeconomic status is associated with IQ (17, 21, 22); by itself, parental socioeconomic status is not the influential variable, but there is an indication that upper-class parents stimulate their children differently than lower-class parents (23). The well-replicated association of family size and child rank with IQ level is probably also mediated by differences in the type of verbal communication and other stimulation provided by the parents (20, 24–26). Fourth, epidemiological data reveal that low IQ may be a risk factor for psychiatric and antisocial disorders and that high IQ may be a protective factor against adversity (27, 28).

Clearly, the study of the interplay between temperament, IQ, and family variables in infancy and preschool years is relevant developmentally to throw light on the intricate interactions between environment and specific child qualities. The investigation of such interactional patterns is also of epidemiological and clinical importance, since temperament and IQ may also be studied as risk and protective factors and thus help us to understand the future appearance of disorders.

In this study, we assessed the relationship between extreme traits of temperament in infancy and intellectual development in preschool years and also took into account the effect of socioeconomic status and certain aspects of family functioning. We were able to control for the effect of family size and the child's rank in the family.

We selected two specific dimensions of family functioning and used the McMaster Model of Family Functioning (MMFF), previously found reliable (12). Parental behavior control measured on the MMFF had previously been found to interact with temperament in middle childhood to predict later behavior disorders (12) and seemed associated with continuity and change of temperament (11). Parental control has also been found to be associated with children's competence in preschool years (29). The MMFF measure of behavior control assesses the clarity of family rules, the consensus between parents about rules, and parental consistency when rules are violated by children (30). We also assessed the MMFF communication dimension, which taps the quantity and quality of communication as well as the clarity and appropriate direction of instrumental and affective messages and found both dimensions to be independent of socioeconomic status ($r = .11$, $p = .25$, and $r = .12$, $p = .30$; unpublished paper).

METHOD

We selected three subgroups of infants from our 1979 birth cohort ($N = 358$). This initial sampling consisted of all babies born in a catchment district within a specific period as officially reported to a community health department of Quebec City (7). The infants were assessed at 4 and at 8 months by means of a French translation of the Carey et al. infant temperament questionnaire (31), which is based on the nine NYLS categories of temperament. We characterized all the infants on our bipolar factor I (principal component analysis), whose stability in infancy and at age 7 and whose similarity with the NYLS easy-difficult typology have been discussed (7). Five traits loaded strongly on factor 1: adaptability, approach/withdrawal, intensity, mood, and distractibility.

The first subgroup of infants displayed extreme traits on the difficult end of the continuum (above the 70th centile on the factor scores distribution) at both the 4- and 8-month measurements. A second subgroup of easiest temperament was composed of infants under the 30th centile on factor 1 at the two occasions. A third subgroup of average temperament consisted of infants situated between the 30th and the 70th centile at both occasions.

The three subgroups were matched for sex and socioeconomic status, which resulted in a total of 29 infants in each subgroup. The selection was made by using research codes; the investigators and parents remained blind to the infant temperament scores. The parents of 80 subjects (92%) agreed to participate. The mean age ± SD of the children at time of follow-up was 4.7 ± 0.10 years; 62% were boys. The socioeconomic statuses (32) for this sample were as follows: classes I and II, 8%; class III, 19%; class IV, 33%; and class V, 40%. There were no significant differences between subgroups in terms of family size, child rank, and maternal depression index (Zung scale).

Temperament was reassessed at age 4.7 by means of a translated Thomas and Chess Parent Temperament Questionnaire (1), which is also based on the NYLS nine categories. The reliability, structure, and demographic characteristics of this questionnaire have been reported (8). When the subjects were 4.5 years old, a first home visit was made to give explanations and obtain a signed consent. Then two other independent home visits permitted 1) an intellectual assessment of the child by means of the Wechsler Preschool and Primary Scale of Intelligence (33) administered by a psychologist (P.B.) and 2) a family assessment through the McMaster's semistructured interview conducted by an experienced investigator (H.B. or J.T.), who then rated behavior control with the McMaster 7-point scale (a global rating and separate ratings for consensus rules clarity, and consistency) and communication (a global rating and separate ratings for instrumental and affective communication). At the time of psychometric assessment, two subjects could not be visited for evaluation because of travel difficulties. As a result of their resistance and lack of cooperation, two other subjects (one of difficult and the other of average temperament when infants) were only assessed with the performance scale, and a third (difficult as an infant) could not be assessed either with the performance scale or the verbal scale; these three subjects did not appear to suffer from any clinical disorder or developmental delay. This reduced the total number of subjects to 77 (88.5%) for the performance IQ and to 75 (86%) for the verbal IQ and full scale IQ. The family interview was audiotaped, independently reviewed, and rated by another investigator, and yielded a satisfactory interrater reliability (r = .79 for behavior control and r = .85 for communication).

With respect to the Wechsler and other standardized developmental indexes, evidence suggests that the norms might be somewhat outdated (34–37), possibly because of the more diverse stimuli available to children during the last decades and the recent social trend toward smaller family size, which is associated with higher IQ. In spite of this, we used the Wechsler to allow comparisons with future assessments in this longitudinal study. In our sample, the score distribution presented in figure 1 is almost symmetric; as expected, we observed a shift of the curve to the right by around 15 points, but we believe this does not preclude comparisons for our three subgroups, given that they were assessed on the same basis.

RESULTS

To look at the association between infant temperament and IQ at age 4.7 years, we first performed Spearman rank correlations on the whole sample. This yielded only –.15 (p = .19) for the verbal IQ, –.22 (p = .06) for the performance IQ, and –.23 (p = .04) for the full scale IQ.

Because of variance heterogeneity, it was not appropriate to test through an analysis of variance (ANOVA) the possible interactions between tempera-

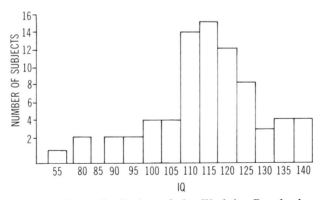

Figure 1. Score distribution of the Wechsler Preschool and Primary Scale of Intelligence Full Scale IQ for 75 4.7-year-old children.

ment and other independent variables. However, we looked at the correlation between temperament and IQ within each socioeconomic status category (table 1). Hollingshead classes I, II, and III were grouped together because of the small numbers in the upper classes. We observed a significant association of temperament with IQ in middle and upper socioeconomic status only ($r_s = -.48$, $p < .05$; the negative sign indicates that difficult infants have higher IQs). We also looked at the relationship between socioeconomic status and IQ in each temperament group as well as in the whole sample (table 2). As replicated in many studies, an overall socioeconomic status effect in the total sample ($r_s = -.34$, $p < .01$) was observed, but strikingly, socioeconomic status showed its strongest effect in the difficult group ($r_s = -.71$, $p < .005$). To test the differences between the correlations found in the different subgroups, Fisher's transformation tests were performed (tables 1 and 2).

We also looked at family communication and family behavior control as control variables (table 1). We observed that infant temperament and IQ at age 4.7 years (both verbal and performance) were significantly correlated in families with superior levels of communication (MMFF score > 4) and furthermore that difficult infants showed a strikingly higher IQ in this type of family. The behavior control dimension showed less effect on the association between temperament and IQ. To some degree, figures 2 and 3 also suggest an interaction of temperament with socioeconomic status and with family communication. The Brown-Forsythe statistic does not point out definite statistical interactions ($p = .09$), but a robust regression approach (38) suggests the presence of such interactions.

We also studied the relationship between temperament assessed at 4.7 years and IQ. First a principal component analysis was run on the temperament mean category scores assessed at 4.7 years: we again found at that age the same five categories strongly loading on factor 1 as in infancy (7) and at age 7 (8). Each subject could then be characterized by a factor score on factor 1 at age 4.7 years. The correlations between this difficult-easy factor score and IQ were nonsignificant ($r \leq .10$). Of the nine temperament categories assessed at 4.7 years, only two (sensory threshold and persistence) correlated with IQ ($r = -.45$ and $r = .32$, respectively). When we looked at the correlations in middle and upper classes, or in families with superior communication, the results were similar.

DISCUSSION

Although extreme infant temperament alone showed little or no main effect on IQ, we found a significant association between infant temperament and IQ assessed at 4.7 years when we took into account social class or certain

Table 1. Correlation Between Infant Temperament and IQ at 4.7 Years in Each Socioeconomic Status Category and Family Functional Level

Subgroup	N	Spearman Rank Correlation (r_s)		
		Verbal IQ[a]	Perform-ance IQ[b]	Full Scale IQ[c]
Total sample	75	−.15	−.22	−.23[d]
Social class				
Hollingshead I, II, III	21	−.52[d]	−.31	−.48[d]
Hollingshead IV	26	−.08	−.19	−.25
Hollingshead V	28	.12	−.15	.02
Family communication[e]				
Dysfunctional (MMFF score<4)	19	.13	.17	.24
Average (MMFF score=4)	16	.19	−.21	−.30
Superior (MMFF score>4)	27	−.50[f]	−.60[g]	−.66[g]
Family behavior control				
Dysfunctional (MMFF score<4)	20	−.15	−.14	−.14
Average (MMFF score=4)	17	−.12	.01	−.15
Superior (MMFF score>4)	38	−.11	−.37[d]	−.34[d]

[a]Significant difference between the correlations for Hollingshead I, II, and III and Hollingshead V (p=.01) and for dysfunctional family communication and superior family communication (p=.02) (Fisher's transformation test).
[b]Significant difference between the correlations for dysfunctional family communication and superior family communication (p=.003, Fisher's transformation test).
[c]Significant difference between the correlations for Hollingshead I, II, and III and Hollingshead V (p=.04) and for dysfunctional family communication and superior family communication (p=.001) (Fisher's transformation test).
[d]p<.05.
[e]Single-parent families (N=13) were excluded because it is impossible to assess adequately MMFF communication in such young families when one parent is absent.
[f]p<.01.
[g]p<.001.

aspects of family functioning. If we consider that we have an index of the behavioral style of young infants, the magnitude of the association found in upper and middle classes and in families with a superior level of communication is striking: the correlations are in the .50–.60 range, especially for verbal IQ, while the IQ mean differences between groups are more than 20 points. Unexpectedly, difficult infants showed a higher IQ.

Table 2. Correlations Between Socioeconomic Status and IQ at
4.7 Years in Each Infant Temperament Group

| Infant Temperament Group | N | Spearman Rank Correlation (r_s) | | |
		Verbal IQ[a]	Performance IQ[b]	Full Scale IQ[c]
Total sample	75	$-.27^d$	$-.33^e$	$-.34^e$
Difficult	23	$-.62^f$	$-.54^e$	$-.71^f$
Average	26	.04	$-.03$	$-.06$
Easy	26	$-.13$	$-.34$	$-.25$

[a]Significant difference between the correlations for difficult and
average infants (p=.01) and for difficult and easy infants (p=.03)
(Fisher's transformation test).
[b]Significant difference between the correlations for difficult and
average infants (p=.03, Fisher's transformation test).
[c]Significant difference between the correlations for difficult and
average infants (p=.003) and for difficult and easy infants (p=.02)
(Fisher's transformation test).
[d]p<.05.
[e]p<.01.
[f]p<.005.

How can difficult infant temperament be an advantage with respect to
intellectual development? It might be that less adaptable infants, withdrawing
from new stimuli, intense in their emotional reactions, not distractible (not
soothable), and negative in mood, solicit to a greater degree the interactions
and opportunities available from a certain category of parents. In order to
quiet the child or to mold the child's style to make it more desirable, parents
would pay greater attention, talk more, or interact more. Such parents would
stimulate the difficult infant more than the extremely easy infant, who is
more readily left to himself. Such special stimulation would favor more rapid
development.

This interactional hypothesis may partially explain why temperament is
associated with IQ only in upper- and middle-class families; because upper-
class parents are different from lower-class parents in their manner of
stimulating children. Some studies have indicated that upper- and middle-
class parents provide more stimulation, especially linguistic stimulation (20,
26, 39–42). Further, empirical data strongly suggest that differences in
linguistic environment have links with children's intellectual development,
even though the mechanism of influence remains to be clarified (23, 43–45).

Conversely, socioeconomic status showed its strongest effect on IQ in the
difficult infant group. The well-demonstrated association of socioeconomic
status with IQ is thus distributed in our sample not equally but differentially,

Figure 2. Effect of socioeconomic status on IQ for each infant temperament group.

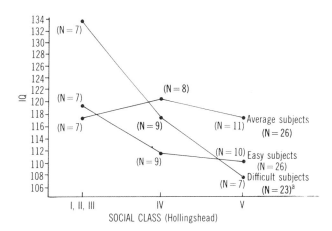

^aFor the difficult group, the mean IQ was significantly higher in Hollingshead classes I, II, and III than in Hollingshead class V (t=3.94, df=8, p<.005; Bonferroni correction, p<.05).

according to the child's temperamental style. Extreme temperament traits possibly provoke and bring to light the observable differences in parental stimulation between upper and middle classes and lower classes, the children with difficult temperament soliciting more of this environmental potentiality, which exists predominantly in upper- and middle-class parents. This indirectly supports the view that the social class effect on the children's intellectual development is mediated in part by the quality and quantity of the stimulation provided.

We also found that difficult infants tended to have higher IQs at age 4.7 years mainly in the families with a superior level of communication. By demanding more attention, difficult children would provoke more interaction available in families with superior communication and thus benefit from the additional stimulation, which speeds up their intellectual development. Since such an opportunity is lacking in other families, the individual differences of temperament would not influence intellectual development. This is compatible with our previous hypothesis that an environment which provides opportunities for stimulation and communication is an important element in the interaction with temperament and IQ.

In addition, our data indicate that temperament has differential interplay with family environment. Temperament seems to interact less with family

Figure 3. Effect of infant temperament on IQ with respect to level of family communication.[a]

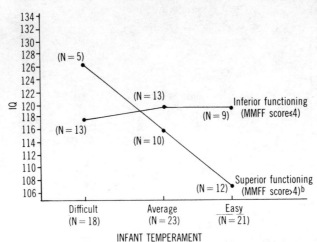

[a]Single-parent families (N=13) were excluded because it is impossible to assess adequately MMFF communication in such young families when one parent is absent.
[b]In families with superior levels of communication, the mean IQ of the difficult infants was significantly higher than that of the easy infants (t=4.34, df=8, p<.002; Bonferroni correction, p<.05).

behavior control (r = −.34) to bring about a significant difference in IQ than with communication (r = −.66), which suggests that appropriate environmental stimulation interacts to a greater extent with temperament to influence development than optimal qualities of behavior control. This result is congruent with previous studies showing an association between IQ change and parental control (46, 47) and suggesting that the early influence on IQ change from the availability of stimulation is greater than that from parental control (48).

Our finding that temperament assessed at 4.7 years correlates little or not at all with IQ at the same age suggests that the cumulative effect of the interaction between early temperament and family variables, built up over several years, has a greater influence on intellectual development than the temperament traits directly observable at the moment of the test. Our data also eliminate the possibility that temperament at 4.7 years influenced importantly the IQ measurement itself.

Some studies (49–51) reported no association between temperament and developmental indexes such as the Bayley in the first 2 years of life. Our results from infancy to 4.7 years are somewhat discrepant with these results. Developmental and methodological reasons might explain this discrepancy. First, these other studies, conducted earlier in the child's life, may have found no association because the progressive and cumulative interactional effect between temperament and environment may take several years to produce a measurable effect on development. Our finding of a strong association between infant temperament and IQ is inconsistent with the results and conclusions of Daniels et al. (49), who found no association between infant temperament and the Bayley scores at 12 and 24 months or any interactional effect. They concluded that their data were adding "growing doubts about the utility of the construct of difficult temperament." We believe that, at the present state of empirical knowledge, such a strong conclusion was premature, especially since their measurement of the NYLS temperament consisted only of a parent's "general impression" scale, which asked only one global question about each temperament trait. Such global impression correlates rather weakly with the multiple items of the infant temperament questionnaire in American samples (31) and in ours and shows less stability from 1 to 3 years than the infant temperament questionnaire (52). Their measurement of temperament and its possible weak validity and specificity may explain their not detecting possible significant associations with various parameters. Daniels et al. (49) and Vaughn et al. (51), in their analyses, did not take into account social class, which presented a strong differential effect in our study, and Bates et al. (50) found little or no interaction of socioeconomic status in their multiple comparisons with fussiness-"difficultness." Considerations about the use of different samplings and their consequences on socioeconomic status representativity may partly explain our different results. Our initial random sample from the general population, which was representative of all socioeconomic statuses, as well as the similar social class representativity of our subsample, may better reflect the full range of the socioeconomic variability of the general population; such a sampling increases the chances of including the two extremes of the socioeconomic continuum of a population and consequently of finding significant social class variations. In addition to the sampling, our satisfactory (although imperfect) rate of response for the initial sample (78%) and for the subsample (86%) tends to diminish a possible bias linked with the use of solicited and volunteer samples or with the fact that a large number of families refuse to collaborate in the process of accumulating subjects for longitudinal studies. Indeed, nonrespondents are different from respondents in epidemiological (53, 54) and clinical (55, 56) studies, and it is probable that volunteers and families willing to participate in a longitudinal study are different from unwilling families with respect to many parental, personal, and social characteristics that may influence the effect on the dependent variables. Our rate of respondents and our selecting extreme subjects from a population-based random sample may partly explain why our results are striking in comparison with results from other studies in which other procedures were used.

We selected the two extremes of the temperament continuum and an average group. Our criteria for difficultness and easiness apply respectively to around 15% of the most difficult and easiest infants in our population. However, we believe that the restriction of not being able to generalize to the whole population (57) is compensated for by the fact that in preventive and clinical settings we face the extreme cases in a population. In addition, our previous data on extreme subjects (12, 58) and the present results support the view that studying extreme subjects may uncover consistent relationships that cannot be detected with around average subjects. Exploratory work on extreme characteristics, either intrinsic or environmental, is less costly because it allows for the use of smaller sample size, an important advantage given the present economic restraints on research funding. The study of extremes complements the studies of variations on the whole continuum. Important new deductive hypotheses for consecutive research might be derived from observations of similarities and dissimilarities in findings between extreme and average subjects.

We must keep in mind that our results are derived from small subsamples and thus need further replication. However, they suggest a strong interplay from infancy to preschool years between extreme temperament and IQ, provided that specific environmental opportunities are present. This interplay may to some degree explain why studies of developmental indexes measured under the age of 18 months (18, 20, 59), without consideration of temperamental differences, show no relation to IQ measured in later years. Our data also support the already expressed hypothesis that the very idiosyncratic patterns of IQ evolution observed for any individual (17, 47) may partially originate from individual temperament differences (20). We cannot eliminate the possibility that our findings could be explained by an intrinsic constitutional link between temperament and IQ; however, at the present state of empirical knowledge, we believe that any constitutional hypothesis is unwarranted. Finally, our present longitudinal data suggest that the extreme temperament traits of difficultness, even if considered undesirable at one time of a child's life, may present advantages at another. The present findings and the emphasis of Thomas and Chess (1) that even extreme temperament traits are not equivalent to deviancy but just one of many aspects of normal human variability help us to keep in mind that in no way do undesirable temperament traits reflect a weakness in the constitutional basis of personality.

REFERENCES

1. Thomas A, Chess S (eds): Temperament and Development. New York, Brunner/Mazel, 1977
2. Rothbart MK: Measurement of temperament in infancy. Child Dev 1981; 52:569–578
3. Matheny AP: Bayley's infant behavior record: behavioral components and twin analyses. Child Dev 1980; 51:1157–1167
4. Bates JE, Bennett Freeland CA, Lounsbury ML: Measurement of infant difficultness. Child Dev 1979; 50:794–803
5. Plomin R, Rowe DC: A twin study of temperament in young children. J Psychology 1977; 97:107–113
6. Torgersen AM, Kringlen E: Genetic aspects of temperamental differences in infants: a study of same-sexed twins. J Am Acad Child Psychiatry 1978; 17:433–445
7. Maziade M, Boudreault M., Thivierge J, et al: Infant temperament: SES and gender differences and reliability of measurement in a large Quebec sample. Merrill-Palmer Quarterly 1984; 30(2):213–226
8. Maziade M. Côté R, Boudreault M, et al: The NYLS model of temperament: gender differences and demographic correlates in a French speaking population. J Am Acad Child Psychiatry 1984; 23:582–587
9. Maziade M, Boudreault M, Côté R, et al: The influence of gentle birth delivery procedures and other perinatal circumstances on infant temperament: developmental and social implications. J Pediatr 1986; 108:134–136
10. Wilson RS: The Louisville twin study: developmental synchronies in behavior. Child Dev 1983; 54:298–316
11. Maziade M, Côté R, Boudreault M, et al: Family correlates of temperament continuity and change across middle childhood. Am J Orthopsychiatry 1986; 56:195–203
12. Maziade M, Capéraà P, Laplante B, et al: Value of difficult temperament among 7-year-olds in the general population for predicting psychiatric diagnosis at age 12. Am J Psychiatry 1985; 142:943–946
13. Maziade M., Boutin P, Côté R, et al: Empirical characteristics of the NYLS temperament in middle childhood: congruities and incongruities with other studies. Child Psychiatry Hum Dev (in press)
14. Ciba Foundation Symposium 89: Temperamental Differences in Infants and Young Children. London, Pittman, 1982
15. Berger M: Temperament and individual differences, in Child and Adolescent Psychiatry: Modern Approaches, 2nd ed. Edited by Rutter M, Hersov L. London, Blackwell Scientific, 1985
16. Vernon PE: Ability factors and environmental influences. Am Psychol 1965; 20:723–733
17. Sameroff AJ: The etiology of cognitive competence: a systems perspective, in Infants at Risk: Assessment of Cognitive Functioning. Edited by Kearsley RB, Sigel IE. New York, John Wiley & Sons, 1979

18. Rutter M, Madge N (eds): Cycles of Disadvantage: A Review of Research. London, William Heinemann Medical Books, 1976
19. Plomin R, DeFries JC: Genetics and intelligence: recent data. Intelligence 1980; 4:15–24
20. Madge N, Tizard J: Intelligence, in Scientific Foundations of Developmental Psychiatry. Edited by Rutter M. London, William Heinemann Medical Books, 1980
21. Rutter M: Social aspects of intellectual and educational retardation, in Education, Health and Behaviour. Edited by Rutter M et al. London, Longman, 1970
22. Hess RD: Social class and ethnic influences upon socialization, in Carmichael's Manual of Child Psychology, 3rd ed, vol II. Edited by Mussen PH, New York, John Wiley & Sons, 1970
23. Quinton D: Cultural and community influences, in Scientific Foundations of Developmental Psychiatry. Edited by Rutter M. London, William Heinemann Medical Books, 1980
24. Oldman D, Bytheway B, Horobin G: Family structure and educational achievement. J Biosoc Sci (Suppl) 1971; 3:81–91
25. Davie R, Butler N, Goldstein H (eds): From Birth to Seven: A Report of the National Child Development Study. London, Longman, 1972
26. Rutter M, Mittler P: Environmental influences on language development, in The Child With Delayed Speech. Edited by Rutter M, Martin JAM. London, William Heinemann Medical Books, 1972
27. Rutter M: Stress, coping and development: some issues and some questions, in Stress, Coping, and Development in Children. Edited by Garmezy N, Rutter M. New York, McGraw-Hill, 1983
28. Richman N, Stevenson J, Graham PJ (eds): Pre-School to School: A Behavioural Study. New York, Academic Press, 1982
29. Baumrind D: Current Patterns of Parental Authority. Developmental Psychology Monograph 1971; 4(1), part 2
30. Bishop DS, Baldwin LM, Epstein NB, et al: Assessment of family functioning, in Functional Assessment in Rehabilitation Medicine. Edited by Granger CV, Gresham GE. Baltimore, Williams & Wilkins, 1984
31. Carey WB, McDevitt SC: Revision of the infant temperament questionnaire. Pediatrics 1978; 61:735–739
32. Hollingshead AD (ed): Two-Factor Index of Social Position. New Haven, Yale University Press, 1957
33. Wechsler D (ed): Manual: Wechsler Preschool and Primary Scale of Intelligence. New York, Psychological Corp, 1967
34. Doppelt JE, Kaufman AS: Estimation of the differences between WISC-R and WISC IQs. Educational and Psychological Measurement 1977; 37:417–424
35. Garfinkel R, Thorndike RL: Binet item difficulty then and now. Child Dev 1976; 47:959–965
36. Ramey CT, Bryant DM, Suarez TM: Preschool compensatory education and the modifiability of intelligence: a critical review, in Current Topics in Human Intelligence. Edited by Detterman D. Norwood, NJ, Ablex Publishers, 1982
37. Schwarting FG: A comparison of the WISC and WISC-R. Psychology in the Schools 1976; 13:139–141
38. Huber PJ (ed): Robust Statistics. New York, John Wiley & Sons, 1981

39. Hinde RA: Family influences, in Scientific Foundations of Developmental Psychiatry. Edited by Rutter M. London, William Heineman Medical Books, 1980
40. Tulkin SR, Kagan J: Mother-child interaction in the first year of life. Child Dev 1972; 43:31–41
41. Newson J, Newson E (eds): Four Years Old in an Urban Community. London, Allen & Unwin, 1968
42. Wootton AJ: Talk in the homes of young children. Sociology 1974; 8:277–295
43. Bing E: Effect of childrearing practices on development of differential cognitive abilities. Child Dev 1963; 34:631–648
44. Jones PA: Home environment and the development of verbal ability. Child Dev 1972; 43:1081–1086
45. Tizard B, Cooperman O, Joseph A, et al: Environmental effects on language development: a study of young children in longstay residential nurseries. Child Dev 1972; 43:337–358
46. McCall RB, Appelbaum MI, Hogarty PS: Developmental Changes in Mental Performance. Monogr Soc Res Child Dev 1973; 38
47. Sontag LW, Baker CT, Nelson VC: Mental Growth and Personality Development: A Longitudinal Study. Monogr Soc Res Child Dev 1958; 23
48. Bradley RH, Caldwell BM: Early home environment and changes in mental test performance in children from 6 to 36 months. Dev Psychol 1976; 12:93–97
49. Daniels D, Plomin R, Greenhalgh J: Correlates of difficult temperament in infancy. Child Dev 1984; 55:1184–1194
50. Bates JE, Olson SL, Pettit GS, et al: Dimensions of individuality in the mother-infant relationship at six months of age. Child Dev 1982; 53:446–461
51. Vaughn BE, Taraldson BJ, Crichton L, et al: The Assessment of Infant Temperament Questionnaire. Infant Behavior and Development 1981; 4:1–17
52. McDevitt SC, Carey WB: Stability of rating vs perceptions of temperament from early infancy to 1–3 years. Am J Orthopsychiatry 1981; 51:342–345
53. Cox A, Rutter M, Yule B, et al: Bias resulting from missing information: some epidemiological findings. Br J Preventive and Social Medicine 1977; 31:131–136
54. Rutter M: Epidemiological/longitudinal strategies and causal research in child psychiatry. J Am Acad Child Psychiatry 1981; 20:513–544
55. Schubert DSP, Patterson MB, Miller FT, et al: Informed consent as a source of bias in clinical research. Psychiatry Res 1984; 12:313–320
56. Spohn HE, Fitzpatric T: Informed consent and bias in samples of schizophrenic subjects at risk for drug withdrawal. J Abnorm Psychol 1980; 89:79–92
57. Moffitt TE, Mednick SA, Cudeck R: Methodology of high risk research: longitudinal approaches, in The Child at Psychiatric Risk. Edited by Tarter RE. New York, Oxford University Press, 1983
58. Maziade M, Côté R, Boutin P, et al: The effect of temperament on longitudinal academic achievement in primary school. J Am Acad Child Psychiatry 1986; 25(5):692–696
59. Bayley N: Development of mental abilities, in Carmichael's Manual of Child Psychology, 3rd ed, vol 1. Edited by Mussen PH. New York, John Wiley & Sons, 1970

18

Home and Mother: Relations with Infant Temperament

Adam P. Matheny, Jr., Ronald S. Wilson,
and Agnes S. Thoben
University of Louisville School of Medicine, Kentucky

Mothers of about 100 toddlers at 12, 18, and 24 months completed the Toddler Temperament Scale. Three other data sets were also available: (a) factors representing lab observations; (b) measures of the mothers who completed the Thurstone Temperament Schedule and ratings made by a social worker of the mother's home; and (c) home measures from Home Observation for Measurement of the Environment and the Family Environment Scale. Direct correlations between the first principal component factor from the Toddler Temperament Scale and the corresponding component from the lab factor were .50, .38, .52, at 12, 18, and 24 months, respectively. Maternal characteristics—emotional stability and social dominance—from the Thurstone Temperament Schedule were related to maternal ratings of the toddler on the Toddler Temperament Scale at all ages (rs = .25 to .46). There were only a few low-order correlations from environmental characteristics. A regression analysis, with lab factors entered first, indicated that, after the lab component was extracted, maternal temperament made a modest but significant contribution to maternal reports of toddler tempera-

Reprinted with permission from *Developmental Psychology*, 1987, Vol. 23, No. 3, 323–331. Copyright 1987 by the American Psychological Association, Inc.

This research was supported, in part, by the United States Public Health Service Research Grants OCD 90-C-922 and HD 14352, and by a research grant from the John D. and Catherine T. MacArthur Foundation.

We are indebted to the many co-workers who have contributed to the research program, including R. Arbegust, P. Gefert, M. Hinkle, J. Lechleiter, B. Moss, S. Nuss, and D. Sanders.

ment. The results are discussed within a model separating objective and subjective components of maternal reports of temperament.

Even though there are instances of infant temperament being assessed by trained observers, the primary source of assessments continues to be parental (usually maternal) reports. That has led to a series of debates about the accuracy of a mother's report in describing her infant's temperament (Bates, 1980; Carey, 1983; Crockenberg & Acredolo, 1983; Hubert, Wachs, Peters-Martin, & Gandour, 1982; Sameroff, Seifer, & Elias, 1982; Thomas, Chess, & Korn, 1982; Vaughn, Deinard, & Egeland, 1980). The theoretical and methodological concerns raised by the debate cannot be reviewed completely here; we address two issues that have appeared recurrently.

The first issue is that comparisons between maternal reports of infant temperament and other objective measures have provided only low-order correlations. The significant instances of validity have been at a modest level, with a median correlation between .30 and .35 (Bates, 1980; Hubert et al., 1982). Bates and Bayles (1984) have pointed out that the correlations are ambiguous in that they have been too small to indicate a pervasive characteristic of the infant expressed reliably across situations, but they have been replicated too often to be ignored.

Others (e.g., Sameroff et al., 1982; Vaughn, Taraldson, Crichton, & Egeland, 1981) have viewed the lack of agreement between maternal reports and direct observations as springing from subjective factors that bias the mother's report. The issue here is the degree to which maternal characteristics, such as personality or social class and education, affect maternal perceptions of infant temperament. Although this subjective component is largely hypothetical, some reports have indicated that maternal reports of infant temperament are correlated more with characteristics of the mother than with direct observations of the infant by trained observers (Bates, Freeland, & Lounsbury, 1979; Sameroff et al., 1982; Vaughn et al., 1981). By implication, the reported temperament of the infant represents more a projection of the mother's personality than an accurate description of the infant's behavior.

Bates and Bayles (1984) proposed a basic model that divided parental reports of temperament into three components: objective, subjective, and psychometric error. In what was described as "aerial survey research," they attempted to partition maternal reports into the objective and subjective components on the assumption that the component due to psychometric error was not specifiable. The maternal reports were obtained from questionnaires completed when the children were 6, 12, 24, and 36 months old.

The various scales were intercorrelated over age and then reduced to eight factor scores. This summary of maternal ratings was then correlated with the following: (a) father's reports, measured at 6 and 36 months; (b) direct observations in the children's homes by trained observers; (c) maternal personality; and (d) background variables, represented by sex and birth order of the child, occupational level of the family, and maternal education.

Among more than 300 correlations between each of the factor scores from maternal reports and all of the other measures, there was evidence for both objective and subjective components. As a whole, ratings by fathers accounted for the largest proportion of the shared variance with factors from the mothers' ratings. Bates and Bayles (1984) recognized that fathers' reports might be influenced by the mothers; but they thought it likely that fathers' reports had an objective (i.e., external) component similar to that of observers. In that regard, observers' ratings accounted for the second largest proportion of variance shared with maternal reports. This was followed by maternal personality variables and background variables.

The broad range of measures employed by Bates and Bayles (1984) seemed to encompass many aspects that would help identify objective and subjective components of maternal reports of infant temperament. However, they suggested that future research could increase the size of the objective component by extending observational measures. Unfortunately, extending direct observations obtained in the home environment may confound features of the infant's temperament with features of the home setting. In this respect laboratory observations of infant temperament become particularly useful.

LABORATORY OBSERVATIONS

Our design of laboratory-based, standardized observations of infant temperament was guided by a concept of temperament as being biologically influenced (Wilson & Matheny, 1986). From that broad perspective, the research was also framed within a theoretical model that treated temperament as a psychobiological concept, originating in the makeup of the organism, and influenced over time by heredity, maturation, and experience (cf. Rothbart & Derryberry, 1981). Temperament was defined as individual differences in reactivity and self-regulation. Reactivity includes such prominent features as motor activity and emotional activity (smiling or crying); self-regulation refers to processes that inhibit or enhance reactivity.

The self-regulatory processes are accomplished chiefly through approach-avoidance behaviors, self-soothing, and attention deployment. Infants differ widely in the predominant emotions expressed—whether irritable or happy— and in how successfully they employ the self-regulatory mechanisms. Both broad aspects of temperament are ultimately rooted in constitutional processes, and, although these constitutional processes may change over age as a function of maturation and experience, some degree of continuity in temperament should be expected.

With the foregoing theoretical considerations as background, a longitudinal study was designed to provide comprehensive lab assessments of the temperament of twin infants and toddlers. The protocol for the lab assessments included opportunities to elicit temperament under standardized interactions (vignettes) to be used by the staff (Matheny & .Wilson, 1981; Wilson & Matheny, 1983a). In essence, the infant or toddler was confronted with a succession of age-related challenges, and the staff used a series of diversionary play activities or soothing techniques, as required. The predominant behavioral style was then reflected in the way in which the child responded to these challenges and, if upset, the degree to which the child was responsive or resistant to being soothed or diverted in play. The sessions were videotaped, and the staff subsequently rated the child's behavior from the videotapes.

The principal ratings were of emotional tone, activity, attentiveness, and social orientation to the staff; each child received a composite rating representing the preponderant reaction during the entire lab assessment. The rating scales were adapted from Bayley's (1969) Infant Behavior Record and they are described more fully in Matheny and Wilson (1981).

Initial analysis of the temperament ratings was performed at 12 months (Wilson & Matheny, 1983a), followed by analyses of the temperament ratings for the same children at 18 and 24 months (Matheny, Wilson, & Nuss, 1984). At each age, the temperament ratings were condensed by factor analysis, from which the first factor identified the core set of lab-temperament variables. Factor scores from the first factor, Lab-Tractability, represented high-scoring toddlers as tending to approach the staff and as being positive in emotional tone, attentive during the tasks within vignettes, and moderately active during play. Low-scoring toddlers by contrast were distressed and resistant to soothing, displayed fleeting attention, withdrew from the staff, and had wider variations in activity level (swinging from constant movement during one period to immobility during the next).

The array of individual differences in Lab-Tractability became increasingly stable over ages: The correlation between the factor scores at 12 and 18 months was .37, and the correlation for 18–24 months increased to .66 (Matheny et al., 1984). The lab measure of temperament thus provided a moderately stable objective measure that could serve as a criterion for appraising the nonsubjective component in maternal ratings of infant temperament.

MATERNAL RATINGS

For the samples of toddlers, ratings of temperament were obtained from mothers who completed the Toddler Temperament Questionnaire (Fullard, McDevitt, & Carey, 1984) when their children were 12, 18, and 24 months old. The nine temperament category scores were condensed by factor analysis performed for each age. The first factor from each factor analysis was loaded heavily for mood, adaptability, approach/withdrawal, and attention/ persistence. Scores from this factor, Questionnaire-Tractability, were used to represent the core dimension of temperament as reported by the mother. High-scoring toddlers were good-humored, adaptable, forward in new situations, and capable of sustained attention. Low-scoring toddlers had the opposite characteristics.

Was the laboratory measure of temperament for each toddler related to the maternal ratings of temperament? The first-factor scores for each data set were correlated at every age, and the resultant correlations were .52 at 12 months, .38 at 18 months, and .52 at 24 months (Matheny et al., 1984).

The significant relation between a dimension of temperament derived from maternal reports and a dimension of temperament derived from laboratory observations indicated that a common core of temperament furnished the bridge between the two sets of observations. Therefore, maternal reports could be confirmed to a substantial degree when laboratory observations served as the objective criterion. In the Bates-Bayles (1984) sense, the objective component of maternal ratings was clearly demonstrable and prominent.

In view of the fact that the objective lab observations moderately confirmed the maternal ratings of temperament, the next question was whether maternal ratings were further associated with personal and temperament characteristics of the mother or with distinctive features of the home environment (components presumably more subjective in nature). To what additional extent was the mother's report of the toddler's temperament colored by her own characteristics or by aspects of the family environment? That is, once the objective correlates of maternal reports of temperament had been identified, did subjective features further determine the ratings from the same reports?

RESEARCH AIM

Since the previous analyses of toddler temperament cited above, the sample size of toddlers had increased, and our study was designed to include a comprehensive assessment of home environment and of maternal characteristics that might affect maternal reports of temperament. It used direct ratings made by a trained social worker who visited the home, as well as the mother's report of the organization and orientation of the family and her self-report ratings of her own temperament.

In addition, the objective measure of infant temperament was available from the laboratory observations, and an independent rating of maternal temperament was available from the home visit. These two measures furnished the criteria for identifying the cross-validated component of temperament in the mother's rating.

METHOD

Subjects

The children in this study were twins who participated in a longitudinal study of temperament (Wilson & Matheny, 1986). At the time of the study, sets of data for child, mother, and family were available for 126 twelve-month-old twins (72 girls, 54 boys), 111 eighteen-month-old twins (61 girls, 56 boys), and 112 twenty-four-month-old twins (64 girls, 48 boys). In a few cases the data were not complete at a given age (e.g., a questionnaire was missing), and the *n* is reported separately for each analysis. Zygosity was not determined at the time of study because, for technical reasons, the twins are not blood-typed until they are at least 3 years old.

The twins were recruited from families representing the entire socio-economic range found in the Louisville metropolitan area. Occupations of heads of household were converted to Duncan's scores for socioeconomic status (Reiss, 1961), and, according to this classification, almost 30% of the families were in the lowest two deciles of the socioeconomic range. The remaining families were distributed in somewhat equal proportions (8–11%) among the other deciles (with the exception of 4% in the highest decile).

Measures

Temperament questionnaire

The mother's report of the child's temperament at each age was assessed by having the mother complete the Toddler Temperament Scale, a question-naire devised by Fullard, McDevitt, and Carey (1984). The questionnaire included 97 items rated on 6-point scales, and the ratings were combined to yield nine scores representing the categories of temperament postulated by Thomas and Chess (1977).

Table 1. First-Factor Loadings for Toddler Temperament Scale
and Laboratory Observations

	First factor loadings		
Measure	12 months	18 months	24 months
Toddler Temperament Scale			
Activity		−.58	−.49
Rhythmicity			
Approach/Withdrawal	.71	.49	.59
Adaptability	.78	.79	.84
Intensity		−.68	−.43
Mood	.66	.72	.77
Attention/Persistence	.65	.47	.48
Distractibility	−.53		
Threshold			
% Total variance	26.4	28.3	26.2
Laboratory observations			
Emotional tone	.92	.91	.93
Activity	.71	.41	.32
Activity: Variability	−.48	−.63	−.68
Attentiveness	.83	.79	.86
Social orientation: Staff	.63	.64	.84
Resistance to restraint		.66	.53
% Total variance	45.5	47.7	52.7

Note. Factor loadings less than .30 omitted. $N > 115$ at each age.

The scores were factor-analyzed (principal-component method) at each age* and two unrotated factors were extracted. As noted in previous studies (Matheny et al., 1984; Wilson & Matheny, 1983a), the first factor incorporated the categories of temperament conceptually akin to the laboratory observations; therefore, only the first factor was used to represent the maternal reports at each age. The unrotated first-factor loadings are presented in Table 1. It will be seen that the loadings remained comparable across age, signifying that a nuclear temperament cluster was reported by the mother at each age. Congruence coefficients (Harman, 1960) were calculated to demonstrate the similarity of the factors. The coefficients were .87, .93, and .88 for 12–18 months, 18–24 months, and 12–24 months, respectively.

The first factor, the temperament core as reported by the mother, was largely defined by the categories of mood, adaptability, approach/withdrawal, and attention/persistence at the three ages. Therefore,

---

*The scoring was inverted on six scales so that high scores would represent the maximum attribute in each category (i.e., high attentiveness, high adaptability, etc.).

the mother's report could be condensed into a primary dimension that had been identified previously (Matheny et al., 1984; Wilson & Matheny, 1983a) and labeled as Questionnaire-Tractability. Factor scores were generated from all infants in this expanded sample as a measure of perceived temperament reported by the mother.

Direct observations

The laboratory assessment has been described in detail elsewhere (Matheny & Wilson, 1981; Wilson & Matheny, 1983a), and it was briefly sketched above. In overview, the toddlers were confronted with a succession of age-related activities and challenges presented in a standardized manner. Some of the vignettes were designed to promote happy, enthusiastic play, whereas others probed for frustration tolerance, reactions to novelty, and responses to goal blocking. For illustration, two of the vignettes used are described here.

Visible barrier (provided at 12 months). The toddler is seated at a feeding table and given an attractive small toy. When the infant proceeds to play with the toy, the toy is taken away, but placed within reach of the infant. As the infant reaches for the toy, a transparent plexiglass screen is placed upright between the infant and the toy. The sequence may be repeated with another toy (time allotted: 2 min).

Mechanical toy (provided at 18 and 24 months). A battery-powered dog that barks and moves is placed in front of the toddler. The controlling mechanism, connected to the dog by a long wire, is held by a staff member who activates the dog and shows the toddler how the toy works. The toddler is offered the control and encouraged to make the dog bark and move. If the toddler does not take the control, it is placed on the floor within the toddler's reach. The toddler is encouraged to get the control, but if no attempt is made within about 10 s, the staff member repeats the procedure (time allotted: 2 min).

Ratings. The laboratory session was videotaped, and ratings were made from the videotape by an independent staff member of each toddler's predominant behavioral style. The primary rating scales for the lab assessment are shown in Table 1 along with the first principal-component loadings at each age.* The congruence coefficients calculated for factor

---

*Interrater reliabilities of the lab ratings are routinely checked by having every fifth case rescored by an independent rater. The percentage of agreement within one point between raters averaged about 90% for the four primary scales rated at 12, 18, and 24 months.

similarity were .95, .99, and .95 for 12–18 months, 18–24 months, and 12–24 months, respectively.

The strong first factor that emerged was anchored primarily by emotional tone, attentiveness, and social orientation to the examiner. At one extreme were toddlers who were positive, attentive, and outgoing; at the opposite extreme were toddlers who were distressed, inattentive, and withdrawn. This factor was designated as Lab-Tractability, and factor scores were generated at each age for all toddlers in this expanded sample.

Maternal temperament

Measures of the mother's temperament were obtained from two sources: a self-report instrument and direct observations of the mother made by a social worker during the home visit, as described below.

Before the toddlers were 12 months old, each mother completed the Thurstone Temperament Schedule for herself (Thurstone, 1953). Although the Thurstone dates from another era, it has continued to enjoy active research use, particularly for examining the psychobiological influences on adult temperament (Loehlin, 1986).

The schedule consisted of 140 items that were answered in yes-?-no format. Seven areas of temperament were appraised: *active* (the tendency to be active and on the go), *vigorous* (liking physical activities and occupations outdoors), *impulsive* (tendency to make quick decisions or change from one activity to another), *dominant* (taking initiative or responsibility, or assuming leadership), *stable* (steady in mood and not easily overwhelmed by distractions or crisis), *sociable* (liking and adapting to other people), and *reflective* (liking quiet work and reflective thinking). The set of seven scores constituted the mother's description of her temperament and it furnished a basis for comparison with her infant's temperament.

Additional measures of the mother were drawn from direct observations made by a trained social worker during a home visit. The home visit was made when the children were about 7 months old (see *Environmental Assessments* below), and, after the visit was completed, the social worker rated the mother on a variety of 7-point scales. For this study, the following ratings were included: sociability, emotional maturity, tension, lability/ stability of temperament, mood, and expressiveness of affect.

Environmental assessments

Given the importance of the home and family environment for psychological development, a comprehensive home-assessment protocol was constructed that was filled out by the social worker during a 2-hr visit to the home. The protocol drew partly on direct observations of the home and the mother, and partly on interview questions answered by the mother. The home visit was made when the twins were 7 months old, in order to obtain a detailed picture of the family environment in which the infants were being raised. The complete selection of 200 items has been presented in Appraisals of Basis Opportunities for Developmental Experiences (ABODE; Matheny, Thoben, & Wilson, 1982). For 21 families, interobserver reliabilities were computed on scores generated by the social worker and a graduate student acting as an independent observer. The mean interobserver reliability for the rating scales was .89.

The items in ABODE were drawn from several sources (Wachs, Uzgiris, & Hunt, 1971; White & Watts, 1973; Yarrow, Rubenstein, & Pedersen, 1975) and were further supplemented by material specifically drawn from interviews with parents of twins (Matheny, Wilson, Dolan, & Krantz, 1981). The items were condensed by a principal-components factor analysis with Varimax rotation. The analysis yielded three factors with eigenvalues greater than 1.00. These factors, with the appropriate loadings for each item, are shown in Table 2.

The first factor pertained to a general dimension termed Adequacy of the Home Environment. The second factor was basically defined by the number of books in the home, but there were additional loadings from several items pertaining to the child's protected personal space; consequently, this factor was labeled Books-Personal Space. The third factor was defined by items characterizing the noise, confusion, and clutter in the household and was labeled Noise-Confusion. Standardized factor scores ($M = 0$, $SD = 1.00$) from these three factors became the first set of measures of the home environment.

Caldwell's HOME scales. In addition, the widely used Home Observation for Measurement of the Environment (HOME; Caldwell, 1978) scales were completed in their entirety by the social worker. The six scales that make up HOME assessed the mother's involvement with the infant and the provision of experiences for the infant. (The title of the six scales are listed in Table 4). Interobserver reliabilities computed on the scales completed by the social worker and a graduate student for 21 families yielded a mean interobserver reliability of .86.

The HOME scales have been frequently reported to capture the qualities of home and mother that have enhanced mental development (Bradley & Caldwell, 1980). Insofar as infant temperament might be affected by these qualities the scales were included to help detect such relations.

Table 2. Factor Loadings for Measures of Home and Neighborhood

	Factor		
Measure	1	2	3
Global rating: Physical environment for adequacy in fostering social development	.88		
Adequacy of indoor play space	.84		
Global rating: Physical environment for adequacy in fostering intellectual development	.83	.41	
Global rating: Total environment for adequacy in fostering intellectual development	.78	.38	
Provision of indoor play materials	.76	.39	
Global rating: Total environment for adequacy in fostering social development	.76		−.32
Parental interest in and control of nutrition	.65		
Provision of children's equipment	.62		.41
Appliance score	.58	.45	
Number of books		.84	
Stimulus shelter: Child's own space	.38	.58	
Ratio of rooms to people	.43	.53	
Decorations in child's room	.33	.51	
Quality of the interior of the home	.35	.51	−.40
Noise and confusion in the home			.78
Cleanliness and lack of clutter in the home	.43		−.66
% Total variance	36.6	16.8	10.8

Note. Factor loadings less than .30 omitted. Factor 1 = Adequacy Home Environment, Factor 2 = Books–Personal Space, and Factor 3 = Noise–Confusion.

Family Environment Scale. The final measure of the home environment was provided by the Family Environment Scale (FES) developed by Moos (1974). The FES consisted of 10 scales that defined the organization of the family, types of interpersonal relations among family members, and general activities and interests of the family. (The scales are listed in Table 4). The FES scales, as completed by parents, have been found to be associated with young children's mental development (Gottfried & Gottfried, 1984; Plomin & DeFries, 1985; Wilson & Matheny, 1983b), temperament (Plomin & DeFries, 1985), and the incidence of childhood psychopathology (Fowler, 1980). Each mother completed the FES before the twins reached their first birthday so that the scales would be sensitive to any family adjustments occasioned by the birth of the twins. Unlike the other environmental measures, the FES depended solely on the mother's report.

RESULTS

Convergent Validity

The first step was to reexamine for this expanded sample ($N > 112$) the relations between objective laboratory measures of toddler temperament and the mother's report of toddler temperament. Using the first-factor scores summarized in Table 1, the correlations were computed between Lab-Tractability scores and Questionnaire-Tractability scores at each age. The correlations were .50, .38, and .52, at 12, 18, and 24 months, respectively (all ps $< .01$). Thus, the mother's report of toddler temperament bore a moderate and significant relation to the toddler's temperament as observed in a controlled laboratory setting. From this perspective, the reports were authenticated by objective criterion measures.

There may, however, be elements in each mother's report that were associated with her own temperament or that covaried with qualities of the home and family environment. Further, the influence of home and family may be progressive and may only become evident later in relations that were not apparent in the first year. Therefore, the link between home-and-mother characteristics and the reported temperament of the toddler was examined at each age.

Maternal Temperament

Thurstone Temperament Schedule. Recalling that the mothers completed the Thurstone Temperament Schedule for themselves when the toddlers were less than 1 year old, the first question concerned whether the mother's temperament was related to her reports of the toddler's temperament at 12, 18, and 24 months. The correlations between the Thurstone scales and the Questionnaire-Tractability scores for the toddler are presented in Table 3. Among all of the correlations it was apparent that at least two aspects of the mother's temperament, as measured by the Thurstone, were associated with the toddler's temperament. Higher scores on the Questionnaire-Tractability factor were associated with mothers who reported themselves more emotionally stable and socially dominant.

Table 3. Correlations of Questionnaire-Tractability Factor With Maternal Characteristics

Maternal measure	Questionnaire-Tractability		
	12 months	18 months	24 months
Thurstone Temperament Schedule			
Active	−.14	−.04	.13
Vigor	.22	.25*	.19
Impulsive	−.01	.28**	.23*
Dominant	.25*	.30**	.39**
Stable	.34**	.40**	.46**
Sociable	.30**	.25*	.13
Reflective	.03	.10	.23*
Home ratings (ABODE)			
Emotional maturity	−.15	−.20	−.24*
Tension	−.14	−.22*	−.23*
Temperament	−.02	.08	.03
Sociability	−.15	−.13	−.22*
Mood	−.13	−.04	−.11
Affect	−.16	−.09	−.24*
Education	.00	.01	.12

Note. $N = 96$ at 12 months; 92 at 18 months; and 90 at 24 months. ABODE = Appraisals of Basic Opportunities for Developmental Experiences.
* $p < .05$. ** $p < .01$.

It is particularly notable that the magnitude of the relations between mother's temperament and toddler's temperament seemed to increase as the toddler became older. The mother's description of herself in the first year was more closely related to her description of the toddler's temperament over a year later than it was to her concurrent description of the toddler. Clearly there was an emergent relation that became somewhat strengthened over age.

It should be noted that the mother's temperament was also related to the lab measures of the toddler's temperament, although at a somewhat lower level (e.g., maternal emotional stability correlated with toddler Lab-Tractability at .38, .26, and .32, for 12, 18, and 24 months, respectively). The lab observations thus showed a confirming link between toddler and mother and verified that the correlations in Table 3 did not arise simply from using the mother as a common reporter for herself and the toddler.

Home ratings. The social worker rated the mother on several dimensions of temperament as perceived during the home visit at 7 months, and these ratings were correlated with the toddler's Questionnaire-Tractability scores. The results are shown in Table 3.

In this case, the significant relations did not clearly appear until 24 months, at which point the toddler's tractability score was correlated with four characteristics of the mother: emotional maturity, freedom from tension, sociability, and warm affect. When the mother had been rated higher on these characteristics by the social worker, the toddler was more likely to be reported by the mother as less tractable at 24 months.

The relations were less robust than for the Thurstone scales, and the direction was reversed from what seemed intuitively reasonable, but the pattern of strengthened relations over age was evident in both data sets. Mother's temperament, whether self-reported or directly rated, became increasingly related to the toddler's temperament as later manifested at 24 months. Incidentally, neither mother's education nor her socioeconomic status (SES) bore any relation to toddler temperament, so there was no tendency for better educated mothers to describe their toddlers as more tractable, or vice versa.

Environmental Characteristics

Each toddler's Questionnaire-Tractability score was correlated with the various measures of the environment, and the results for all scales are presented in Table 4.

Among the large number of entries, only eight of the correlations reached significance and they did not fall into a discernible pattern. Unlike maternal temperament, the qualitative features of home and family life bore no systematic relation to toddler temperament. In particular, the measures from ABODE and HOME were notably devoid of significant correlations, in contrast to their clearly significant relations with early mental development (Wilson & Matheny, 1983b). In this perspective mental development seemed more sensitive to distinctive home-and-family characteristics than did toddler temperament. The Noise-Confusion factor did emerge as a significant sharpener variable.

The few significant relations were found among the scores from the FES, which was completed by the mother in the first year. Two scales, independence and conflict, showed the strongest relations with toddler temperament, and conflict was the only scale that seemed to show a progressive trend over age. (Toddlers from high-conflict families were reported as less tractable by their mothers at 24 months.)

Table 4. Correlations of Questionnaire-Tractability Factor with Environmental Characteristics

Measure	Questionnaire-Tractability		
	12 months	18 months	24 months
Home environment factors (ABODE)			
Adequacy of Home Environment	−.03	−.12	−.21*
Books–Personal space	.04	.02	.08
Noise–Confusion	.08	−.23*	−.07
Home environment scores (HOME)			
Emotional–Verbal responsivity	−.13	.00	−.11
Avoidance of restriction	−.08	−.10	−.15
Organization of environment	.05	−.01	−.05
Provision of play materials	.03	.16	.10
Maternal involvement	−.03	.02	.08
Opportunities for variety	.09	.14	−.08
Family Environment Scale (FES)			
Cohesion	.15	.09	.16
Expressiveness	.10	−.09	.10
Conflict	−.10	−.21*	−.26*
Independence	.27**	.00	.12
Achievement	.10	−.09	−.04
Intellectual–Cultural	.15	.05	.15
Active–Recreational	.10	.20	.19
Moral–Religious	−.13	−.09	−.22*
Organization	.06	.21*	.14
Control	−.23*	−.05	.00
Socioeconomic status	−.09	.07	−.02

Note. $N = 96$ at 12 months; 92 at 18 months; and 90 at 24 months. ABODE = Appraisals of Basic Opportunities for Developmental Experiences. HOME = Home Observation for Measurement of the Environment.
* $p < .05$. ** $p < .01$.

On balance, the mother's report about family structure and values had a limited bearing on her ratings of toddler's temperament. To the extent that subjective factors might be expected to exert a common bias on the mother's report of family structure and her toddler's temperament, it was a modest effect at best.

Multiple Regression Analyses

We now return to an earlier query: How might the mother's report of toddler temperament be separated into objective and subjective components? The objective component would reflect the component that was validated by some external criterion measure, and the subjective component would represent the distinctive characteristics of the mother that jointly affected the ways in which she rated the toddler and described herself.

For this analysis, Questionnaire-Tractability was selected as the dependent measure of toddler temperament. The predictor variables were entered into a hierarchical multiple regression analysis in the following order: first, the most objective and direct measure of the toddler's temperament (the Lab-Tractability score); second, the set of measures of mother's temperament, both self-reported and directly observed; and third, the set of environmental measures.

The regression program examined each variable in the set and extracted those that made a significant contribution ($p < .05$) to the multiple correlation. Once a significant predictor variable was included in the multiple regression equation other variables sharing variance with that significant predictor were removed by the program because their apparent contribution had been accounted for. The multiple regression analysis was carried out for 12, 18, and 24 months, and the results are presented in Table 5.

At 12 months the external criterion measure, Lab-Tractability, accounted for the largest proportion of variance, as expected from its original correlation with the questionnaire factor. Once it was removed, however, the mother's temperament as directly observed and as self-reported helped to improve prediction of the toddler's reported temperament. The family characteristics of independence then entered as a final sharpening variable.

At 18 and 24 months the remarkable feature was that the first four predictor variables were exactly the same. After Lab-Tractability was removed, the mother's report of her own emotional stability was the next largest contribution to the ratings of toddler tractability. The social worker's rating of maternal tension further improved the prediction, and the Noise-Confusion factor from the home assessment added extra refinement. In

Table 5. Hierarchical Regression Analysis of All Variables with Temperament Questionnaire Factor

Predictor variable	Original r	Partial r	R
12 months			
Lab–tractability	.50	—	.50
Maternal–Sociability (ABODE)	−.15	−.28	.55
Maternal–Sociable (Thurstone)	.30	.26	.59
Maternal–Vigor (Thurstone)	.22	.22	.62
Maternal–Temperament (ABODE)	−.02	−.24	.64
Independence (FES)	.27	.21	.66
18 months			
Lab–tractability	.38	—	.38
Maternal–Stable (Thurstone)	.40	.33	.49
Maternal–Tension (ABODE)	−.22	−.23	.53
Noise–Confusion Factor (ABODE)	−.23	−.30	.59
Maternal–Impulsive (Thurstone)	.28	.25	.62
24 months			
Lab–tractability	.52	—	.52
Maternal–Stable (Thurstone)	.46	.38	.61
Maternal–Tension (ABODE)	−.23	−.24	.64
Noise–Confusion Factor (ABODE)	−.07	−.23	.66
Maternal–Affect (ABODE)	−.24	−.24	.69

Note. ABODE = Appraisals of Basic Opportunities for Developmental Experiences. Thurstone = Thurstone Temperament Schedule. FES = Family Environment Scale.

aggregate, these four common predictors generated a multiple correlation of .66 at 24 months for the toddler's temperament as reported by the mother.

When the signs of the partial correlations are taken into account, toddlers that scored higher on the tractable factor from the questionnaire were more likely (a) to be tractable in the lab setting, (b) to have mothers who reported themselves to be steady in mood and not easily upset, (c) to have mothers who were rated as tense by the social worker, and (d) to be from relatively quiet, well-organized homes. By contrast, toddlers depicted as more distressed and intractable by the questionnaire were more likely (a) to be upset in the lab setting, (b) to have mothers who reported themselves as labile and emotionally sensitive, (c) to have mothers who were rated as relatively relaxed at home, and (d) to be from homes characterized by noise and confusion.

The predictor variables were taken out in hierarchical sequence, so the variables in b, c, and d accounted for additional aspects of the toddler's temperament score not fully explained by the objective laboratory measure. For example, mothers who rated themselves as more labile in temperament also tended to rate their toddlers as less tractable (after the toddlers had been equalized on the objective laboratory measure). This would seem to be a genuinely subjective factor, because a characteristic of the mother entered into both sets of ratings in an intuitively reasonable way.

The next predictor, however, ran counter to intuition, in that mothers who were rated as more tense by the social worker tended to describe their toddlers as more tractable, whereas mothers rated as more relaxed described their toddlers as less tractable. Incidentally, this contribution depended on a different subset of mothers and toddlers than the preceding relation because the previous set of mothers' self-reported lability was uncorrelated with social workers' ratings of the mother's tension ($r = -.10$). The relation also gave expression to the earlier finding that four related maternal characteristics— emotional maturity, freedom from tension, warm affect, and sociability— were negatively correlated with infant tractability (cf. Table 3).

In order to discover the basis of this counterintuitive link, the records were reviewed for the mothers rated by the social worker as quite tense during the visit, as opposed to those mothers who were rated more comfortable and relaxed. It became apparent that the highly tense mothers often seemed to hold a somewhat idealized view of the way that their toddlers should behave; consequently, these mothers were inclined to rate toward a more tractable ideal. Mothers rated as more relaxed at home, however, seemed more realistic in regard to their toddler's behavior and could acknowledge less tractable behavior if it was evident. Thus, their ratings more directly portrayed the toddler, even when the portrait was unfavorable, than the ratings from tense mothers with an ideal of the perfect child.

Finally, when the previously used variables were partialed out, there was a significant association between reported intractability and the noise-confusion level in the home. This association was enhanced when the lab and maternal measures were equalized; thus, it represented a suppressed relation that became significant only when all other factors were accounted for. Given two toddlers of equal temperament, whose mothers were matched for lability and tension, the toddler from the home that was scored higher on the Noise-Confusion factor would be described as less tractable.

The regression analysis extracted one last maternal temperament factor as the final significant predictor (a different one at 18 and 24 months), but at this stage of analysis it is not stable enough to warrant interpretation. The four previous predictors that were replicated at both ages, however, clearly represented a stable core of predictors that included objective and subjective components. The way in which the mother described her toddler's temperament could be confirmed by objective, verifiable behavior, but, once that component was taken into account, the remaining nuances were influenced by characteristics of mother and home.*

DISCUSSION

From a theoretical perspective, these results can be interpreted within the context of the objective-subjective dichotomy hypothesized for maternal reports (Bates & Bayles, 1984). The objective component is self-evident from the associations provided by the laboratory observations at all three ages. By contrast, aspects of the mother's temperament and the noise-confusion level in the home could be designated as factors more subjectively coloring the mother's report of her toddler's temperament.

The thrust of dichotomizing maternal reports of temperament into two components has been to argue that the subjective components represent a source of bias or distortion in the mother's report; in effect, the subjective component would represent inaccuracies within the data set. Although Bates (1980) has argued that the subjective component deserves study in its own right, other investigators (e.g., Sameroff et al., 1982; Vaughn et al., 1981) have viewed the subjective aspect as swamping any objective utility in maternal reports. These results, however, demonstrate that maternal reports are connected to a wide variety of presumably subjective characteristics and objective assessments.

Because this study provides a lab-based assessment of the toddler's temperament, it adds to the findings of Daniels, Plomin, and Greenhalgh (1984). In their study maternal reports of difficult temperament for adopted

---

*A reviewer pointed out that twins are not independent cases and suggested that only a single twin from each pair be used in these analyses. When that was done, Lab-Tractability continued to come out as the significant basal predictor at each age ($r > .51$). Two maternal predictors were added at 24 months (maturity and stability) yielding $R = .68$. The other maternal variables plus noise-confusion did not reach significance as independent predictors with this reduced sample. With the current emphasis on nonshared environmental influences that may foster differences among offspring in the same family (Rowe & Plomin, 1981), it seems less informative to discard cases and data by splitting the total sample of toddlers. However, one should be cautious in interpreting the correlations until larger samples are available.

and nonadopted children at 12 and 24 months were correlated with characteristics of mother and the home environment. Maternal characteristics were measured by the extraversion and neuroticism factors from the Sixteen Personality Questionnaire (16-PF test, Cattell, Eber, & Tatsuoka, 1970), the EASI Temperament Survey (Buss & Plomin, 1975), and observer ratings pertaining to the mother's characteristic mood. Environmental measures were determined by using the HOME (Caldwell, 1978) and the FES (Moos, 1974). In general, only a few significant correlations were found between the child's temperament and characteristics of mother, and, among these correlations, none reached .30. There were no significant correlations between the HOME and temperament at either 12 or 24 months, a finding also replicated in our study.

If there is a strong social-desirability bias in maternal reports of child temperament, that bias should be evident in the links with maternal reports of the family and home life. For example, the FES contains items pertaining to family disputes, interactions among family members, shared responsibilities, and so forth. Given the opportunity to portray child, home, and family in the best (or worst) manner, one might expect a pervasive connection between the reports on the child and the reports on the child's environment. The findings in Daniels et al. (1984) and in this study, however, show only a marginal connection between the two sets of reports, even though both sets came from the same source, the mother. In this regard, Rothbart (1986) reported no consistent relations between a mother's report of infant temperament and her behavior toward the infant while the mother and infant were being observed at home at 3, 6, and 9 months. Apparently, the subjective component is not so pervasive that it enters into all reports or behaviors of the mother.

One surprising result was the very modest link between toddler temperament and the direct observations of the home environment. It might be that the home assessment during infancy had no bearing on toddler temperament because the measures of the home environment were not stable, even over an interval of less than 1 year. Offsetting this possibility is the fact that many of the measures employed in this study have been shown to be moderately to strongly stable over a 12-month interval (e.g., Caldwell, 1978; Wachs, 1979). A follow-up assessment of the home environments at 36 months is in progress; when it is completed the issue of stability can be addressed directly.

It is intriguing that there was a trend for the relations between maternal characteristics and the toddler's temperament to increase between 12 and 24 months. The mother's temperament, which was assessed in the first year, was somewhat more strongly related to the toddler's reported temperament at 24 months than at 12 months. Thus, it was only with increasing age that the toddler's temperament tended to become more similar to that of the mother. From this longitudinal perspective, some apparent transformation in the toddler's temperament was bringing it into closer concordance with maternal temperament.

This trend evokes the question of whether the mother has conditioned the toddler to become more like her in respect to temperament or whether there has been a maturational change that activated inherited components of temperament. These data do not permit a separation of effects, and any analysis must quickly acknowledge a significant role for conditioning, particularly when the fit between mother's and toddler's temperament is antagonistic or troublesome.

However, a possible role for developmental genetic processes in this relationship might be inferred from other data. It is already apparent that infant intelligence increasingly resembles parental education and IQ by 24 months of age, after being virtually uncorrelated in the first year (Wilson & Matheny, 1983b). Adoption studies show stronger parent-offspring relations for temperament and personality among natural families than among adoptive families, who only share a common home environment (Plomin & DeFries, 1985). In another study of temperament, identical twins became progressively more similar in emotional tone over the first 2 years and displayed synchronized changes in emotional tone over age, whereas fraternal twins became less concordant (Wilson & Matheny, 1986). These results all seem to be consonant with a prospective role for "developmental genetic processes that determine the increasing degree of resemblance of offspring and parent . . . during the first years of life" (McClearn, 1970, p. 68). When our sample has been bloodtyped, this issue can be pursued in greater detail.

REFERENCES

Bates, J. E. (1980). The concept of difficult temperament. *Merrill-Palmer Quarterly, 26,* 299–319.

Bates, J. E., & Bayles, K. (1984). Objective and subjective components in mothers' perceptions of their children from age 6 months to 3 years. *Merrill-Palmer Quarterly, 30,* 111–130.

Bates, J. E., Freeland, C. A., & Lounsbury, M. L. (1979). Measurement of infant difficultness. *Child Development, 50,* 794–803.

Bayley, N. (1969). *Bayley scales of infant development.* New York: Psychological Corporation.

Bradley, R. H., & Caldwell, B. M. (1980). Home environment, cognitive competence and IQ among males and females. *Child Development, 51,* 1140–1148.

Buss, A. H., & Plomin, R. (1975). *A temperament theory of personality development.* New York: Wiley-Interscience.

Caldwell, B. M. (1978). *Home observation for the measurement of the environment.* Little Rock: University of Arkansas.

Carey, W. B. (1983). Some pitfalls in infant temperament research. *Infant Behavior & Development, 6,* 247–254.

Cattell, R. B., Eber, H. W., & Tatsuoka, M. M. (1970). *Handbook for the sixteen personality questionnaire (16 PF).* Champaign, IL: Institute for Personality and Ability Testing.

Crockenberg, S., & Acredolo, C. (1983). Infant temperament ratings: A function of infants, of mothers, or both? *Infant Behavior and Development, 6,* 61–72.

Daniels, D., Plomin, R., & Greenhalgh, J. (1984). Correlates of difficult temperament in infancy. *Child Development, 55,* 1184–1194.

Fowler, P. C. (1980). Family environment and early behavioral development: A structural analysis of dependencies. *Psychological Reports, 47,* 611–617.

Fullard, W., McDevitt, S. C., & Carey, W. B. (1984). Assessing temperament in one- to three-year-old children. *Journal of Pediatric Psychology, 9,* 205–217.

Gottfried, A. E., & Gottfried, A. W. (1984). Home environment and mental development in middle-class children in the first three years. In A. W. Gottfried (Ed.), *Home environment and early cognitive development: Longitudinal research* (pp. 329–342). New York: Academic Press.

Harman, H. H. (1960). *Modern factor analysis.* Chicago: University of Chicago Press.

Hubert, N. C., Wachs, T. D., Peters-Martin, P., & Gandour, M. J. (1982). The study of early temperament: Measurement and conceptual issues. *Child Development, 52,* 571–600.

Loehlin, J. C. (1986). Heredity, environment and the Thurstone Temperament Schedule. *Behavior Genetics, 16,* 61–73.

Matheny, A. P., Jr., Thoben, A. S., & Wilson, R. S. (1982). Appraisals of basic opportunities for developmental experiences (ABODE): Manual for home assessments of twin children. *JSAS, Catalog of Selected Documents in Psychology, 12,* 31. (Ms. #2472)

Matheny, A. P., Jr., & Wilson, R. S. (1981). Developmental tasks and rating scales for the laboratory assessment of infant temperament. *JSAS, Catalog of Selected Documents in Psychology, 11,* 81–82. (Ms. #2367)

Matheny, A. P., Jr., Wilson, R. S., Dolan, A. B., & Krantz, J. Z. (1981). Behavioral contrasts in twinships: Stability and patterns of differences in childhood. *Child Development, 52,* 579–588.

Matheny, A. P., Jr., Wilson, R. S., & Nuss, S. M. (1984). Toddler temperament: Stability across settings and over ages. *Child Development, 55,* 1200–1211.

McClearn, G. E. (1970). Genetic influences on behavior and development. In P. H. Mussen (Ed.), *Carmichael's manual of child psychology* (Vol. 1, pp. 39–76). New York: Wiley.

Moos, R. H. (1974). *Preliminary manual for Family Environment Scale, Work Environment Scale, and Group Environment Scale.* Palo Alto, CA: Consulting Psychologists Press.

Plomin, R., & DeFries, J. C. (1985). *Origins of individual differences in infancy: The Colorado adoption project.* New York: Academic Press.

Reiss, A. J. (1961). *Occupations and social status.* New York: Free Press of Glencoe.

Rothbart, M. K. (1986). Longitudinal observation of infant temperament. *Developmental Psychology, 22,* 356–365.

Rothbart, M. K., & Derryberry, D. (1981). Development of individual differences in temperament. In M. Lamb & A. Brown (Eds.), *Advances in developmental psychology* (Vol. 1, pp. 37–86). Hillsdale, NJ: Erlbaum.

Rowe, D. C., & Plomin, R. (1981). The importance of nonshared (E_1) environmental influences in behavioral development. *Developmental Psychology, 17,* 517–531.

Sameroff, A. J., Seifer, R., & Elias, P. K. (1982). Sociocultural variability in infant temperament ratings. *Child Development, 53,* 164–173.

Thomas, A., & Chess, S. (1977). *Temperament and development.* New York: Brunner/Mazel.

Thomas, A., Chess, S., & Korn, S. (1982). The reality of difficult temperament. *Merrill-Palmer Quarterly, 28,* 1–20.

Thurstone, L. (1953). *Examiner manual for the Thurstone Temperament Schedule* (2nd ed.). Chicago, IL: Science Research Associates.

Vaughn, B., Deinard, A., & Egeland, B. (1980). Measuring temperament in pediatric practice. *Journal of Pediatrics, 96,* 510–514.

Vaughn, B., Taraldson, B. J., Crichton, L., & Egeland, B. (1981). The assessment of infant temperament. *Infant Behavior and Development, 4,* 1–17.

Wachs, T. D. (1979). Proximal experience and early cognitive-intellectual development: The physical environment. *Merrill-Palmer Quarterly, 25,* 3–41.

Wachs, T. D., Uzgiris, I., & Hunt, J. McV. (1971). Cognitive development in infants of different age levels and from different environmental backgrounds. *Merrill-Palmer Quarterly, 17,* 283–317.

White, B., & Watts, J. (1973). *Experience and environment: Major influences on the development of the young child* (Vol. 1). Englewood Cliffs, NJ: Prentice Hall.

Wilson, R. S., & Matheny, A. P., Jr. (1983a). Assessment of temperament in infant twins. *Developmental Psychology, 19,* 172–183.

Wilson, R. S., & Matheny, A. P., Jr. (1983b). Mental development: Family environment and genetic influences. *Intelligence, 7,* 195–215.

Wilson, R. S., & Matheny, A. P., Jr. (1986). Behavioral genetics research in infant temperament: The Louisville Twin Study. In R. Plomin & J. Dunn (Eds.), *The study of temperament: Changes, continuities, and challenges.* Hillsdale, NJ: Erlbaum.

Yarrow, L. J., Rubenstein, J., & Pedersen, F. (1975). *Infant and environment.* New York: Wiley.

19

Temperament and Home Environment Characteristics as Causal Factors in the Early Development of Childhood Psychopathology

Felton Earls and Kenneth G. Jung

Washington University School of Medicine, St. Louis, Missouri

Results are reported of a 2-year prospective, longitudinal study of young children representing a general population sample. Temperament and home environment characteristics measured at age 2 and again at 3 are used to predict behavioral problems at age 3. The findings indicate that the temperament characteristics of poor adaptability and high intensity of emotional expression more powerfully predict behavior problems than do indices of the interpersonal and material home environment. Beyond the influence of temperament, marital discord operates rather selectively in boys to heighten the risk for a poor outcome.

Using epidemiological strategies, the Martha's Vineyard Child Health Survey has addressed a series of questions on the prevalence, types, duration, and correlates of behavior problems in preschool children. The preschool period was chosen because many of the disorders common in older children have derivatives early in life making it possible to study the pathogenesis of

Reprinted with permission from the *Journal of the American Academy of Child and Adolescent Psychiatry,* 1987, Vol. 26, No. 4, 491–498. Copyright 1987 by the American Academy of Child and Adolescent Psychiatry.

This research was supported by NIMH Grant MH-37044 and by The John D. and Catherine T. MacArthur Foundation, Network III on Risk and Protective Factors in the Major Mental Disorders.

these disorders prospectively. Examining children in a general population context, as the study has done, eliminated the biases associated with selecting clinical samples and permitted an analysis of the complete range of hypothesized causal factors and outcomes.

So far, the findings of the study reflect three specific concerns all tested in a sample of children born in 1974 and 1975; (1) validation of a method of selecting preschool children at high risk of developing psychiatric disorders, (2) follow-up to determine patterns of change and persistence in psychiatric problems as children grew into middle childhood, and (3) determination of the types of factors that appear to be most strongly associated with the emergence of psychiatric disorders early in life. This paper examines prospectively, in a new sample drawn from the same general population base, factors previously shown to correlate with behavior problems in 3-year-olds (Baron and Earls, 1984). Because the earlier findings indicated that behavior problems in 3-year-old children were already taking on the appearance of psychiatric disorders seen in older children, the objective of this longitudinal study was to explore factors that might be causally related.

A considerable part of the first few years of this project was devoted to establishing the validity of a method to select children with behavioral and emotional problems of clinical significance. The method used, the Behavioral Screening Questionnaire (BSQ), had been developed in the United Kingdom where an initial validation study preceded its use in a general population study of 3-year-olds (Richman and Graham, 1971; Richman et al., 1975). Based on a count of the number and severity of psychiatric symptoms occurring in 3-year-olds, a cutting point was established to identify children who were at high risk of having a psychiatric disorder. Subsequently, a comparison was made of children from two different ethnic groups living in the same area of London (Earls and Richman, 1980a,b), and a study comparing British and American samples of 3-year-olds was also conducted to examine how well the method worked cross-nationally (Earls, 1980a). The results of both studies confirmed the generalizability of the method by indicating that the proportion of children selected from general population samples and the types of problems described were similar (Earls, 1982a).

Two other steps were taken to validate the BSQ. First, children selected as probable cases on the basis of having high scores on the questionnaire were compared with all other children in the population sample. Using the clinical judgments of an expert panel as a criterion for the presence of a disorder, the sensitivity and specificity of the BSQ were found to be well within acceptable limits for a screening test (Earls et al., 1982). Secondly, DSM-III criteria were used to diagnose the criterion group (Earls, 1982b). Diagnostic criteria for attention-deficit disorder with hyperactivity, oppositional disorder, pica, and separation anxiety were met in this group.

The originators of the BSQ adopted the custom of referring to psychiatric symptoms and disorders as behavior problems to reflect their reservation about the clinical significance of these phenomena (Richman and Graham, 1971). In the first place it was not clear which of the various problems included in the BSQ were primarily of developmental significance and which represented early signs of psychiatric disorder, even though many items had been eliminated from the instrument because they did not discriminate cases from noncases. Secondly, at the outset of these studies, it was believed that the development of behavior problems occurred in response to environmental stressors of various types. Yet, a process explaining how such stressors produced behavior problems had not been described based on an empirical study. Two types of studies were proposed to address these issues: a follow-up study to examine the stability and change of behavior problems from the preschool period to school age and a longitudinal study beginning in infancy to examine mechanisms involved in the origins of behavior problems.

A 3-year follow-up study was carried out with the results showing that 54% of the children identified at age 3 continued to manifest high levels of symptoms in first grade (Garrison and Earls, 1985). This degree of stability appeared to be a function of the informant and setting from which the child's behavior was rated, however. The stability was present only when the mother was the informant at both points in time. Little consistency was obtained between mother's reports of problems in 3-year-olds and teacher's reports of children's behavior in the first-grade classroom. This suggests that much of the variance in psychiatric problems in this age group is explained by factors that are situationally specific.

Another step in the project was to examine various social and biological correlates of behavior problems in 3-year-olds (Barron and Earls, 1984). A number of putative causal factors were examined cross-sectionally in the original sample: psychiatric disorder in the parents, martial discord and other acute and chronic stressors occurring in families, prenatal and perinatal events known to damage the developing brain, and temperamental characteristics of the children. Contrary to expectations, stressful home experiences were less powerfully associated with disorders than were the temperamental characteristics of children. The contribution of prenatal and perinatal factors was negligible by the age of 3. Recognizing that the relationship between temperament and behavior problems could be confounded. a subsequent step in the project was planned to investigate longitudinally from birth the same social and biological factors that were found to be correlates in the cross-sectional data. Because relatively crude measures of the home environment were used in the first study, the plan called for in this study was to incorporate a more detailed and sensitive method. This paper reports the findings of this phase of the project.

METHOD

Sample Selection and Experimental Design

The location for this study, Martha's Vineyard, was chosen because of its geographical demarcation and relatively low out-migration of families with young children. As important was the enthusiastic support provided by medical and school personnel on the island for a general population study of children. Although there is a special character and history to the island, its permanent, year-round population is representative of many other rural communities (Mazer, 1976). The traditional industries of farming and fishing in this community have been overtaken by tourism and house construction in the past two decades. The two major ethnic groups are Old Americans and Portuguese Americans, each making up about 45% of the population. Much smaller groups of blacks and native Americans constitute the remainder.

A longitudinal design incorporating multiple cohorts was used as a strategy for sampling and interviewing families with infants and toddlers. A birth register consisting of all births to permanent residents living in this island community was compiled and used as a sampling frame. The total number of children born during a 3-year-period between 1978 and 1980 to parents who were permanent residents of the island community were eligible to participate. The number of children born in each of these 3 years were considered members of three separate birth cohorts. Interviewing was carried out between 1980 and 1983 when the children were between 6 and 36 months old. The sampling design is illustrated in Figure 1. Children in the 1978 cohort were interviewed once when they were 36 months old; those in the 1979 cohort were interviewed twice in 1981 and 1982 when the children were 18 to 24 months and 36 months old; and children in the 1980 cohort were interviewed three times during their first, second, and third years after birth. This report is based on an analysis of data on children in waves I and II of the 1979 cohort and waves II and III of the 1980 cohort. These segments cover the same 2-year interval during the children's second and third years of life. Wave I of the 1980 cohort and the single wave of the 1978 cohort represent segments that will be used to extend the findings of this core sample.

A sample of 95 families serves as the basis for this report. Each family contributed one child in the designated age range to serve as the index child. This resulted in a sample of 48 boys and 47 girls. These 95 families were

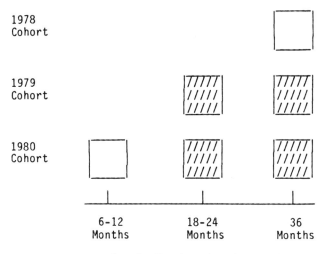

Figure 1. Convergent longitudinal design including three birth cohorts and multiple waves of interviewing. Slanted lines in boxes indicate those cohorts and waves that serve as the basis for the analyses included in this report.

selected because they have complete data on all variables included in the analysis. They represent 71% of the 134 families who participated in the 1979 and 1980 cohorts. Index children in the 39 families who participated in both interviews but for whom incomplete data were obtained did not differ from those included in the analysis on any of the behavioral variables. Over the 2-year period of the study the combination of refusals and sample attrition led to a loss of 21 families. Thus, the families included in the analysis represent 61% (95 of 155) of the total population of families in the community who had children in the age range. Some demographic characteristics of this sample are shown in Table 1.

Assessment Procedures

The procedures for assessing the family environment and children's behavior were composed of three parts. Mothers were chosen to be the informants for each segment because a previous study in this project demonstrated them to be the most valid informants on children's behavior problems (Earls, 1980b). The first part consisted of a section covering

Table 1. Demographic Characteristics of the Sample[a]

Characteristics	Values (%)
Father's employment	
Nonmanual	27.3
Manual	72.6
Father's education	
High school	36.6
Some college	26.9
College graduate	36.5
Mother's education	
High school	35.1
Some college	26.2
College graduate	37.8
Marital status	
Married, living together	90.5
All other arrangements	9.5
Mother's age	
<25	4.5
25 to 29	30.4
30 to 34	40.1
≥35	25.0
Number of children in family	
1	20
2	50.5
3+	29.5

[a] $N = 95$.

demographic characteristics of the family and the pre-and perinatal history of the child. This was followed by a section covering the occurrence of acute and chronic stressors and social supports in the family over the 12 months before the interview. The mental status of the mother and the quality of the parents' marriage were also assessed in this section. The structure of the interview was adapted from the work of Brown and Harris (1978) and has been discussed in an earlier report (Garrison and Earls, 1983).

The second part of the assessment was an evaluation of the children's temperaments using a series of age graded questionnaires developed by McDevitt and Carey (1978) and Fullard (1978). Two separate questionnaires were used: one for toddlers between 12 and 24 months old and one for children who were 3 years old. Each questionnaire was developed from the same item pool but reworded to reflect age appropriate behaviors. They consisted of 80 to 95 descriptive statements that were scored on a 7-point scale to indicate the degree to which they were characteristic of the child.

Items belonging to each of the nine temperament categories (activity level, approach-withdrawal, adaptability, mood, rhythmicity, intensity of emotional expression, persistence, distractibility, and threshold to sensory stimuli) were then summed to produce category scores.

The family interview and temperament questionnaire were given to all mothers at each wave. A third component, the Preschool Behavior Checklist, was given only to mothers of 3-year-olds. It is a self-administered form of the Behavior Screening Questionnaire. The validity of PBCL has been checked against several sources of information, including a direct comparison with the BSQ, and has been found to produce high levels of agreement (McGuire and Richman, 1986; Richman, 1977). The PBCL consists of 22 behavioral problem items rated on a 0 to 2 scale, where 0 indicates the absence of the problem, 1 indicates the infrequent occurrence of the problem, and 2 indicates the frequent occurrence of the problem. For purposes of this study, the 12 items that were found to maximally discriminate between children with and without disorders on the BSQ were used as the outcome variable (Richman and Graham, 1971).

In this study the questionnaire was used to measure behavioral adjustment as a dimensional, rather than a categorical, variable, as originally done. When used as a categorical variable, the summing of items in the questionnaire determines whether a child has a score above or below the cutoff value. Those with scores at or above the cutoff score are defined as having a behavior problem. In other respects, however, the PBCL can be properly thought of as a general scale that samples a wide range of behavior problems. Used in this way, scores place a child on a dimension of severity in behavioral adjustment. It is assumed that a child with a score of 8, for instance, is less well adjusted than a child with a score of 6, although both have scores that are below the cutoff value for a categorically defined behavior problem.

The distinction between dimensional and categorical approaches represents a recurring debate in psychiatry (Earls, 1985). The measure is used as a dimensional scale in this report because we are interested in the fundamental issue of how dimensions of temperament and the home environment are related, over a short time interval in early development, to dimensions of behavioral adjustment. However, as the analysis proceeds we do treat the items composing the scale in a categorical way, reflecting broad diagnostic types.

The range of PBCL scores was from 0 to 24. As shown in Table 2, the scores for boys and girls were similar. It should also be noted that the prevalence of behavior problems, using cutoff scores of 9 and 10, was 22% and 10.5%, proportions that are similar to those reported for an earlier sample (Earls, 1980a; Earls et al., 1982).

Table 2. Means and Standard Deviations of Independent and Dependent Variables Included in the Research Design

	First Interview at Age 2	Second Interview at Age 3
Independent variables		
Temperament characteristics		
Activity level	3.93 ± 0.62	3.63 ± 0.61
Adaptability	3.06 ± 0.65	2.71 ± 0.57
Approach/withdrawal	2.77 ± 0.90	3.01 ± 0.75
Rhythmicity	2.78 ± 0.64	2.90 ± 0.60
Intensity	3.89 ± 0.68	4.28 ± 0.54
Persistence	3.56 ± 0.68	3.11 ± 0.64
Mood	2.95 ± 0.58	3.30 ± 0.62
Distractibility	4.17 ± 0.59	3.90 ± 0.58
Threshold	3.98 ± 0.75	3.78 ± 0.51
Home environment characteristics		
Rating of marital discord	0.83 ± 0.68	0.94 ± 0.68
Number of maternal depressive symptoms	0.24 ± 0.73	0.30 ± 0.46
Adversity index	3.54 ± 2.0	3.76 ± 1.98
Total number of life events in past year	6.60 ± 3.42	10.09 ± 5.34
Weighted life events index	60.39 ± 40.12	79.20 ± 49.74
Dependent variable		
Preschool behavior checklist score		
Boys, $N = 48$		6.42 ± 2.86
Girls, $N = 47$		6.30 ± 2.52
Prevalence of behavior problems		
Using a cutoff score of 9		22.1%
Using a cutoff score of 10		10.5%

Data Analysis

The data were edited to form a list of variables of prime interest in testing the hypothesis that behavior problems are a reaction to environmental stress. These variables are (1) the total number of life events occurring over the past year, (2) a cumulative weighted index of life events, (3) an index of chronic adversity, (4) an index of marital discord, (5) an index of maternal depressive symptoms, and (6) the nine temperament categories. Mean and standard deviations for each of these variables are provided in Table 2.

The analysis of data proceeded in three steps. First, the stability of temperament and home environment characteristics between ages 2 and 3 were examined using product-moment correlations. Second, the univariate relationships between these two sets of independent variables and behavior problem scores were examined at ages 2 and 3. This gives a picture of the predictive relationship over a 1-year period and the concurrent relationship of the variables. Finally, several multiple regression analyses were performed to assess the independent and combined effects of temperament and home environment on the behavior problems score.

RESULTS

Stability of Temperament and Home Environment Characteristics

The correlations between each temperament characteristic measured at ages 2 and 3 are presented in Table 3. The correlations range from 0.56 to 0.26 with a median value of 0.39, indicating a moderate level of stability in temperament over a 1-year period. In order to ascertain whether differences in stability by sex of child were greater than that expected by chance, Fisher's *r* to *z* transformation was used. Two of the nine categories show significant sex differences in stability. Boys show a higher degree of stability in rhythmicity than girls ($z = -2.26, p < 0.05$), whereas girls demonstrate more consistency in ratings of mood ($z = -2.46, p < 0.05$). The finding with regard to rhythmicity may reflect a more rapid rate of maturation in girls in the biological functions tapped by this category during early childhood. The correlations of the home environment variables from age 2 to 3 are shown in Table 4. Stability was assessed for both the total sample and by sex. As expected, the adversity index shows the highest degree of stability, with the other variables showing lower, although still statistically significant, degrees of stability with the exception of the total number of events occurring over a 12-month period.

To assess the combined effects of temperament and home environment characteristics on behavior problems, a 3-step process was used. First, each of the nine temperament scales and five home environment characteristics were correlated with the behavior problems score. This was done for the total sample and by sex. Sex differences were assessed using Fisher's *r* to *z* transformation. The predictive relationship between temperament and home environment characteristics at age 2 and behavior problems at age 3 is presented in Table 5. The temperament characteristics of high activity, low adaptability, high intensity, and negative mood at age 2 are significantly related to behavior problems at age 3. Although high activity more strongly

Table 3. Stability of Temperament from Age 2 to 3

Temperament characteristics	Total Sample, $N = 95$ (r)	Boys, $N = 48$ (r)	Girls, $N = 47$ (r)	(z)
Activity level	0.56***	0.54***	0.58***	−0.27
Adaptability	0.50***	0.56***	0.46**	0.64
Approach/withdrawal	0.55***	0.53***	0.57**	−0.27
Rhythmicity	0.26**	0.47**	0.03	2.26*
Intensity	0.39***	0.28	0.49***	−1.17
Persistence	0.36***	0.20	0.47***	−1.45
Mood	0.43***	0.20	0.62***	−2.46*
Distractibility	0.38***	0.43**	0.36**	0.39
Threshold	0.31***	0.31*	0.24	0.33

* $p < 0.05$; ** $p < 0.01$; *** $p < 0.001$.

Table 4. Stability of Home Environment Characteristics from Age 2 to 3[a]

Home Environment Characteristics	Total Sample, $N = 95$ (r)
Marital discord	0.30**
Maternal depressive symptoms	0.37***
Adversity index	0.51***
Total number of life events in past year	0.18
Weighted life events index	0.34**
	($N = 80$)

** $p < 0.01$; *** $p < 0.001$.
[a] No sex differences observed.

predicted behavior problems for boys, and negative mood more strongly predicted behavior problems for girls, none of the temperamental characteristics had such wide discrepancies by sex to reach a level of statistical significance as reflected in the z score. Contrary to expectation, none of the home environment characteristics were found to predict behavior problems at age 3.

The concurrent relationships between temperament and home environment characteristics at age 3 and the behavior problems score at the same age are presented in Table 6. With the exception of distractibility and threshold, all the temperament categories were significantly related to the behavior problems score. Characteristics of the current home environment, with the exception of the life event scores, were also significantly related to the behavior problems score. In addition, a significant differential prediction by sex emerged for marital discord ($z = 1.97$, $p < 0.05$), with marital discord being more related to behavior problems in boys than in girls.

Consideration was given to the possibility that home environmental influences operating when the children were age 2 might have had an effect on specific types of problems for boys and girls, an effect that might have been masked by the overall behavior problems score. The BCL was decomposed into two shorter scales for this purpose; an externalizing scale, which included the overt behavioral symptoms of hyperactivity, poor concentration span, frequent temper tantrums, and aggressivity; and an internalizing scale, which included more emotional symptoms such as marked fears and worries, overdependency, poor appetite, and sleeping difficulties. The association of the five home environment variables with each of the two scales was then reexamined separately for boys and girls. The results, shown in Table 7, were illuminating. Marital discord and maternal

Table 5. Relationship of Temperament Characteristics and Home Environment Characteristics at Age 2 to Behavior Problems at Age 3

	Total Sample, N = 95 (r)	Boys, N = 48 (r)	Girls, N = 47 (r)	(z)
Temperament characteristics				
High activity level	0.32**	0.45**	0.20	1.33
Low adaptability	0.47***	0.40**	0.55***	-0.91
Low approach	0.11	0.09	0.13	-0.19
Low rhythmicity	0.17	0.06	0.31*	-1.23
High intensity	0.45***	0.36**	0.55***	-1.14
Low persistence	-0.02	-0.20	0.18	-1.81
Negative mood	0.27**	0.13	0.43**	-1.55
High distractibility	0.02	0.00	0.05	-0.24
Low threshold	0.06	0.22	-0.08	1.43
Home environment characteristics				
Marital discord	0.07	0.23	-0.10	1.57
Maternal depression	0.15	0.21	0.11	0.48
Adversity index	0.08	0.21	-0.06	1.29
Total number of life events in past year	0.01	0.09	-0.10	0.90
Weighted life events index	0.03 (N = 80)	0.20 (N = 41)	-0.22 (N = 39)	1.95

* $p < 0.05$; ** $p < 0.01$; *** $p < 0.001$.

Table 6. Relationship of Child Temperament and Home Environment at Age 3 to Behavior Problems at Age 3

	Total Sample, N = 95 (r)	Boys, N = 48 (r)	Girls, N = 47 (r)	(z)
Temperament characteristics				
High activity level	0.41***	0.49***	0.34*	0.86
Low adaptability	0.62***	0.58***	0.67***	-0.70
Low approach	0.27**	0.15	0.41**	-1.34
Low rhythmicity	0.25*	0.23	0.28	-0.25
High intensity	0.31**	0.35*	0.29*	0.31
Low persistence	0.27**	0.17	0.35**	-0.91
Negative mood	0.57***	0.66***	0.53***	0.96
High distractibility	0.14	0.07	0.22	-0.73
Low threshold	0.15	0.29*	0.05	1.17
Home environment characteristics				
Marital discord	0.3***	0.53***	0.17	1.97*
Maternal depression	0.26**	0.45**	0.11	1.77
Adversity index	0.29**	0.33*	0.25	1.10
Total number of life events in past year	-0.06	0.00	-0.12	-0.57
Weighted life events index	0.08 (N = 94)	0.24 (N = 48)	-0.04 (N = 46)	1.34

* $p < 0.05$; ** $p < 0.01$; *** $p < 0.001$.

Table 7. Relationship of Home Environment Characteristics at Ages 2 and 3 to Externalizing and Internalizing Types of Behaviors at Age 3

Home Environment Characteristics	Boys		Girls	
	Internalizing	Externalizing	Internalizing	Externalizing
Marital discord at age 2	0.07	0.31*	-0.32*	-0.21
Maternal depression at age 2	-0.01	0.28*	0.20	-0.08
Adversity index at age 2	0.12	0.27	-0.17	-0.10
Total number of life events in past year at age 2	-0.08	0.26	0.03	-0.16
Marital discord at age 3	0.33*	0.42**	0.04	0.10
Maternal depression at age 3	0.25	0.29*	0.01	0.05
Adversity index at age 3	0.13	0.30*	0.20	0.07
Total number of life events in past year at age 3	-0.08	0.07	-0.04	-0.39**

$* p < 0.05; ** p < 0.01.$

depression at age 2 were significantly related to the externalizing scale score for boys ($r = 0.31$, $p < 0.04$, $r = 0.28$, $p = 0.05$). The data show a very different effect for girls. Marital discord appears to have an inhibiting effect, especially on the development of internalizing problems ($r = -0.32$, $p < 0.03$). By age 3, marital discord is shown to have a significant effect on both the internalizing and externalizing scales for boys. Maternal depression and the stress indices have a more limited effect on the externalizing scale only. No significant effects in these variables were observed for girls.

In the next step of the analysis, a simultaneous multiple regression procedure was used to assess the independent effects of the temperament characteristics on behavior problems for the sample as a whole. This mode of analysis takes into account the fact that the independent variables are intercorrelated. The first multiple regression equation includes those temperament characteristics at age 2 that significantly predicted child behavior at the univariate level. "Low adaptability" and "high intensity" were the only two temperament variables that significantly accounted for unique variance in child behavior problems from age 2 to 3. No significant two-way interactions emerged. These two temperament characteristics accounted for 30% of the variance in the behavior problems score ($p < 0.0001$).

The second multiple regression equation includes those temperament characteristics at age 3 that were significantly related to behavior problems at the univariate level. Of the six temperament variables that were significantly related to behavior problems based on the zero-order correlations reported earlier, only high activity, low adaptability, and negative mood explain unique variance in the behavior problems score. These three temperament characteristics accounted for 54% of the variance ($p < 0.0001$). No significant two-way interactions emerged.

These analyses reflect the overriding importance of temperament in the origins of behavior problems. To separately assess the power of the home environment variables, they were entered alone as independent variables in a hierarchical regression equation. The hierarchical mode of analysis was warranted because of the inclusion of the sex by marital discord interaction term. This term was included in the regression equation based on the differential sex effect of marital discord on behavior problems reported in Tables 6 and 7. By hierarchically ordering the sex and marital discord main effects before the sex by marital discord cross-product term, the appropriate test of the interaction is achieved (Cohen and Cohen, 1975). Twenty-three percent variance is explained with the significant predictors being the adversity index and the sex by marital discord interaction term.

A similar analysis to assess the power of the home environmental variables taken at age 2 to predict behavior problems scores at 3 was not done, because none of the home environment variables had a statistically significant association with the behavior problems score. Limitations imposed by sample size precluded completing separate regression analyses by sex and for the externalizing and internalizing types of behavior problems, but it can be anticipated that stronger environment effects would have been observed for boys than for girls.

Finally, the combined effects of the home environment characteristics *and* temperament characteristics at age 3 were included in a single multiple regression equation. Only the three temperament variables, high activity, low adaptability, and negative mood, contributed significantly to unique variance in predicting behavior problems. Again, because of sample size limitations, this kind of analysis was not done using temperament and home environment data at age 2. Given findings of the bivariate relationships, a meaningful finding would only be anticipated for boys in this connection, however.

DISCUSSION

The major objective of this study was to investigate the contribution that characteristics of the home environment make to the origins of child psychiatric disorders. For this purpose a particular effort was made to make a detailed assessment of stressful circumstances characterizing the home environment over a 2-year period. Compared with these characteristics, however, temperament characteristics had a stronger predictive and concurrent relationship with the index of the number and severity of behavior problems manifested by the child. At first sight this is a less interesting result than finding support for the hypothesized relationship between stress and behavior problems would have been, because temperament and behavior problems are confounded. Both of these variables represent measures of behavior and emotional expression, although different connotations are attached to each.

In previous work using statistical approaches we were able to demonstrate that despite their confounding affect, temperament still appeared to make an important contribution to behavior problems (Barron and Earls, 1984; Earls, 1981). However, it has remained for this prospective study to be able to demonstrate a temporal relationship. We interpret this finding to mean that certain temperament characteristics represent an initializing step in the early development of psychiatric disorders.

As shown in Table 5, only two of the temperament characteristics measured at age 2, low adaptability and high intensity, uniquely predicted high behavior problems scores at 3. When these variables were examined concurrently at age 3, only three of the nine temperament characteristics independently explained variance in the behavior problems score. These are the same characteristics found by previous investigators to represent a vulnerability to develop later psychiatric disorders (Graham et al., 1973; Maziade et al., 1985; Rutter et al., 1964; Thomas et al., 1968). To signify the risk inherent in the particular features of temperament, children so characterized are commonly referred to as "difficult."

Despite this growing body of evidence supporting the important role of temperament in early development, there still exists considerable debate on issues related to its meaning and measurement (Bates, 1980; Rothbart and Goldsmith, 1985). Most researchers assume that there are both genetic and environmental contributions to temperament, although determining the proportion of variance accounted for by these domains has proved difficult. Goldsmith and Gottesman (1981) concluded a comprehensive review examining twin, adoption, and family study designs by suggesting that genes probably contribute no more than 50% variance to personality. It may be that temperament characteristics vary in the degree to which they are mutable to the environment. Our findings point to the characteristics of adaptability, intensity of emotional expression, and mood as most important in studying psychiatric disorders.

The other important finding of this study is the demonstration that sex differences in the development of behavior problems are emerging by the second year of life. This result extends downward in age findings from a large scale British epidemiological study of children from 3 to 8 years (Richman et al., 1982; Stevenson et al., 1986). In that study, although sex differences in the prevalence of behavior problems did not exist at age 3, boys proved to have more persisting problems than girls and had a higher incidence of problems over the 5-year follow-up period. By age 8, the male:female ratio in prevalence of psychiatric disorder had reached 2:1. In our own follow-up study (Garrison and Earls, 1985) sex differences in the frequency of clinically significant problems were not prominent, although predictable differences did exist in the types of problems present. Another source of support for the early emergence of sex differences in the development of psychopathology is in the work of Lewis et al. (1984) These investigators demonstrated that mother-child attachments classified as insecure (either anxious or avoidant) in infancy resulted in higher symptoms on The Child Behavior Checklist for boys than for girls by age 6. Thus, sex differences in behavior problems arise from processes that are operating quite early in development.

Because we found few significant sex differences in temperament but rather striking differences in the types of behavior problems that were linked to stressful environments, we suggest that different causal mechanisms are involved for boys and girls. For boys, temperament characteristics appear important initially, but once they are established, stressful home environment characteristics, and particularly marital discord, become most important in determining the severity and persistence of problems. A plausible explanation, suggested by Maccoby and Jacklin (1974), is that boys receive more intense socialization experiences than girls. Under conditions of family stress, the higher activity level of boys may predispose them to become targets of more punishment and restrictions than girls. Others who have observed a differential impact of marital discord in producing psychiatric problems in boys and girls have explained this phenomenon on the basis of other socialization phenomena (Emery and O'Leary, 1982; Wallerstein and Kelly, 1975). Certainly, this is an important area for future research.

A number of caveats are necessary to make in interpreting the results of this study. First, the idea is now widely accepted that preschool children can have psychiatric disorders that meet formal diagnostic criteria (Earls, 1982b; Kashani, 1984). Separation of behavior items into externalizing and internalizing scales was illustrative of the importance of this distinction, because sex differences were apparent only after considering these types of problems. Nevertheless, because the PBCL was primarily used as a dimensional scale in these analyses, it would be desirable to reexamine these findings in a larger sample using more specific diagnostic criteria.

Second, basing the measurement of temperament on parent reports, as was done in this study, opens the way for a systematic bias to confound other measures dependent on parents. Observational measures offer a way around this problem, but they, too, are enveloped by difficulties such as those related to time sampling and targeting salient behaviors for coding. At the moment there continues to be interest in the use of parent report measures, because some studies examining the relationship between such reports and direct observations, confirm that characteristics of parent-child interaction as observed are a function of differences in temperament as reported (Dunn and Kendrick, 1980; Lee and Bates, 1985).

We have considered factors that appear to be causally related to the generation of common types of psychiatric disorders originating in the first few years of life. Our results underscore the earlier findings of the New York Longitudinal Study (Thomas et al., 1968) and principles of developmental psychopathology set forth by the authors of this study (Thomas and Chess, 1980). The point of view this supports is that many types of childhood behavioral and emotional disorders evolve as deviations in personality development. These deviations are set in motion by temperamental characteristics of the child, such as being poorly adaptable or reacting too intensely to changing environmental demands. In this regard boys are particularly susceptible to developing a disorder in a context of stressful family relationships. It is conceivable that girls possess a similar vulnerability but have a higher threshold to respond deviantly to stressful home environment characteristics. Alternatively, the psychopathological effects that become obvious in boys during early childhood may have a more delayed effect in girls, or the vulnerability possessed by girls may become manifest at a later developmental period.

In planning for the prevention of psychiatric disorders in children, it will be essential to take into account the child's sex and temperament and the quality of family relationships early in the child's life. It is worth emphasizing that although certain temperamental characteristics are important as a first step in the development of psychopathology, environmental characteristics may become more important in determining the persistence and course of a disorder once it is set in motion (Earls, 1986). In fact, this kind of result has been recently reported as a long-term outcome of the New York Longitudinal Study in which parental conflict measured at age 3, rather than temperament characteristics, was significantly associated with mental health in young adulthood (Chess et al., 1983).

REFERENCES

Barron, A. & Earls, F. (1984), The relation of temperament and social factors to behavior problems in 3-year-old children. *J. Child Psychol. Psychiat.,* 25:23–33.

Bates, J. (1980), The concept of difficult temperament. *Merrill-Palmer Quart.,* 26:299–319.

Brown, G. & Harris, T. (1978), *Social Origins of Depression: A Study of Psychiatric Disorder in Women.* London: Tavistock Press.

Chess, S., Thomas, A., Korn, S., Mittelman, M. & Cohen, J. (1983), Early parental attitudes, divorce and separation, and young adult outcome: findings of a longitudinal study. *This Journal,* 22:47–51.

Cohen, J. & Cohen, P. (1975), *Applied Multiple Regression/Correlation Analysis for the Behavioral Sciences,* Hillsdale, N.J.: Lawrence Erlbaum Associates, p. 295.

Dunn, J. & Kendrick, C. (1980), Studying temperament and parent-child interaction: comparison of interview and direct observation. *Develpm. Med. Child Neurol.,* 22:484–496.

Earls, F. (1980a), The prevalence of behavior problems in three-year-old chldren: a cross-national replication. *Arch. Gen. Psychiat.,* 37:1153–1157.

_____ (1980b), The prevalence of behavior problems in three-year-old children: comparison of the reports of fathers and mothers. *This Journal,* 19:439–452.

_____ (1981). Temperament characteristics and behavior problems in three-year-old children. *J. Nerv. Ment. Dis.,* 169:367–373.

_____ (1982a), Cultural and national differences in the epidemiology of behavior problems of preschool children. *Cult. Med. Psychiat.,* 6:45–56.

_____ (1982b), Application of DSM-III in an epidemiological study of preschool children. *Amer. J. Psychiat.,* 139:242–243.

_____ (1985), Epidemiology of psychiatric disorders in children and adolescents. In: *Psychiatry,* Vol. 3, gen. ed. J. O. Cavenar, Jr. Philadelphia: J. B. Lippincott.

_____ (1986), A developmental perspective on psychosocial stress in childhood. In: *Family Stress and Coping: A Systems Perspective,* ed. M. W. Yogman & T. B. Brazelton. Cambridge, Mass.: Harvard University Press, pp. 29–41.

_____ Jacobs, G., Goldfein, D., Silbert, A., Beardslee, W. & Rivinus, T. (1982), Concurrent validation of a behavior problems scale to use with three-year-olds. *This Journal,* 21:47–57.

_____ Richman, N. (1980a), The prevalence of behavior problems in three-year-old children of West Indian-born parents living in London. *J. Child Psychol. Psychiat.,* 21:99–107.

_____ _____ (1980b), Behavior problems in preschool children of West Indian-born parents: a re-examination of family and social factors. *J. Chlid Psychol. Psychiat.,* 21:108–117.

Emery, R. E. & O'Leary, R. D. (1982). Children's perception of marital discord and behavior problems in boys and girls. *J. Abnorm. Child Psychol.,* 10:11–24.

Fullard, W. (1978), *The Toddler Temperament Scale.* Unpublished manuscript, Temple University, Department of Educational Psychology.

Garrison, W. & Earls, F. (1983), Life events and social supports in families with a two-year-old: methods and preliminary findings. *Compr. Psychiat.,* 24:439–452.

_____ _____ (1985), Change and continuity in behavior problems from the pre-school period through school entry: an analysis of mothers' reports. In: *Recent Research in Developmental Psychopathology,* ed. J. E. Stevenson, A Book Supplement to the Journal of Child Psychology and Psychiatry, No. 4, series ed. M. Berger & E. Taylor. Oxford: Pergamon Press, pp. 51–65.

Goldsmith, H. & Gottesman, I. I. (1981), Origins of variation in behavioural style: a longitudinal study of temperament in young twins. *Child Develpm.,* 52:91–103.

Graham, P., Rutter, M. & George, S. (1973). Temperament characteristics as predictors of behavior disorders in children. *Amer. J. Orthopsychiat.,* 43:328–339.

Kashani, J. H., Ray, J. S. & Carlson, G. A. (1984), Depression and depressive-like states in preschool-age children in a child development unit. *Amer. J. Psychiat.,* 141:1397–1402.

Lee, C. L. & Bates, J. E. (1985), Mother-child interaction at age two and perceived difficult temperament. *Child Develpm.,* 56:1314–1325.

Lewis, M., Feiring, C., McGuffog, C. & Jaskir, J. (1984), Predicting psychopathology in six-year-olds from early social relations. *Child Develpm.,* 55:123–136.

Maccoby, E. E. & Jacklin, C. N. (1974), *The Psychology of Sex Differences.* Stanford, Calif.: Stanford University Press, p. 348.

Mazer, M. (1976), *People and Predicaments.* Boston: Harvard University Press.

Maziade, M., Caperaa, P., LaPlante, B., et al. (1985), Value of difficult temperament among 7-year-olds in the general population for predicting psychiatric diagnosis at age 12. *Amer. J. Psychiat,* 142:943–946.

McDevitt, S. C. & Carey, W. B. (1978), Measurement of temperament in 3- to 7-year-old children. *J. Child Psychol. Psychiat.,* 19:245–253.

McGuire, J. & Richman, N. (1986), Screening for behaviour problems in nurseries: the reliability and validity of the Preschool Behaviour Checklist. *J. Child Psychol. Psychiat.,* 27:7–32.

Richman, N. (1977), Is a behaviour checklist for preschool children useful? In: *Epidemiological Approaches to Child Psychiatry,* ed. P. J. Graham. London: Academic Press, pp. 125–136.

_____ Graham, P. J. (1971), A behavioral screening questionnaire for use with three-year-old children: preliminary findings. *J. Child Psychol. Psychiatr.,* 15:5–33.

_____ Stevenson, J. & Graham, P. J. (1975), Prevalence of behaviour problems in 3-year-old children: an epidemiological study in a London borough. *J. Child Psychol. Psychiatr.,* 16:277–287.

―――― ―――― ―――― (1982), *Pre-school to School: A Behavioural Study.* London: Academic Press.

Rothbart, M. K. & Goldsmith, H. H. (1985), Three approaches to the study of infant temperament. *Developm. Rev.,* 5:237–260.

Rutter, M., Birch, H., Thomas, A. & Chess, S. (1964), Temperamental characteristics in infancy and the later development of behavioural disorders. *Brit. J. Psychiat,.* 110:651–661.

Stevenson, J., Richman, N. & Graham, P. (1986), Behavioural problems and language abilities at three years and behavioural deviance at eight years. *J. Child Psychol. Psychiat.,* 26:215–230.

Thomas, A. & Chess, S. (1980), *Dynamics of Psychological Development.* New York: Brunner/Mazel.

Thomas, A., Chess, S. & Birch, H. (1968), *Temperament and Behavior Disorders in Children.* New York: New York University Press.

Wallerstein, J. S. & Kelly, J. B. (1975), The effects of parental divorce: experiences of the preschool child. *This Journal,* 14:600–616.

Part VI
CLINICAL ISSUES

By coincidence, two substantial papers on childhood accidents from widely separated countries have appeared this year. One is by Matheny, from the University of Louisville, Kentucky, and the other by Nyman, from the University of Helsinki, Finland. The two studies were anterospective and complemented each other on the issues upon which they focus. Both reports did find a significant correlation with the children's temperament. Matheny's group showed a correlation in one cohort, aged one to three years, with low adaptability, low rhythmicity, low/high persistence, and intensity but also negative mood. Their second cohort, aged six to nine years, showed high activity and low adaptability, low rhythmicity, and high distractibility. Nyman's subjects, on whom temperament ratings were obtained at six to eight months and correlated with accidents under the age of five, found significant correlations with high activity, persistence, and high intensity. The two investigators, in other words, found some similar temperamental correlations but also differences that may be due to methodological and/or cultural factors. Matheny also concentrates on family characteristics and Nyman reports on the relationship between temperament and hospitalization in general. Both papers make useful contributions to the identification of accident-prone children.

The paper by Dalton and associates examines the problems involved in the psychiatric hospitalization of preschool children. Their clinical findings are clearly documented and provide a realistic presentation of a difficult psychiatric problem—namely, how to give appropriate and time-limited inpatient treatment to preschoolers and how the availability or unavailability of appropriate posthospitalization resources skews discharge plans.

The paper by Lee also deals with preschool children but within the context of a military psychiatric clinic. The author describes succinctly and clearly an innovative method of assessing the psychiatrically referred child, which highlights the value of clinical strategies that are not tied to conventional child guidance clinic procedures. It has been emphasized by others, but it is well worth repeating, that the diagnostic and treatment methods should be shaped by the facts of life of the patient and his or her family.

An extensive body of literature has emerged regarding posttraumatic stress disorder (PTSD) among adults. Fewer studies have been reported among children, though there is a growing recognition that children, also, may suffer from PTSD following specific events of severe trauma. The paper by Lyons provides an up-to-date component and systematic review of this important issue, including methods of evaluation, age and sex differences, treatment, and implications for prevention and future research.

Fragile-X syndrome is a recently described X-linked disorder that ranks second to Down's syndrome as the most prevalent chromosomal form of mental retardation. Bregman and his associates provide a clear, authoritative, and comprehensive review of the genetic factors and multiple manifestations of behavioral dysfunction. The possible relationship to autism is of special interest.

20

Psychological Characteristics of Childhood Accidents

Adam P. Matheny, Jr.
University of Louisville, Kentucky School of Medicine

Research on the psychological characteristics of children injured inadvertently has been beset by criticisms reflecting partly concerns about research methodology and partly a view that the research may detract from the wide-scale public health approaches to injury prevention. Moreover, the research has often led to the too general application of the notion of accident proneness, presumably reflecting a trait. Because of these criticisms, the search for systematic psychological factors affecting children's injuries has been disparaged. A longitudinal research program is described that concentrates on the behaviors of children in conjunction with injury history. Extended data incorporating measures of parents, home environments, and children demonstrate that injury liability is associated with psychological characteristics of the child, but the association is qualified by age and sex of the child, as well as by attributes of the parents and the home. The accumulation of evidence shows that psychological characteristics of the child enter into the injury equation and there is a need for psychologists to trace them along developmental lines.

Reprinted with permission from the *Journal of Social Issues, 1987, Vol. 43, No. 2, 45–60.* Copyright 1987 by the Society for the Psychological Study of Social Issues.

This report was supported in part by the USPHS research grants HD 03217 and HD 14352, and by a research grant from the John D. and Catherine T. MacArthur Foundation (R. S. Wilson, principal investigator). A research grant from the Graduate School, University of Louisville fostered the completion of data collection and analyses. The assistance of R. Arbegust, J. Henry, M. Hinkle, J. Lechleiter, B. Moss, S. Nuss, D. Sanders, and A. Thoben is gratefully acknowledged.

Examination of the statistics on the unintentional injuries of children consistently indicates that the risks for injuries are not randomly distributed but vary systematically. For example, boys are injured more than girls, poisonings are more common among toddlers, and pedestrian injuries are more common among children of school age. These examples illustrate sex and developmental differences, but other differences have been sought among the many characteristics of the child that might be associated with the systematic variations in childhood injuries. The guiding premise for these efforts has been that children's characteristics, including individual differences in behavior, contribute to the factors related to childhood injury liability (Matheny & Fisher, 1984).

The past research literature shows that the search for and the identification by psychological characteristics of injury-liable individuals have always been of some interest (for examples, see Haddon, Suchman, & Klein, 1964). In fact, during a long period around World War II, psychological research on injuries was a significant enterprise. During this same period, the concept of *accident proneness* was widely applied as accounting for injury liability, but gradually became tarnished because it implied an intrinsic and relatively immutable trait, it seemed to blame the victim, and it was thought to deflect attempts to render environments less hazardous to everyone. The history of the development of the concepts and its eventual use in the literature on children's injuries have been traced elsewhere (Matheny & Fisher, 1984; Shaw & Sichel, 1971); one will note that for reasons both theoretical and pragmatic, the concept has been largely abandoned (Langley, 1982).

The shift of attention away from the concept of accident proneness, as well as the limitations and methodological problems of behavioral studies on childhood injuries (Haddon et al., 1964), eventually fostered the impression that behavioral research was of little importance. Nevertheless, in more recent years, interest in the behavioral aspects of childhood injuries has been revived, primarily within the context of general behavioral methods to foster health-related activities (Roberts, Elkins, & Royal, 1984).

Methods to modify children's behaviors so as to prevent injuries are illustrated throughout the contributions to this volume. For example, children can be taught to carry out practices such as crossing streets safely, remaining in their auto seat restraints, and carrying out safer practices during home emergencies (Roberts, Fanurik, & Layfield, 1987). Obviously, the unifying principle guiding these exercises is that children's behavior is unsafe at one or more ages, or in one situation or another, and the behavior can be modified. But it is also evident that children are not all alike in their safe or unsafe practices; moreover, they are certainly not alike in being "modifiable." Some children do not protest being placed in an auto seat restraint, others do;

some children easily learn to take a companion's hand at a street crossing, others continue to rush heedlessly into the street even after repeated instructions and discipline. In short, there are individual differences among children for safe and unsafe behavior. Whether the differences accrue from developmental, biogenic, social, or other factors is largely unknown. Nevertheless, professionals must take them into account when attempting to understand and to prevent injuries. We can illustrate this point by citing a few large-scale longitudinal studies of childhood injuries.

Manheimer and Mellinger (1967) conceptualized two behavioral domains as underlying children's injury liability: behaviors that govern exposure to hazards and behaviors that impair coping with hazards. After examining the personality characteristics of about 700 children who were categorized according to the frequency of medically attended injuries, they found that injury liability was related to characteristics such as activity, extraversion, and roughhousing—presumably increasing exposure to hazards. Children with more injuries were also reported to be more aggressive, impulsive, and inattentive—these being among the characteristics that might impair coping with hazards.

Later investigations (Langley, McGee, Silva, & Williams, 1983; Langley, Silva, & Williams, 1980; Matheny, Brown, & Wilson, 1971) examined the history of children's injuries and found somewhat similar sets of behaviors related in injury liability. Taken as a whole, the results indicated that children who were more active, emotionally reactive or temperamental, inattentive or distractible, or who posed management problems tended to have more injuries than children rated as having contrasting characteristics.

In overview, the studies cited simply illustrated that children's injuries were systematically related to children's behaviors. However, because of the importance attributed to parents and home for the safety of the child, it is not clear that characteristics of the child make any additional contribution to childhood injuries once the characteristics of parents and home have been accounted for. The Louisville Twin Study has recently addressed these issues, but the background for these efforts will be reviewed first.

EARLY STUDIES OF CHILDHOOD INJURIES

Our own systematic longitudinal research on the developmental-behavioral aspects of children's injuries began almost 15 years ago with semistructured interviews routinely made when parents brought their twins to the research center. The twin pairs were recruited as infants and seen periodically for 15 years.

During each of the visits, parents were interviewed and asked to compare the behaviors of one twin with those of the other, and to provide health and injury histories for each twin. One initial exercise in relating injury liability to children's behavior depended on linking the difference within twin pairs for histories of injuries with differences reported for the twins' behaviors. This approach yielded an association between frequent temperamental outbursts, irritability, inattentiveness and activity, and injury liability for a longitudinal sample ranging in age from 1 to 6 years (Matheny et al., 1971). The same co-twin method was applied in a later investigation that contrasted twins on characteristics of temperament. The twin with a higher liability for injuries was likely to be more negative in mood, less adaptable in the face of environmental changes, and more avoidant or withdrawn from persons and novel events (Matheny, 1985).

The co-twin method highlighted the subtle within-pair behavioral differences related to injuries because so many other factors, by being common to both twins, were controlled. Despite its power, the method permitted only within-pair (or within-family) contrasts to be examined; the contrasts among children from different families did not enter into the analyses. Consequently, the relevance of contributions from variations in socioeconomic factors, attributes of the parents, and conditions of home life could not be established.

Matheny (1980) ignored the twin situation, and examined the relation between children's attention deployment and the injuries reported for the children during the age range from 6 to 9 years. Attention deployment was indirectly measured by the errors made when children were given the perceptual-exploration task devised by Elkind and Weiss (1967). Errors on the task given to six-year-olds provided low-order but significant correlations with children's injuries within the following 3 years. Socioeconomic status of the children's families and the children's IQ scores were also examined, but neither measure was related to the children's liability for injury.

The previous results from the Louisville Twin Study illustrate in one form or another the behavioral characteristics of the child that were linked with reports of injuries. In general, children who were active, temperamental, and deployed attention less optimally appeared more liable to injury than children who were less active, more easygoing, and more attentive to some types of visual-environmental features. Apparently, the characteristics of the child entered into the ordering of injury liability. However, the developmental component and the contributions from factors extrinsic to the child were not fully appreciated.

RESULTS FOR AN EXPANDED LONGITUDINAL SAMPLE

Since the analyses outlined above, the data set has been expanded to include measures of the parent and home, and additional measures of child temperament. Samples of children from the longitudinal study were divided into two contrasting cross sections: one group of children followed over the first three years of life (Cohort I), and one group of children followed for an interval from 6 to 9 years (Cohort II).

Samples

The children in both cohorts were selected from pairs of twins participating in the Louisville Twin Study. The selection was made on the basis of the children having completed the period of study for their respective age groups, and complete sets of measures being available for all children, parents, and home situations. On this basis there were 96 children (49 boys, 47 girls) in Cohort I and 76 children (42 boys, 34 girls) in Cohort II.

The children's families represented the entire socioeconomic range found in the Louisville metropolitan area. Occupations of the heads of household were converted to Duncan's scores for socioeconomic status (Reiss, 1961). The distribution of the scores indicated that the families of Cohort I and Cohort II were closely matched on socioeconomic status.

Injury Criterion

The reports of the children's injuries obtained from the interviews with parents could be specified in many ways—e.g., the type and severity of trauma, and circumstances surrounding the injury. For this report, the classification used was whether medical attention had been received. A child was denoted as having received medical attention if the child's injury was brought to the attention of any person(s) providing health care services in the metropolitan area, even if the child was not seen or treated by a physician. For example, when a parent called a poison control center about a child's ingestion of some substance, and the medical advice was tended only by telephone, the incident was counted as a medically tended injury. Moreover, injuries to teeth and gums cared for only by dentists were counted as medically attended injuries.

For Cohort I (1–3 years old), injuries obtained by parental interviews at 18, 24, 30, and 36 months represented the injury history for the two-year period. For Cohort II (6–9 years old), injuries reported during the interviews at 7, 8, and 9 years represented the injury history for the three-year period.

According to the history of injuries reported for each of the two cohorts, the children were assigned to one of two groups representing injury liability. A child in Cohort I or Cohort II reported to have had two or more injuries, with at least one of the injuries receiving medical attention, was categorized in the "higher liability" group. A child in Cohort I or Cohort II who had injuries not receiving medical attention or no injuries at all was categorized in the "lower liability" group. Injuries from animal bites were not counted. Injuries related to motor vehicles were counted only if the child was a pedestrian.

The circumstances surrounding injuries and the types of injuries received were not included in the analyses because of sample size; however, several trends among these aspects of the children's injuries should be sketched in a general fashion. The majority of the injuries in Cohort I, medically attended or not, resulted from falls—off furniture, down steps, against objects, and upon toys. In Cohort II, injuries from sports equipment, riding toys, and household utensils became more likely, but falls still accounted for almost half of the injuries. For the most part, injuries in both cohorts took place within the child's home or on the property around the home. Usually the location of injury was the head or the upper extremities, head injuries being more typical of the children in Cohort I. Most of the head injuries receiving medical attention required stitches or dental repair.

According to the scheme used for classifying injuries, there were 30 children assigned to the higher liability group and 66 children assigned to the lower liability group of children in Cohort I. Assignment for Cohort II yielded 28 children and 48 children in the higher and lower liability groups, respectively.

Parental Characteristics

Mothers and fathers independently completed the Thurstone Temperament Schedule (Thurstone, 1953). The Thurstone scores represent seven aspects of adult temperament defined by the following: active (participates in active engagements with the world), vigorous (is physically active and engaged in energetic occupations), impulsive (makes quick decisions, or changes from one activity to another), dominant (takes initiative, responsibility, or leadership), stable (is emotionally steady in mood and not overwhelmed by crisis), sociable (seeks and adapts to others), and reflective (likes quiet work and reflective thinking).

In addition, the years of schooling completed by the mother and the father were included as an indirect indication of each parent's realized intellectual attainments.

Characteristics of the Home Environment

In view of the fact that most injuries to young children take place within or about the child's home, a comprehensive home assessment was conducted by a social worker during a two-hour visit to the home. The home visit for the children in Cohort I was made when the children were between 6 and 9 months old; for Cohort II the visit was made when the children were about 6 years old.

The home assessment contained items presented in ABODE (Appraisals of Basic Opportunities for Developmental Experiences; Matheny, Thoben, & Wilson, 1982). Although most items were age independent, some items were adjusted to reflect features of the home environment appropriate either for infants or for children of an older age.

The items from ABODE were condensed by two principal-components factor analyses with Varimax rotation. The first analysis applied to the items scored from the home visit of the infant children and the second analysis applied to the items completed during the home visits of older children.

The analysis applicable to Cohort I yielded three factors with eigenvalues ≥ 1.00. The first factor pertained to a general dimension, termed "Adequacy of the Home Environment," which represented the social and material features of the home. The second factor was defined by the number of books in the home, but there were additional loadings from several items representing the amount of a child's protected personal space; consequently, this factor was labeled "Books—Personal Space." The third factor was defined by items characterizing the noise, confusion, and clutter in the household, and was labeled "Noise-Confusion."

The factor analysis of the items from the home visits for Cohort II yielded a first factor virtually equivalent to the one extracted for Cohort I and, therefore, was also labeled "Adequacy of the Home Environment." A second factor was not used for further analyses because it did not represent a clearly specifiable dimension and accounted for only 8% of the total variance.

The second set of measures of the home was obtained from the Family Environment Scale (FES) developed by Moos and Moos (1981). The FES consists of 10 subscales representing cohesion (support shared among families), expressive (degree to which family members are free to express themselves), conflict (amount of anger and hostility in the family), independence (self-assertion of family members), achievement (competitive striving), intellectual-culture orientation, active-recreational orientation (interest in social and recreational activities), moral-religious (emphasis on ethical and religious issues), organization (emphasis on planning family activities), and control (extent to which procedural rules govern family life).

The FES was completed by the mothers for Cohort I when the children were infants. For Cohort II, the mothers completed the FES when the children were about 6 years of age.

Finally, socioeconomic status, as determined by the occupation of the head of household (Reiss, 1961), was added as a distal measure of the resources within the family.

Characteristics of the Child

Temperament. The child's temperament for each cohort was assessed by having the mother complete temperament questionnaires. For Cohort I, the questionnaire given to the mother was the Toddler Temperament Scale devised by Fullard, McDevitt, and Carey (1984). It includes 97 ratings combined to yield nine categories of temperament postulated by Thomas and Chess (1977): activity level, rhythmicity (regularity of sleeping, eating), approach (movement toward novel persons or events), adaptability, intensity, mood, persistence/attention, distractibility, and threshold of reaction (level of stimulation required to evoke a reaction).

Because the mother completed the Toddler Temperament Scale each time the child was seen at the research center, there were four complete questionnaires available to represent each child's temperament from 1 to 3 years. Several methods for condensing the four scales were considered; however, in view of the fact that previous analyses had shown stability of the temperament measures by 2 years (Wilson & Matheny, 1986), the Toddler Temperament Scale completed at 2 years was used as the temperament measure for the period from 1 to 3 years.

For Cohort II, the most appropriate temperament questionnaire, also completed by the mother, was the Behavioral Style Questionnaire (McDevitt & Carey, 1978). The Behavioral Style Questionnaire was devised to rate the same categories of temperament found on the Toddler Temperament Scale; therefore, the two questionnaires are conceptually equivalent. Because the Behavioral Style Questionnaire was given at several ages, an arbitrary decision was made to use the questionnaire completed at 6 years as the single measure of the child's temperament for Cohort II.

Mental development. For Cohort I, the child's abilities were measured by the Mental Development Index (Bayley, 1969). The score obtained at 2 years was used to represent the child's relative status in development for the period from 1 to 3 years. For Cohort II, the full-scale IQ score from the Wechsler Preschool and Primary Scale of Intelligence (Wechsler, 1967) obtained at 6 years was used to represent the child's developmental status.

Sex of the child. The sex of the child is not a behavioral variable, but it presumably mediates a number of behavioral attributes. Therefore, the influence of the sex of the child was examined by introducing sex as an independent variable.

EXPANDED RESULTS

Cohort I

The direct correlations between the sets of measures—child, parents, or home environment—and injury liability for Cohort I are shown in Table 1. It is apparent that several characteristics from all sets of measures made modest but significant contributions to the two-way classification of children's injuries between 1 and 3 years of age.

An overview of the correlations indicates that the children with one or more injuries receiving medical attention were characterized by the following measures, according to source:

Parental characteristics. Mothers who portrayed themselves more emotionally stable, more actively engaged with the world, more energetic, or more reflective were mothers whose children were reported to have a lower liability for injuries. For the same children, fathers depicted themselves as being more social and taking more initiative. In addition, both mothers and fathers who were better educated had children with lower injury liability, but the correlation was significant only for the mothers.

Characteristics of home environment. Children with lower liability tended to be found in households where it was directly observed that there was less noise and confusion, and more adequate provisions for child development. The FES also indicated that families stressing active involvement and independence had children with lower injury liability. Not unexpectedly, families with higher socioeconomic status had children with lower liability.

Child characteristics. Children reported to be more adaptable, positive in mood, regular in sleeping and eating habit, persistently attentive, or less intense were less likely to be categorized within the group with higher injury liability. As found for previous studies (Matheny, 1987), boys were more likely than girls to receive the injuries requiring medical attention.

Cohort II

For the children in Cohort II, the same or equivalent sets of measures as used for Cohort I provided a different pattern. The correlations in Table 2 indicate that characteristics of the parents contributed little to the correlations with injury liability of children between 6 and 9 years. The only linkage found was that the children of more impulsive fathers were more likely to belong to the higher liability group. On the other hand, features of the home environment and the children themselves continued to play a role.

Table 1. Children's Injury Liability During 1–3 Years: Correlations with Characteristics of Parents, Home, and Child[a]

Parents		Home environment		Child	
Mother: Thurstone		ABODE factors		Sex of Child	.20[b]
Activity	-.23[b]	I Adequacy of the home environment	-.21[b]		
Vigor	-.20[b]	II Books–personal space	-.15		
Impulsive	.10	III Noise–confusion	.32[c]		
Dominant	.15			Toddler Temperament Scale	
Stable	-.28[c]	Family Environment Scale		Activity	.04
Social	.05	Cohesion	.11	Rhythmicity	-.23[b]
Reflective	-.25[b]	Expressive	-.17	Approach	-.09
		Conflict	.12	Adaptability	-.31[c]
Father: Thurstone		Independence	-.23[b]	Intensity	.23[b]
Activity	.07	Achievement	.02	Mood	-.27[c]
Vigor	-.15	Intellectual	-.16	Persistence	-.21[b]
Impulsive	.01	Activity	-.33[c]	Distractibility	.08
Dominant	-.23[b]	Moral	.16	Threshold	-.07
Stable	-.14	Organization	-.01		
Social	-.27[c]	Control	.17		
Reflective	.07				
Parental education		Socioeconomic status	-.25[b]	Bayley Mental Index	-.04
Mother	-.29[c]				
Father	-.19				

[a]Injury liability classified with 1, lower liability; 2, higher liability. Sex is classified with 1, female; 2, male.
[b]$p \leq .05$.
[c]$p \leq .01$.

Table 2. Children's Injury Liability During 6–9 Years: Correlations with Characteristics of Parents, Home, and Child[a]

Parents		Home environment		Child	
Mother: Thurstone		ABODE factor		Sex of child	.34[c]
Activity	.13	I Adequacy of the home environment	−.23[b]		
Vigor	.09			Toddler Temperament Scale	
Impulsive	−.07	Family Environment Scale		Activity	.45[c]
Dominant	−.04	Cohesion	−.25[b]	Rhythmicity	−.30[c]
Stable	−.02	Expressive	−.17	Approach	−.17
Social	−.07	Conflict	.10	Adaptability	−.23[b]
Reflective	.08	Independence	−.15	Intensity	−.01
		Achievement	.06	Mood	−.20
Father: Thurstone		Intellectual	.24[b]	Persistence	−.02
Activity	.20	Activity	.03	Distractibility	.23[b]
Vigor	.15	Moral	−.15	Threshold	.10
Impulsive	.29[b]	Organization	−.22		
Dominant	.05	Control	−.31[c]	IQ score	.05
Stable	−.02				
Social	−.05	Socioeconomic status	−.06		
Reflective	.15				
Parental education					
Mother	−.10				
Father	−.06				

[a]Injury liability classified with 1, lower liability; 2, higher liability. Sex is classified with 1, female; 2, male.
[b]$p \leq .05$.
[c]$p \leq .01$.

Characteristics of the home environment. As before, families with more adequate provisions for child development were marked by lower injury liability. From the FES, the families depicted as more cohesive and more governed by procedural rules had fewer children's injuries. For these children in this age range, socioeconomic status had no association with injury liability.

Child Characteristics. Child temperament, as reported by the mother, entered into the relation with injury liability in several direct ways: children who were more active, less adaptable, less regular in sleeping and eating habits, or more distractable were likely to belong to the group with higher liability for injuries. It is also evident that the children with higher liability were likely to be boys.

Multiple Regression Analyses

Since almost all of the significant correlations in Tables 1 and 2 were low, the next step was to see what combination of measures could maximize the prediction of injury liability. A multiple regression program was used to identify the set of variables making independent contributions to the prediction. The measures were entered in hierarchical order with the presumption that first, parental characteristics, and second, features of the home environment, would be more influential than child characteristics in predicting injury liability. For both cohorts, parental education and family socioeconomic status were considered as background variables, and placed last in the analyses.

The results for the regression analyses applied to Cohort I and II are presented in Table 3. It is evident that the multiple correlations for both cohorts are substantially improved over the correlations provided by each measure considered singly. It is equally evident that there were overlaps among some of the measures entering into the predictive correlations; when some measures were entered, other measures did not make independent contributions to the prediction. For example, several of the child measures obtained for Cohort I had higher correlations with injury liability than the measures of parents or home provided; however, once the latter measures were entered first, many of the child measures provided no additional independent contributions.

For Cohort I, higher injury liability was clearly associated with a number of measures that, in combination, produced a multiple $R = 0.64$. The combination of (1) a less active and less emotionally stable mother, (2) a less sociable and more impulsive father, (3) noise and confusion in the home, and

Table 3. Multiple Correlations of Parent, Home, and Child: Variables with Child Injury Liability in Cohorts I and II

Step no.	Assigned level of entry	Variables and source	Original R	Partial R	Multiple R
		Cohort I (1–3 years)			
1	1	Mother: stability (Thurstone)	−.28	—	.28
2	1	Father: social (Thurstone)	−.28	−.23	.35
3	1	Mother: activity (Thurstone)	−.23	−.21	.41
4	2	Home: noise–confusion factor	.32	.37	.53
5	3	Child: rhythmicity (Toddler Temperament Scale)	−.23	−.25	.57
6	1	Father: impulsive (Thurstone)	.10	.21	.60
7	3	Child: intensity (Toddler Temperament Scale)	.23	.28	.64
		Cohort II (6–9 years)			
1		Child: activity (Behavioral Style Questionnaire)	.45	—	.45
2		Home: control (Family Environment Scale)	−.31	−.37	.56
3		Sex of child	.34	.37	.64
4		Child: rhythmicity (Behavioral Style Questionnaire)	−.30	−.24	.66

(4) a child irregular in sleeping or eating habits, and intensely reactive to stimulation, predicted a higher liability for injuries.

For Cohort II, the contributions from the child measures to the prediction of injury liability became more evident. Active boys who were irregular in sleeping and eating habits, and who were from homes in which family members were less subject to rules, were more liable to injuries receiving medical attention. Unlike Cohort I, in which parent and home measures contributed more to the predictive composite, the composite of predictive measures in Cohort II could be made almost entirely from measures of the child.

Supplementary analyses were run to see if the order of entry of the measures affected the selection of the measures independently contributing to the predictive composites. Except for minor variations in the final ordering of the measures, the supplementary analyses yielded virtually the same results as in Table 3.

DISCUSSION

This exercise has illustrated the importance of behavioral measures, and especially those obtained for children, for understanding systematic differences in children's injury liability. Within two cross-sectional samples, representing two widely separated periods of childhood, behavioral differences among children were linked to differences in the reported presence or absence of injuries receiving medical attention. Generalizations across studies of childhood injuries are risky; nevertheless, the present results confirm general trends apparent among a variety of studies reviewed elsewhere (Matheny, 1987): injuries during childhood vary systematically; and the variations can be connected with the age and sex of the child, and individual differences in activity level, temperamental behaviors, and attention span or distractibility. These attributes of children have been highlighted as contributors to children's (and adults') injuries and one is sorely pressed to find any consistent evidence that injuries are linked to behaviors of an opposite sort (see Matheny, 1987).

We did not anticipate that rhythmicity or regularity of a child's habits, such as sleeping and eating, would distinguish between levels of injury liability. In view of these behaviors' biological aspects, including genetic influences (Matheny, Wilson, Dolan, & Krantz, 1981), one should consider the possibility that constitutional factors contribute to injury liability. However, it was also evident that higher liability for injuries was linked to family situations marked by disorganized features. Therefore, it is easy to imagine that the chaotic situations as described fostered disruptions in the child's routines for sleep and other habits.

The unique aspect of the present exercise is that the child's behaviors were considered within the larger context of attributes assessed for parents and the home environment. Thereby, the few strands connecting the child's behaviors to injuries became part of a larger tapestry with an evolving pattern: (1) in early childhood, with the strands woven by a composite of characteristics of parents, home, and child; and (2) at the beginning of the school years, with the weave more closely patterned by the characteristics of the child.

The available evidence (Langley et al., 1983, Manheimer & Mellinger, 1967; Matheny, 1980) has already indicated that the behaviors of the older child are more associated with injury histories. But the increase in the child's contribution to injuries is defined, of course, by the characteristics measured. Because the present and previous studies did not assess attributes of persons and environments beyond the family, it could be that the child's injury-related behaviors are no more (or no less) important at later ages than during the years of the toddler. Unfortunately, the techniques for assessing the child's world beyond the family are limited, particularly if applied to large groups of children.

Injury Prevention

Injuries involve multiple causes, with mutual interactions, and the understanding of the injury equation requires us to identify the important variables and their interactions (McFarland, 1963). Many important hazards, especially those in the environment, have been identified and some hazards have been controlled, as reflected in the decrease of childhood mortality rates. Successes in that direction have been so striking that it is tempting to assume that wide-scale, public health approaches will be the ultimate "fix" for the injury problem (Rivara & Mueller, 1987; Wilson & Baker, 1987). However, at some point, the application of injury prevention measures, whether passive or active (Haddon, 1974), falters at the threshold of individual actions. Most of the nonlethal injuries of children are not due to the vehicular collisions, poisonings, or other occurrences that receive so much attention and demand passive improvements because of their serious outcomes. Rather, the nonlethal injuries occur within situations not so susceptible to engineered improvements on a large scale. One might argue that these relatively less serious injuries are of little consequence, perhaps the injury equivalent of the common cold; however, if nothing else, the economic costs are considerable. For example, we crudely estimated that the children with higher injury liability in Cohorts I and II incurred average medical costs of about $2000 for their injuries. If one were to generalize this estimate to the U.S. population of children of similar ages, the estimated medical bill would be many millions of dollars.

For the purposes of injury prevention, our focus on the child and the more immediate aspects of the child's world is important. First, the results suggest, as common sense would dictate, that the primary factors pertaining to the toddler's injury liability are those of parents and homes. Therefore, for ordinary household injuries, our attention should be directed not only toward early and repeated cautions given to all parents, but especially to those at higher risk (see also Peterson, Farmer, & Mori, 1987). In this context, higher risk simply refers to the composites of those characteristics of parents and households that match the characteristics outlined in this report. Our impression of these families is that they are less assertive or energetic in dealing with many aspects of family life, including the guidance of their young children. For these families, a more assertive stance may have to be taken by the health professionals if one expects the parents to budge from the status quo. Although we are just beginning to collect data to support this impression, the observations we have indicate that the parents must be taught or shown that, for example, furniture can be moved out of the way, objects can be placed out of reach, unsteady furniture can be anchored, and railings in stairwells can be lowered so that a child can grasp them.

Among the older children, the guidance and cautions could be best directed, as we see it, to the primary agent—the child. In this instance, parents, teachers, television, or any other conduit may carry the message; yet the ultimate effect desired is for a child to act more safely. No doubt some children who are overly active, impulsive, or the like may require carefully calibrated behavioral methods (see Roberts et al., 1987). In most other instances parents or others may have to assure that safe behaviors are modeled. Nevertheless, the child has to get the message.

If it appears we are advocating active psychological approaches for understanding injurious circumstances and for preventing injuries, we have made our point. Such approaches can be effective, although some critics might disagree (see Rivara & Mueller, 1987). For example, simply examine the emergent success of the active individualized efforts to improve one's own health—now a national industry. Apparently, repeated messages nurtured by the climate of opinion that health can be improved by changes in day-to-day behavior (Nightingale, 1981) have had a cumulative effect on behaviors related to smoking, diet, alcohol consumption, exercise, and stress. Moreover, behavioral changes have come about by the repeated reminders that some lifestyles are less healthy than others (Wiley & Camacho, 1980). Behavioral research on childhood injuries points in the same direction. With further research to refine what safe or unsafe lifestyles entail for children, we will be in a position to address the question, If health sells, why not safety?

REFERENCES

Bayley, N. (1969). *Bayley scales of infant development.* New York: Psychological Corp.

Elkind, D., & Weiss, J. (1967). Studies in perceptual development III: Perceptual exploration. *Child Development, 38,* 1153–1163.

Fullard, W., McDevitt, S. C., & Carey, W. B. (1984). Assessing temperament in one-to three-year-old children. *Journal of Pediatric Psychology, 9,* 205–217.

Haddon, W. (1974), Strategy in preventive medicine: Passive versus active approaches to reducing human wastage, *Journal of Trauma, 14,* 353–354.

Haddon, W., Suchman, E. A., & Klein, D. (1964). *Accident research methods and approaches.* New York: Harper & Row.

Langley, J. (1982). The "accident prone" child—The perpetration of a myth. *Australian Paediatric Journal, 18,* 243–246.

Langley, J., Silva, P. A., & Williams, S. (1980). A Study of the relationship of ninety background, developmental, behavioural and medical factors to childhood accidents. A report from the Dunedin Multidisciplinary Child Development Study. *Australian Paediatric Journal, 16,* 244–247.

Langley, J., McGee, R., Silva, P., & Williams, S. (1983). Child behavior and accidents. *Journal of Pediatric Psychology, 8,* 181–189.

Manheimer, D. E., & Mellinger, G. D. (1967). Personality characteristics of the child accident repeater. *Child Development, 38,* 491–513.

Matheny, A. P., Jr., (1980). Visual-perceptual exploration and accident liability in children. *Journal of Pediatric Psychology, 5,* 351–353.

Matheny, A. P., Jr. (1985, April). *Toddler temperament and accident liability within twinships.* Paper presented at the biennial meeting of the Society for Research in Child Development, Toronto.

Matheny, A. P., Jr. (1987). Accidents and injuries. In D. Routh (Ed.), *Handbook of pediatric psychology* (pp. 108–134), New York: Guilford Press.

Matheny, A. P., Jr., & Fisher, J. E. (1984). Behavioral perspectives on children's accidents. In M. Wolraich & D. Routh (Eds.). *Advances in behavioral pediatrics* (Vol. V, pp. 221–262). Greenwich, CT: JAI Press.

Matheny, A. P., Jr., Brown, A., & Wilson, R. S. (1971). Behavioral antecedents of accidental injuries in early childhood: A study of twins. *Journal of Pediatrics, 79,* 122–124.

Matheny, A. P., Jr., Thoben, A. S., & Wilson, R. S. (1982). Appraisals of basic opportunities for developmental experiences (ABODE): Manual for home assessments of twin children. *JSAS Catalog of Selected Documents in Psychology, 12,* 31. (Ms. No. 2472)

Matheny, A. P., Jr., Wilson, R. S., Dolan, A. B., & Krantz, J. Z. (1981). Behavioral contrasts in twinships: Stability and patterns of differences in childhood. *Childhood Development, 52,* 579–588.

McDevitt, S. C., & Carey, W. B. (1978). The measurement of temperament in 3–7 year-old children. *Journal of Child Psychology and Psychiatry, 19,* 245–253.

McFarland, R. A. (1963). A critique of accident research. *Annals of New York Academy of Science, 107,* 686–695.

Moos, R. H., & Moos, B. S. (1981). *Family environment scale.* Palo Alto, CA: Consulting Psychologists Press.

Nightingale, E. (1981). Prospects for reducing mortality in developed countries by changes in day-to-day behavior. In *International population conference* (pp. 207–233). Liege, Belgium: International Union for the Scientific Study of Population.

Peterson, L., Farmer, J., & Mori, J. (1987). Process analysis of injury situations: A complement to epidemiological methods. *Journal of Social Issues, 43* (2), 33–44.

Reiss, A. J. (1961). *Occupations and social status.* New York: Free Press of Glencoe.

Rivara, F. P., & Mueller, B. A. (1987). The epidemiology and causes of childhood injuries. *Journal of Social Issues, 43* (2), 13–31.

Roberts, M. C., Elkins, P. D., & Royal, G. P. (1984). Psychological applications to the prevention of accidents and illness. In M. C. Roberts & L. Peterson (Eds.), *Prevention of problems in childhood: Psychological research and applications* (pp. 173–199). New York: Wiley Interscience.

Roberts, M. C. Fanurik, D., & Layfield, D. A. (1987). Behavioral approaches to prevention in childhood injuries. *Journal of Social Issues, 43* (2), 10–118.

Shaw, L., & Sichel, H. S. (1971). *Accident proneness: Research in the occurrence, causation and prevention of road accidents.* New York: Pergamon.

Thomas, A., & Chess, S. (1977). *Temperament and development.* New York: Brunner/Mazel.

Thurstone, L. L. (1953). *Examiner manual for the Thurstone Temperament Schedule* (2nd Ed.). Chicago, IL: Science Research Associates.

Wechsler, D. (1967). *Wechsler preschool and primary scale of intelligence.* New York: Psychological Corp.

Wiley, J. A., & Camacho, T. C. (1980). Life style and future health: Evidence from the Alameda County study. *Preventive Medicine, 9,* 1–21.

Wilson, M., & Baker, S. (1987). Structural approach to injury control. *Journal of Social Issues, 43* (2), 73–86.

Wilson, R. S., & Matheny, A. P., Jr. (1986). Behavior genetics research in infant temperament: The Louisville Twin Study. In R. Plomin & J. Dunn (Eds.), *The study of temperament: Changes, continuities, and challenges* (pp. 81–98). Hillside, NJ: Lawrence Erlbaum.

21

Infant Temperament, Childhood Accidents, and Hospitalization

Göte Nyman
University of Helsinki, Finland

The role of infant temperament in predicting the incidence of hospitalization and accidents of children under the age of 5 was studied in a prospective follow-up study. Temperament type and profile was originally measured for 1,855 infants (6 to 8 months of age). We obtained data for 270 who had later been hospitalized because of accidents or illnesses. Of these, the temperament of 35 who had suffered a contusion, poisoning, burns, or other accidents were more closely analyzed. The results show that a disproportionate number of all hospitalized children had earlier been characterized as "difficult" in their temperament. This was typical, however, for both the accident group and other hospitalized children. The hospitalized children had a significantly more negative mood and higher intensity of responses to normal everyday life situations. The accident group differed from other hospitalized children in being mainly more persistent but also showed a tendency to higher activity level and negative reactions to new situations. The results do not support a straightforward hypothesis of an early accident

Reprinted with permission from *Clinical Pediatrics,* 1987, Vol. 26, No. 8, 398–404. Copyright 1987 by J. B. Lippincott Co.

I thank Dr. Matti Huttunen for collaboration in many phases of this work and Nina Sajaniemi, MA for collecting the data in the children's hospital.

Editors' Note: One reviewer commented as follows: "This interesting paper reports a relationship between infant temperament measured at 6–8 months and accidents and hospitalizations occurring up to the age of 5 years. It is extraordinary that behavioral data at that early age were able to predict these physical problems so much later, although the temperament itself shows only moderate stability over the same time period. These findings are valuable. It is important that one hospital serves the whole study population, so few cases were lost."

prone temperament but point out the significance of temperament
in the processes of hospitalization and accidents.

In the United States accidents cause more child deaths than pneumonia, meningitis, cardiovascular diseases, and cancer combined.[1-4]. It has been suggested that by proper application of available preventive methods one-third of the injuries could be prevented.[5]

One of the key questions in the preventive work has been, whether it is possible to predict the accident susceptibility of individual children on the basis of their personal characteristics and, if so, which are the critical personal traits that should be considered. It has been suggested that accidentally poisoned children, especially accident repeaters, typically have a hyperactive temperament.[5-10] Aggressive, overactive, or impulsive reactions[11-15] have also been suggested as predisposing factors for injuries. The validity of such correlations has been challenged by referring to studies which show that there are also other significant predisposing factors that are related to family history and maternal well-being.[16-18] Furthermore, it has been argued that applying the concept of accident susceptibility is hazardous to accident prevention because it implies that prevention is either useless or extremely difficult.[19]

Despite this controversy, some personality traits are known to be associated with a higher than normal risk for childhood accidents. Significant correlations have been established in a large study[20] including over 8,000 children, which showed that injuries correlate with extroversion and aggressiveness. This has been confirmed lately by another retrospective study with 12,000 children, which showed that aggressive and overactive behavior are significant predictors for accidents, even when social class, crowding, maternal stress, age, and marital status have been controlled.[21] Of course, the existence of such correlations does not prove a direct casual relationship between personality and accidents; it is possible that they only reflect the nature of the relationship between the child and her environment or guardian. An aggressive or extroverted child, for example, can easily evoke continuous conflicts in the family and, consequently, increase the accident risk.

The knowledge of the role of personality in the accident process can help to develop better and more practical models for diagnostic and preventive work. Most earlier studies that have estimated the role of the child's personality in predicting her involvement in accidents, have done this retrospectively by measuring the child's personality after the accidents have taken place. Many types of bias are likely to occur in such studies because the experienced accidents can change the behavioral habits of the children involved and especially the attitudes of the parents and teachers who are usually the source of the information about the child.[20,21] These changes can lead to selective observations of the child's behavior and biased interpretation of his or her behavior during the time after the accident. To avoid such bias, it is better to study the children's personal characteristics before the accidents have taken place.

We had earlier collected temperament data on 1,855 children whose temperaments were estimated by the mother or the guardian when the babies were at the age of about 6–8 months.[22] We were interested in determining if these early temperamental traits would have any value in estimating the child's risk for later accidents. Because early temperament as defined in the original studies by Thomas *et al.*[23] and Carey[24] describes the energetic nature of the child's behavior without direct reference to the context and without complex interpretations of its meanings, it was expected to be a fruitful source of predictive information.

For the purpose of our study we looked up children in our 6–8 month old patient sample who, later in their first 5 years of life had become hospitalized because of accidents or illnesses. It was hoped that in a prospective follow-up, we might gain reliable information about possible temperamental characteristics that are related to accident susceptibility.

METHOD

Assessment of Temperament

Temperament profiles of 1,855 children born during 1975–1976 in Helsinki were collected by asking the mother or the baby's guardian to describe the baby's behavior and character by completing the translated Infant Temperament Questionnaire.[23-24] This contains 70 three-alternative items that describe the infant's responses and behavior in typical everyday life situations (during sleep, play, feeding, and daily care). On the basis of this description the infant's temperament was determined in nine temperament dimensions. The names of the dimensions and the scoring used are given within the parentheses:

1. Amount of activity
   (Activity)   (0 = high 2 = low)
2. Regularity of habits
   (Regularity)   (0 = high 2 = low)
3. First reactions to
   new situations
   (First reaction)   (0 = approach 2 = avoid)

4. Adaptation
    capability
    (Adaptability)   (0 = high 2 = low)
5. Sensory threshold
    (Threshold)   (0 = high 2 = low)
6. Intensity of
    responses
    (Intensity)   (0 = high 2 = low)
7. Positive or negative
    mood (Mood)   (0 = posit. 2 = negat.)
8. Concentration
    ability
    (Distractibility)   (0 = low 2 = high)
9. Persistence during
    activity
    (Persistence)   (0 = high 2 = low)

The questionnaire includes nine extra items in which the mother gave her own view about the child's temperament on the same nine dimensions that form the temperament profile. In our total sample (N = 1,855), the correlations between the nine temperament dimensions obtained by scoring the questionnaire and these dimensions as estimated by the mother varied from .41 (Threshold) to .72 (Regularity).[22]

Because the nine temperament dimensions describe the energetic and adaptive nature of the infant's behavior without direct reference to the context of the behavior, they can be expected to bear a close relationship to the child's way of dealing with many normal situations, such as play and handling toys and exploring new places and things. Whether or not there is a direct causal relationship between the incidence of accidents and the infant temperament, we expected that children with "difficult" temperaments would be more likely than others to be involved with accidents.

The term "difficult" temperament is characterized by five critical temperament features: irregularity, negative first reactions, negative mood, poor adaptability, and high intensity. These have been successfully used as a basis for diagnosing children who have a "risk" temperament[23-24] and they are closely related to the hyperactive type of behavior which has been suggested to increase the risk for accidents.[10] Some of these temperament features seem likely to produce risky behavior; this will be analyzed later in the "discussion."

Using the criteria described by Carey[24] the children were divided into three different diagnostic groups called "easy," "difficult," and "intermediate."

Although the connotations of these terms involve several value judgments, the terms as used here (and originally) refer only to the category of temperament. By "difficult" we mean an infant who has in 4–5 of the above mentioned five critical temperament dimensions a score that is towards the difficult end of the temperament dimension (irregular, negative first reactions, poor adaptability, intensive reactions, and negative mood), and in at least 2 of them, a score more than 1 Standard Deviation (SD) above the mean of the total sample.

SELECTION OF THE CHILDREN TO THE STUDY

Of the 1,855 children of our original sample, 270 (15%) were hospitalized in the Helsinki City Hospital (Aurora) during 1975–1980. Of these, we could get information on about 35 (1.9%) who had suffered some kind of an accident (contusion, poisoning, burns, wounds, or fractures) that was severe enough to cause hospitalization. Two hundred thirty-five were hospitalized because of a suspected or diagnosed illness. The average age of the children who had been involved in accidents and were hospitalized was 2.25 years. The social class distribution of the hospitalized children did not differ from that of the families belonging to the corresponding age group and having children in Helsinki.

RESULTS

Temperament Profile of the Accident Group

The average temperament profiles of the children in the total sample, including the accident cases (N = 1,855) and the accident group (N = 35), proved to be different. As Table 1 shows, the children in the accident group had, on average, higher intensity of responses (p < .001), more negative mood (p < .005) and negative first reactions (p < .05), more persistence (p < .05), and a tendency to a higher activity level (p < .1) than the babies in the total material. Three of these temperament dimensions (First reaction, Intensity, Mood) belong to those five critical features which have been used as a basis for defining the general temperament type of the child.[23]

These differences in observed temperament do not necessarily mean that certain temperament features would be directly connected with a higher accident susceptibiity. They might simply reflect a higher probability of hospitalization. For example, a child with a negative mood and high intensity of responses will probably show stronger and more alarming responses to injuries or illnesses, which in turn increases the probability of hospitalization.

Table 1. Temperament Profile of the Hospitalized Children

Temperament Dimension	Total Sample (I) (N = 1,855)		Accident Group (II) (N = 35)		Other Hospitalized Children (III) (N = 235)		T-test (I vs. II)	T-test (II vs. III)
	x	sd	x	sd	x	sd	p	p
Activity	.49	.26	.43	.25	.49	.26	<.10	<.10
Regularity	.56	.42	.65	.46	.59	.42	N.S.	N.S.
First reaction	.55	.29	.65	.35	.55	.28	<.1	<.05
Adaptability	.35	.24	.40	.31	.37	.24	N.S.	N.S.
Threshold	.94	.33	.93	.32	.92	.28	N.S.	N.S.
Intensity	.81	.24	.67	.25	.70	.28	<.001	N.S.
Mood	.55	.19	.66	.21	.65	.19	<.005	N.S.
Distractibility	.37	.21	.41	.34	.35	.21	N.S.	N.S.
Persistence	.90	.30	.99	.32	.87	.31	<.05	<.05

In retrospective studies, such behavioral differences in individual response patterns might also affect the accuracy of mother's recall of these incidents and thus cause spurious correlations.

Indeed, the average scores of the accident group and the other hospitalized group (illnesses) proved rather similar with only some exceptions. Slight differences remained between these two groups in Persistence ($p < .05$), Activity ($p < .1$), and First reaction ($p < .1$).

On average, children having an active or persistent temperament or tendency to negative reactions in new situations, appear more frequently in the accident group. It seems possible that negative mood and intensive responses give extra weight to the child's symptoms,which in turn increases the probability of hospitalization. If negative mood *and* intensive responses are interpreted as a sign of aggression, then this might also partly explain why Bijur *et al.* (1986) found in their large material that overactivity was associated with injuries that did not result in hospitalization, whereas aggression was significantly associated with both hospitalized and non-hospitalized injuries.

The temperament score for each dimension was obtained as the mean score of the items that belong to the dimension concerned. It turned out that in four out of six items that described the infant's sleep behavior, the children in the accident group had an average score that was significantly different from the total sample. The four items describe how easily the child adapts to a new time or place of sleep, what her mood is like when put to bed and waking up, and how much she moves during her sleep. A similar trend was observed for the items that dealt with the feeding of the infant. Apparently these two factors are diagnostically significant and would require further study.

Accidents, Hospitalization, and the "Difficult" Temperament Type

Originally, we expected the "difficult" temperament type to be connected with a higher risk for accidents, simply because it is characterized by a behavior that is more difficult for the parents to predict and control.[25] The average scores on the nine temperament dimensions showed, however, that the observed temperamental differences were not typically in the five critical diagnostic temperament features that define the "difficult" temperament type. Still, it might be that the distribution of accidents among the three different temperament types (easy, intermediate, difficult) would better reveal a possible connection between accidents and temperament type.

To see if this is so, we calculated the number of children who had had accidents in each of these groups (for definitions, see "method") and the data are shown in Table 2 and Table 3. It turned out that in the accident group, the relative proportion of "difficult" children was approximately twice the proportion observed in the total material and the distributions differed significantly as shown by chi-square analysis (χ^2 = 8.27, p < .02). Furthermore, the proportion of "easy" children who had suffered accidents was less than about half of that observed in the total sample

This result, however, might suggest a higher probability of hospitalization, so accident susceptibility of the "difficult" babies was compared to the corresponding probability of all the children in our sample. Indeed, this was confirmed by a similar comparison between the accident group and the other hospitalized babies; there the observed and expected frequencies of the temperament types did not significantly differ statistically (χ^2 = .750, N.S.) even though both groups differed from the total material.

Because the total number of patients who had suffered accidents was only 35, the proportions of different accident types are not statistically reliable. Their distribution into cases of contusions, burns, and poisonings have been included in Table 3, however, to show the trends involved. Figure 1 shows the relative proportions of different temperament types in the total material (N = 1,855), the accident group (N = 35), and other hospitalized children (N = 235).

MOTHER'S VIEW OF THE CHILD

It could be suggested that it is not the temperamental features as such that determine the baby's risk for accidents but rather the parents' views and interpretation of the baby's behavioral character. It is reasonable to assume that all parents have developed a "cognitive scheme" of their child's personality and behavior habits and that the prediction of the child's behavior and possible risks involved in different situations are based on this scheme. Mothers with an unrealistic or strongly biased view of the child could be

Table 2. Temperament Type and Proportion of Accidents

Temperament Type	Total Sample (N = 1,855)	Accident Group (N = 35)
Difficult	14.6% (270)	31.4% (11)
Intermediate	53.4% (990)	48.6% (17)
Easy	32.0% (595)	20.0% (7)
Total	100.0%	100.0%

(χ^2 = 8.27, p < .02)

Table 3. Temperament Type, Hospitalization and Accidents

Temperament Type	Accident Group (N = 35)	Other hospitalized Babies (N = 235)	Contusions	Burns	Poisoning	Others
Difficult	31.4% (11)	24.7% (58)	41.2% (7)	33.3% (3)	(1)	(—)
Intermediate	48.6% (17)	53.6% (126)	41.2% (7)	44.5% (4)	(5)	(1)
Easy	20.0% (7)	21.7% (51)	17.6% (3)	22.2% (2)	(1)	(1)
Total	100.0%	100.0%	100.0%	100.0%		

(χ^2 = .750, N.S.)

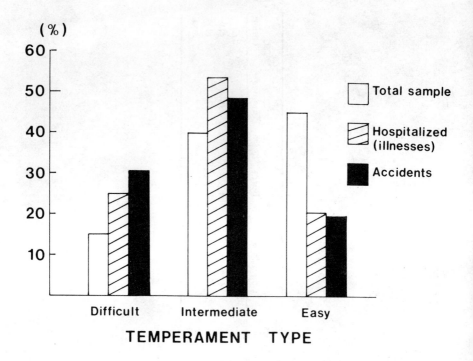

Figure 1. Relative proportions of the three temperament types in the accident group (N = 35), other hospitalized children (N = 235) and the total sample (N = 1,855). The proportion of "difficult" infants of the accident group and of the other hospitalized children is larger than would be predicted from the total sample. There is also a relatively smaller number of easy infants in these two groups.

expected to allow more risky situations for the child or to be incapable of predicting them.

To see if the general impression that the mothers of the accident group had of their children differed from that of the total sample, we calculated the correlations between the nine temperament scores and the items by which the mothers estimated the baby on the same nine temperament dimensions. Furthermore, they were asked to choose a general temperament category ("easy," "intermediate," or "difficult") that best described the baby.

The correlations between the temperament scores obtained and the mothers' estimations on same dimensions are seen in Table 4.

It was somewhat surprising to see that the mothers in the accident group obtained several higher correlations than were found in the total sample. In

Table 4. Correlations Between the Scores of the Temperament Test and Mothers' Estimation of the Same Temperamental Dimensions

	Activity	Regul	First r	Adapt	Thres	Inten	Mood	Distr	Persist
Total Sample (N = 1,855)	.70	.72	.44	.55	.41	.40	.46	.50	.51
Accident Group (N = 35)	.74	.83	.61	.59	.67	.25	.43	.51	.35

other words, they were more accurate in estimating their babies. The temperament dimensions for which this was observed, were: Activity, Regularity, First reaction, Adaptability, and Threshold. However, in estimating the Persistence of the baby, the correlation in the accident group was clearly lower than in the total sample (.35 vs .51). Even though the interpretation of these correlations is not straightforward, the finding suggests that mothers of the accident group are not less accurate in estimating the activity (amount of movement) or the type of reactions their children typically show. This is contrary to the hypothesis that the mothers of the accident group would be less observant or unrealistic in interpreting the risky temperament of the child. However, in the accident group the mothers described their child as "difficult" significantly more often than in the total sample ($\chi^2 = 116.89$, p < .001).

DISCUSSION

Our results show that children under 5, who have been hospitalized because of accidents are more likely to have a temperament type which is characterized by negative mood, high intensity of responses, persistence, high level of activity, or negative reactions to new situations. However, it seems that this temperament type is also associated with a higher probability of hospitalization for medical reasons.

It has been shown (Bijur *et al.,* 1986) that aggressiveness and overactivity are associated with a higher risk of injuries in children under 5. However, from clinical practice it is known that the temperament of the child gives weight to her symptoms caused by an injury or an illness. Such a tendency was also shown in our material by the high significance of negative mood (p < .005) and intensity of responses (p < .001) in differentiating the hospitalized group from the total material.

Persistence, a tendency to high activity, and avoidance reactions were more directly connected with the incidence of accidents, because these features were typical of the accident group alone. However, it was not possible to define a specific temperamental composition which would best describe the children at risk for accidents because of the rather weak effects observed and the small number of accident cases (N = 35) available. Interestingly, sleep and feeding behavior seemed diagnostically important sources of information about those temperamental characteristics which are connected with hospitalization. It is likely that problems in sleep and feeding become very quickly stressful to the mother and the family, which makes these disturbances rather alarming.

The parental rating that we have used is not ideal for studying those personal properties that might predict accidents in later childhood. Nevertheless, our results confirm other retrospectively obtained results suggesting that some individual characteristics at a relatively early age are related to later hospitalization and accidents. Because the temperament measurements were conducted before the accidents had taken place, the mother's interpretation of the baby's behavior and temperament had not been affected by the experiences of the accidents or hospitalization.

We found only partial support of the hypothesis that very active temperament is connected with an increased risk of accidents. The children in the accident group had a tendency to high activity but also to withdrawal (negative first reactions to new situations such as new food, new persons or places). Furthermore, they had a significantly higher persistence than other hospitalized children. The incidence of accidents was not associated with a higher sensory threshold or deviance in adaptability which could have been expected on the assumption that such characteristics indicate a weak ability to perceive risk factors. Neither did we find a difference between the average distractibility of the accident group and the controls which would have been suggestive of poor perception of accidental situations.

Our data show that the mothers of the accident group were even more aware of the children's temperamental character than were the mothers in our total sample. The mothers of the accident group had a higher correlation between their estimations and that of the questionnaire score. It is understood that other information is necessary to estimate how objective they were in estimating the child's behavioral type.

The study of very young children, as in our study, involves many complications, and the results show how intimately hospitalization and infant temperament are linked with parental interpretation of the child's personality and behavior. In order to analyze the connections between the accident process and personal characteristics of the child, it might prove more profitable to approach the problem by observing near-accidents and risk-taking behavior, instead of the serious cases that lead to hospitalization. Such an approach has been applied in the study of work safety and accident prevention.[26] This would better allow the study of individual behavior patterns and their role in risk situations and it could also be applied with reasonable costs in prospective studies of childhood accidents. It might also give more practical hints for the design of preventive actions in the environment.

428

Annual Progress in Child Psychiatry and Development

REFERENCES

1. Jones M. The child accident repeater. Clin Pediatr 1980;19:284.
2. Feldman KW. Prevention of childhood accidents: recent progress, Pediatr. Rev. 1980;2:75.
3. Greensher J. Prevention of childhood injuries. Pediatrics 1984;74:970.
4. O'Shea JS, Collins EW, Butler CB. Pediatric accident prevention. Clin Pediatr 1982;21:290.
5. Rivara FP. Traumatic deaths of children in the United States: Currently available prevention strategies. Pediatrics 1985;75:456.
6. Wehrle PF, DeFreest L, Penhollow J, Harris VG. The epidemiology of accidental poisoning in an urban population. Pediatrics 1961;27:614.
7. Sobel R, Margolis JA. Repetitive poisoning in children: a psychosocial study. Pediatrics 1965;35:641.
8. Baltimore CL, Meyer RJ. A study of storage, child behavioral traits, and mother's knowledge of toxicology in 52 poisoned families and 52 comparison families. Pediatrics 1968;42:312.
9. Angle CR, McIntire MS, Meile RL. Neurologic sequelae of poisoning in children. J Pediatr 1968;73:531.
10. Stewart MA, Thach BT, Freidin MR. Accidental poisoning and the hyperactive child syndrome. Dis Nerv Syst 1970;31:403.
11. Krall V. Personality characteristics of accident-repeating children. J Abnorm Soc Psychol 1953;48:99.
12. Mellinger GD, Manheimer DI. An exposure-coping model of accident liability among children. J Health Soc Behav 1967;8:96.
13. Bakwin H, Bakwin RM. Behavior disorders in children. Philadelphia: W. B. Saunders, 1972.
14. Matheny AP, Brown AM, Wilson RS. Behavioral antecedents of accidental injuries in early childhood: a study of twins. J Pediatr 1971;79:122.
15. Ackerman NW, Chidester I. Accidental self injury in children. Clin Pediatr 1936;53:711.
16. Shaw MTM. Accidental poisoning in children: A psychosocial study. NZ Med J 1977;85:269.
17. Brown GW, Davidson S. Social class, psychiatric disorder of mother, and accidents to children. Lancet 1978;1:378.
18. Klein D. Social influences on childhood accidents. Accident Anal Prevent 1980;12:275.
19. Langley MA, Silva PA, Williams S. A study of the relationship of ninety background, developmental, behavioral and medical factors to childhood accidents. Aust Paediatr J 1980;16:244.
20. Mannheimer DI, Mellinger GD. Personality characteristics of the child accident repeater. Child Dev 1961;38:491.
21. Bijur PE, Stewart-Brown S, Butler N. Child behavior and accidental injury in 11,966 preschool children. Am J Dis Child 1986;140.
22. Nyman G, Nyman M, Huttunen MO. Measurement of infant behavior and temperament: the Helsinki Longitudinal Study. Psychiat Fenn 1982;47.
23. Thomas A, Chess S, Birch HG, Korn S. Behavioral individuality in early childhood. New York: New York University Press, 1963.

24. Carey WB. A simplified method for measuring infant temperament. J Pediatr 1970;77:188.
25. Huttunen MO, Nyman G. On the continuity, change and clinical value of infant temperament in a prospective epidemiological study. In: Temperamental differences in infants and young children. Ciba Foundation Symposium 89. London: Pitman, 1982.
26. Tarrants WE. The measurement of safety performance. New York: Garland, 1980.

22

Psychiatric Hospitalization of Preschool Children: Admission Factors and Discharge Implications

Richard Dalton, Marc A. Forman, George C. Daul, and Dorothy Bolding

Tulane University School of Medicine and New Orleans Adolescent Hospital, New Orleans, Louisiana

The psychiatric hospitalization of 18 preschool children is examined. Behavioral, diagnostic, developmental, family, and community factors contributing to the admissions are reviewed and discussed. Implications for treatment and discharge planning are noted.

The treatment of psychiatrically disturbed preschool children has been a focus of child psychiatry for many years. Therapists have addressed issues of play therapy, parent counseling, and behavior management as they relate to this population (Brody, 1980; Walder, 1933; Wolpe, 1973). Much has been written about the issues of attachment and separation in the psychological development of the very young child (Bowlby, 1958; Fraiberg, 1969; Mahler et al., 1965). Recently, the occurrence of depression in preschool children has been studied (Earls, 1982; Kashani et al., 1984; Kashani and Ray, 1983). Curiously little, however, has been written about the psychiatric hospitalization of this population. Buffet-Arinal and Mazet (1982) discussed the role of psychiatric hospitalization for preschool patients. They described how children transfer to staff members their feelings about their own family

The authors wish to acknowledge the Department of Health and Human Resources of Louisiana for its support of this study.

members and situations. They concluded that such a hospitalization could be successful if it repairs, at a vital time in the child's development, an impaired level of functioning and relating that would otherwise contribute significantly to subsequent psychopathology. Although some investigators have examined the day-hospital treatment for psychiatrically disturbed preschool children (Richer et al., 1974) and others the issues of outpatient therapy (Beitchman et al., 1981; Feldman et al., 1974; Havelkova, 1968; Mahler et al., 1965), no researchers have directly addressed the issues involved in the psychiatric hospitalization of preschool children. That this is an underinvestigated group is seen in the statistic that 1,000 preschoolers were hospitalized in 1975 in private and public psychiatric facilities. The admission rate was 3 per each 100,000 preschool children in the U. S. (Sowder et al., 1981).

This report examines the developmental, family, and community factors that contribute to the hospitalization of preschool children. Information regarding symptom presentation, diagnosis, family situation, and demographic considerations about 18 preschool psychiatric inpatients is presented. Implications for discharge planning and the appropriateness of psychiatric hospitalization for preschool children are discussed.

METHOD

All of the preschool children ($N = 18$) who were admitted to either New Orleans Adolescent Hospital (a state facility for children and adolescents) or the Tulane University Hospital Children's Neuropsychiatric Unit during a period from August 1982 through May 1985 comprise the study population. Two patients (P and Q) were admitted to Tulane University Hospital after they were referred by family physicians. The remainder were referred to New Orleans Adolescent Hospital by special multidisciplinary, interagency, regional panels that review all requests for state-subsidized hospitalization in Louisiana. These panels, comprising physicians, psychologists, social workers, and educators, review outpatient psychiatric and medical examinations and psychological testing and make recommendations for the level of care (hospitalization, group home, foster care, outpatient therapy, and so forth) most appropriate for the patient.

The patients were diagnosed via structured interviews by the unit child psychiatrist. The patients' mothers were diagnosed by the unit child psychiatrist or, in four cases (G, H, M, N), by their treating psychiatrists. We were not able to ascertain systematic, baseline data regarding all 18 patients' behaviors because, in five cases (F, G, J, K, M), there was no one who could provide reliable data at the time of admission. Structured, baseline data regarding family functioning of all of the patients was not gathered because five children (E, G, J, M, N) had lived outside of the family home for at least 1 year. Furthermore, four patients (G, H, I, N) had been permanently removed from parental custody.

Developmental scales (Developmental Profile II, Vineland Adaptive Scales) were used to assess each child's self-help, social, and communication skills and to monitor his or her progress in these areas during the hospitalization. The socioeconomic status of each family was determined according to Hollingshead and Redlich (1958). A compilation of symptomatic behaviors either presented in the history or observed in the hospital is shown in Table 1. Diagnoses and demographic data are presented in Table 2.

RESULTS

The major presenting complaints and observed behaviors are listed in Table 1. These patients' symptoms are not unlike those found by Beitchman et al. (1981) in a preschool outpatient population. Hyperactivity (found in 47% of their patients), aggression (36%), tantrums (37%), language delays (32%), short attention span (21%), and destructiveness (17%) were primary presenting complaints described in their study. Each of these symptoms, in addition to several other symptoms not mentioned by Beitchman, occurred in a high percentage of our patients, apparently reflecting the level of disorganization within the inpatient group.

There were basically two groups of preschool children who were hospitalized, as shown in Table 2. The first group, comprising the four children who suffer with autism (A, B, C, D), were hospitalized for comprehensive diagnostic evaluations and subsequent treatment planning. Community resources were lacking and thorough outpatient evaluations were not obtained. These patients came from families who were not socially isolated and who were able to advocate for their children.

The second group of 14 patients had several common findings. In 9 of 14 cases the following tetrad was present: the mothers suffered with major psychiatric disorders, the fathers were not living in the homes, alternative placements (foster homes and other family homes) before hospitalization were unsuccessful in containing the children's behaviors, and the children suffered with conduct disorder. In two of the remaining cases, the only part of the tetrad that was missing was that prehospital, alternative placements had not been tried. In two other cases, the fathers lived within the homes but the other parts of the tetrad were present.

Although behaviors of all of the nonautistic patents fit the DSM-III criteria for conduct disorder, several diagnostic clusters were apparent within the group. Four patients were depressed. Each presented with an observable

Table 1. Observed Symptomatic Behaviors

Patients	A	B	C	D	E	F	G	H	I	J	K	L	M	N	O	P	Q	R	Total No.	%
Short attention span	X	X	X	X	X	X	X	X	X	X			X	X	X	X	X	X	16	89
Aggression	X	X			X	X	X	X	X	X	X	X	X	X	X		X	X	15	83
Temper trantrums	X	X	X		X	X	X	X	X	X	X	X	X		X	X		X	15	83
Destructiveness					X	X	X	X	X		X	X	X	X	X			X	11	61
Impulsivity	X	X	X	X		X	X		X	X						X	X		10	56
Unpredictable mood shifts	X	X	X	X		X	X				X	X	X					X	10	56
Hyperactivity	X	X	X	X			X		X	X						X	X		9	50
Language delays	X	X	X	X					X	X			X	X	X	X	X		8	44
Self-destructive acts						X	X		X		X	X	X	X				X	7	39
Enuresis	X	X		X	X	X	X	X	X										7	39
Sleep distrubance					X	X	X	X								X	X		6	33
Dysphoric mood					X	X		X	X						X				5	28
Fire setting					X	X						X							4	22
Encopresis			X				X		X				X					X	4	22
Psychomotor retardation					X			X							X				4	22
Auditory hallucations							X		X										2	11

Table 2. Demographic Data and Diagnoses

Patients	A	B	C	D	E	F	G	H	I	J	K	L	M	N	O	P	Q	R
Age at admission	4	5.5	4.5	5.5	5	3.5	3.5	4	4.5	4.5	5	4.5	5	4.5	5	5	4.5	4
Sex	M	F	F	M	M	M	F	M	M	M	F	M	F	M	M	M	M	M
Race	B	B	W	B	W	W	W	W	W	B	W	B	W	W	B	W	W	B
Socioeconomic status	4	4	3	5	4	5	N/A	N/A	N/A	5	4	4	5	N/A	5	3	4	5
Intelligence	30+	50	50+	30+	115	75	72	100	100	50	80+	80+	50	70+	72	70+	70+	80+
Previous placement		X			X	X	X	X	X	X	X		X	X				X
Father not in home				X	X	X	X		X	X	X	X	X					
Mother with major psychiatric disorder					X	X	X	X	X	X	X	X	X					X
History of seizures	X									X	X	X				X		
Abuse/neglect					X	X	X	X	X	X	X	X		X	X		X	X
Patient in state custody				X	X	X	X	X	X	X	X			X	X			
Length of hospitalization (days)	230	500	200	120	270	870	630	500	a	520	370	a	440	360	a	120	80	a
Conduct disorder					X	X		X	X	X	X	X		X	X	X	X	X
Major affective disorder					X	X		X							X			
Borderline personality										X	X	X	X					X
Attention deficit disorder																X	X	
Mental retardation moderate-severe	X	X	X	X									X					
Autism	X	X	X	X														
Schizophrenia							X		X									

a Patient still hospitalized.

dysphoric affect, sleep problems, psychomotor retardation, oppositional behavior, and appetite changes. The four children with borderline features exhibited unpredictable aggression toward themselves and others: K impulsively pulled out handfuls of hair, L endangered himself with fires, M gouged her eyes and banged her head, and R aggressively attacked peers. Three patients had attention deficit disorders. Although several patients presented with impulsivity, hyperactivity, and short attention spans, this diagnosis was limited to three patients because these symptoms in other patients were due to other illnesses. Both schizophrenic patients were distinguished by the presence of auditory hallucinations.

Within these families, maternal illnesses included: schizophrenia ($N = 6$), major affective disorder-depression ($N = 3$), borderline personality disorder ($N = 4$), and mental retardation ($N = 2$). Most of the families of the nonautistic patients were socially isolated, and extended family members were either not available or not able to help significantly. The 11 alternative, prehospital placements (3 with grandmothers, 7 in foster care, 1 in a group home) were unsuccessful because of a lack of support and supervised training with such disturbed children for the surrogate parents.

Case Reports

Case 1. B, a 5-year-old black girl, was admitted to New Orleans Adolescent Hospital with an extensive history of language and developmental delays, short attention span, hyperactivity, and aggression. The patient's mother felt that she had never had a warm relationship with her daughter, who preferred stuffed animals to people. At 17 months of age the patient began to use the word "mama" but did not progress beyond that. She demonstrated untoward anxiety and aggression in the face of change and was frequently echolalic and perseverative. The patient was taken to a series of doctors and finally to a mental health center in her community. Diagnoses ranged from severe anxiety to schizophrenia. Treatment planning included psychotropic medication and day care. When the patient's mother was not satisfied with her daughter's course, she was referred for hospitalization. The child was admitted; after extensive testing a diagnosis of autism was made and structured therapy was begun. The patient's discharge from the hospital was delayed by several months because of the difficulty in arranging for appropriate language, educational, and behavioral therapy on an outpatient basis.

Case 2. I, a 4½-year-old white boy, was admitted to New Orleans Adolescent Hospital in transfer from a residential facility where he had been previously admitted because of aggressive behavior, temper tantrums that could not be controlled, continual encopresis, short attention span, and destructive behavior. The patient had been abused before his placement in the residential facility and had witnessed the abuse of his mother by a series of live-in friends. The patient's mother suffered with a serious substance abuse disorder as well as a borderline personality disorder. She was unable to place limits on her son and was also unable to provide the consistent warmth and nurturance that he needed. The patient's mother had very few social supports and the family had had no contact with the patient's father for several years. When the patient's destructiveness escalated to the point that his mother responded with physical abuse, the state intervened, took custody, and placed the patient in a local residential facility.

After several months of out-of-control behavior in that facility the patient was transferred to the hospital. It quickly became obvious that this neurologically competent patient was totally unable to repress primary process thinking. He frequently suffered with auditory hallucinations. For months he insisted that he was riding on a fire truck with his pet dog and that the unit staff were "people on the street" watching as the truck passed. At times he became agitated, shouting at imaginary characters; at other times the agitation led to disorganized, destructive behavior. He was treated 5 times per week with alliance-building psychotherapy, a consistent milieu therapy program, and pharmacotherapy. Because of severe extrapyramidal side effects, various antipsychotic and antocholinergic medicines were tried. When the severe dystonic reactions did not remit, continual use of the neuroleptics was stopped. The medicines were then used on a short-term basis to manage the patient's acutely destructive episodes.

After several months, as the patient formed relationships in therapy and on the unit, he became more organized and able to participate in social discourse. Play therapy themes underscored his desire for closeness and fear of engulfment. In spite of improvements, the hallucinations continued intermittently. After 2 years the patient remains in the hospital because a suitable placement cannot be found.

DISCUSSION

This population ($N = 18$) represents the preschool children who were psychiatrically hospitalized in Louisiana during the previously noted period. The regional panels reviewed all of the requests for hospitalization in the public sector and referred the appropriate candidates to New Orleans Adolescent Hospital. Furthermore, Tulane University Hospital was the only private facility in Louisiana that admitted preschoolers during the period of the study.

The data reflect the fact that most of the preschoolers were hospitalized because their severe symptoms could be neither contained nor successfully treated within their disturbed and unsupported family settings and they were not able to be managed in less restrictive, out-of-home settings. In short, there were no other options. These data also reflect the view that serious maternal psychopathology and family chaos are associated with psychopathology within young children (Richman, 1976; Rutter, 1966; Wolff, 1961).

During hospitalization each nonautistic child sought a primary relationship and once this relationship was established, the presenting symptoms began to remit. No child's self-help, social, and communication skills began to improve until a relationship had been established.

The four hospitalized, autistic children do not represent all of the autistic, preschool children in Louisiana. Most of these children respond to educational and outpatient therapeutic approaches. These four patients were hospitalized because of the severity of their symptoms and because each diagnosis was not obvious but was made after extensive testing and observation. Each child responded positively to the hospitalization with a diminution of the presenting symptoms.

Whether the identified diagnostic clusters within the nonautistic group have predictive value remains to be seen. Most of the children (except P and Q) demonstrated very regressed, unrealistic behavior in response to stress at some point in their hospitalization. This is not unusual for children their age. The presence of auditory hallucinations is a pernicious sign at any age, however, and those two patients' (G, I) symptoms met the DSM-III criteria for schizophrenia. The patients with borderline personality features were not unlike the "symbiotic" children described by Mahler (1955). They established relationships on the unit and acted out attachment and separation themes in therapy. They were certainly more organized than the schizophrenic patients. Their self-destructive tendencies, however, exceeded what one expects from children who suffer with conduct disorder alone. Some might diagnose these four children (K, L, M, R) as suffering with children onset pervasive developmental disorder. The children with attention deficit disorder, treated with stimulant medication and consistent milieu therapy, were more able to integrate their positive experiences and decrease negative behaviors than the other patients. Three of the depressed patients (E, F, H) developed symptoms when children with whom they had formed an alliance were discharged. Their dysphoria was unmistakable. The symptoms remitted without medication 3 to 7 weeks after they developed. Each had been given by his mother to his maternal grandmother early in life. This then became a nidus of conflict between each mother and grandmother. One mother suffered with schizophrenia, one seriously abused alcohol, and one was in prison. The other patient (O) became depressed when told he would be returning home. His mother suffered with schizophrenia and was emotionally withdrawn.

The fact that hospitalization was the only option for these children (because of the severity of their symptoms and the limited family and community resources) had serious implications for discharge planning. The average length of stay for the 10 nonautistic, discharged children was 410 days. The discharges for all but two of these patients (E, Q) were each delayed by at least 60 days because suitable posthospital placements could not be found. Residential facilities and community agencies, in a state beset with economic problems and social service cutbacks, were reluctant to accept these patients who had previously failed in out-of-hospital settings into their programs. Further complicating the picture was the treatment team's ambivalence about the patients' discharge criteria. As each patient became more organized and as the goals set in the treatment plan were approximated, discharge became a consideration. This created a conflict within the team. Some thought that because the symptoms had remitted and the child was developmentally on track, it was time for the child to be moved to a less restrictive setting. Others thought that the disruption of the primary relationship at such an important point during the patient's development would create another loss and would ultimately be destructive. This underscores the major problem with the hospitalization of this population. The remission of psychiatric symptoms is dependent on, among other things, the development of a primary relationship, but the time required to develop a stable, ongoing, primary relationship with an adult is often too extensive for contemporary hospital resources. These conflicts, plus the unavailability of less restrictive, out-of-home, postdischarge placements, complicate the discharge process.

These lengths of stay and delays of discharge have special meaning for this population because it is in these early, formative years when the issues of attachment to, and separation from, the primary caregivers play such an important role in personality development (Bowlby, 1958; Fraiberg, 1969; Mahler et al., 1965). Our experience shows that when a preschool child is psychiatrically hospitalized the unit on which the child is treated must provide for the child's normal developmental needs in addition to the special, psychiatric needs that initially prompted the admission. The treatment setting requires a carefully designed milieu and structured program that includes a primary caregiving system that fosters the development of a special and primary relationship between the patient and a staff member.

Because of the needs of these patients and the conflicts around issues of discharge, the optimal treatment setting, in our opinion, is a small group home for this age group, which is managed by house parents and which offers psychiatric care. Such units are expensive, however, and the present economic climate makes their development unlikely. Psychiatric admissions of very disturbed preschoolers to hospitals will probably continue. For those preschool children who are admitted, four factors are necessary for a successful hospitalization and discharge: (*1*) a special program specifically designed to meet both the child's developmental and psychiatric needs is essential; (*2*) the hospital must be prepared for an extended hospitalization, and plans for discharge must be based on both the resolution of the psychiatric symptoms and the state of the child's special relationship; (*3*) the posthospital placement must adequately meet the child's special relationship needs and psychiatric needs; and (*4*) the implementation of the discharge plan must take into account the time required for adequate separation from the hospital.

REFERENCES

Beitchman, J., Murray, C. & Minty, G. (1981), A survey of referral problems to a psychiatric preschool program: patient characteristics and therapeutic considerations. *Canad. J. Psychiat., 26:323–328.*

Bowlby, J. (1958). The nature of the child's tie to mother. *Int. J. Psychoanal.,* 39:350–373.

Brody, J. P. (1980), Behavior therapy. In: *Comprehensive Textbook of Psychiatry,* ed. H. Kaplan, A. Freedman & J. Sadock. Baltimore: Williams & Wilkins, p. 2143.

Buffet-Arinal, Y. & Mazet, P. (1982), Psychopathologie du premier age-l'experience d'hospitalisation dans une Unité de Soins psychiatriques pour jeune enfant. *Neuropsychiat. Enfance Adolesc.,* 30:219–223.

Earls, F. (1982), Application of DSM-III in an epidemiological study of preschool children. *Amer. J. Psychiat.,* 139:242–243.

Feldman, R., Solomon, M., Levinson, E. & Lasry, J. (1974). Treatment of the seriously disturbed preschool child. *Canad. Psychiat. Assn. J.,* 19:127–128.

Fraiberg, S. (1969), Libidinal object constancy and mental representation. In: *The Psychoanalytic Study of the Child,* Vol 14. New York: International Universities Press.

Havelkova, M. (1968), Psychiatry and the pre-school age child. *Canad. Psychiat. Assn. J.,* 13:327–334.

Hollingshead, A. B. and Redlich, F. C. (1958), *Social Class and Mental Illness.* New York: Wiley.

Kashani, J. H. & Ray, J. S. (1983), Depression related symptoms among preschool-age children. *Child Psychiat. Hum. Developm. 13:233–238.*

———— ———— & Carlson, G. A. (1984), Depression and depressive-like states in preschool-age children in a child development unit. *Amer. J. Psychiat.,* 141:1397–1402.

Mahler, M. & Gosliner, B. (1955), On symbiotic child psychosis: genetic, dynamic, and restitutive aspects. In: *Selected Papers of Margaret S. Mahler,* New York: Jason Aronson.

_____ Pine, F., & Bergman, A. (1965), *The Psychological Birth of the Infant.* New York: Basic Books.

Richer, S., Lecompte, F., Collerette, J., Fouchard, D. & LeClerc, P. (1974), La maternelle therapeutique: philosophie de traitment. *Rev. Neuropsychiat. Infant. Hyg. Ment. Enfance* 22:335–350.

Richman, N. (1976), Depression in mothers of preschool children. *J. Child Psychol. Psychiat.,* 17:75–78.

Rutter, M. (1966), *Children of Sick Parents.* [Maudsley Monograph]. London: Oxford University Press.

Sowder, B., Burt, M., Rosenstein, M. & Milazzo-Sayre, L. (1981), *Use of psychiatric facilities by children and youth, United States, 1975.* (U. S. Department of Health and Human Resources No. (ADM) 81–1142). Washington, D. C.: U. S. Government Printing Office.

Walder, R. (1933), Psychoanalytic theory of play. *Psychoanal. Quart.,* 2:208–224.

Wolff, S. (1961), Social and family background of preschool children attending a child guidance clinic. *J. Child Psychol. Psychiat.,* 2:260–268.

Wolpe, J. (1973), *The Practice of Behavior Therapy,* Ed. 2. New York: Pergamon.

PART VI: CLINICAL ISSUES

23

Multidisciplinary Evaluation of Preschool Children and Its Demography in a Military Psychiatric Clinic

Bernard J. Lee

Tripler Army Medical Center, Honolulu, Hawaii

This report presents the methods and results of psychiatric evaluation in a military psychiatric clinic of preschool children by a multidisciplinary team consisting of a child psychiatrist, a developmental pediatrician, a speech pathologist, an occupational therapist, and a social worker. Five or six children were evaluated in three weekly sessions. A cluster of symptoms concerning behavior problems was most frequently reported by the parents. About 40% of the children had developmental disorders. Most of the children evaluated needed only brief intervention. Seventy-five percent were seen in fewer than 10 sessions and half of the children had improved at the time of closing.

In order to meet the increasing demand of preschool children referrals to the Child and Adolescent Psychiatry Service, Tripler Army Medical Center, Hawaii, we opened a multidisciplinary diagnostic team clinic, the Child Study Group (CSG). This report presents the composition, function, schedule, evaluation method, and results of the CSG.

Reprinted with permission from the *Journal of the American Academy of Child and Adolescent Psychiatry,* 1987, Vol. 26, No. 3, 313–316. Copyright 1987 by the American Academy of Child and Adolescent Psychiatry.

The opinions and assertions contained herein are the private views of the author and are not to be construed as official or as reflecting the views of the Department of the Army or the Department of Defense.

CHILD STUDY GROUP

The CSG evaluates all children, ages 5 and under, who are referred to the child psychiatric service. This clinic is free to all eligible dependents of active duty and retired military personnel living in Hawaii. The clinic is scheduled weekly, three mornings every month. The evaluation team consists of a child psychiatrist, a developmental pediatrician, a speech pathologist, an occupational therapist, and a social worker. A first-year child psychiatry fellow is assigned to the clinic for a 6-month period. A PGY-III psychiatric resident also participates. The children are divided into two groups, ages 4 and 5, and age 3 and younger, with five or six children in each group. Once a child is referred to the CSG, he or she is assigned to a child psychiatrist, a child psychiatry fellow, or a PGY-III resident under staff supervision, who becomes the primary physician responsible for parent interview, chart keeping, and follow-up.

The evaluation begins with a history-taking interview with one or both parents. After the initial interview, the child is scheduled for the appropriate age group while the parents are scheduled in a group setting with a social worker to discuss child-rearing practices and problems. Before the CSG begins, the team meets briefly to discuss the cases scheduled.

The evaluation begins in the waiting room with observation of child-parent interaction and the separation process. Once the children are introduced to each other and to the staff, we observe how they cope with strange situations and mingle with each other. The children start to play or draw pictures. The team members intermingle and start formal evaluation of the children. The developmental pediatrician gives developmental tests, usually the McCarthy Screening Test (adapted from McCarthy Scales of Children's Ability), the Gesell Developmental Test, or a combination of these. The occupational therapist tests for gross and fine motor coordination by using parts of the Denver Developmental Screening Test, Erhardt Test for Prehension Skill, Peabody Motor Development Test, and the Child Observation by Jean Ayres. The speech pathologist listens to the children and, if appropriate, selects a child for speech evaluation using Zimmermen's Preschool Language Skill, Peabody Picture Vocabulary Test, Arizona Articulation Proficiency Scale, or Sequence Inventory of Communication Development. The child psychiatrist observes and participates in the children's activities. The child psychiatry fellow or the PGY-III resident may observe and give some diagnostic tests. The social worker conducts the parents' group in another room during the time the children are being evaluated in the playroom. In this way all team members assume the roles of observer, participant, evaluator, and therapist.

After 40 minutes, juice and cookies are served and the child can engage in a lively discussion. Each session lasts 1 hour.

Through these three sessions we familiarize ourselves with every child in the group in the areas of motor development, language development, adaptive and cognitive development, social behavior, and the emotional aspect of personality development. After each session, team members gather to synthesize the information each has gathered. At the end of the third session, each child is discussed by the team members to formulate diagnoses according to DSM-III and offer recommendations, depending upon the needs of each child. Parents are usually seen again a week later for a feedback session, at which time the results of the CSG evaluation are shared with them.

DEMOGRAPHY

From January through December 1984, 129 preschool children were referred to the CSG clinic. The following report is the demographic study of the CSG during that period.

Population and Clinic Setting

The Tripler Child and Adolescent Psychiatry Service is located in Honolulu, Hawaii and is responsible for the psychiatric care of all military dependents in Hawaii under age 18. The total population of active-duty dependents under age 18 is 38,793; 19,837 are male and 18,956 are female. Each branch of service is represented in the following manner: Army 34%, Navy 34%, Air Force 17%, Marine Corps 14%, and Coast Guard 1%. Officers' children represent about 20% and enlisted children 80% (U. S. Army Health Services Command, 1984).

Data Collection

Data for this study were obtained from an Intake Form filled out by the parents before the initial interview, psychiatric evaluation notes from the CSG, and the closing summary sheet in the chart. All patients referred to the CSG between January and December 1984 were included in the study. The total number of children referred was 129, which represented 20% of the entire child psychiatric referrals (641 patients).

The variables in this study included age; sex; sponsor's branch of service and rank; the number of months the family had been living in Hawaii;

whether the child lives with the natural parents, stepparents, or others; referral sources; presenting problems; precipitating event; diagnoses; recommendations; number of sessions seen in the clinic; reason for closing; and condition of patient at closing.

RESULTS

Age and Sex

Of the total child psychiatric clinic population, 20% were preschool children. School-age children represented 53% and adolescents 27%. The age and sex distribution of the CSG population is shown in Figure 1. Among the preschool referrals, 60% were boys and 40% were girls (1.5:1 ratio). This sex distribution was similar to the latency age group, whereas the adolescents had an equal number of boys and girls. There were only three referrals in the 1- to 2-year age group and all three were boys.

Rank and Branch of Service of the Sponsor

The referrals, according to branch of service, were Army 51%, Navy 29%, Air Force 13%, Marine Corps 5%, and Coast Guard 2%. This overrepresen-

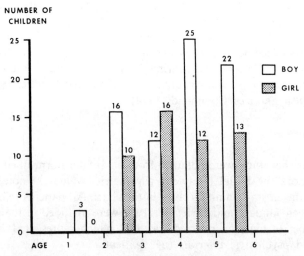

Figure 1. Age and sex distribution of Child Study Group population.

tation of the Army is probably due to more communication with the Army Pediatric Clinic. Eighty-eight percent of the patients evaluated in the CSG were children of enlisted parents, and 12% were children of officers. The distribution of rank was Specialist 4 and under (20%), Sergeant and Staff Sergeant (68%), Sergeant First Class and above (6%), and officers (12%).

Status of Parents

Among the many variables of family constellation, only one variable was evaluated in the study: whether the child referred was living with natural parents, stepparents, or other. Seventy-five percent of the children were living with both natural mother and father. The stepfamily constituted 12%, and 10% were living with a single, enlisted, active-duty mother.

Referral Sources

About 54% of all referrals were initiated by medical services, including pediatric clinic, speech pathology, and family practice. Thirty percent of the referrals were initiated by parents who contacted the clinic directly, and 8% were referred from school. It is important to note that about 6% of the children were referred by a parent's psychiatrist with concerns about the child's mental health or disciplinary problems or both. Three percent of the children were referred from Child Protective Services or related agencies.

Presenting Problems

Presenting problems in order of frequency are shown in Table 1. A cluster of symptoms concerning behavior problems was most frequently reported by the parents. In all of these items (difficult to manage, temper tantrums, hyperactive, aggressive, stubborn, poor relationships with peers and siblings, and school-behavior problems), boys outnumbered the girls about twice in frequency.

The only item that occurred more frequently in girls was "sad, unhappy mood, or depressed." Delayed speech development and "child not talking" were presented in 20% of the children with an equal number of boys and girls represented.

Some items were presented less frequently than expected, including sleeping problems, eating problems, fear, phobia, worries, anxiety, and somatic complaints (Earles, 1980). A few presenting problems not listed in

Table 1. Frequency of Presenting Problems Reported by Parents

Behavior Items	Boys (N = 78)	Girls (N = 51)	Total (N = 129)
Difficult to manage/control	35	20	55
Temper tantrums	21	9	30
Overactive/hyperactive	17	8	25
Aggressive/destructive	17	7	24
Sad/unhappy mood/depressed	8	12	20
Oppositional/stubborn	11	8	19
Delayed speech development	9	10	19
Enuresis	7	6	13
Poor relationships with peers/sibs	7	3	10
School behavior problems	7	3	10
Not talking	4	5	9
Sleeping problems	6	3	9
Withdrawn/shy	6	2	8
Poor impulse control	6	0	6
Encopresis	5	1	6
Dependency/attention seeking	3	2	5
Eating problem	4	1	5
Pulling hair	2	2	4
Poor learning	2	2	4
Lies	3	1	4
Steals	2	0	2
Sexual play	3	0	3
Anxious/nervous	2	1	3
Phobia/fears	1	1	2
Somatic complaints	0	2	2
Cruel to animals	2	0	2

Table 1 occurred only once: head-banging, breath holding, threat to run away, fire setting, and bulimia.

Precipitating Event and/or Stresses in the Child's Life

In about 40% of the cases, the parents noted possible stressors in the child's life that might have precipitated the child's problem. Suspected child abuse and neglect (SCAN) and sexual abuse were noted in almost 10% of the children. Divorce of parents was cited in 7% of the cases and the father's absence in 5%. Other items cited as precipitating events were birth of sibling (6%), parental illness (4%), severe marital problems (4%), and moving to Hawaii (3%).

Diagnoses

The different diagnostic categories rendered at the end of the third CSG session are summarized in Table 2. Adjustment disorder of infancy and childhood was most frequently diagnosed (18 boys, 14 girls). Disruptive Behavior Disorder included Attention Deficit Disorder (12 boys, 0 girl), Oppositional Disorder (5 boys, 5 girls), and Conduct Disorder (4 boys, 0 girl). Almost an equal number of enuretic boys (6) and girls (5) was seen. Encopresis occurred more frequently in boys (5) than in girls (1). The Parent-Child Problems were reserved for the cases in which the child was free of psychiatric problems but the parents had parenting difficulties, including child abuse and neglect. Other diagnoses included Separation Anxiety Disorder (1 boy, 1 girl), Dysthymia (2 boys, 1 girl), Sleep Terror Disorder (3 boys, 1 girl), Elective Mutism (1 boy, 1 girl), Bulimia (1 girl), and Post-traumatic Stress Disorder (1 girl). A relatively large number of children with Trichotillomania was diagnosed (2 boys, 2 girls).

About 40% of the children had developmental disorders and received Axis II diagnoses. Specific Developmental Disorders included Speech and Language Disorder (8 boys, 7 girls), Academic Skill Disorder (3 boys), and Motor Skill Disorder (2 boys). Global Developmental Delay was diagnosed when there were delays in more than one area of development. Mental Retardation was included in this group. One quite unexpected finding was that a large number of children had Pervasive Developmental Disorder. Eleven children were diagnosed with either having Autistic Disorder (1 boy, 4 girls) or Atypical Pervasive Developmental Disorder (3 boys, 3 girls). The

Table 2. Summary of Diagnoses

	%
Adjustment Disorder of Infancy and Childhood	35
Disruptive Behavior Disorder	25
Disorder of Elimination	15
Specific Developmental Disorder	18
Global Developmental Delay	13
Pervasive Developmental Disorder	10
Parent-Child Problems	10
Other	16

Pervasive Developmental Disorder is reported as three times more common in boys than in girls and more frequent in the upper socioeconomic class (DSM-III), but in our group seven were girls. However, three of 15 officers' children were autistic.

Recommendations

Parent counseling was recommended in 50% of the cases evaluated, individual psychotherapy in 20%, and preschool group therapy in 15%. Psychopharmacotherapy was recommended in about 10% of the cases. Nine children were given Ritalin. Two patients with severe nightmares were given Valium, and one child with autistic disorder was tried on Mellaril. About 20% of the patients were referred to the Department of Education for further evaluation and proper class placement. About 10% were referred to other departments, including Pediatrics, Occupational Therapy, and Speech Pathology, and another 10% to other treatment facilities outside the hospital.

Number of Sessions in the Clinic

Fourteen percent of referrals were never seen in evaluation. About 50% of the children were seen in one to six sessions, which was the basic evaluation time. Thirteen percent required an additional three to five sessions, whereas 16% needed six to 15 sessions, and 6% needed 16 to 50 additional sessions. Children who required more than seven sessions were seen for various types of therapy, including parent counseling, individual or group therapy, or psychopharmacotherapy. One child was seen in more than 80 sessions for twice weekly psychotherapy.

Closing a Case

The reasons for closing a case were failure to keep evaluation appointment (14%), failure to keep follow-up appointment (20%), moving from Hawaii (20%), referral to other agencies (10%), and improvement of condition (25%). There were 11 patients still in weekly therapy at the time of this study (December 1985).

Condition of Patient at Closing

About half of the patients were improved and the other half were either unchanged or their condition was unknown at the time of closing. Only two cases were reported as "condition worse." Both children were diagnosed as having Attention Deficit Disorder and Conduct Disorder and were referred for hospitalization.

DISCUSSION

This presentation of psychiatric evaluation and demographic study of preschool children in a military child psychiatry clinic is unique—no similar report is available for comparison. The first 5 years of life are universally accepted to be of profound importance to human emotional development. Yet less psychiatric intervention occurs in this period (Kirz, 1980) than in any other. Evaluating preschool children and their parents in group settings by a multidisciplinary team was not only time-saving but also effective as a vehicle for the evaluation process and intervention. In our experience, developmental, occupational, and speech evaluations were an important part of the psychiatric evaluation of preschool children because 40% of the children evaluated had developmental disorders.

The multidisciplinary team approach also provided a rich learning experience for the child psychiatry fellows by their active participation in the evaluation processes performed by the different specialists.

The other advantages of seeing children in a group setting were shortening of waiting period and the therapeutic value of the evaluation process. Most of the children referred to the CSG were seen in the group within a month's time. Most children evaluated in the CSG needed only brief intervention, and 75% were seen in fewer than 10 sessions. Fifty percent were reported as having improved at the time of closing.

Some questions were raised by reviewing the CSG evaluation process and demography of the children. The most frequently presented problem was the difficult to manage child. Possibly, this is related to the parents' occupation where military discipline might be extended to family life. The higher percentage of children with pervasive developmental disorder seen in the clinic and its preponderance of female over male was unexpected and unexplained.

SUMMARY

One rather unique way of evaluating preschool children has been presented together with a brief demographic study of these children seen at a military child psychiatric clinic during 1984. We found that evaluating preschool children and their parents in a group setting was not only possible but economical and effective. This is our first attempt to present the CSG. We hope to continue to work with preschoolers and share our results again in the future.

REFERENCES

Earles, F. (1980), Prevalence of behavior problems in three-year-old children. *Arch. Gen. Psychiat.* 37:1153–1157.
Kirz, R. H. (1980), The preschool child. *Psychiat. Clin. North Amer.,* 3:547–561.
U.S. Army Health Services Command (1984), Fiscal Year, 1984 Population Estimates. Fort Sam Houston, Texas 78234–6000.

24

Posttraumatic Stress Disorder in Children and Adolescents: A Review of the Literature

Judith A. Lyons

Veterans Administration Medical Center and Tufts University School of Medicine, Boston, Massachusetts

Recently, an extensive body of literature has begun to emerge regarding posttraumatic stress disorder (PTSD) among adults, particularly in combat veterans. Fewer studies of PTSD in children have been reported. However, there is growing recognition of the fact that discrete events can have a severe and lasting impact on children, and clinicians are becoming increasingly sensitive to the psychological needs of young survivors of traumatic events. Examples of this awareness are seen in the fact that clinical intervention programs were organized immediately for Concord, New Hampshire, schoolchildren after the televised loss of teacher Christa McAuliffe aboard the space shuttle Challenger in January 1986, and for children involved in the May 1986 hostage-taking and bombing at an elementary school in Cokeville, Wyoming.

The goal of the present paper is to address some of the central issues pertaining to PTSD in children and adolescents, using pertinent research and clinical reports for illustration. The paper is divided into sections on theory,

---

Reprinted with permission from *Developmental and Behavioral Pediatrics,* 1987, Vol. 8, No. 6, 349–356. Copyright 1987 by Williams & Wilkins Co.

This work was supported by a Veterans Administration Merit Review Award to Terence M. Keane, Ph.D. The views expressed in this paper are solely those of the author and do not necessarily reflect those of the Veterans Administration or Tufts University.

The author would like to thank Terence Keane, John Fairbank, Ollie McClendon, Danny Kaloupek, and Jessica Wolfe for their comments on an earlier draft of this manuscript.

diagnosis, age and sex differences, treatment, and future directions. Clinical issues regarding assessment and intervention are the primary focus.

THEORIES REGARDING POSTTRAUMATIC STRESS DISORDER

Two recent reviews of the theoretical literature regarding posttraumatic stress disorder (PTSD) are available. Terr[1] presents a historical review of our understanding of children's responses to trauma. She traces the literature from the basic framework set by Freud at the turn of the century, through the early retrospective psychoanalytic cases, to more recent studies on children's responses to war and natural disaster. A more general summary of the major theoretical models of PTSD is presented by Fairbank and Nicholson[2] in a paper on PTSD among Vietnam veterans.

Early psychodynamic formulations regarding trauma were primarily based on the concept of "energy overload," in which the individual's "stimulus barrier" became overwhelmed. More recent psychodynamic formulations have been based on the concept of "information overload." The contemporary models postulate that, because traumatic events are outside the realm of usual experience, the individual has no schemata to assimilate or accommodate the new information. The inability to process the event cognitively is said to create anxiety, which is further compounded by subjective interpretations of threat. Psychodynamic models (e.g., Horowitz[3]) generally propose a phasic response in which the individual alternates between (1) denial of the incongruous/incomprehensible situation—what Freud[4] referred to as the negative effects of trauma, and (2) intrusive reexperiencing of the vividly encapsulated traumatic imagery—what Freud referred to as positive effects. Both the early and the more recent psychodynamic models incorporate the idea that the impact of the trauma is related to the individual's developmental stage. Symptomatology is often discussed in terms of regression or disruption of psychosocial development.

Alternatively, the behavioral model commonly used in conceptualizing PTSD[5,6] is based on two-factor learning theory. The model incorporates both classical/Pavlovian and instrumental/operant conditioning theories. In classical conditioning, involuntary responses are elicited by inherently neutral stimuli (conditioned stimuli, CS) through the repeated pairing of the neutral stimuli with stimuli that naturally elicit the reflexive response (unconditioned stimuli, USC). The textbook example of this phenomenon is Pavlov's conditioning of salivary responses in dogs. By sounding a bell (CS) each time he gave meat (UCS) to the dogs, Pavlov developed a conditioned response in the dogs, such that they salivated whenever they heard the bell, even if no food was present. The behavioral model of PTSD postulates that similar classical conditioning takes place when an individual is traumatized. The individual is reflexively distressed by the threatening aspects of the traumatic event (UCS). Other inherently neutral cues (CS) present at the time of the trauma become classically conditioned such that they too come to elicit anxiety, even though they represent no inherent danger. Thus, if a girl is attacked in the woods by a middle-aged male stranger, she may become anxious whenever near any wooded areas or when approached by any middle-aged man (even a friend or relative), since these cues are now associated with the traumatic event.

The second of the behavioral theory's two factors incorporates instrumental/operant conditioning, in which the individual learns to voluntarily behave in such a way as to bring about a desired consequence. In PTSD, the desired consequence is usually relief from anxiety. The individual learns that avoidance of or escape from the trauma-associated cues (both UCS and CS) minimizes anxiety level. In the example above, the little girl might change her route to school to avoid going near any woods and might try to avoid contact with her father and uncles. Such actions take her away from trauma-related cues and thereby reduce her anxiety. Thus, according to the behavioral model, some symptoms (e.g., sleep disturbance, nightmares, startle response) are viewed as involuntary anxiety responses associated with the UCS/CS whereas other symptoms (e.g., behavioral avoidance, emotional numbing) are seen as instrumentally conditioned avoidance responses.

ASSESSMENT OF POSTTRAUMATIC STRESS DISORDER

The Diagnostic and Statistical Manual of Mental Disorders (DSM-III)[7] is based on a person/environment interaction model in which both an extreme situation and a symptom-laden response to that situation are required for an individual to be considered "traumatized." Thus, for example, not all child-snatching or abuse victims develop posttraumatic stress disorder (PTSD). Some percentage of such children develop no disorder, some develop something other than PTSD, and some develop PTSD.[8,9] Clarity in the literature has been greatly sacrificed by use of the term "traumatized" to describe any pathological response to an extreme event, a situation due in part to the fact that PTSD has been available as a diagnostic category only since 1980. Briefly summarized, the diagnostic criteria for PTSD include the following: (1) exposure to an event that could be traumatic, (2) intrusive reexperiencing of the trauma, (3) numbing of responsiveness to or reduced involvement with the external world, and (4) at least two of a variety of other symptoms, including hyperalertness/startle, sleep disturbance, survivor guilt, impaired memory/concentration, behavioral avoidance of trauma-related cues, and intensification of symptoms when exposed to trauma-related cues. The first two criteria (identification of a traumatic event, and intrusive reexperiencing) are most critical in making a differential diagnosis, and will be discussed in detail.

Identification of the Stressor

Individuals who have been traumatized generally present to a clinician in one of two ways. In some cases, the clinician is informed directly regarding the occurrence of a potentially traumatic event and is asked to assess and/or treat the physical/psychological sequelae of that event. In many other cases, however, the client is referred on the basis of physical/psychological symptoms, and no mention is made of traumatic events in the child's history. In such cases, the burden is on the clinician to uncover information regarding the traumatic event, so as to diagnose and treat the PTSD.

Identification of traumatic events thus requires that clinicians be alert for a possible history of trauma and that they, as a matter of course, enquire regarding reexperiencing of any unpleasant events. Routine use of questionnaires assessing stressful life events is advocated by some clinicians.[10]

There is controversy in the literature as to what constitutes a traumatic event.[11-14] DSM-III[7] stipulates that, to qualify as a traumatic event, the identified stressor must generally be "outside the range of such common experiences as simple bereavement, chronic illness." Terr[14] further clarifies that the experience is generally "surprising, unanticipated, and piercingly intense" and "must be real, not imagined." It is important to note, however, that it *is* possible for individuals to be traumatized by events at which they are not actually present. Generally, such cases of PTSD occur when an individual perceives a "near miss" or strongly identifies with an individual who did suffer loss or injury in the event. For example, Terr[1] describes the development of PTSD in a boy who was let off a schoolbus just before all the children aboard the bus were kidnapped. The boy's symptomatology was not as extensive or severe as that of the children who had actually been kidnapped, yet significant symptoms were still evident 4 years after the event. Similarly, individuals can be traumatized by acts they commit themselves, which violate their value system (as in the case of soldiers who have committed atrocities), or by events that they witness as a bystander, as well as by events that actually threaten their personal safety.

A number of factors often interact to impede detection of traumatic events. First, parents, teachers, and clinicians often deny or downplay the impact that distressing events have on children.[15,16] For example, Burke and colleagues[17] studied the effects of a disastrous blizzard and flood. They compared parental ratings of specific child behaviors reported after the event with ratings done by the parents prior to the disaster. Parents identified more behavior problems after the event. When asked their subjective impression of the impact the disaster had on their child, however, all parents denied that their child's behavior had been affected. Harrison et al[18] found a similar phenomenon when they examined staff perceptions of the impact of President Kennedy's assassination on children on an inpatient psychiatry unit. In spite of documented behavior changes, staff members generally reported that the children were unaffected by the event. Eth et al[19] suggest that such apparent insensitivity on the part of adults may stem from the adults' own conflicts regarding their inability to protect the child from the event that occurred.

A second factor that may cause the clinician and other adults to underestimate the incidence of traumatization in children is an inaccurate perception of the frequency with which potentially traumatizing events occur. For example, one survey has shown that 27% of women and 16% of men report having been sexually abused as a child,[20] and approximately 10% of murders[21] and rapes[22] are reportedly witnessed by a child. Thus, a large percentage of children experience events that could potentially lead to the development of PTSD. This, in fact, was the primary conclusion drawn in an elaborate 8-year follow-up study comparing the adjustment of abused children versus child accident victims versus matched control children.[23] Basically, the study found no group differences in functioning, not because the abuse and accident victims had fared so well, but because so many of the control children also had suffered traumatic events during the 8-year follow-up interval.

An additional complication in the assessment of PTSD is the fact that individual perception plays a critical role in determining whether or not a given event is traumatic.[24-26] In light of Yamamoto's[27] data suggesting a lack of convergence between the events children report as stressful and the events adults perceive as being stressful for children, it is important that clinicians not overlook the importance a *child* places on a given event. The fact that children often do not report traumatic events to anyone[20,28] contributes further to the potential for under-diagnosing PTSD.

Reexperiencing

In addition to having experienced an extreme stressor, in order to qualify for a DSM-III diagnosis of PTSD, an individual must repeatedly and intrusively reexperience the traumatic event through nightmares, recurrent and unbidden waking recall, and/or flashback experiences during which the individual actually acts or feels as if the event is recurring. Such reexperiencing is the hallmark symptom of PTSD, the core symptom that generally sets PTSD apart from other psychiatric disorders. The reexperiencing in PTSD usually recreates the traumatic event as it occurred, with little symbolic transformation. Thus, for example, it stands in stark contrast to the nightmares of children who fear fantasized monsters.[23]

It appears that children rarely experience the type of dissociative flashbacks that adults do.[14] Instead, children's reexperiencing more often takes the form of nightmares, volitional behavioral reenactment of the event, or posttraumatic play. In repeating the themes of the traumatic event in play or other daily behavior, children often strive to master the event. However, such counterphobic behavior can be very maladaptive, particularly if it causes individuals to place themselves in additional life-threatening situations.[14,29,30] Terr,[14] for example, cites the case of Leslie, a 7-year-old girl who was among the 26 children whose schoolbus was hijacked in Chowchilla, California, in 1976. The children were driven at gunpoint for hours, then buried alive for 16 hours. For years after the kidnapping, Leslie continued to dream of the event and she reenacted the experience repeatedly in play. Eventually, at age 10, Leslie ran away from home and began hitching rides from strangers. When later questioned, Leslie appeared oblivious to the seriousness of the risks she had taken and argued that hitchhiking was not like being kidnapped since, in hitchhiking, she persuaded people to take her where *she* wanted to go rather than being forced to go where she did *not* want to go.

Additional Criteria

The final two sets of criteria for diagnosing PTSD require that the individual show evidence of reduced responsiveness/involvement with the external world, and exhibit at least two of a variety of other symptoms such as hyperalertness/startle response, sleep disturbance, guilt, memory/concentration impairment, avoidance of traumatic cues, and increased symptomatology in the presence of traumatic cues. Careful historytaking is therefore necessary to contrast the child's pre- and posttrauma functioning.

DSM-III-R

The diagnostic criteria for PTSD are currently under revision.[31] The proposed changes, however, do not alter the basic symptoms which are viewed as differentiating PTSD from other disorders. Instead, the revisions are largely conceptual in focus, reorganizing the diagnostic criteria more coherently along the dimensions of intrusive reexperiencing, numbing/

avoidance, and increased arousal. The addition of a new symptom, "sense of a foreshortened future," has been proposed, based on work with children involved in the Chowchilla bus kidnapping.[1]

Differential Diagnosis

Other diagnoses which often closely resemble PTSD include adjustment disorder, major depression, and closed head injury. Krener[32] reviewed the cases of 22 treated incest victims and found that the most common diagnosis in the children's charts was adjustment disorder. By Krener's report, several of those patients actually met criteria for a diagnosis of PTSD, but had not been diagnosed as such. Similarly, cases diagnosed as major depressive disorder[33,34] may also meet PTSD criteria, with psychotic-like features reflecting reexperiencing of the event. A concurrent diagnosis of PTSD should be considered in many cases of closed head injury, as well. Symptoms that might otherwise be attributed to brain injury may, in fact, be related to the psychological trauma resulting from the auto crash,[35] child abuse,[36] or other event in which the child was injured.

"Contagion" or "secondary traumatization" is a phenomenon commonly reported in children. Rosenheck and Nathan[37] cite the case of a boy whose father had PTSD secondary to combat in Vietnam. Even though the boy had never experienced combat, he had witnessed his father's combat flashbacks and nightmares. The boy manifested numerous PTSD-like symptoms, including preoccupation with war games and combat fantasies. Terr[14] refers to a number of examples of such contagion of symptoms. The fact that children can display various PTSD-like symptoms without having personally experienced the traumatic event has important implications for diagnosis. In the cases cited by Rosenheck and Nathan[37] and Terr,[1,14] it was known which individuals had experienced the traumatic event and which had not. In some situations, that distinction might not be as clear. Rimsza and Niggemann,[38] for example, emphasize that assailants often sexually abuse more than one child, and that efforts should be made to identify friends and siblings who may also have been abused. However, awareness of the possibility that PTSD-like symptoms can be acquired through "contagion" makes it clear that a clinician cannot safely assume that a second child has been victimized simply because the second child exhibits PTSD-like symptomatology. (It is diagnostically important to note that, in the cases of "contagion" described above, none of the children claimed to have experienced the traumatic event.) Efforts must be made to distinguish true cases of PTSD in which children may be traumatized through identification with the actual trauma survivor even though they were not themselves present at the traumatic event versus cases in which various PTSD-like symptoms are acquired through contagion.

Multimethod Evaluation

Because differential diagnosis of PTSD can be difficult in cases such as those outlined above, a multimethod assessment procedure is recommended.[16,39,40] The child's self-report regarding the traumatic event and its sequelae, observation of the child's behavior, and information reported by collaterals (parents, teachers, etc.) can provide much of the information needed. Structured play, puppetry, story-telling, and art activities can facilitate young children's ability to express their thoughts and feelings. Archival information such as school records documenting past and present functioning can also be helpful. The development of standardized interviews and psychometric tests specifically for the assessment of PTSD in children may provide useful sources of diagnostic information in the future.

AGE DIFFERENCES IN VULNERABILITY TO POSTTRAUMATIC STRESS DISORDER

Apparently, there is no age at which individuals are immune to the effects of traumatic events. Reports on holocaust survivors show that even infants were affected by the experience,[41] and posttraumatic stress disorder (PTSD) symptoms have been reported in response to attacks by animals in children as young as 20–36 months old.[42,43] However, it appears that the effects of some types of events—such as the death of a significant other, or sexual abuse— may involve high levels of cognitive mediation such that very young children may lack the capacity to be traumatized by these events.[8,44,45] There is also evidence in the literature on combat veterans suggesting that, as individuals enter adulthood, they develop greater capacities to deal with stressful situations and therefore are less likely to be traumatized.[46] However, studies such as that of Ruch and Chandler[47] report greater symptomatology among adult assault victims than among children. Further research is needed to clarify whether or not individuals are especially vulnerable to the effects of specific types of events at specific ages.

AGE DIFFERENCES IN POSTTRAUMATIC STRESS DISORDER SYMPTOMATOLOGY

Theoretically, it has been suggested that the way in which posttraumatic stress disorder (PTSD) symptoms will be manifested depends in part on the developmental stage the individual is in at the time of the trauma.[48] Although some research indicates that symptomatology is relatively independent of age at traumatization,[1] other clinical reports support the hypothesis that symptomatology is linked to level of psychosocial development. For example, trauma victims of all ages report difficulty reestablishing trust after the event,[49] but children appear to be especially vulnerable to a collapse of both basic trust and autonomy.[14] Such results are consonant with an Eriksonian model of psychosocial stages,[50] according to which basic trust and autonomy would be expected to be less consolidated in young children than in adults. Similarly, traumatized adolescents have been described as having impaired identity formation as a result of disruption of their psychosocial development during the critical years when individual identity generally is established.[32,51,52]

Several studies have reported a fairly consistent pattern of additional age differences in symptomatology following potentially traumatic events, although it should be noted that the children studied were not formally diagnosed as having PTSD. Infants' responses were found to be characterized by irritability, sleep problems, diarrhea, and frequent illnesses.[53,54] High levels of dependency and separation anxiety, as well as irritability and sleep disturbance, were noted among preschool children.[51,53,54] Additionally, pre-school children were observed to reenact traumatic situations in their play.[51] Elementary school children began to show more of the behaviors typically associated with PTSD: nightmares, preoccupation with the traumatic event, complex reenactments of the event, appreciation of the irreversibility of the event, hyperarousal and hypervigilance, numbing of affect, vacillation between withdrawal/friendliness/aggressive outbursts, fears, and avoidance behaviors.[45,51,53,54] Somatization appears to be a less frequent response once children reach school age.[45] Adolescents were reported to become either very compliant and withdrawn, or aggressive, to abuse substances, and act out sexually.[45,51,55] Guilt was a more salient feature among adolescents than among younger trauma victims, and adolescents were often secretive about the traumatic event.[51,53,54]

Terr[1,14,56,57] has drawn a number of contrasts between PTSD symptoms in adults and children. Unlike many adults, children do not show evidence of psychogenic amnesia, or the same degree of numbing as do traumatized adults. Children often openly relive the traumatic event through thematic play and direct reenactment, as well as through dreams and waking intrusive recall. Flashbacks such as those often seen in adult PTSD patients are not common among children. Cognitive-perceptual distortions regarding the event, as evidenced particularly by skewed recall of the sequencing of events and a belief that unheeded omens warned of the coming trauma, are particularly characteristic of children. Many children report dreams in which they experience their own death, a phenomenon not generally seen among adult PTSD patients. It is also common for traumatized children to have a very limited view of themselves existing in the future and a consequent inability to make plans for their lives. Deterioration in job performance is often seen in adult PTSD, but reports are inconsistent as to whether children's school performance suffers following a traumatic experience.[1,14,17,32,51] The effect of stress on children's school achievement may vary as a function of IQ, with performance being impaired only in children with lower IQ scores.[58]

SEX DIFFERENCES IN SYMPTOMATOLOGY

The limited data that exist suggest that boys may show a more symptomatic response to potentially traumatic events than do girls. Burke et al[17] found that boys' anxiety scores increased from pre- to postdisaster, whereas girls' scores actually showed a decrease. Maternal reports collected by Jaffe et al[59] regarding children's reactions to the mother being beaten by her partner also indicate a more symptomatic response among boys. It should be noted, however, that neither of these studies actually focused on children diagnosed as having posttraumatic stress disorder.

TREATMENT OF POSTTRAUMATIC STRESS DISORDER

Convincing a family to obtain treatment for a traumatized child can represent a major clinical task in itself. Even when the child is seen for an initial evaluation (e.g., in an emergency room) and psychotherapy is recommended, many families fail to pursue treatment for the child.[1,32,60] It is important, therefore, to take the initiative in arranging treatment. Bringing therapy to the client by going to the school[19,61-63] is one way to increase the child's opportunity to receive treatment.

A number of treatment approaches are available for working with traumatized individuals, including behavioral deconditioning, hypnosis, play therapy, psychodynamic psychotherapy, group therapy, family therapy, and pharmacotherapy.[2,8,14,40,62,64-67] To date, no treatment outcome studies have been published which evaluate the relative efficacy of various treatment strategies for use with traumatized children. Therefore, general treatment principles, rather than discrete techniques, will be discussed.

Central to virtually all treatment strategies is an emphasis on reexposing the individual to the traumatic cues in a structured and supportive manner.[2,40] Particularly with younger children, techniques such as semi-structured art activities, writing, story telling, music, and puppetry can facilitate such a focus.[8,19,55,61,62,68,69] Given that controlled reexposure to traumatic cues is the apparent treatment of choice, it is important that clinicians undertaking such cases be prepared to work through the traumatic memories in their entirety without shying away from aspects that may be particularly upsetting either to the child *or* to the clinician. Temporary increases in symptomatology are to be expected when traumatic memories are initially focused on, and parents should be alerted to this possibility. Such exacerbations are not indicative of a negative response to treatment. Instead, they signal that an increased range of traumatic cues is being reexperienced. According to Keane et al,[6] reexposure to all facets of the traumatic memory is required for extinction of the traumatic response. If reexposure is incomplete, conservation of anxiety is likely.

It has been suggested that the strongest outcome predictor for a traumatized child is the ability of significant adults, such as parents and teachers, to deal with the traumatic event.[15,70] It is well documented that such adults are often very reluctant to discuss the event with the child, and that they often oppose reexposing the child to traumatic cues.[1,18,19,62] Such avoidance reinforces the child's fear that the event is not masterable and deprives the child of much-needed social support.[61] Therefore, teaching parents and teachers ways to address the event honestly and openly with the child can be an important treatment goal. Modeling and direct instruction can both be useful in this regard.[62]

In the face of an apparently uncontrollable situation, self-blame is one coping strategy which trauma victims may use in an effort to minimize their sense of helplessness and restore a feeling of control.[1,24,71] Thus, guilt is often a major symptom in PTSD. Some treatment programs place a heavy emphasis on persuading the child that they had no responsibility for the events that took place. As Lamb[72] points out, such arguments are unlikely to convince the child for very long, and may actually jeopardize the child's sense of efficacy. A more effective strategy may be to try to shift the child's self-blame away from global characterological condemnations—"I'm a horrible person"—toward self-blame for specific behaviors—"I should not have gotten into the car with a stranger."[24] It may also be therapeutic to emphasize the fact that the child may not have had sufficient life experience at the time to know how to handle the situation. The child can then plan ways to deal with possible future stressors and know that different choices could be made if the event were to recur.[62,72]

A sense of self-efficacy can also be promoted by providing the child with active coping strategies to help deal with the intrusive reexperiencing. For example, teaching children and their families to anticipate anniversary reactions and increases in symptomatology in response to other reminders of the traumatic event can reduce feelings of helplessness and discouragement when such reactions occur.[73] Relaxation training has also been reported to be effective in the treatment of traumatized children.[62]

FUTURE DIRECTIONS

The literature on adult posttraumatic stress disorder (PTSD) has grown exponentially over the past several years, and research paradigms have become increasingly refined. The literature on children's PTSD lags behind the adult literature, but is steadily progressing, and increased awareness of PTSD as a diagnostic entity is becoming evident.

The greatest return for our research efforts will come from studies that include systematic documentation of observed behavior and comprehensive psychiatric diagnoses of the children involved. As research on PTSD evolves, it is becoming increasingly evident that not all survivors of extremely stressful events meet the diagnostic criteria for PTSD. It is, therefore, critical in future research to differentiate children who develop PTSD from children who respond to the same or a similar stressor by developing other symptom patterns, as well as from children who show no psychopathology following such a stressor.

The development of multimethod assessment protocols specifically for the diagnosis of PTSD in children is needed to enable clinicians at various sites to conduct standardized evaluations of children who experience various stressful events. Some follow-up studies have been conducted,[1,23] but more longitudinal work needs to be done to study the time course of children's PTSD symptomatology. Treatment-outcome studies are needed, and sex and age differences require further investigation.

One of the difficulties in conducting research on the effects of trauma is that the traumatic event may be embedded in a long series of stressors. Physical and sexual abuse of children, for example, are often associated with parental separations, financial hardship, parental substance abuse, and foster placement.[59,60,74-78] Similarly, after the death of a family member, families often break up, change associates, or relocate.[21,79] It may be difficult to discriminate the effect of the traumatic event itself from the effects of preexisting or ensuing stressors. Such variables must therefore be controlled either statistically or through careful research design.[47,80]

A second difficulty, encountered in both clinical practice and research with this population, is reluctance to reexpose children to cues associated with the trauma. It is difficult to imagine, for example, an ethics review board approving psychophysiological assessment procedures in which children's physiological reactivity would be monitored while they watched videotapes of situations similar to the trauma they had endured, even though such procedures have been found to be effective in evaluating PTSD symptomatology among combat veterans.[81] The desire to protect children from further discomfort by shielding them from trauma-related cues is well-intentioned, but it is not always in the children's best interest. In working with traumatized children, a willingness to discuss the traumatic situation openly and to assist the child in dealing with *all* disturbing aspects of the event without shying away from any of the traumatic cues is critical, not only to produce positive treatment gains, but also to avoid the potential iatrogenic effects of signaling to the child that the traumatic memories are too horrible to face and master.

The difficulties involved in conducting therapy and research with this population should not be overlooked, but neither should they preclude further advancement in this area. PTSD in children and adolescents promises to be a field in which we can expect numerous theoretical and clinical advances in the next several years.

REFERENCES

1. Terr LC: Chowchilla revisited: The effects of psychic trauma four years after a school-bus kidnapping. Am J Psychiatry 140:1543–1550, 1983
2. Fairbank JA, Nicholson RA: Theoretical and empirical issues in the treatment of posttraumatic stress disorder in Vietnam veterans, J Clin Psychiatry 43:44–55, 1987
3. Horowitz MJ: Stress Response Syndromes. New York, Jason Aronson, 1976
4. Freud S: Moses and monotheism, in Strachey J (ed): The Standard Edition of the Complete Psychological Works of Sigmund Freud, vol 23. London, Hogarth Press, 1939, pp 1–137
5. Keane TM, Fairbank JA, Caddell JM, et al: A behavioral approach to assessing and treating post-traumatic stress disorder in Vietnam veterans, in Figley CR (ed): Trauma and Its Wake. New York, Brunner/Mazel, 1985, pp 257–294
6. Keane TM, Zimering RT, Caddell JM: A behavioral formulation of posttraumatic stress disorder in Vietnam veterans. Behav Therapist 8:9–12, 1985
7. American Psychiatric Association: Diagnostic and Statistical Manual of Mental Disorders, 3rd ed. Washington, DC, American Psychiatric Association, 1980
8. Frederick CJ: Children traumatized by catastrophic situations, in Eth S, Pynoos RS (eds): Post-traumatic Stress Disorder in Children. Washington, DC, American Psychiatric Press, 1985, pp 71–99
9. Terr, LC: Child snatching: A new epidemic of an ancient malady. J Pediatr 103:151–156, 1983
10. Green JW, Walker LS, Hickson G, et al: Stressful life events and somatic complaints in adolescents. Pediatrics 75:19–22, 1985
11. Heimberg RG: What makes traumatic stress traumatic? Behav Ther 16:417–419, 1985

12. Keane TM: Defining traumatic stress: Some comments on the current terminological confusion. Behav Ther 16:419–423, 1985
13. Saigh PA: On the nature and etiology of traumatic stress. Behav Ther 16:423–426, 1985
14. Terr, LC: Psychic trauma in children and adolescents. Psychiatr Clin N Am 8:815–835, 1985
15. Benedek EP: Children and disaster: Emerging issues. Psychiatry Ann 15:168–172, 1985
16. Benedek EP: Children and psychic trauma: A brief review of contemporary thinking, in Eth S, Pynoos RS (eds): Post-traumatic Stress Disorder in Children, Washington, DC. American Psychiatric Press, 1985, pp 1–16
17. Burke JD, Borus JF, Burns BJ, et al: Changes in children's behavior after a natural disaster. Am J Psychiatry 139:1010–1014, 1982
18. Harrison SI, Davenport CW, McDermott JF: Children's reactions to bereavement: Adult confusions and misperceptions. Arch Gen Psychiatry 17:593–597, 1967
19. Eth S, Silverstein S. Pynoos RS: Mental health consultation to a preschool following the murder of a mother and child. Hosp Community Psychiatry 36:73–76, 1985
20. Associated Press: Poll says 22% were sexually abused as children. Clarion Ledger/Jackson Daily News. Jackson, MS, Aug 25, 1985, p 3A
21. Turkington C: Support urged for children in mourning. APA Monitor, December 1984, pp 16–17
22. Pynoos RS, Eth S: Children traumatized by witnessing acts of personal violence: Homicide, rape or suicide behavior, in Eth S, Pynoos RS (eds): Post-traumatic Stress Disorder in Children. Washington, DC, American Psychiatric Press, 1985, pp 17–43
23. Elmer E: A follow-up study of traumatized children. Pediatrics 59:273–279, 1977
24. Janoff-Bulman R: The aftermath of victimization: Rebuilding shattered assumptions, in Figley CR (ed): Trauma and Its Wake. New York, Brunner/Mazel, 1985, pp 15–35
25. Lazarus RS, DeLongis A, Foldman S, et al: Stress and adaptational outcomes: The problem of confounded measures. Am Psychol 40:770–779, 1985
26. Veronen LJ, Kilpatrick DG: Stress management for rape victims, in Meichenbaum D, Jaremko ME (eds): Stress Reduction and Prevention. New York, Plenum Press, 1983, pp 341–374
27. Yamamoto K: Children's ratings of the stressfulness of experiences. Dev Psychol 15:581–582, 1979
28. Lister ED: Forced silence: A neglected dimension of trauma. Am J Psychiatry 139:872–876, 1982
29. de Young M: Counterphobic behavior in multiply molested children. Child Welfare 63:333–339, 1984
30. Nir Y: Post-traumatic stress disorder in children with cancer, in Eth S, Pynoos RS (eds): Post-traumatic Stress Disorder in Children. Washington, DC, American Psychiatric Press, 1985, pp 121–132
31. American Psychiatric Association: DSM-III-R in Development, 2nd draft (8/1/86). Washington, DC, American Psychiatric Association, 1986
32. Krener P: After incest: Secondary prevention? J Am Acad Child Psychiatry 24:231–234, 1985

33. Frances A, Petti TA: Boy with seriously ill mother manifests somatic complaints, withdrawal, disabling fears. Hosp Community Psychiatry 35:439–440, 1984
34. Senior N, Gladstone T, Nurcombe B: Child snatching: A case report. J Am Acad Child Psychiatry 21:579–583, 1982
35. Jacobson MS, Rubenstein EM, Bohannon WE, et al: Follow-up of adolescent trauma victims: A new model of care. Pediatrics 77:236–241, 1986
36. Bergman AB, Larsen RM, Mueller BA: Changing spectrum of serious child abuse. Pediatrics 77:113–116, 1986
37. Rosenheck R, Nathan P: Secondary traumatization in children of Vietnam veterans. Hosp Community Psychiatry 36:538–539, 1985
38. Rimsza ME, Niggemann EH: Medical evaluation of sexually abused children: A review of 311 Cases. Pediatrics 69:8–14, 1982
39. Keane TM, Wolfe J, Taylor KL: Post-traumatic stress disorder: Evidence for diagnostic validity and methods of psychological assessment. J Clin Psychol 43:32–43, 1987
40. Garmezy N, Rutter M: Acute reactions in stress, in Rutter M, Hersov L (eds): Child Psychiatry: Modern Approaches, 2nd ed. Oxford, Blackwell Scientific Publications, 1985, pp 152–176
41. Eaton WW, Sigal JJ, Weinfeld M: Impairment in holocaust survivors after 33 years: Data from an unbiased community sample. Am J Psychiatry 139:773–777, 1982
42. Gislason IL, Call JD: Dog bite in infancy: Trauma and personality development. J Am Acad Child Psychiatry 21:203–207, 1982
43. MacLean G: Addendum to a case of traumatic neurosis. Can J Psychiatry 25:506–508, 1980
44. Faravelli C, Webb T, Ambonetti A, et al: Prevalence of traumatic early life events in 31 agoraphobic patients with panic attacks. Am J Psychiatry 142:1493–1494, 1985
45. Gomes-Schwartz B, Horowitz JM, Sauzier M: Severity of emotional distress among sexually abused preschool, school-age, and adolescent children. Hosp Community Psychiatry 36:503–508, 1985
46. van der Kolk BA: Adolescent vulnerability to posttraumatic stress. Presented at the 135th annual meeting of the American Psychiatric Association, Toronto, Canada, May 1982
47. Ruch LO, Chandler SM: The crisis impact of sexual assault on three victim groups: Adult rape victims, child rape victims, and incest victims. J Soc Serv Res 5:83–100, 1982
48. Wilson JP, Smith WK, Johnson SK: A comparative analysis of PTSD among various survivor groups, in Figley CR (ed): Trauma and Its Wake. New York, Brunner/Mazel, 1985, pp 142–172
49. Glover H: Themes of mistrust and the posttraumatic stress disorder in Vietnam veterans. Am J Psychother 37:445–452, 1984
50. Erikson EH: Childhood and Society, 2nd ed. New York, WW Norton, 1963
51. Eth S, Pynoos RS: Developmental perspective on psychic trauma in childhood, in Figley CR (ed): Trauma and Its Wake. New York, Brunner/Mazel, 1985, pp 36–52
52. Wilson JP: Conflict, stress and growth: The effects of war and psychosocial development among Vietnam veterans, in Figley CR, Leventman S (eds): Strangers at Home: Vietnam Veterans Since the War. New York, Praeger, 1980

53. Alessi JJ, Hearn K: Group treatment of children in shelters for battered women, in Roberts AR (ed): Battered Women and Their Families: Intervention Strategies and Treatment Programs. New York, Springer, 1984, pp 49–61
54. Ayalon O: Children as hostages. Practitioner 226:1773–1781, 1982
55. Newman J: Children of disaster: Clinical observation at Buffalo Creek, Am J Psychiatry 133:306–312, 1976
56. Terr LC: Psychic trauma in children: Observations following the Chowchilla school-bus kidnapping. Am J Psychiatry 138:14–19, 1981
57. Terr LC: Children traumatized in small groups, in Eth S, Pynoos RS (eds): Posttraumatic Stress Disorder in Children, Washington, DC, American Psychiatric Press, 1985, pp 45–70
58. Garmezy N, Masten AS, Tellegen A: The study of stress and competence in children: A building block for developmental psychopathology. Child Dev 55:97–111, 1984
59. Jaffe P, Wolfe D, Wilson SK, et al: Family violence and child adjustment: A comparative analysis of girls' and boys' behavioral symptoms. Am J Psychiatry 143:74–77, 1986
60. Byrne JP, Valdiserri EV: Victims of childhood sexual abuse: A follow-up study of a noncompliant population. Hosp Community Psychiatry 33:938–940, 1982
61. Crabbs MA: School mental health services following an environmental disaster. J Sch Health 51:165–167, 1981
62. Klingman A, Eli ZB: A school community in disaster: Primary and secondary prevention in situational crisis. Prof Psychol 12:523–533, 1981
63. Turkington C: Good Grief program helps those at risk. APA Monitor, December 1984, p 17
64. Saigh P: In vitro flooding of a childhood posttraumatic stress disorder. Sch Psychol Rev (in press)
65. Saigh P: In vitro flooding of an adolescent posttraumatic stress disorder. J Clin Child Psychol 16:147–150, 1987
66. Saigh P: In vitro flooding of childhood posttraumatic stress disorders: A systematic replication, Prof Sch Psychol 2:135–146, 1978
67. Valdiserri EV, Byrne JP: Hypnosis as emergency treatment for a teen-age rape victim. Hosp Community Psychiatry 33:767–769, 1982
68. Alger I, Linn S, Beardslee W: Puppetry as a therapeutic tool for hospitalized children. Hosp Community Psychiatry 36:129–130, 1985
69. Kelley SJ: Drawings: Critical communications for sexually abused children. Pediatr Nurs 11:421–426, 1985
70. Black D: Children and disaster. Br Med J 285:989–990, 1982
71. De Jong AR: The medical evaluation of sexual abuse in children. Hosp Community Psychiatry 36:509–512, 1985
72. Lamb S: Treating sexually abused children: Issues of blame and responsibility. Am J Orthopsychiatry 56:303–307, 1986
73. Koocher GP: Psychosocial care of the child cured of cancer. Pediatr Nurs 11:91–93, 1985
74. Donaldson MA, Gardner R: Diagnosis and treatment of traumatic stress among women after childhood incest, in Figley CR (ed): Trauma and Its Wake. New York, Brunner/Mazel, 1985, pp 356–377

75. Green AH: Children traumatized by physical abuse, in Eth S, Pynoos RS (eds): Post-traumatic Stress Disorder in Children. Washington, DC, American Psychiatric Press, 1985, pp 133–154

76. Jaffe P, Wolfe D, Wilson S, et al: Similarities in behavioral and social maladjustment among child victims and witnesses to family violence. Am J Orthopsychiatry 56:142–146, 1986

77. Orzek AM: The child's cognitive processing of sexual abuse. J Child Adolesc Psychother 2:110–114, 1985

78. Truesdell DL, McNeil JS, Deschner JP: Incidence of wife abuse in incestuous families. Soc Work 31:138–140, 1986

79. Cain AC, Fast I: Children's disturbed reactions to parent suicide. Am J Orthopsychiatry 36:873–880, 1966

80. Monroe SM, Steiner SC: Social support and psychopathology: Interrelations with preexisting disorder, stress, and personality. J Abnorm Psychol 95:29–39, 1986

81. Malloy PF, Fairbank JA, Keane TM: Validation of a multimethod assessment of posttraumatic stress disorders in Vietnam veterans. J Consult Clin Psychol 51:488–494, 1983

25

Fragile-X Syndrome: Variability of Phenotypic Expression

Joel D. Bregman and Elisabeth Dykens
Yale University, New Haven, Connecticut
Michael Watson
Washington University, St. Louis, Missouri
Sharon I. Ort and James F. Leckman
Yale University, New Haven, Connecticut

Fragile-X syndrome is a recently described X-linked disorder that ranks second to Down syndrome as the most prevalent chromosomal form of mental retardation. Affected male individuals manifest a variable clinical phenotype that includes distinctive facial features, macroorchidism, cognitive and language impairments, and an impressive prevalence of attention deficit disorder and infantile autism. A sizable proportion of female carriers are similarly affected. The molecular basis for these phenotypic features has not been established, nor have the factors mediating the variable expression of the syndrome in vulnerable individuals. However, improved behavioral functioning in prepubertal children may result from early identification and folate supplementation.

Since the nineteenth century it has been appreciated that significantly more male than female individuals experience serious intellectual handicaps (Penrose, 1963). In recent years, the importance of genetic factors has been recognized. It is estimated that X-linked genes alone may account for 20% of

Reprinted with permission from the *Journal of the American Academy of Child and Adolescent Psychiatry,* 1987, Vol. 26, No. 4, 463–471. Copyright 1987 by the American Academy of Child and Adolescent Psychiatry.

This research was supported in part by the John Merck Fund, NIH grants HD03008 and RR00125, and by Yale Mental Health Clinical Research Center grant MH30929.

468

male individuals with significant degrees of intellectual impairment (Turner and Turner, 1974).

During the past 40 years, numerous reports have appeared in the literature describing families in which mental retardation has been transmitted in an X-linked manner. Martin and Bell (1943) reported the first such kindred, which included 11 mentally retarded male members within two generations. In 1969, Lubs described a pedigree demonstrating the X-linked transmission of intellectual impairment and facial dysmorphism. Cytogenetic analyses on cultured lymphocytes from affected male and female subjects revealed an unusual secondary constriction involving the distal segment of the long arm of the X chromosome, termed "a marker X" by Lubs (1969). Since this pivotal discovery, 17 fragile sites have been identified in the human karyotype (Sutherland and Hecht, 1985). However, the fragile-X site (fra(X) q 27.3) is the only one that has been consistently associated with a specific mental retardation syndrome. It now is apparent that the fragile-X syndrome is the most common identifiable form of X-linked mental retardation (XLMR), accounting for more than 50% of such cases. The estimated population prevalence of 0.73 to 0.92 per 1,000 male individuals places this syndrome second only to Down syndrome as the leading cause of mental retardation associated with a chromosomal abnormality (Herbst and Miller, 1980; Webb et al., 1986).

During the past 10 years, clinical and research interest in the fragile-X syndrome has grown substantially. One of the most intriguing findings has been an appreciation for the significant degree of cytogenetic and phenotypic variability present within the syndrome.

This report will review our current knowledge of the genetic and phenotypic characteristics of the fragile-X syndrome focusing upon the range of phenotypic expression within and across families.

GENETIC FACTORS

Cytogenetics

Fragile sites are chromosomal loci susceptible to breakage under specific tissue culture conditions. Although somewhat variable in appearance, fragile sites most often present as nonstaining gaps occurring at predictable chromosomal locations for a given individual and family. Inheritance characteristics typically follow classic Mendelian patterns.

Currently, there are four identified types of fragile sites that differ in the tissue culture conditions necessary for reliable expression. The fragile X site is one of 14 folate-sensitive sites that require a growth environment lacking in thymidine and folate for optimal expression. Several biochemical techniques known to interrupt thymidine metabolism are often adopted in order to enhance the expression of these sites, including the addition of methotrexate (MTX) (Mattei et al., 1981a) and 5-fluorodeoxyuridine (FUdR) (Glover, 1981) to the tissue culture media.

Diagnosis

At the present time, the diagnosis of fragile-X syndrome is based largely upon results of cytogenetic assessment. Demonstration of the fragile site in a small proportion of the X chromosomes is sufficient for diagnosis; however, a review of pedigree data is often necessary for the putative identification of obligate male and female carriers, because cytogenetic findings are often negative or inconclusive among these individuals.

Affected male individuals invariably express the fragile site more consistently than do female carriers, and individuals with mental retardation are more likely to express the site than are those with normal intelligence (the latter is particularly true of female individuals). The highest rates of expression have been recorded for affected male subjects, 99% of whom express the fragile site in 15 to 40% of cells (rarely in greater than 50%). Fragile-X male subjects without mental retardation, however, demonstrate a much lower frequency of expression (Froster-Iskenius et al., 1986a).

Fragile-X expression is most variable among female carriers. Of the one third who manifest intellectual impairment, approximately 95% express the marker in greater than 4% of cells. This contrasts sharply with the frequency of fragile-X expression found among the two thirds of obligate carriers who have normal intelligence. Most studies suggest that fewer than 50% of the normal female carriers express the fragile site.

In an effort to improve case identification and carrier detection, a major research focus has been directed toward the discovery of chromosomal linkage patterns among DNA polymorphic markers flanking the fragile site. Several closely linked markers have been identified thus far (Murphy et al., 1985; Oberle et al., 1985) and have proved quite helpful in the identification of carriers and in prenatal diagnosis (Murphy et al., 1986).

During the past several years, investigators have reported successful prenatal identification using cultured amniocytes (Schmidt and Passarge, 1986), fetal blood cells (Shapiro et al., 1984), and chorionic villous cells (Tommerup et al., 1985). Interpretation of findings is problematic, however, because false negative and false positive errors may result. In view of the occurrence of phenotypically normal carriers and the problems encountered in accurate prenatal diagnosis, care must be exercised when current cytogenetic techniques are relied upon for prenatal decision making.

Population Genetics

The fragile-X syndrome has been reported in individuals of diverse geographic and racial background. The true incidence of the syndrome is not known, because valid and reliable data are unavailable at the present time. In the only methodologically sound study performed to date, Sutherland and Hecht (1985) evaluated 3,090 consecutive newborns and found none to carry the fragile-X chromosome; however, because of the relatively small sample size, definitive conclusions cannot be drawn. Indirect methods also have been used and suggest an incidence of 0.67 to 0.92 per 1,000 male newborns (Gustavson et al., 1986; Herbst and Miller, 1980).

Investigators have explored the prevalence of the fragile-X syndrome within the mentally retarded population. Of those studies that screened at least 200 male and 100 female subjects and included mental retardation as the only ascertainment criterion, 2 to 7% of male subjects and 0.3 to 10% of intellectually impaired female subjects were found to carry the fragile-X chromosome (Jacobs et al., 1986; Webb et al., 1986).

Segregation Analysis

Sherman et al. (1984, 1985) performed a segregation analysis of the fragile-X syndrome using data from 206 pedigrees. Among fragile-X male subjects, a segregation ratio of 0.406 ± 0.028 was found. This differs significantly from the 0.5 value expected of a disorder segregating along classic Mendelian lines. The investigators offered several explanations for this apparent 20% underrepresentation of affected male subjects, including selective male fetal loss, non-Mendelian inheritance, variable expressivity, and incomplete penetrance. The current literature supports the hypothesis of incomplete penetrance, which posits transmission of the syndrome to successive generations through men who carry the gene but express neither the complete clinical phenotype nor the fragile site. Among female subjects, a segregation ratio of 0.28 ± 0.24 was reported (Sherman et al., 1984, 1985), indicating that only 56% of carriers are detected by the presence of intellectual impairment or by the identification of the fragile site. This finding is misleading, because obligate carriers may be of normal intelligence and fail to express the fragile-X chromosome.

Using their segregation analysis data, Sherman et al. (1985) calculated a mutation rate in sperm of 7.2×10^{-4} loci per generation, one of the highest rates reported for a human disorder. However, when adjustments are made to account for the reproductive advantage experienced by intellectually impaired female carriers (increased rates of fertility and twin pregnancies, Fryns, 1986) and the significant frequency of nonpenetrant male subjects, the mutation rate becomes more realistic, similar to that found in Duchennes Muscular Dystrophy (Vogel, 1984).

Genetic Counseling

The presence of genotypic and phenotypic variability significantly affects the development of strategies for genetic counseling. Because of deviations from classical Mendelian X-linked inheritance, the fragile-X syndrome presents several problems to the genetic counselor, making it essential that pedigree information be collected from both maternal and paternal branches of the family. The segregation analyses of Sherman et al. (1985) represent an initial set of parameters from which risk figures may be generated and appropriate counseling offered. These preliminary data suggest that the likelihood of clinical expression varies with the intellectual phenotype of the carrier parent. In cases where the carrier is an *unaffected father,* all daughters will be carriers but very few will be affected clinically. For families in which a clinically *unaffected female carrier* transmits the gene, sons inheriting the fragile site have a 75% chance of being affected clinically, whereas daughters have a 30% chance. If, however, the carrier is an *intellectually impaired mother,* one half of the daughters and all of the sons who inherit the fragile site will be affected. Sherman's data also suggest that clinically unaffected male subjects are unlikely to carry the gene. As can be seen, genetic counseling is a difficult undertaking and is best reserved for those experienced with this disorder.

PHENOTYPIC EXPRESSION

Physical Characteristics

The majority of mentally retarded male subjects with the fragile-X syndrome manifest a characteristic physical phenotype that includes enlarged genitalia and a set of facial features characteristic of a connective tissue dysplasia.

General growth and development

Investigators have studied the pattern of growth and development exhibited by male subjects with fragile-X syndrome. Findings indicate that increases in weight, height, and head circumference (macrocephaly) are present during childhood relative to general population norms and control samples (Partington, 1984; Sutherland and Hecht, 1985). These findings are significant, because most newborns and children with chromosomal abnormalities are of low weight and small stature. During adulthood weight and height parameters normalize; however, the proportion of affected male individuals with macrocephaly increases, perhaps reflecting the CNS pathology responsible for the high prevalence of seizures (occurring in 15% of fragile-X male subjects; see Figure 1). This association has not been demonstrated empirically, however.

Facial characteristics

Several facial features have been associated consistently with the fragile-X syndrome. These include the presence of an elongated facial contour, a high forehead, prominent supraorbital ridges, midfacial hypoplasia, a broad nasal root, a prominent mandible, and enlarged, underdeveloped ears (see Figure 1). Meryash et al. (1984) and Brondum-Nielsen et al. (1982) have documented the specificity of these physical features for the fragile-X syndrome by performing systematic measurements on both affected individuals and control subjects (including both intellectually normal and mentally retarded, fragile-X negative subjects). Furthermore, Shapiro et al. (1982) were able to increase the yield of positive chromosomal analyses by using facial and ear lengths as screening factors.

Hagerman et al. (1984), Hagerman and Synhorst (1984), and Opitz et al. (1984) have hypothesized that a connective tissue dysplasia may underlie many of the physical stigmata exhibited by fragile-X patients. Characteristic features include joint hyperextensibility; macroorchidism; high arched palate; enlarged ears; pes planus; velvety, hyperelastic skin; and mitral valve prolapse.

An increasing number of studies have focused upon identification of the phenotypic attributes manifested by female carriers. The current literature suggests that the features characteristic of affected male individuals occur commonly among carriers with intellectual impairment yet only occasionally among those with average intelligence (Fryns, 1986; Hagerman et al., 1984; Partington, 1986). Fryns, for instance, studied the physical phenotype of 125 obligate female carriers and discovered that characteristic facial stigmata

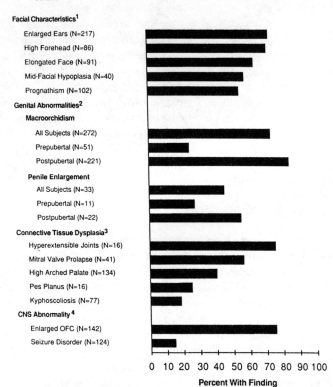

Figure 1. Physical phenotype of the fragile-X syndrome in male subjects. The data for this figure were obtained from these references: Brondum-Nielsen et al. (1983); Cantu et al. (1976, 1978); Carpenter et al. (1983); Fryns et al. (1982); Hagerman and Synhorst (1984); Hagerman et al. (1984); Hecht et al. (1983); Jacobs et al. (1980); Jennings et al. (1980); Kaiser-McCaw and Hecht (1980); Labrisseau et al. (1982); Loehr et al. (1986); Lubs (1969); Mattei et al. (1981b); McDermott et al. (1983); Meryash et al. (1984); Opitz et al. (1984); Partington (1984); Pueschel et al. (1983); Pyeritz et al. (1982); Renier et al. (1983); Rhoads et al. (1982); Richards et al. (1981); Schmidt (1982); Shapiro et al. (1982); Turleau et al. (1979); Ven der Hagen et al. (1983); Van Roy et al. (1983); Venter et al. (1981).

were present in 28% of subjects. An impressive relationship was noted between phenotypic expression and the degree of cognitive impairment; whereas 55% of those with mental retardation manifested the facial stigmata, only 42% of those with borderline intellectual functioning and 14% of those with normal intelligence did so.

Macroorchidism and other genital abnormalities

Macroorchidism is the most consistent and reliable physical feature identified among fragile-X men. Men with fragile-X syndrome regularly present with testicular volumes in excess of 40 ml (25 ml is generally accepted as the upper limit of normal) (Zachman et al., 1974). Twenty-seven studies reporting on the fragile-X phenotype were reviewed by the present authors. Macroorchidism was noted among 72% of the 226 men examined (see Figure 1). Twenty-four percent of the prepubertal subjects and 84% of the postpubertal subjects demonstrated this characteristic, suggesting the presence of a developmental phenomenon. A similarly impressive frequency of macroorchidism has been reported in studies of fragile-X men ascertained without reference to testicular volume (Sutherland, 1983). Macroorchidism is not entirely specific for the fragile-X syndrome, however. As many as 20% of institutionalized, mentally retarded men without fragile-X syndrome exhibit enlarged testicular volumes (Brondum-Nielsen et al., 1982).

Testicular biopsies from 12 patients (one prepubertal and 11 postpubertal subjects) have revealed an essentially normal histological pattern (Cantu et al., 1976, 1978; McDermott et al., 1983; Ruvalcaba et al., 1977; Shapiro et al., 1982). Other genital abnormalities have been reported, however. Meryash et al. (1983), for instance, have noted a 30- to 50-fold increase in the incidence of hypospadias and cryptorchidism among male fragile-X syndrome subjects.

Neuroendocrine Functioning

The presence of abnormalities in genital maturation and development among fragile-X male subjects has generated interest in the regulation of gonadal functioning. The hypothalamic-pituitary-testicular axis of fragile-X male subjects has been evaluated. The majority of studies report normal baseline FSH, LH, and testosterone levels, normal pulsatility of pituitary LH and FSH release, normal hypothalamic-pituitary responsiveness (as assessed by the LHRH stimulation test) and normal Leydig cell reserve (as assessed by the HCG stimulation test) (Berkovitz et al., 1986; Cantu et al., 1976; McDermott et al., 1983; O'Hare et al., 1986; Ruvalcaba et al., 1977; Shapiro et al., 1982; Turner et al., 1975). However, gonadal dysfunction may be present among a subset of fragile-X male individuals. McDermott et al. (1983), Shapiro et al. (1982), and Turner et al. (1975) have reported that up to one third of subjects exhibit elevated baseline LH and FSH levels in association with depressed testosterone levels and evidence of decreased spermatogenesis in biopsy specimens.

Although there have been no reports of formal endocrine evaluation among heterozygous female subjects, neuroendocrine dysfunction is suggested by the presence of high rates of fertility and twinning (Fryns, 1986). This intriguing finding warrants further study.

The recognized association of hypothyroidism with macroorchidism has led to the study of thyroid function among fragile-X male individuals. Normal thyroxine and TSH levels have been reported by several investigators (Brondum-Nielsen et al., 1982; McDermott et al., 1983; O'Hare et al., 1986; Ruvalcaba et al., 1977; Shapiro et al., 1982; Wilson et al., 1983). Studies of the hypothalamic-pituitary regulation of thyroid metabolism also have been reported. Wilson et al. (1983) and O'Hare et al. (1986) performed TRH stimulation tests on 18 subjects and found that 16 exhibited a blunted TSH response. Therefore, although fragile-X male subjects appear to be clinically euthyroid, subtle abnormalities in the hypothalamic-pituitary control of thyroid functioning may be present.

Behavioral Functioning

During the past several years investigators have become increasingly interested in identifying the cognitive, linguistic, and behavioral features of the fragile-X syndrome.

Cognitive functioning

Within the fragile-X population there exists a significant degree of heterogeneity with regard to cognitive functioning. Although the majority of male individuals with fragile-X syndrome experience moderate intellectual dysfunction (Chudley, 1984; de la Cruz, 1985), the range of impairment is quite broad. Male subjects with normal intelligence as well as those with profound mental retardation have been shown to transmit the marker. Heterozygous female subjects also demonstrate variability in cognitive functioning, although their overall abilities are usually higher than those of their male counterparts. Approximately one third of carriers experience cognitive deficits of a mild to moderate degree (Fryns, 1986; Partington, 1986; Venter et al., 1986), whereas as many as one half experience some type of diagnosable learning disability (Fishburn et al., 1983). The pattern of cognitive growth and development among fragile-X male subjects has been studied by several investigators. Hagerman et al. (1983) and Paul et al. (1984) have reported that progressive growth during childhood is followed by a plateau or actual decline in intellectual performance during adolescence. In addition, certain cognitive functions may be more sensitive to developmental influences. Herbst et al. (1981), for instance, reported that receptive vocabulary improves with age in contrast with nonverbal reasoning, numerical memory, and drawing ability.

Investigators have attempted to identify characteristic patterns of cognitive dysfunction within the fragile-X population. One strategy has been the comparison of scores on verbal and performance subtests of the WISC-R or WAIS. However, conflicting results have been reported for both male subjects and carrier female subjects. Several studies have noted superior verbal ability (Miezcjeski et al., 1984 for female subjects; Theobald and Hay, 1982 for male subjects); whereas others have noted superior performance ability (Chudley, 1984, for male subjects; Uchida and Joyce, 1982, for female subjects). Another strategy has been the examination of performance profiles on WISC-R or WAIS subtests. Fragile-X male subjects have revealed deficits in short-term numerical memory (Theobald and Hay, 1982) and in numerical reasoning and abstraction (Herbst and Miller, 1980). These deficits may not be specific for the fragile-X syndrome, however. Dykens et al. (in press) found the performance of institutionalized fragile-X men was equivalent to that of an institutionalized control group (matched for chronological and mental age) on tasks of numerical reasoning and memory.

A rather consistent pattern of cognitive dysfunction has been reported for female carriers. Deficient performance on the arithmetic, block design, and digit span subtests of the Weschler scales suggest specific deficits in numerical calculation and visual-spatial perspective (Kemper et al., 1986; Miezcjeski et al., 1984).

Speech and language functioning

Abnormalities in speech and language functioning have been described. Frequent findings include dysfluent, dyspraxic, poorly articulated speech (Herbst, 1980; Paul et al., 1984), with jocular, "litany-like" phraseology (Turner et al., 1980). In addition, echolalia and palilalia also have been described (Newell et al., 1983). Handon et al. (1986) performed a systematic speech and language analysis of 10 fragile-X boys with normal intelligence. The speech of nine subjects was characterized by a rapid rate, an erratic rhythm, and a disorganized, repetitious style. This pathological speech pattern has been termed cluttering. The investigators also noted relatively strong receptive language skills in the presence of relatively weak auditory memory and processing skills.

Although it is clear that speech and language deficits are common among fragile-X individuals, the actual pattern of dysfunction may not be specific to fragile-X syndrome. In a recent study of receptive and expressive language ability, Paul et al. (in press) found no significant differences in the performance of institutionalized fragile-X male subjects and a group of control subjects matched on chronological and mental age.

Adaptive functioning

In recent years, considerable importance has been placed upon assessing the level of adaptive functioning achieved by mentally retarded individuals. Accurate diagnostic and prognostic judgments depend upon the degree of personal independence and social responsibility demonstrated by the intellectually impaired (Grossman, 1983). Despite this, there is a relative paucity of data regarding the adaptive functioning of individuals with fragile-X syndrome.

Herbst et al. (1981) observed that their fragile-X patients demonstrated "reasonably good independence skills" but did not report results of formal assessments. In another study, "social adaptability" was noted to correlate positively with intellectual ability (Herbst, 1980). A more complete evaluation of adaptive ability was performed by Dykens et al. (in press) using the Vineland Adaptive Behavior Scales (Sparrow et al., 1984). Institutionalized fragile-X male subjects exhibited adaptive behavior that surpassed expectations based upon mental age. However, the functioning of fragile-X subjects did not differ significantly from that of control subjects matched for chronological and mental age who resided at the same institution.

Behavioral functioning

Several investigators have reported that fragile-X individuals experience relatively normal emotional and behavioral functioning, presenting with a pleasant, cheerful, and cooperative demeanor (Chudley, 1984; de la Cruz, 1985; Herbst et al., 1981). However, other researchers have described the frequent occurrence of hyperactivity, attention deficits, stereotypy, and gaze aversion, as well as of aggressive and self-injurious behavior (Brown et al., 1982; Hagerman and Smith, 1983; Mattei et al., 1981b; Turner et al., 1980). Attention deficits and hyperactivity appear to be particularly common among fragile-X male subjects. Three recent studies found that 41 of 50 subjects

(82%) demonstrated these behavioral difficulties (Finelli et al., 1985; Fryns et al., 1984; Largo and Schinzel, 1985).

The presence of gaze aversion, communication deficits (e.g., perseverative and echolalic speech), and behavioral atypicalities (e.g., stereotypic and self-injurious behavior) among many fragile-X individuals has generated interest in the relationship between the fragile-X syndrome and infantile autism. In 1982, Brown and colleagues reported that 5 of 27 (18.5%) fragile-X male subjects had been diagnosed previously as having autism. Since that initial report, numerous researchers have noted the frequent association of these two syndromes (Table 1). Levitas et al. (1983) reported that more than 60% of their fragile-X patients met DSM-III criteria for infantile autism. In a more recent study by the same investigators, 23 of 50 fragile-X male subjects (46%) received a DSM-III diagnosis of infantile autism, full syndrome or residual state (Hagerman et al., 1986b). However, even among those for whom a definitive diagnosis could not be made, autistic symptomatology was present more frequently than among a group of mentally retarded control subjects. A somewhat less impressive association has been noted by Fryns et al. (1984). Of 21 individuals with fragile-X syndrome, only 3 (14%) received an autistic diagnosis (specific diagnostic criteria were not noted). Some investigators question whether autistic features are, in fact, especially prevalent among fragile-X individuals. Chudley (1984) noted an absence of autistic characteristics within his fragile-X cohort, whereas Dykens et al. (in press) reported a similar occurrence of autistic symptomatology among mentally retarded men with and without fragile-X syndrome. In a recent study, Brown et al. (1986b) evaluated the frequency of autism among 434 fragile-X male subjects and found that 92 (21.2%) received autistic diagnoses. Of 150 subjects personally

Table 1. Frequency of Autism Among Male Subjects with Fragile-X Syndrome

Study	Fra-X (*N*)	Autism (*N*)	Autism (%)
Brown et al. (1982)	27	5	19
Fryns et al. (1984)	21	3	14
Brown et al. (1986b)			
Total subjects	434	91	21
Subjects examined	150	24	17
Literature review	284	67	24
Hagerman et al. (1986b)	50	23	46
Total	532	122	23

examined by the investigators, 24 (17.3%) met DSM-III criteria for infantile autism. This compares with 24% of the 284 subjects reported in a review of the literature.

There have been few published surveys addressing the frequency of emotional and behavioral problems among female carriers. Fryns (1986) evaluated 134 obligate carriers and found that psychiatric disorder (primarily of a psychotic nature) was present among 20% of the 46 intellectually impaired subjects and 10% of the 88 intellectually normal subjects. Partington (1986) reported a much lower prevalence of psychiatric disorder among 83 heterozygotic female subjects. Only two (2.4%) of the women experienced significant psychiatric difficulties (drug-induced psychosis and personality disorder). Female relatives within a four-generational fragile-X kindred were assessed by Reiss et al. (1986) using the Schedule for Affective Disorders—Lifetime Version (SADS-L) semistructured interview. The three obligate carriers in the family demonstrated a significant degree of psychopathology. Psychiatric diagnoses included major depressive disorder, bipolar disorder, and schizoaffective disorder. Pervasive developmental disorders appear to be uncommon among female carriers. Among their large fragile-X population, Hagerman et al. (1986c) have reported only two female subjects who meet DSM-III criteria for infantile autism.

Researchers also have explored the frequency of fragile-X syndrome among children and adults with infantile autism in an effort to identify a possible etiological determinant of the autistic syndrome (Table 2). Several studies screened relatively large numbers of autistic individuals. Findings have been reported from a Swedish multicenter study, which involved the participation of 101 autistic male subjects diagnosed according to DSM-III criteria (Wahlstrom et al., 1986). Sixteen (16%) of the subjects expressed the fragile-X site on cytogenetic assessment. This percentage proved to be 3 to 4 times higher than the frequency of marker expression among nonautistic, mentally retarded individuals (Blomquist et al., 1982, 1983).

Brown et al. (1986b) performed cytogenetic screenings on 183 autistic male subjects diagnosed according to DSM-III criteria and found 24 (13.1%) to be fragile-X positive. This compared with a frequency of 20.6% for a group of 254 nonautistic, mentally retarded individuals who were also evaluated (Fisch et al., 1986). In an American study, Watson et al. (1984) screened 76 subjects with infantile autism, as defined by DSM-III criteria, who were residing in institutional, group residential, and home settings. Within the total study population, four subjects (5.3%) demonstrated the chromosomal marker in cultured lymphocytes. All four were among the group of 40 autistic male subjects residing in the institutional setting.

Table 2. Frequency of Fra(X) Among Male Subjects with Autism

Study	Autism (N)	Fra-X (N)	Fra-X (%)
Chudley (1984)	16	1	6.3
Watson et al. (1984)	76	4	5.3
Mikkelsen (1984)	20	1	5.0
Turner (1984)	70	1	1.4
Goldfine et al. (1985)	37	0	0
Pueschel et al. (1985)	18	0	0
Blomquist et al. (1985) and Wahlstrom et al. (1986)	101	16	15.8
Brown et al. (1986b) and Fisch et al. (1986)	183	24	13.1
McGillivray et al. (1986)	33	3	9.1
Venter et al. (1986)	40	0	0
Total	594	50	8.4

Other investigators have reported a lower prevalence of the fragile-X syndrome within the autistic population. The fragile-X site was demonstrated in only three of 201 autistic male subjects evaluated by Chudley (1984), Goldfine et al. (1985), Mikkelsen (1984), Pueschel et al. (1985), Turner (1984), and Venter et al. (1986). As presented in Table 2, 50 of 594 autistic male subjects (8.4%) reported in 10 studies were shown to have fragile-X syndrome. This figure contrasts with the negative findings reported for autistic female subjects. Of 46 female subjects with autism, none were found to demonstrate the fragile-X site (McGillivray et al., 1986; Venter et al., 1986; Wahlstrom et al., 1986).

Pharmacological Approaches to Treatment

The use of folic acid in the treatment of patients with fragile-X syndrome was initially described by Lejeune (1981). The rationale for these clinical trials was the assumption that the in vitro sensitivity of the fragile-X site reflects an intrinsic abnormality in folate metabolism. Both researchers reported that folic acid induced substantial behavioral improvement and decreased marker expression in affected male and heterozygous female subjects. Subsequently, several research groups studied folate metabolism in cell lines cultured from fragile-X male subjects and carrier female subjects and found no intrinsic metabolic defects (Branda et al., 1983; Wang and Erbe,

1984). Interest generated by the success of the early clinical trials, however, led to the initiation of several controlled studies assessing folate efficacy in pre- and postpubertal fragile-X patients. Four double-blind, crossover studies involving a total of 14 prepubertal subjects have been reported (Brown et al., 1984; Carpenter et al., 1983; Froster-Iskenius et al., 1986b; Hagerman et al., 1986a.) Across these studies, the daily folic acid dosage ranged from 10 mg orally to 1.6 mg/kg intravenously and the treatment period ranged from 2 weeks to 12 months. Despite these methodological differences, similar findings were reported in all four studies, including a significant attenuation of hyperactive behavior and a concomitant increase in attentional ability. Although one study reported improvements in expressive language (Brown et al., 1984), none of the other studies noted changes in either intellectual functioning or language ability. There also have been four double-blind, crossover studies involving 40 postpubertal subjects (Brown et al., 1984, 1986a; Froster-Iskenius et al., 1986b, Hagerman et al., 1986a). The daily folate dosage ranged from 10 to 250 mg orally and the treatment period ranged from 2 weeks to 12 months. Only one of the 40 subjects demonstrated improvements in intellectual and linguistic functioning, and only two exhibited improvements in activity level and attention span.

These studies suggest that folic acid may decrease the symptomatology associated with attention deficit disorder among prepubertal children with fragile-X syndrome.

DISCUSSION

During the past 10 years, investigators and clinicians have begun to recognize the importance of the fragile-X syndrome as a major cause of mental retardation and psychiatric disability. Prevalence studies, pedigree analyses, and careful physical and psychological assessments have contributed to our appreciation for the breadth of the syndrome's influence. Although a significant body of research has already emerged, many questions remain unanswered regarding the genetic and phenotypic characteristics of the syndrome.

Since the fragile site was first identified, much has been learned about the biochemical pathways involved in fragile site expression. However, the specific molecular lesion responsible for the cytogenetic finding has not yet been elucidated. Research evidence suggests that the abnormality may involve regions of DNA (of one or more genes) that are particularly susceptible to fluctuations within nucleotide pools, perhaps as a result of viral integration. A relative deficiency of thymidine or deoxycytidine would result in a nucleotide imbalance that, ultimately, may lead to abnormal chromosomal condensation and faulty replication and transcription. Confirmation of this hypothesis awaits further research in the molecular genetics laboratory.

It is intriguing that of all the currently identified fragile sites, that located at Xq27 is the only one associated with a recognizable set of clinical features. This finding may be related to the effects of chromosomal location or to the unique molecular characteristics of the fragile-X site, itself.

Current knowledge indicates that the presence of the fragile-X site is associated with a variable clinical phenotype that involves a spectrum of physical and behavioral features. Common physical findings among affected male subjects include a distinctive facial phenotype (elongated facial contour, high forehead, prominent mandible, and enlarged ears), joint hyperelasticity, and macroorchidism. Frequent behavioral attributes include cognitive impairment, language disability, and psychiatric disorder. An appreciable number of female carriers also are affected and display a variable phenotype that may include some of the physical stigmata, as well as mild mental retardation and behavioral disturbance. Of particular interest to the psychiatrist is the impressive incidence of attention deficit disorder and infantile autism among fragile-X male subjects. The association between fragile-X syndrome and autism is particularly significant. Studies indicate that fragile-X male subjects are at a much greater risk of developing autism than male individuals in the general population. The converse is also true; autistic individuals express the fragile site much more frequently than those without autism. This finding suggests that the fragile-X site may play an etiological role in the development of the autistic syndrome in some individuals. Patients who present with the clinical spectrum described above should be suspected of manifesting the fragile-X syndrome and considered for a more complete diagnostic assessment, including a careful family history, cytogenetic screening, and, if indicated, linkage analysis.

It is significant that the characteristics frequently associated with the syndrome are present to varying degrees among affected male subjects and female carriers. The individual characteristics themselves do tend to cluster with similar prominence in those affected, however (e.g., individuals with moderate to severe mental retardation are likely to manifest a significant degree of facial dysmorphism, macroorchidism, and psychiatric impairment). The occurrence of such phenotypic heterogeneity is most intriguing, especially because the locus of genetic abnormality appears to be quite circumscribed. Current knowledge suggests that a predictable relationship exists between the degree of cytogenetic expression and the presence of clinical characteristics (e.g., gender, intellectual impairment, and to a lesser extent, age (Sutherland, 1979)). Identification of the constitutional and environmental factors that modify the phenotypic expression of the syndrome will require careful evaluations of large fragile-X pedigrees.

The performance of thorough physical and neuroendocrine evaluations of affected individuals and their families will be central to this undertaking. Emphasis should be placed upon assessment of heterozygous females and of the process of pubertal development (through longitudinal studies). Future research also should include neuropsychiatric examinations of fragile-X families in an effort to uncover the factors underlying psychiatric vulnerability and to determine whether a characteristic pattern of psychopathology is, in fact, present: one that distinguishes the fragile-X syndrome from nonspecific forms of mental retardation.

Specific genetic mechanisms have been hypothesized to underlie the variability observed in clinical presentation. Pembrey et al. (1986) have offered an explanation for the inheritance pattern present within families of transmitting male subjects, those phenotypically normal men—up to 20% of the male fragile-X population—who transmit the clinical syndrome to their grandchildren through intellectually normal daughters (Froster-Iskenius et al., 1986a; Webb et al., 1981). These investigators suggest that a premutation (rather than an actual mutation) may be inherited and transmitted by such nonpenetrant men. A premutation consists of a harmless DNA change that becomes activated to produce a definitive mutation following X chromosomal recombination in the ova of unaffected daughters. Differential frequencies of recombination across the fragile site have been hypothesized to underlie the phenotypic heterogeneity present among fragile-X families (Brown et al., 1986c).

Other genetic mechanisms also may be responsible for the presence of phenotypic variability. Autosomal genes, for instance, may serve to modify the expression of the fragile site. In addition, polygenic factors (such as those responsible for intelligence) may contribute to the intrafamilial heterogeneity that has been observed. Clarification of these hypotheses will be aided by research in molecular genetics (e.g., the study of linkage analysis and restriction length polymorphisms).

Environmental factors such as dietary and pharmacological exposures also may play a role in clinical variability. Inborn metabolic disorders such as the aminoacidurias (e.g., PKU) and organic acidemias (e.g., methylmalonic acidemia) serve as examples of the dramatic influence that offending environmental agents may have upon phenotypic expression. Folic acid is one agent that may play a significant role in the cytogenetic and phenotypic expression of the fragile-X syndrome. The current body of data suggests that folate may be of value in ameliorating the behavioral deficits associated with the syndrome. Future studies should focus primarily upon prepubertal subjects, because this group appears to benefit most from folate therapy. In addition, therapeutic trials using prenatal supplementation may become warranted.

The future holds much promise for advances in our understanding of fragile sites and of the fragile-X syndrome in particular. Ultimately, this knowledge will contribute to our appreciation of the relationship between chromosomal abnormality and clinical disease.

REFERENCES

Berkovitz, G. D., Wilson, D. P., Carpenter, N. J., Brown, T. R. & Migeon, C. J. (1986), Gonadal function in men with the Martin-Bell (fragile-X) syndrome. *Amer. J. Med. Genet.,* 23:227–239.

Blomquist, H. K., Gustavson K. H., Holmgren, G., Nordenson, I. & Palsson-Strae, U. (1983), Fragile X syndrome in mildly mentally retarded children in a northern Swedish county. A prevalence study. *Clin. Genet.,* 24:393–399.

———— ———— ———— ———— Sweins, A. (1982), Fragile site X-chromosomes and X-linked mental retardation in severely retarded boys in a northern Swedish county. A previous study. *Clin. Genet.,* 21:209–214.

Branda, R. F., Arthur, O. C. & King, R. A. (1983), Fragile X patients have normal folate metabolism. *Clin. Res.,* 31:290A.

Brondum-Nielsen, K., Tommerup, N., Dyggve, H. V. & Schoa, C. (1982), Macroorchidism and fragile X in mentally retarded males. Clinical, cytogenetic, and some hormonal investigations in mentally retarded males including the fragile site at Xq28, fra(X) (q28). *Hum. Genet.,* 61:113–117.

———— Tommerup, N. & Mikkelsen, M. (1983), Clinical and cytogenetic findings in 26 mentally retarded males with the fragile X. *Clin. Genet.,* 23:241.

Brown, W. T., Jenkins, E. C., Friedman, E. et al. (1982), Autism is associated with the fragile X syndrome. *J. Aut. Develpm. Disord.,* 12:303–307.

———— ———— ———— et al (1984), Folic acid therapy in the fragile X syndrome. *Amer. J. Med. Genet.,* 17:289–297.

———— Cohen, I. L., Fisch, G. S., et al. (1986a), High dose folic acid treatment of fragile X males. *Amer. J. Med. Genet.,* 23:263–271.

———— Jenkins, E. C., Cohen, I. L., et al. (1986b), Fragile X and autism. *Amer. J. Med. Genet.,* 23:341–352.

———— Gross, A. C., Chan, C. B. & Jenkins, E. C. (1986c), DNA linkage studies in the fragile X syndrome suggest genetic heterogeneity. *Amer. J. Med. Genet.,* 23:643–664.

Cantu, J. M., Scaglia, H. E., Medina, M. et al. (1976), Inherited congenital normofunctional testicular hyperplasia and mental deficiency. *Hum. Genet.,* 33:23–33.

———— Scaglia, H. E., Gonzalez-Diddi, M. et al. (1978), Inherited congenital normofunctional testicular hyperplasia and mental deficiency, a corroborative study. *Hum. Genet.,* 41:331–339.

Carpenter, N. J., Leichtman, L. G. & Say, B. (1982), Fragile X-linked mental retardation. A survey of 65 patients with mental retardation of unknown origin. *Amer. J. Dis. Child,* 136:392–398.

_____ Barber, D. H., Jones, M., Lindley, W. & Carr, C. (1983), Controlled six-month study of oral folic acid therapy in boys with fragile X-linked mental retardation. *Amer. J. Med. Genet.,* 35:82A.

Chudley, A. (1984), Behavior phenotype. In: *Conference Report: International Workshop on the Fragile X Syndrome and X-Linked Mental Retardation,* ed. A. Chudley & G. Sutherland. *Amer. J. Med. Genet.,* 17:45–53.

de la Cruz, F. (1985), Fragile X syndrome. *Amer. J. Ment. Defic.,* 90:119–123.

Dykens, E., Leckman, J., Paul, R. & Watson, M. (in press), Cognitive, behavioral and adaptive functioning in fragile X and non-fragile X retarded males. *J. Aut. Develpm. Disord.*

Finelli, P., Pueschel, S. M., Padre-Mendoze, T. & O'Brien, M. (1985), Neurological findings in patients with the fragile-X syndrome. *J. Neurol. Neurosurg. Psychiat.,* 48:150–153.

Fishburn, J., Turner, G., Daniel, A. & Brookwell, R. (1983), The diagnosis and frequency of X-linked conditions in a cohort of moderately retarded males with affected brothers. *Amer. J. Med. Genet.,* 14:713–724.

Fisch, G. S., Cohen, I. L., Wolf, E. G., Brown, W. T., Jenkins, E. C. & Gross, A. (1986), Autism and the fragile X syndrome. *Amer. J. Psychiat.,* 143:71–73.

Froster-Iskenius, U., McGillivray, B. C., Dill, F. J., Hall, J. G. & Herbst, D. S. (1986a), Normal male carriers in the fragile (X) form of X-linked mental retardation (Martin-Bell Syndrome). *Amer. J. Med. Genet.,* 23:619–631.

_____ Bodeker, K., Oepen, T., Matthes, R., Piper, U. & Schwinger, E. (1986b), Folic acid treatment in males and females with fragile-(X)-syndrome. *Amer. J. Med. Genet.,* 23:273–289.

Fryns, J. P. & Van Den Berghe, H. (1982), Transmission of fragile (X)(q27) from normal male(s). *Hum. Genet.,* 61:262–263.

_____ Jacobs, J., Kleczkowska, A. & Van den Berghe, H. (1984), The psychological profile of the fragile X syndrome. *Clin. Genet.,* 25:131–134.

_____ (1986), The female and the fragile X. A study of 144 obligate female carriers. *Amer. J. Med. Genet.,* 23:157–169.

Glover, T. W. (1981), FUdR induction of the X chromosome fragile site: evidence for the mechanism of folic acid and thymidine inhibition. *Amer. J. Hum. Genet.,* 33:234–242.

Goldfine, P. E., McPherson, P. M., Heath, G. A., Hardesty, V. A., Beauregard, L. J. & Gordon, B. (1985), Association of fragile X syndrome with autism. *Amer. J. Psychiat.,* 142:108–110.

Grossman, H., ed. (1983), *Classification in Mental Retardation.* Washington, D.C.: American Association of Mental Deficiency.

Gustavson, K. H., Blomquist, H. K. & Holmgren, G. (1986), Prevalence of the fragile-X syndrome in mentally retarded boys in a Swedish county. *Amer. J. Med. Genet.,* 23:581–587.

Hagerman, R. J. & Smith, A. C. M. (1983), The heterozygous female. In: *The Fragile X Syndrome: Diagnosis, Biochemistry, and Intervention,* ed. R. Hagerman & P. M. McBogg. Dillon, Colo.: Spectra Publishing, pp. 83–94.

_____ Synhorst, D. P. (1984), Mitral valve prolapse and aortic dilatation in the fragile-X syndrome. *Amer. J. Med. Genet.,* 17:123–131.

—— VanHousen, K., Smith, A. C. M. & McGavran, L. (1984), Consideration of connective tissue dysfunction in the fragile-X syndrome. *Amer. J. Med. Genet.*, 17:111–121.

—— Jackson, A. W., Levitas, A. et al. (1986a), Oral folic alcid versus placebo in the treatment of males with the fragile-X syndrome. *Amer. J. Med. Genet.*, 23:241–262.

—— Jackson, A. W., III, Levitas, A., Rimland, B. & Braden, M. (1986b). An analysis of autism in fifty males with the fragile-X syndrome. *Amer. J. Med. Genet.*, 23:359–374.

—— Chudley, A. E., Knoll, J. H., Jackson, A. W., III, Kemper, M. & Ahmad, R. (1986c), Autism in fragile-X females. *Amer. J. Med. Genet.*, 23:375–380.

Hanson, D. M., Jackson, A. W., III & Hagerman, R. J. (1986), Speech disturbances (cluttering) in mildly impaired males with the Martin-Bell/fragile-X syndrome. *Amer. J. Med. Genet.*, 23:195–206.

Hecht, J. T., Scott, C. I., Butler, I. J. & Moore, C. M. (1983), X-linked mental retardation with fragile site at band Xq 2800. *Lancet* 1:986.

Herbst, D. S. (1980), Nonspecific X-linked mental retardation I: a review with information from 24 new families. *Amer. J. Med. Genet.*, 7:443–460.

—— & Miller, J. (1980), Nonspecific X-linked mental retardation II: the frequency in British Columbia. *Amer. J. Med. Genet.*, 7:461–470.

—— Dunn, H., Dill, F., Kalousek, D & Krywanick, L. (1981), Further delineation of X-linked mental retardation. *Hum. Genet.*, 58:366–372.

Jacobs, P. A., Glover, T. W., Mayer, M. et al. (1980), X-linked mental retardation: a study of 7 families. *Amer. J. Med. Genet.*, 7:471–489.

—— Mayer, M. & Abruzzo, M. A. (1986), Studies of the fragile-X syndrome in populations of mentally retarded individuals in Hawaii. *Amer. J. Med. Genet.*, 23:567–572.

Jennings, M., Hall, J. G. & Hoehn, H. (1980), Significance of phenotypic and chromosomal abnormalities in X-linked mental retardation (Martin-Bell or Renpenning Syndrome). *Amer. J. Med. Genet.*, 7:417–432.

Kaiser-McCaw, B. & Hecht, F. (1980), The fragile-X: no dysmorphic syndrome, but a marker. *Amer. J. Hum. Genet.*, 32:114a.

Kemper, M. B., Hagerman, R. J., Ahmad, R. S. & Mariner, R. (1986), Cognitive profiles and the spectrum of clinical manifestations in heterozygous fra(x) females. *Amer. J. Med. Genet.*, 23:139–156.

Labrisseau, A., Jean, P., Messier, B. & Richer, C-L. (1982), Fragile-X chromosome and X-linked mental retardation. *Canad. Med. Assn. J.*, 127:123–126.

Largo, R. H. & Schinzel, A. (1985), Developmental and behavioral disturbances in 13 boys with Fragile-X syndrome. *Eur. J. Pediat.*, 143:269–275.

Lejeune J. (1981), Metabolism of monocarbons and fragile-X syndrome. *Bull. Acad. Natl. Med.* (Paris), 165:1197–1206.

Levitas, A., McBogg, P. & Hagerman, R. (1983), Behavioral dysfunction in the fragile X syndrome. In: *Diagnosis, Biochemistry, and Intervention*, ed. R. Hagerman & P. McBogg. Dillon, Colo.: Spectra Publishing, pp. 153–173.

Loehr, J. P., Synhorst, D. P., Wolfe, R. R. & Hagerman, R. J. (1986), Aortic root dilatation and mitral valve prolapse in the fragile-X syndrome. *Amer. J. Med. Genet.*, 23:189–194.

Lubs, H. A. (1969), A marker X chromosome. *Amer. J. Hum. Genet.*, 21:231–244.

Martin, J. & Bell, S. (1943), A pedigree of mental defect showing sex linkage. *J. Neurol. Psych.,* 6:154–157.

Mattei, M. H., Mattei, J. F., Vidal, I. & Giraud, F. (1981a), Expression in lymphocyte and fibroblast culture of the fragile X chromosome: a new technical approach. *Hum. Genet.,* 59:166–169.

Mattei, J. F., Mattei, M. H., Mattei, M. G., Aumeras, C., Auger, M. & Giraud, F. (1981b), X-linked mental retardation with the fra(x). A study of 15 families. *Amer. J. Med. Genet.,* 59:281–289.

McDermott, A., Walters, R., Howell, R. T. & Gardner, A. (1983), Fragile-X chromosome: clinical and cytogenetic studies on cases from seven families. *Amer. J. Med. Genet.,* 20:169–178.

McGillivray, B. C., Herbst, D. S., Dill, F. J., Sandercock, H. J. & Tischler, B. (1986), Infantile autism: an occasional manifestation of fragile-X mental retardation. *Amer. J. Med. Genet.,* 23:353–358.

Meryash, D. L., Hazen, R. & Gerald, P. S. (1983), Fragile-X syndrome and genital abnormality (abstract). *Pediatr. Res.,* 17:215A.

—— Cronk, C. E., Sachs, B. & Gerald P. S. (1984), An anthropometric study of males with the fragile-X syndrome. *Amer. J. Med. Genet.,* 17:159–174.

Miezejeski, C. M., Jenkins, E. C., Hill, A. L., Wisniewski, K. & Brown, W. T. (1984), Verbal vs. nonverbal ability, fragile X syndrome, and heterozygous carriers. *Amer. J. Hum. Genet.,* 36:227–229.

Mikkelsen, M. (1984), Behavior phenotype. In: *Conference Report: International Workshop on the Fragile-X and X-linked Mental Retardation,* ed. J. M. Opitz & G. R. Sutherland, *Amer. J. Med. Genet.,* 17:5–53.

Murphy, P. D., Kidd, J. R., Breg, W. R., Ruddle, F. H. & Kidd, K. K. (1985), An anonymous single copy X-chromosome clone, DX579, from Xq26-Xq28, identifies a moderately frequent RFLP [HGM 8 provisional no. DX579]. *Nucleic Acids Res.,* 13/8:3015.

—— Watson, M. S., Kidd, K. K. & Breg, W. R. (1986), Molecular approaches to carrier detection and prenatal diagnosis of the fragile X syndrome. *Pediatr. Res.,* 20:269A.

Newell, K., Sanborn, B. & Hagerman, R. (1983), Speech and language dysfunction in the fragile X syndrome. In: *The Fragile X Syndrome: Diagnosis, Biochemistry, and Intervention,* ed. R. Hagerman & P. M. McBogg, Dillon, Colo.: Spectra Publishing, pp. 175–200.

Oberle, I., Drayna, D., Camerino, G., White, R. & Mandel, H. L. (1985), The telomeric region of the human X chromosome long arm: presence of a highly polymorphic DNA marker and analysis of recombination frequency. *Proc. Natl. Acad. Sci.* (U.S.A.), 82:2824–2828.

O'Hare, J. P., O'Brian, I. A. D., Arendt, J. et al. (1986), Does melatonin deficiency cause the enlarged genitalia of the fragile-X syndrome? *Clin. Endocrinol.,* 24:327–333.

Opitz, J. M., Westphal, J. M. & Daniel, A. (1984), Discovery of a connective tissue dysplasia in the Martin-Bell syndrome. *Amer. J. Med. Genet.,* 17:101–109.

Partington, M. W. (1984), The Fragile-X syndrome II: preliminary data on growth and development in males. *Amer. J. Med. Genet.,* 17:175–194.

—— (1986), Female relatives in families with the fragile X syndrome. *Amer. J. Med. Genet.,* 23:111–126.

Paul, R., Cohen, D., Breg, R., Watson, M. & Herman, S. (1984), Fragile-X syndrome: its relation to speech and language disorders. *J. Speech Hear. Disord.,* 49:328–332.

―――― Dykens, E., Leckman, J., Watson, M., Breg, R. & Cohen, D. (in press), A comparison of language characteristics of mentally retarded adults with fragile X syndrome and those with non-specific mental retardation. *J. Aut. Devlpm. Disord.*

Pembrey, M. E., Winter, R. M. & Davies, K. E. (1986), Fragile X mental retardation: current controversies. *TINS,* Feb:58–62.

Penrose, L. S. (1963), *The Biology of Mental Defect.* New York: Grune and Stratton.

Pueschel, S. M., Hays, R. M. & Mendoze, T. (1983), Familial X-linked mental retardation syndrome associated with minor congenital anomalies, macroorchidism, and fragile-X chromosome. *Amer. J. Ment. Defic.,* 87:372–376.

―――― Herman, R. & Groden, G. (1985), Brief Report: Screening children with autism for fragile-X syndrome and phenylketonuria. *J. Aut. Devlpm. Disord.,* 15:335–338.

Pyeritz, R. E., Stamberg, J., Thomas, G. H., Bell, B. B., Zahka, K. G. & Bernhardt, B. A. (1982), The marker Xq28 syndrome ("fragile-X syndrome") in a retarded man with mitral valve prolapse. *Johns Hopkins Med. J.,* 151:231–245.

Reiss, A. L., Feinstein, C., Toomey, K. E., Goldsmith, B., Rosenbaum, K. & Caruso, M. A. (1986), Psychiatric disability associated with the fragile-X syndrome. *Amer. J. Med. Genet.,* 23:393–401.

Renier, W. O., Smeets, D. F. C. M., Scheres, J. M. J. C. et al. (1983), The Martin-Bell Syndrome: a psychological, logopaedic, and cytogenetic study of two affected brothers. *J. Ment. Defic. Res.,* 27:51–59.

Rhoads, F. A. (1982), X-linked mental retardation and fragile-X or marker-X syndrome (letter), *Pediatrics,* 69:668–669.

―――― Oglesby, A. C., Mayer, M. & Jacobs, P. A. (1982), X syndrome in an Oriental family with probable transmission by a normal male. *Amer. J. Med. Genet.,* 12:205–217.

Richards, B. W., Sylvester, P. E. & Broker, C. (1981), Fragile X-linked mental retardation: the Martin-Bell syndrome. *J. Ment. Defic. Res.,* 25:252–256.

Ruvalcaba, R. H. A., Myhre, S. A., Roosen-Runge, E. C. & Beckwith, J. B. (1977), X-linked mental deficiency megalotestes syndrome. *J. Amer. Med. Assn.,* 238:1646–1650.

Schmidt, A. (1982), Fragile site Xq27 and mental retardation. Clinical and cytogenetic manifestations in heterozygotes and hemizygotes of 5 kindreds. *Hum. Genet.,* 60:322–327,

―――― Passarge, E. (1986), Differential expression of fragile site Xq27 in cultured fibroblasts from hemizygotes and heterozygotes and its implications for prenatal diagnosis. *Amer. J. Med. Genet.,* 23:515–525.

Shapiro, L. R., Hasen, J., Gordon, G., Southren, A. L., Wilmont, P. L. & Brenholz, P. (1982), Testicular insufficiency and disordered thyroid metabolism in the fragile-X chromosome syndrome. *Amer. J. Hum. Genet.,* 34:110A.

―――― Wolmot, P. L. & Brenholz, P. (1984), The fragile X syndrome: experience with prenatal diagnosis (abstract). *Amer. J. Hum. Genet.,* 36:196S.

Sherman, S. L., Morton, N. E., Jacobs, P. A. & Turner, G. (1984), The marker (X) chromosome: a cytogenetic and genetic analysis. *Ann. Hum. Genet.,* 48:21–37.

_____ Jacobs, P. A., Morton, N. E. et al. (1985), Further segregation analysis of the fragile X syndrome with special reference to transmitting males. *Hum. Genet.,* 69:289–299.

Sparrow, S., Balla, D. & Cicchetti, D. (1984), Vineland Adaptive Behavior Scales. Circle Pines, Minn.: American Guidance Service.

Sutherland, G. R. (1979), Heritable fragile sites on human chromosomes. I. factors affecting expression in lymphocyte culture. *Amer. J. Hum. Genet.,* 31:125–135.

_____ (1983), The fragile-X chromosome. *Int. Rev. Cytol.,* 81:107–143.

_____ Hecht, F. (1985), Fragile sites on human chromosomes. New York: Oxford University Press, pp. 163–177.

Theobald, T. & Hay, D. (1982, June), *Behavior correlates of the fragile-X syndrome.* Paper presented at the Twelfth Annual Meeting of the Behavior Genetic Association, Fort Collins, Colo.

Tommerup, N., Sondergaard, F., Tonnesen T., Kristensen, M., Arveiler, B. & Schinzel, A. (1985), First trimester prenatal diagnosis of a male fetus with fragile X. *Lancet,* 1:870.

Turleau, C., Czernichow, P., Gorin, R., Royer, P. & DeGrouchy, J. (1979), Debilite mentale life au sexe, visage parlticulier, macroorchide et zone de fragilite de l'X. *Annales de Genetique,* 22:205–209.

Turner, G. & Turner, B. (1974), X-linked mental retardation. *J. Med. Genet.,* 11:109–113.

_____ Eastman, C., Casey, J., McLeary, A., Procopis, P. & Turner, B. (1975), X-linked mental retardation associated with macro-orchidism. *J. Med. Genet.,* 12:367–371.

_____ Brookwell, R., Daniel, A., Selikowitz, M. & Zilibowitz, M. (1980), Heterozygous expression of X-linked mental retardation and the marker X: fra(X)(q27). *New Eng. J. Med.,* 303:662–664.

_____ (1984), Behavior phenotype. In: *Conference Report: International Workshop on the Fragile-X and X-linked Mental Retardation,* ed. J. M. Opitz and G. R. Sutherland. *Amer. J. Med. Genet.,* 17:45–53.

Uchida, I. & Joyce, E. M. (1982), Activity of the fragile-X in heterozygous carriers. *Amer. J. Hum. Genet.,* 34:286–293.

Van der Hagen, C. B., Orstavik, K. H., Bakke, J. & Berg, K. (1983), Monozygous male triplets with mental retardation and a fragile-X chromosome. *Clin. Genet.,* 23:232.

Van Roy, B. C., DeSmedt, M. C., Rues, R. A., Leroy, J. G. & Dumon, J. E. (1983), Fragile-X syndrome transmitted through males. *Clin. Genet.,* 23:219.

Venter, P. A., Gericke, G. S., Dawson, B. & Op't Hof. J. (1981), A marker X chromosome associated with non-specific male mental retardation. The first South African cases. *S. Afr. Med. J.,* 60:807–811.

_____ Op't Hof, J. & Coetzee, D. J. (1986), The Martin-Bell Syndrome in South Africa. *Amer. J. Med. Genet.,* 23:597–610.

Vogel, F. (1984), Mutation and selection in the marker (X) syndrome: a hypothesis. *Ann. Hum. Genet.,* 48:327–332.

Wahlstrom, J., Gillberg, C., Gustavson, K. H. & Holmgren, G. (1986), Infantile autism and the fragile-X. A Swedish multicenter study. *Amer. J. Med. Genet.,* 23:403–408.

Wang, J. C. & Erbe, R. W. (1984), Folate metabolism in cells from fragile-X syndrome patients and carriers. *Amer. J. Med. Genet.,* 17:303–310.

Watson, M. S., Leckman, J. F., Annex, B. et al. (1984), Fragile-X in a survey of 75 autistic males (letter). *New Eng. J. Med.,* 310:1462.

Webb, G. C., Rogers, J. G., Pitt, D. B., Halliday, J. & Theobald, T. (1981), Transmission of fragile (X)(q27) site from a male. *Lancet,* 2:1231–1232.

Webb, T. P., Bundey, S. E., Thake, A. I. & Todd, J. (1986). Population incidence and segregation ratios in the Martin-Bell Syndrome. *Amer. J. Med. Genet.,* 23:573–580.

Wilson, D. P., Carpenter, N. J., Berkovitz, G. P., Brown, T. R. & Migeon, C. F. (1983), Thyroid function in fragile X-linked mental retardation. *Amer. J. Hum. Genet.,* 35:122A.

Zachman, M., Prader, A., Kind, H. P., Hafliger, H. & Budliger, H. (1974), Testicular volume during adolescence cross-sectional and longitudinal studies. *Helv. Paediat. Acta,* 29:61–72.

Part VII

AUTISM

In the 45 years that have elapsed since Kanner first described "Autistic Disturbances of Affective Contact," afflicted children have continued to fascinate both clinicians and researchers to an extent far in excess of their frequency of occurrence in the population. Once considered to be of psychogenic origin, autism is now classified in DSM-III-R as a Pervasive Developmental Disorder characterized by major deficits in the development of both reciprocal social interaction and verbal and nonverbal communicative skills, occurring together with a markedly restricted repertoire of activities and interests.

In the first paper in this section, Prior points out that more progress has been made in describing and measuring behavioral deficits than in solving the puzzle of its etiology. Although the available evidence clearly indicates that autistic symptoms may be correlates of numerous biologically based disorders affecting the central nervous system, our understanding of its mechanism remains speculative. The building and testing of neuropsychological models has been hampered both by limitations in knowledge of brain physiology and of the functional relationships between brain and behavior and by the selection of heterogeneous samples of autistic children for study. Increasingly, the evidence suggests that Autism is not a specific disorder but can occur in many different types of children with many different underlying problems. If the search for etiological factors is to be more productive in the future, it will be necessary to focus on children who are behaviorally homogeneous. The increased specificity of DSM-III-R criteria for the diagnosis of Autistic Disorder may well provide a much-needed basis for the selection of more appropriate research samples.

The social behavior of autistic children has received less attention in the empirical literature than have the cognitive and linguistic deficits that are also characteristic of the disorder. Snow and her co-workers address this relatively neglected area of investigation in their systematic examination of emotional expression of autistic children as it occurs spontaneously in a social context. The data are quantitatively consistent with clinical observation. Young autistic children, videotaped in naturalistic interaction with three different partners, were found to display significantly less positive affect than control children matched for mental and chronological age. When they did smile or laugh, it was just as likely to be a random, self-absorbed way as it was to be related to social interaction. Although the group differences in affective expression were striking, the authors point out that they do not reflect a polarized all-or-none phenomenon. The data suggest that it is not the case that autistic children are uniformly flat in affect or that the affect they do express is always inappropriate or unrelated to the interpersonal context. The autistic children did on occasion display clear episodes of smiling and laughing that were related to the behavior of their partners. Although the frequency of episodes is far lower than is the case with nonautistic children with comparable developmental delays, appropriate, partner-related smiling and laughing does occur in young autistic children.

26

Biological and Neuropsychological Approaches to Childhood Autism

Margot R. Prior
La Trobe University, Bundoora, Victoria, Australia

There is growing conviction that childhood autism is a biologically based disorder. The evidence that has accrued in a variety of areas pertaining to biological abnormality in autism suggests that, with the possible exception of genetic factors, very few data are available that illuminate the autistic disorder specifically. Neurological models which might be useful in guiding further research are discussed and reasons for the slow progress in this important aspect of the study of autism are identified.

Early childhood autism, which traditionally has been considered to be the earliest form of childhood psychosis, has been the subject of a quantity of research greatly out of proportion to its incidence in the population. It is a severe disorder, beginning probably from birth, characterised by major deficits in cognitive and social functioning. In its purest form, autism occurs in less than two children in 10,000 (Lotter, 1966); in its more diluted form, i.e. when diagnostic criteria are less stringent, the incidence is still only about four in 10,000. Its interest to clinicians, researchers and lay people alike is perhaps due to the very mysteriousness of the condition, the fact that most of the children given this diagnosis tend to be attractive and appealing in appearance without outward physical signs of the very serious handicap it entails, and the fact that it is a disorder which is manifest from a very early age.

Early infantile autism was first delineated by Kanner in the early 1940s and is characterised by the following symptoms: extreme aloneness or self-

Reprinted with permission from the *British Journal of Psychiatry*, 1987, Vol. 150, 8–17. Copyright 1987 by the Royal College of Psychiatrists.

isolation and withdrawal from social contact from very early in development, an obsessive need for sameness in the environment and in daily routine, a preoccupation with objects which are often used in peculiar non-functional ways, ritualistic and stereotyped behaviours such as rocking, spinning or manipulation of objects, extreme resistance to new learning, severe language disability which for more than half of cases means muteness and in most of those who do speak, bizarre non-functional language including echolalia, perseverative and stereotyped speech, idiosyncratic use of pronouns and sometimes metaphorical language.

The use of gestures to communicate, and symbolic play are notably absent in infancy (Ricks & Wing, 1976; Prior, 1979). Although Kanner claimed in his original formulations that these children had 'good cognitive potential', it has now been demonstrated repeatedly that most autistic children are moderately or severely retarded and that only a small minority (about one-fifth) show evidence of normal intellectual ability, albeit of a rather uneven and idiosyncratic kind. Autistic children with measured IQs below 40 or 50 have a very poor prognosis (DeMyer *et al*, 1973). Data on intellectual functioning levels together with results of many experimental studies suggest that the disorder is primarily cognitive rather than emotional and consequently the direction of basic research has been adapted to this conceptualisation of the disorder (Rutter, 1983).

In the most recent DSM-III classification of disorders of childhood and adolescence (American Psychiatric Association, 1980), infantile autism is now categorised as a 'pervasive developmental disorder'. This reclassification of autism involves a shift from a perception of the disorder as a psychosis to a perception of a disorder which involves failure to follow the normal developmental process in social, cognitive and psychological spheres.

Psychodynamic aetiology was stressed by Kanner and other early workers, although paradoxically at the same time it was asserted that the disorder was 'inborn' (Kanner, 1943, 1944). On the basis of his observations of the parents of autistic children, Kanner believed that they were 'refrigerator'-type parents—cold, intellectual, obsessive, highly educated people who had been unable to form the normal bonds of attachment with their child. Happily, little credence is given now to this proposition. A number of studies have supported the counter claim, that where it is found that a majority of parents of autistic children are intelligent and highly educated (and this has indeed been the case in a number of studies [e.g. Lotter, 1966; Prior *et al*, 1976]), this has most likely been the result of referral artefacts (Schopler *et al*, 1979; Wing, 1980).

The current consensus of opinion is very much towards a biological basis for childhood autism (Rutter, 1974; Schopler, 1983). However, very much more progress has been made in describing and measuring the behavioural deficits in the disorder than in solving the puzzle of its aetiology. In this paper, research aimed at revealing biologically based abnormalities in autism will be reviewed briefly as a preface to a discussion of current neuropsychological models which might be helpful in guiding future research of an aetiological type.

BIOLOGICAL FACTORS

Because of the rarity of the syndrome, genetic studies are necessarily scant. However, there is accumulating evidence of some kind of genetic influence, albeit of a non-specific kind. The rate of autism and of milder cognitive and language disorders in siblings of autistic children is notably in excess of population-based rates (Lotter, 1966; Spence, 1976; Folstein & Rutter, 1977; August *et al,* 1981; Minton *et al,* 1982).

Ritvo and his colleagues (1982, 1985) have mounted a major study of genetic influences in autism and are investigating families with more than one autistic child in the USA, Canada and France. Although they report that their data are consistent with autosomal recessive inheritance of the disorder, it may not be possible to generalise the results from these very unusual families. In fact, the nature of inheritance is unknown at this stage and only a general influence can be identified. The raised risk of perinatal stress, especially in twin studies, dilutes the force of the genetic hypothesis (Folstein & Rutter, 1977). Furthermore, the well documented excess of males with the disorder has not been explained by any of the genetic theories.

A number of studies have reported significantly more perinatal complications in children who developed autism and childhood psychosis (Kolvin *et al,* 1971; Harper & Williams, 1975; Prior *et al,* 1976; Finegan & Quarrington, 1979; Links *et al,* 1980; Tsai & Stewart, 1983). However, without detailed and accurate records of pregnancy and birth histories, we are hampered by reliance on retrospective reporting by parents which may be particularly suspect when reasons for the severe abnormalities of autism are being sought. Gillberg & Gillberg (1983) have circumvented this problem in their report of a Swedish population study based on extensive and systematic official birth history data. They found high scores for 'reduced optimality' (i.e. pre, post- and neonatal factors which are related to risk) in their sample of autistic children, thus supporting some influence of birth risk factors in at least a proportion of cases.

Major areas of research effort in the search for physiological abnormalities in autism have been neurobiological investigations and EEG, sleep, and evoked potential studies. These areas are replete with methodological difficulties. Despite this the importance of neurobiological factors in the aetiology of autism is argued strongly. Although earlier it was held that autistic children were free from overt signs of brain damage (indeed, in the past this has been one of the exclusionary criteria for the diagnosis of autism), more recent research concerned with neurobiological factors has supported biologically based aetiology. Kolvin *et al* (1971) and Lobascher *et al* (1970) concluded that at least half of their cases showed organic signs, whilst DeMyer *et al* (1972) found that only 14% of their autistic sample were within normal limits on brain dysfunction indices.

Motor milestones are often reported as slow (Kolvin *et al*, 1971; Ornitz *et al*, 1978; DeMyer *et al*, 1981), and DeMyer (1976) has claimed that gross motor abilities involving the lower limbs are at a retarded level although less handicapped than fine motor and ball-handling skill. She sees autistic children as a neurologically disabled group and has described them as 'dyspraxic' (see also Jones & Prior, 1985).

Delayed development of hand preference in autistic children is of a similar order to that reported for retarded children (Colby & Parkinson, 1977) and this has been interpreted as suggestive of neurobiological dysfunction or delay (but see McCann, 1981). Lower levels of functioning have been found in autistic children with mixed handedness compared with those with established dominance (Tsai, 1983; Fein *et al*, 1984b). A review of 13 studies of handedness by Fein *et al* (1984a) showed only two with a real increase in left-handedness, although overall they concluded that left-handedness was about twice as common as in a normal population and almost exactly the same as in retarded and epileptic populations (Satz, 1973). A proportion of neurodevelopmental findings are undoubtedly the result of inclusion of children with a variety of biologically based disorders in which autism is part of the symptoms; nevertheless there does seem good evidence to support the significance of abnormalities in this area. Damasio & Maurer (1978) have emphasised the motor deficits of autistic children and suggested that, in particular, they may implicate basal ganglia structures in the aetiology.

The incidence of reported EEG abnormalities in autistic children ranges from 10 to 83% with an average of 52% (DeMyer *et al*, 1981). However, there are no EEG abnormalities which are unique to the disorder and there is minimal evidence concerning localisation of any EEG abnormalities; most commonly they are distributed diffusely (Waldo *et al*, 1978). Tsai *et al* (1981) have reported a significantly greater incidence of epilepsy and abnormal EEGs in autistic girls as compared with autistic boys, attesting to the greater severity of the disorder in females. Unsurprisingly, cases with normal EEG are likely to have a better long-term outcome (Tsai *et al*, 1985). However, on the basis of a thorough review of psychophysiology in 'early onset psychosis',

James & Barry (1980) could only conclude that "characteristic spontaneous EEG irregularities, indicating some CNS disability *may* exist". The question of interpretation of abnormalities as indicating under- or over-arousal remained unresolved according to their review, although maturational factors were seen as influential. Evidence related to cardiovascular, respiratory and electrodermal activity was similarly inconsistent and inconclusive. Sleep studies (e.g. Ornitz *et al,* 1969; Tanguay, 1977) suggest immaturity in REM sleep but no unique abnormality.

Brainstem dysfunction in autistic children has been explored using brainstem auditory evoked potentials (BAEPs) (Skoff *et al,* 1980; Fein *et al,* 1981; Gillberg *et al,* 1983a). Longer brainstem transmission time and a suggestion of greater abnormalities on the left side of the brain are reported. However, a significant proportion of cases show no abnormalities at all, and some studies do not find prolonged transmission times (Courchesne *et al,* 1984).

A number of researchers have postulated specific brainstem abnormalities as basic to autism. These include Rimland (1964), who suggested the reticular formation, Ornitz (1978), who suggested the vestibular system, MacCulloch & Williams (1971), a dorsal brainstem lesion around the nucleus of the tractus solitarius, Simon (1975), a specific lesion in the inferior colliculi, and Rosenblum *et al* (1980), "neurological dysfunction in the auditory system at the brainstem level". Empirical data to support these hypotheses have not been forthcoming. Tanguay *et al* (1982) have proposed a relationship between abnormal auditory evoked responses, implicating auditory processing deficits in some children, and the maldevelopment of neural substrates at critical early periods. This suggestion is supported by the conclusions of Niwa *et al* (1983) who investigated the P300 component of evoked response potentials in a pitch-discrimination task in autistic subjects. However, the influence of attention deficits and/or auditory processing problems on findings in this area has been investigated insufficiently to allow anything but speculation at this stage.

Biochemical research was reviewed by Piggott in 1979 and found to offer equivocal and inconsistent findings. Variation in biochemical research techniques, lack of normative and developmental data (Ritvo, 1979) and the uncertain influence of mental retardation on reported data contribute to this unsatisfactory state of affairs. There has been much focus on serotonin function areas in the central nervous system because of the theory that abnormalities of serotonin metabolism are related to psychotic disorders (e.g. Ritvo *et al,* 1970; Piggott *et al,* 1975; Yuwiler *et al,* 1975). Hyperserotoninaemia has been reported in approximately one-third of autistic children but is similarly found in many medical and neuropsychiatric disorders and in mental retardation. Its relationship to central nervous system functioning, or to any symptom or behaviour is uncertain (Kuperman *et al,* 1985). DeMyer *et al* (1981) have concluded that 'blood serotonin levels are more strongly related to intellectual status than to psychiatric diagnosis'. Neuroendoncrino-logical studies (Yamazaki *et al,* 1975), immunological studies (Stubbs, 1976; Stubbs *et al,* 1977) and enzyme studies (e.g. Jackson & Garrod, 1978) have also produced some evidence for non-specific abnormalities but no coherent pattern related to a diagnosis of autism has emerged. Gillberg's group reported inferential evidence for the importance of abnormalities of mono-amine metabolism in at least some autistic children (Gillberg *et al,* 1983b).

Wing's claim (1981) that autism is not a single disorder but occurs in combination with many other developmental and organic disorders is consistent with the evidence noted above, i.e. many physiological and biochemical disturbances seen in some autistic children are also seen in children with a wide range of disturbed functioning.

AUTISM ASSOCIATION WITH OTHER DISORDERS

It appears that one of the possible causes of autism may be a viral infection either early in life, or, as an effect later in development of a 'slow virus'. The incidence of autism in rubella children is much in excess of that in the normal population (412 in 10,000 *vs* 2–4 cases per 10,000) (Chess, 1971, 1977) suggesting a specific link between the rubella virus and the development of autism. Chess (1971) has suggested that autism may be one consequence of the invasion of the central nervous system by the rubella virus in the same way as autistic behavioural disturbance can be produced by viral encephalitis. However, any form of brain damage such as that produced by the rubella virus, may increase the risk of the development of behavioural and cognitive handicaps such as those found in autism.

Autism or autistic behaviour is also associated with some other organically based disorders involving retardation, most strongly with tuberous sclerosis, phenylketonuria and encephalitis. It has also been associated with coeliac disease, congenital syphilis, histidinaemia, toxoplasmosis, purine disorder, infantile spasms, Cornelia de Lange syndrome, congenital cytomegalovirus (Stubbs *et al,* 1984), neurofibromatosis (Gillberg & Forsell, 1984) and the fragile X syndrome (Meryash *et al,* 1982; August & Lockhart, 1984). However, the association may be between retardation and autism rather than any relationship with specific syndromes. Study of the symptoms associated with these disorders serves to illustrate the fact that autistic behaviour can be a consequence of various kinds of insults to the nervous system as well as developing without apparent organic origin.

Consideration of these kinds of data suggests a somewhat perturbing trend in biological research in autism. In the eagerness to discover biological markers, a wide variety of cases whose *primary diagnosis* is not autism but who have autistic behaviour is being investigated. Whilst this shows clearly that autistic symptoms may be correlates of numerous biologically based disorders, it does not contribute to our understanding of the basis for autism in the original Kannerian sense of the syndrome. It is important to focus research efforts on the children with no other obvious disorders if we are to contribute to knowledge of aetiological significance in autism. Thus, out of a multitude of studies, little has emerged to illuminate the puzzle of the aetiology of autism. Of the areas considered, genetics seems to offer the most promise for productive further exploration. However, the development of some theoretical underpinning to guide further research may be essential if wasteful 'fishing expeditions' are to be avoided. One approach to such an effort is to take a neuropsychological view of the handicaps of autism and to consider whether this has any advantages in guiding further research.

NEUROPSYCHOLOGICAL APPROACHES

There have been some attempts in recent speculations concerning the causes of autism to formulate some neurological models which can subsume findings in the area so far. For example, an early study by Hauser *et al* (1975) using pneumoencephalography showed enlargement in the ventricular system in a proportion of a sample of autistic children. They suggested a deficiency of substance in the left hemisphere of the brain. Unfortunately their group was a heterogeneous one precluding conclusions specific to autism.

DeLong (1978) concedes that autism probably has multiple aetiologies but suggests that at least for a subgroup a neuropsychological interpretation is relevant. He draws attention to the similarities between symptoms in autism and in the Kluver-Bucy syndrome. This disorder occurs in man as a consequence of bilateral surgical ablations of medial temporal lobes or following herpes simplex encephalitis. "Deficits in the Kluver-Bucy syndrome have been described as an incapacity for adaptive social behaviour, and a loss of recognition of the significance of persons and events. Such patients show an empty blandness, an absence of emotion or concern for family or other persons, and pursue no sustained purpose in activity" (DeLong, 1978). This description does suggest a strong parallel with the most severe and more retarded cases of autism but is less generally apt for the higher functioning group. In addition, autistic children do sometimes show extreme concern for particular (idiosyncratic) events or activities and, at least in middle childhood, for particular people, i.e. empty blandness does not characterise their behaviour in situations important to them, and this may be observed even in the most severe cases.

DeLong also comments on some similarities between autistic behaviour and some features of Korsakoff's psychosis; however, the work of Boucher & Warrington (1976) which was concerned with this issue did not provide convincing evidence for relating the amnesic syndrome to autism. Drawing on the neurological data relating to Korsakoff's psychosis, DeLong (1978) suggested that a left unilateral medial temporal lesion, which impairs verbal learning, and an intact right hemisphere might produce the pattern (which is seen in autism) of adequate learning of places, faces and nonsense patterns together with impaired social interaction and language. The problem of lack of transfer of damaged left hemisphere function to the intact right hemisphere (which would normally be expected in lesions sustained early in life) is accounted for by suggesting that such transfer only occurs when the lesion involves specific left hemisphere cortical areas. DeLong has suggested, as have Prior and her colleagues (Prior, 1979; Hoffman & Prior, 1982), that for the majority of severely retarded cases, where intellectual and social functioning is extremely impaired, damage would have to be bilateral with no right hemisphere compensation or normal development. The idea of unilateral and bilateral damage in accounting for the considerable differences between high and low functioning cases is attractive; however, the clinical picture is not sufficiently clear cut, nor are the neuropsychological data yet compelling enough to consider this idea more than an hypothesis worthy of further investigation. Furthermore, comparisons between ablated monkeys, Kluver-Bucy syndrome adults, alcohol-induced brain damage and a developmental disorder like autism must be considered as tenuous to say the least.

These hypotheses have been evaluated further by Hetzler & Griffin (1981) who have suggested bilateral neuropathology of the temporal lobes of the brain as a significant aetiological factor in autism. Their model is based not only on the Kluver-Bucy amnesic syndrome data but also incorporates evidence relating to developmental dysphasia and Geschwind's (1965) 'disconnection syndrome', as well as a variety of reported organic factors. However, these authors concede the difficulties involved in developing this proposition. Such a model would not account satisfactorily for the high functioning autistic sub-group.

Neurological Models

A speculative neurological model for autism was elucidated by Damasio & Maurer in 1978. Beginning with the observation that the abnormal behaviour in autism is comparable to that seen in brain damaged adults, especially those with frontal lobe, basal ganglia or limbic system damage, they propose that "autism is consequent to dysfunction in a complex of bilateral CNS structures that include mesial frontal lobes, mesial temporal lobes, basal ganglia. . .and thalami. . ." (1978). As evidence for this theory they cite the motility disturbances, abnormalities of muscular tone, posture, gait and akinesia as signs of dysfunction of the basal ganglia, especially the neostriatum and of closely related structures of the medial aspects of the frontal lobes (see also Tsai *et al,* 1981). This also fits with the disturbances of communication, attention and perception which can occur as a result of mesial frontal lobe lesions and basal ganglia abnormalities and which are characteristic of autism. The ritualistic and compulsive behaviours commonly observed in autism are also seen in patients with damaged frontal lobes, especially those with early sustained lesions. The inability to learn by experience, to adapt to changing environments and to organise appropriate responses are common to both autistic and frontal lobe patients. Perseverance, lack of initiative, concreteness, shallow affect and lack of empathy similarly can be observed in individuals with autism and damage to the frontal lobe. Hoffman & Prior (1986) have attempted to explore this hypothesis by administering tests purported to be sensitive to frontal lobe dysfunctioning. Autistic children did indeed show deficits in behaviour mediated by the frontal lobe, e.g. on the Milner Maze Test, where their performance was characterised by inability to form plans or strategies, considerable perseverance, inability to profit from feedback concerning errors and lack of affective response to either correct or incorrect choices. Their performance on the Wisconsin Card Sorting Test suggested impaired conceptualisation abilities, and again perseverance responses were common.

Whilst these hypotheses deserve further investigation, the leap from behavioural observation to physiological abnormality is large and in view of the lack of evidence for lesions in autistic patients the proposed connection between frontal lobe damage and autistic behaviour remains tenuous. It would be encouraging if there were some evidence of structural abnormalities consistent with neuropsychological hypotheses. However, recent computerised axial tomography studies (Hier *et al,* 1979; Damasio *et al,* 1980; Campbell *et al,* 1982; Gillberg & Svendsen, 1983; Prior *et al,* 1984) have offered little support. Although abnormalities are sometimes reported in a proportion of samples, they seem to be characteristic of those children with severe retardation and other organic signs and thus say little specifically about autism. No abnormalities have been observed in high functioning cases (Prior *et al,* 1984). Of course the problem may be biochemical rather than structural, but again there is no evidence to support any hypothesised abnormality.

The speculative nature of these neurological models is well illustrated by the fact that, whilst using the same kind of behavioural evidence, Damasio & Maurer (1978) implicate older cortical structures, whilst Tanguay (1977) suggested the neocortex as the locus of abnormality. Tanguay's suggestion is that autism may be the result of dysfunction in the "frontolimbic system" and that autistic behaviour may be a later reaction to a major early insult. He emphasised the importance of timing in the effects of any neural insult—a theoretically critical issue which can only be investigated properly with comprehensive developmental research (Tanguay & Edwards, 1982). Geschwind & Galaburda (1985) have speculated recently on cerebral lateralisation, biological mechanisms and pathology of various kinds, including developmental disorders such as autism. Whilst their arguments are too complex to be summarised here, the nub of their thesis in relation to autism concerns links between anomalies of handedness, differential rates of development of the right and left cerebral hemispheres and aspects of the immune system. An interesting suggestion is that the worsening of conditions at or near puberty (as, for example, the increase in fits seen in autism) argues for a major role for the sex hormones. They also suggest that the higher incidence of developmental learning disorders (of which autism might be an extreme form) in males may be related to testosterone possibly interacting with genetic influences.

A limbic system model proposed by Lamondella in 1977 has received surprisingly little attention in the autism literature. Lamondella suggests that the limbic system may be the site of dysfunction in autism. This suggestion had in fact been made in 1960 by Schain & Yannet and a related hypothesis had been proposed again in modified form by Deslauriers & Carlson in 1969. Since the limbic system is responsible for arousal, social interaction, emotion, sensory thresholds, attention to novel stimuli, as well as basic communication functions, Lamondella (1977) suggests "intrinsically or extrinsically triggered limbic malfunctions as the cause of early infantile autism". Limbic epilepsy may also be proposed as the cause of the increase in fits in adolescent and young adult autistic cases. Derryberry & Rothbart (1983) have noted that the limbic system seems to be significant in controlling information processing within the cortex via the reticular system and that "direct cortical projections from the limbic systems may serve to alert central processing mechanisms to the presence of a motivationally-relevant stimulus, and to direct attention toward that stimulus".

Lamondella offers a model which divides the limbic system into subsystems that correspond to levels of forebrain organisation all of which are relevant to communicative functions. Level 1 involves primary sign behaviour, Level 2 visceral sign complexes, Level 3 somatic sign schemata and somatovisceral sign learning, Level 4 signal communication, and Level 5 propositional communication. It is hypothesised that in autism there is a breakdown around Level 4 (thalamic level) or in some cases even lower in the system. The thalamus is said to be influential in neocortical speech systems and thus this is relevant to the fact that a universal symptom in autism is language abnormality (Prior *et al*, 1976). Such a model also fits well with Hermelin's (1982) conceptualisation of autism as a failure to develop adequate communication in either thought *or* feeling as a consequence of developmental deficits in genetically preprogrammed capacities for non-verbal as well as verbal communication. The interesting question of critical periods for the development of limbic functions is also pertinent since it brings in the notion of the ability to compensate for damaged limbic components. This factor is unknown in human subjects but data from monkeys suggest that compensation is only possible up to the age of 1 or 2 years. After that time limbic damage has permanent effects on behaviour. Given the belief that autism is supposed to have its onset before the age of 2 or 3 years, it is of interest to speculate on the relationship between age of onset and plasticity in the limbic system. It is claimed that other structures may take over limbic system functions in congenital damage cases.

Although Lamondella's model is difficult to test and lacks support from any extant physiological or neurological studies, it appears worthy of further exploration since it fits well with behavioural observations of autistic children, it incorporates the notions of critical periods and plasticity, it covers the most critical and basic aspects of autism, the social, motivational and communication deficits, and it is not weakened by the findings so far of no particular structural defects in the brains of autistic individuals. It also allows for some heterogeneity in symptoms and could conceivably be elaborated to include some explanation of the fact that a proportion of autistic children do show normal intelligence, can develop language and can make a reasonable adjustment in later life. However, imperfect understanding of the structures and the functions of the limbic system, its relationship with other brain functions and the connexion between structure and function in the individual almost certainly means that we may wait some time before being able to explore this hypothesis productively.

At a somewhat different level of brain organisation are the proposals of Prior and Hoffmann (Prior, 1979, 1984; Hoffmann & Prior, 1982). Drawing together behavioural, psychometric, neurophysiological and experimental evidence, they have suggested that it appears that much of the behaviour of higher functioning autistic children, at least, reflects mediation or control of function by the right hemisphere of the brain. Hoffman & Prior (1982) have presented evidence which shows that higher functioning autistic children perform according to their chronological age level on tests purporting to assess right brain functions but are grossly handicapped, in fact perform more poorly than mental age-matched (and therefore younger) controls, on tests purporting to assess left brain functions. In addition, there is some evidence from dichotic listening studies (Prior & Bradshaw, 1975) and from evoked potential data suggesting abnormal lateralisation of function (Dawson *et al,* 1982, 1986). It is not yet clear whether this pattern of performance in autistic children reflects immaturity (with right hemisphere and less mature strategies being used in all cognitively demanding situations) or whether there is in fact selective damage to the left hemisphere in a subgroup of autistic children who may have been able to compensate for such damage by greater development of the right hemisphere permitting the attainment of quasi-normal intelligence except on tests of high language content.

There are a number of theoretical problems with this model, especially since, if autism has its onset early in life, there ought to be more effective compensation for lateralised damage in the infant brain. Bilateral damage would have to be proposed for the low functioning majority of autistic children who share many of the behavioural symptoms while lacking the intellectual and language attainments of the high functioning group. If it were considered that the two groups represent different disorders, of course this problem would be resolved in part at least. Reference to Kanner's early discussions of the disorder suggest that early cases of infantile autism did not show the degree of global retardation which characterises so many of the cases now called autistic. Despite these caveats, there is some further support for the proposals in a study of lower functioning autistic children using the Halstead-Reitan Neuropsychological Test Battery for Children (Dawson, 1983), where results essentially similar to those of Hoffman & Prior (1982) were found with significantly greater left than right hemisphere dysfunction. However, Dawson was careful to note that only five autistic children showed left hemisphere impairment alone, while the remaining five showed involvement of both hemispheres. Failure to develop the usual symbolic functions of the left hemisphere, in particular language and gesture, is hardly surprising since autistic children appear to be detached from normal social, cognitive and linguistic experiences during the early developmental period. Thus, atypical hemisphere functioning is perhaps to be expected.

Lamondella has suggested that the two hemispheres may process limbic input differentially. This allows some connecting threads to be drawn between his model and the hemispheric dysfunction proposals. Lamondella notes support for the hypothesis of differential interaction of right and left hemispheres with limbic functions and suggests that integration of the two functional areas may occur via systems which could in turn be part of the limbic system. Further exploration of such a hypothesis may well be very profitable. Fein *et al* (1984*a*) have been critical of the hypothesis of left hemisphere dysfunction on the grounds that it lacks corroborative anatomical and physiological data, and are sceptical regarding its applicability to low functioning cases and the perceived overemphasis of the language disorder in autism with de-emphasis of the social impairments. They also note the marked individual differences across cases and the likelihood of similar variation in the biological/neural substrates of the disorder. However, this does not mean that investigations permitted by more sophisticated techniques of measurement of brain function at various levels will not prove illuminating on this proposal.

It is also helpful to consider Luria's (1973) model of brain function, which is based on the idea of three zones—primary, secondary and tertiary—each zone being dependent on adequate development of the preceding structures and functions. Abnormality in the primary functional area leading to inadequacy in processing of sensory information will in turn affect higher cortical processes. The development and interaction of these zones in young children is seen as a 'bottom-upwards' process, with intact lower zones necessary for adequately functioning higher zones—the secondary and tertiary areas. Thus multiple impairments in a number of areas can occur as a consequence of insult or deficits in a single primary area. This principle of hierarchical development of the brain could then explain the varying consequences of early damage to the limbic system (see also Tanguay & Edwards, 1982).

CONCLUSIONS

Consideration of the research concerned with biological factors in childhood autism shows that we appear to have made little progress in the search for specific aetiologies. It seems that we may not be very much closer to finding causes than we were 40 years ago when the search began. There are some obvious reasons for this lack of progress despite considerable quantities of research. In summary, they are:

(a) the use of heterogeneous samples of autistic children who, whilst they all exhibit autistic behaviour, do so for many different and sometimes obvious reasons;

(b) methodological and measurement problems in biological research which make findings difficult to replicate and to interpret;

(c) lack of normative developmental data in most of the areas studied making comparisons between autistic and other groups difficult to interpret;

(d) failure to take account of retardation factors in sample selection and measurement;

(e) the primitive nature of our knowledge of brain physiology and of the functional relationships between brain and behaviour.

It certainly appears at this stage that a search for a unique cause for autism may be fruitless. A variety of neuropathological conditions may produce broadly defined behaviour symptoms. Wing (1981) and others argue strongly, and many researchers who work with autistic children imply, that autism may not be a specific disorder but can occur in many very different types of children with many different underlying problems. If the search for aetiological factors in childhood autism is to be more productive in future, it will be necessary to focus on 'pure' cases (as far as this is possible), who are preferably high functioning, thus minimising the influence of retardation. Equally important is hypothesis-testing on the basis of theoretical models that could account for the core features of the disorder and that arise from, and are consistent with, current neuropsychological data.

REFERENCES

August, G. & Lockhart, L. (1984) Familial autism and the fragile-x chromosome. *Journal of Autism and Developmental Disorders, 14,* 197–204.

———, Stewart, M. & Tsai, L. (1981) The incidence of cognitive disabilities in the siblings of autistic children. *British Journal of Psychiatry, 138,* 416–422.

Boucher, J. & Warrington, E. K. (1976) Memory deficits in early infantile autism: some similarities to the Amnesic Syndrome. *British Journal of Psychology, 67,* 73–87.

Campbell, M., Rosenbloom, S., Perry, R., George, A., Kricheff, I., Anderson, L., Small, A. & Jennings, S. (1982) Computerized axial tomography in young autistic children. *American Journal of Psychiatry, 139,* 510–512.

Chess, S. (1971) Autism in children with congenital rubella. *Journal of Autism and Childhood Schizophrenia, 1,* 33–47.

——— (1977) Follow-up report on autism in congenital rubella. *Journal of Autism and Childhood Schizophrenia, 7,* 68–81.

Colby, K. M. & Parkinson, C. (1977) Handedness in autistic children. *Journal of Autism and Childhood Schizophrenia, 7,* 3–9.

Courchesne, E., Kilman, B., Galambos, R. & Lincoln, A. (1984) Autism: processing of novel information assessed by event-related brain potentials. *Electroencephalography and Clinical Neurophysiology, 59,* 238–248.

Damasio, A. R. & Maurer, R. G., (1978) A neurological model for childhood autism. *Archives of Neurology, 35,* 777–786.

Damasio, H., Maurer, R. G., Damasio, A. R. & Chui, H. C. (1980) Computerized tomographic scan findings in patients with autistic behaviour. *Archives of Neurology, 37,* 504–510.

Dawson, G. (1983) Lateralized brain dysfunction in autism: Evidence from the Halstead-Reitan Neuropsychological Battery. *Journal of Autism and Developmental Disorders, 13,* 269–286.

——, Warrenburg, S. & Fuller, P. (1982) Cerebral lateralization in individuals diagnosed as autistic in early childhood. *Brain and Language, 15,* 353–368.

——, Finley, C., Phillips, S. & Galpert, L. (1986) Hemispheric specialization and the language abilities of autistic children. (In press).

DeLong, G. R. (1978) A neuropsychologic interpretation of infantile autism. In *Autism: A Reappraisal of Concepts and Treatment* (eds M. Rutter and E. Schopler). New York: Plenum.

DeMyer, M. (1976) Motor, perceptual-motor and intellectual disabilities of autistic children. In *Early Childhood Autism* (ed. L. Wing). 2nd ed., Oxford: Pergamon Press.

——, Barton, S. & Norton, J. A. (1972) A comparison of adaptive, verbal and motor profiles of psychotic and nonpsychotic subnormal children. *Journal of Autism and Childhood Schizophrenia, 2,* 359–377.

——, ——, DeMyer, W., Norton, J., Allen, J. & Steele, R. (1973) Prognosis in autism: a follow-up study. *Journal of Autism and Childhood Schizophrenia, 3,* 199–246.

——, Hingtgen, J. N. & Jackson, R. K. (1981) Infantile autism reviewed: a decade of research. *Schizophrenia Bulletin, 7,* 388–451.

Derryberry, D. & Rothbart, M. (1983) Emotion, attention and temperament. In *Emotion, Cognition and Behavior* (eds C. Izard, J. Kagan and R. Zajonc) New York: Cambridge University Press.

Deslauriers, A. & Carlson, C. (1969) *Your Child is Asleep.* Illinois: Dorsey.

Fein, D., Skoff, B. & Mirsky, A. (1981) Clinical correlates of brainstem dysfunction in autistic children. *Journal of Autism and Developmental Disorders, 11,* 303–315.

——, Humes, M., Kaplan, E., Lucci, D. & Waterhouse, L. (1984*a*) The question of left hemisphere dysfunction in infantile autism. *Psychological Bulletin, 95,* 258–281.

——, Waterhouse, L., Lucci, D., Snyder, D. & Humes, M. (1984*b*) Cognitive functions in left and right-handed autistic children. Paper presented at the meeting of the International Neuropsychological Society, Houston, Texas.

Finegan, J. & Quarrington, B. (1979) Pre-, peri-, and neonatal factors and infantile autism. *Journal of Child Psychology and Psychiatry, 20,* 119–128.

Folstein, S. & Rutter, M. (1977) Infantile autism: a genetic study of 21 twin pairs. *Journal of Child Psychology and Psychiatry, 18,* 297–322.

Geschwind, N. (1965) Disconnection syndromes in animals and man. *Brain, 88,* 237–294.

Geschwind, N. & Galaburda, A. (1985) Cerebral lateralization. Biological mechanisms, association, and pathology: I A hypothesis and a program for research. *Archives of Neurology, 42,* 428–459.

Gillberg, C. & Gillberg, J. (1983) Infantile autism: a total population study of reduced optimality in the pre-, peri-, and neonatal period. *Journal of Autism and Developmental Disorders, 13,* 153–166.

—— & Svendsen, P. (1983) Childhood psychosis and computed tomographic brain scan findings. *Journal of Autism and Developmental Disorders, 13,* 19–32.

—— & Forsell, C. (1984) Childhood psychosis and neurofibromatosis—more than a coincidence. *Journal of Autism and Developmental Disorders, 14,* 1–8.

_____, Rosenhall, U. & Johansson, E. (1983*a*) Auditory brainstem responses in childhood psychoses. *Journal of Autism and Developmental Disorders, 13,* 181–195.

_____, Svennerholm, L. & Hamilton-Hellberg, C. (1983*b*) Childhood psychosis and monoamine metabolites in spinal fluid. *Journal of Autism and Developmental Disorders, 13,* 383–396.

Harper, J. & Williams, S. (1975) Age and type of onset as critical variables in early infantile autism. *Journal of Autism and Child Schizophrenia, 5,* 25–36.

Hauser, S. L., DeLong, G. R. & Rosman, N. P. (1975) Pneumographic findings in the infantile autistic syndrome. *Brain, 98,* 667–688.

Hermelin, B. (1982) Thoughts and feelings. *Australian Autism Review, 1,* 10–19.

Hetzler, B. & Griffin, J. (1981) Infantile autism and the temporal lobe of the brain. *Journal of Autism and Developmental Disorders, 11,* 317–330.

Hier, D. B., LeMay, M. & Rosenberger, P. B. (1979) Autism and unfavorable left-right asymmetries of the brain. *Journal of Autism and Developmental Disorders, 19,* 153–159.

Hoffmann, W. & Prior, M. (1982) Neuropsychological dimensions of autism in children: a test of the hemispheric dysfunction hypothesis. *Journal of Clinical Neuropsychology, 4,* 27–42.

_____ & _____ (1986) Frontal lobe deficits in autistic children. In preparation.

Jackson, M. J. & Garrod, P. J. (1978) Plasma, zinc, copper and amino acid levels in blood of autistic children. *Journal of Autism and Childhood Schizophrenia, 8,* 203–208.

James, A. L. & Barry, R. J. (1980) A review of psychophysiology in early onset psychosis. *Schizophrenia Bulletin, 6,* 506–525.

Jones, V. & Prior, M. (1985) Motor imitation abilities and neurological signs in autistic children. *Journal of Autism and Developmental Disorders, 15,* 37–46.

Kanner, L. (1943) Autistic disturbances of affective contact. *Nervous Children, 2,* 217–250.

_____ (1944) Early infantile autism. *Journal of Pediatrics, 25,* 211–217.

Kolvin, I., Ounsted, C., Humphrey, N. & McNay, A. (1971) Six studies in the Childhood Psychoses. II—Phenomenology of Childhood Psychoses. *British Journal of Psychiatry, 118,* 385–395.

Kuperman, S., Beeghly, J., Burns, T. & Tsai, L. (1985) Serotonin relationships of autistic probands and their first-degree relatives. *Journal of the American Academy of Child Psychiatry, 24,* 186–190.

Lamondella, J. (1977) The limbic system in human communication. In *Studies in Neurolinguistics (eds H. Whitaker and H. A. Whitaker). New York: Academic Press.*

Links, P. S., Stockwell, M., Abichandani, F. & Simeon, J. (1980) Minor physical anomalies in childhood autism. 1: Their relationship to prenatal and perinatal complications. *Journal of Autism and Developmental Disorders, 10,* 273–285.

Lobascher, M., Kingerlee, P. & Gubbay, S. (1970) Childhood autism: aetiological factors in 25 cases. *British Journal of Psychiatry, 117,* 525–529.

Lotter, V. (1966) Epidemiology of autistic conditions in young children. I. Prevalence. *Social Psychiatry, 1,* 124–137.

Luria, A. R. (1973) *The Working Brain.* London: Penguin.

MacCulloch, M. & Williams, C. (1971) On the nature of infantile autism. *Acta Psychiatrica Scandinavia, 47,* 295–314.

McCann, B. S. (1981) Hemispheric asymmetries and early childhood autism. *Journal of Autism and Developmental Disorders, 11,* 401–411.

Meryash, D., Szymanski, L. & Park, S. (1982) Infantile autism associated with the Fragile-X syndrome. *Journal of Autism and Developmental Disorders, 12,* (3), 295–301.

Minton, J., Campbell, M., Green, W., Jennings, S. & Samit, C. (1982) Cognitive assessment of siblings of autistic children. *Journal of the American Academy of Child Psychiatry, 21,* 256–261.

Niwa, S., Ohta, M. & Yamazaki, K. (1983) P300 and stimulus evaluation process in autistic subjects. *Journal of Autism and Developmental Disorders, 13,* 33–42.

Ornitz, E. (1978) Neurophysiologic studies. In *Autism: A Reappraisal of Concepts and Treatment* (eds M. Rutter & E. Schopler). New York: Plenum Press.

——, Ritvo, E., Brown, M., La Franchi, S., Parmelee, T. & Walter, R. (1969) The EEG and rapid eye movements during REM sleep in autistic and normal children. *Electroencephalography and Clinical Neurophysiology, 26,* 167–175.

——, Guthrie, D. & Farley, A. (1978) The early symptoms of childhood autism. In *Cognitive Deficits in the Development of Mental Illness* (ed. G. Serban). New York: Brunner/Mazel.

Piggott, L. R. (1979) Overview of selected basic research in autism. *Journal of Autism and Developmental Disorder, 9,* 199–217.

——, Frohman, C., Ward, V. & Gottlieb, J. (1975) The effect of plasma from psychotic children on tryptophan uptake in chicken erythrocytes. *Neuropsychobiology, 1,* 284–295.

Prior, M. (1979) Cognitive abilities and disabilities in infantile autism: A review. *Journal of Abnormal Child Psychology, 7,* 357–380.

—— (1984) Developing concepts of childhood autism: The influence of experimental cognitive research. *Journal of Consulting and Clinical Psychology, 52,* 4–16.

—— & Bradshaw, J. L. (1975) Hemispheric functioning in autistic children. *Cortex, 15,* 73–81.

——, Gajzago, C. & Knox, D. (1976) An epidemiological study of autistic and psychotic children in the four eastern states of Australia. *Australia and New Zealand Journal of Psychiatry, 10,* 173–184.

——, Tress, B., Hoffmann, W. & Boldt, D. (1984) Computed tomographic study of children with classic autism. *Archives of Neurology, 41,* 482–484.

Ricks, D. M. & Wing, L. (1976) Language, communication and the use of symbols. In *Early Childhood Autism* (ed. L. Wing). New York: Pergamon Press.

Rimland, B. (1964) *Infantile Autism.* New York: Appleton-Century-Crofts.

Ritvo, E. (1979) *Autism: Diagnosis, Current Research and Management.* New York: Spectrum.

Ritvo, E., Yuwiler, A., Geller, E., Ornitz, E., Saeger, K & Plotkin, S. (1970) Increased blood serotonin and platelets in early infantile autism. *Archives of General Psychiatry, 23,* 566–572.

——, Ritvo, E. C. & Brothers, A. M. (1982) Genetic and immunohematological factors in autism. *Journal of Autism and Developmental Disorders, 12,* 109–114.

——, Spence, A., Freeman, B., Mason-Brothers, A., Mo, A. & Marazita, M. (1985) Evidence for autosomal recessive inheritance in 46 families with multiple incidences of autism. *American Journal of Psychiatry, 142,* 187–192.

Rosenblum, S., Arick, J., Krug, D., Stubbs, E., Young, N. & Pelson, R. (1980) Auditory brainstem evoked responses in autistic children. *Journal of Autism and Developmental Disorders, 10,* 215–226.

Rutter, M. (1974) The development of infantile autism. *Psychological Medicine, 4,* 147–163.

—— (1983) Cognitive deficits in the pathogenesis of autism. *Journal of Child Psychology and Psychiatry, 24,* 513–532.

Satz, P. (1973) Left-handedness and early brain insult: An explanation. *Neuropsychology, 11,* 115–117.

Schain, R. J. & Yannet, H. (1960) Infantile autism: An analysis of 30 cases and a consideration of certain neurophysiological concepts. *Journal of Pediatrics, 57,* 560–567.

Schopler, E. (1983) New Developments in the definition and diagnosis of autism. In *Advances in Clinical Child Psychology* (ed. A. Kazdin) Vol. 6. New York: Plenum.

———, Andrews, C. & Strupp, K. (1979) Do autistic children come from upper-middle-class parents? *Journal of Autism and Developmental Disorders, 9,* 139–152.

Simon, N. (1975) Echolalic speech in childhood autism: Consideration of possible underlying loci of brain damage. *Archives of General Psychiatry, 32,* 1439–1446.

Skoff, B., Mirsky, A. & Turner, D. (1980) Prolonged brainstem transmission time in autism. *Psychiatry Research, 2,* 157–166.

Spence, M. A. (1976) Genetic studies. In *Autism: Diagnosis, Current Research and Management* (ed. E. Ritvo). New York: Halstead/Wiley.

Stubbs, E. (1976) Autistic children exhibit undetectable hemagglutination-inhibition antibody titers despite previous rubella vaccination. *Journal of Autism and Childhood Schizophrenia, 6,* 269–274.

———, Crawford, M., Burger, D. & Vanderbart, A. (1977) Depressed lymphocyte responsiveness in autistic children. *Journal of Autism and Childhood Schizophrenia, 7,* 49–55.

———, Ash, E. & Williams, C. (1984) Autism and Congenital Cytomegalovirus. *Journal of Autism and Developmental Disorders, 14,* 183–190.

Tanguay, P. (1977) Clinical and electrophysiological research. In *Autism: Diagnosis, Current Research and Management* (ed. E. Ritvo). New York: Spectrum.

——— & Edwards, R. M. (1982) Electrophysiological studies of autism: The whisper of the bang. *Journal of Autism and Developmental Disorders, 12,* 177–184.

———, Edwards, R., Buchwald, J., Schwafel, J. & Allen, V. (1982) Auditory brainstem evoked responses in autistic children. *Archives of General Psychiatry, 39,* 174–180.

Tsai, L. Y. (1983) The relationship of handedness to the cognitive, language and visuo-spatial skills of autistic patients. *British Journal of Psychiatry, 142,* 156–162.

——— & Stewart, M. A. (1983) Etiological implication of maternal age and birth-order in infantile-autism. *Journal of Autism and Developmental Disorders, 13,* 57–65.

———, Stewart, M. & August, G. (1981) Implication of sex differences in the familial transmission of infantile autism. *Journal of Autism and Developmental Disorders, 11,* 165–173.

———, Tsai, M. & August, G. (1985) Brief report: Implication of EEG diagnosis in the subclassification of Infantile Autism. *Journal of Autism and Developmental Disorders, 15,* 339–344.

Waldo, M., Cohen, D., Caparulo, E., Young, J., Prichard, J. & Shaywitz, B. (1978) EEG profiles of neuropsychiatrically disturbed children. *Journal of the American Academy of Child Psychiatry, 17,* 656–670.

Wing, L. (1980) Childhood autism and social class: A question of selection? *British Journal of Psychiatry, 137,* 410–417.

——— (1981) Sex ratios in early childhood autism and related conditions. *Psychiatry Research, 5,* 129–137.

Yamazaki, K., Saito, Y., Okada, F., Fujieda, T. & Yamashita, I. (1975) An application of neuroendocrinological studies in autistic children and Heller's syndrome. *Journal of Autism and Childhood Schizophrenia, 5,* 323–332.

Yuwiler, A., Ritvo, E. R., Geller, E., Glousman, R., Schneiderman, G. & Matsuno, D. (1975) Uptake and efflux of serotonin from platelets of autistic and nonautistic children. *Journal of Autism and Childhood Schizophrenia, 5,* 83–98.

PART VII: AUTISM

27

Expression of Emotion in Young Autistic Children

Margaret Ellis Snow, Margaret E. Hertzig, and Theodore Shapiro

Cornell University Medical College, New York, New York

Expression of emotion was examined in a group of 10 preschool-aged autistic children and a control group of 10 developmentally delayed children matched for chronological and mental age. Each child was videotaped for 15 minutes of interaction with the mother, a child psychiatrist, and the nursery school teacher. Affective expression was recorded using a behavior checklist. The autistic child was found to display less positive affect than the delayed children (p < 0.01). In addition, the positive affect displayed by the autistic children was less likely to be partner-related and more likely to be related to self-absorbed activity than was the case with the delayed children (p < 0.001). The groups were not found to differ in the frequency of negative affect.

In his original statement, Kanner (1943) described the hallmark of infantile autism as "an innate inability to form the usual, biologically provided affective contact with people" (p. 250). Although this deficit in social relatedness has remained the most salient clinical feature of autism, it has received less attention in the empirical literature than the cognitive and linguistic deficits that are also typical of the disorder. Most of what is now known about autistic children's cognitive and language deficits derives from precise research findings, whereas documentation of certain aspects of these children's social functioning remains based on clinical anecdote.

Reprinted with permission from the *Journal of the American Academy of Child and Adolescent Psychiatry*, 1987, Vol. 26, No. 6, 836–838. Copyright 1987 by the American Academy of Child and Adolescent Psychiatry.

This discrepancy is probably related to the fact that over the past two decades autism has been viewed primarily as a cognitively based disorder, in which social deviance emerges secondarily (Hermelin and O'Conner, 1970; Reichler and Schopler, 1971; Rutter, 1978). In addition, it has been the case in psychological research in general that more sophisticated methods were available for studying cognition and language than for examining social and emotional functioning. Recently, however, advances in videotape technology have presented the opportunity for a much more sophisticated approach to studying social and emotional functioning. Along with these methodological advances have come a renewed interest in the social deficits of autism and a developing conception of these social deficits as being more than just epiphenomena of a primary cognitive disorder (Fein et al., 1986) It should no longer be the case that our descriptions of the many complex aspects of autistic children's social functioning be without grounding in systematically collected data.

One facet of social relatedness that has been anecdotally described as deviant in autism is the expression of emotion, or affect. In normal babies, emotional expression has been demonstrated to play a crucial role in establishing and regulating adaptive interpersonal contact from the earliest months of life (Bretherton et al., 1986). Young autistic children on the other hand, have been described as being markedly underresponsive, labile, and/or inappropriate in their expression of affect. The literature is lacking in naturalistic investigations of autistic children's facial expression of emotion; however, the few studies that have examined older autistic subjects' ability to identify and imitate affective expression in controlled task situations have found significant deficits in these skills (Hertzig and Snow, 1985; Hobson, 1986; Jennings, 1973; Langdell, 1978, 1981). It was the goal of the present study to further explore this neglected area by examining affective expression in young autistic children as it occurred spontaneously in a social context.

A group of autistic children was compared with a matched sample of nonautistic, developmentally delayed children in an effort to determine whether any perceived deficits in affective expression might simply be the expectable outcome of developmental immaturity. Children were videotaped in naturalistic interaction with three different partners, and the frequency of expressed affect, as well as its relatedness to aspects of the interpersonal context, were measured.

METHOD

Subjects

Subjects were randomly selected from a therapeutic nursery school associated with The New York Hospital Department of Psychiatry. Their socioeconomic backgrounds ranged from working class to upper-middle-class. The two groups consisted of 10 children each, matched for chronological age and nonverbal mental age (as measured by the Adaptive Scale of the Gesell Developmental Examination, Knobloch et al., 1980). Each group consisted of 9 boys and 1 girl. The children ranged in age from 2 years, 6 months, to 4 years. Their mental ages ranged from 1 year to 3 years, 6 months. The mean chronological age was 3 years, 4 months in both groups (Autistic groups S.D., 4.71; Delayed group S.D., 5.34). The mean mental age was 2 years, 3 months in both groups (Autistic group S.D., 8.85; Delayed group S.D., 8.28). Gesell developmental quotients for nonverbal intelligence ranged from moderately retarded to average in both groups, with means in the mildly retarded range. Although children were not matched for language levels, the mean language ages (as measured by the Gesell) did not differ significantly in the two groups. All Autistic children met DSM-III criteria for the disorder as judged by psychiatrists who were not involved in the study. The Delayed group included five children with mental retardation and five with specific developmental disorders, as defined by DSM-III. They, too, were diagnosed by psychiatrists not involved in the study.

Procedure

Data used in the present study were extracted from a more extensive videotaped session, routinely done for evaluation and research purposes in the therapeutic nursery. In that session, children were observed interacting with three different partners: the mother, an unfamiliar child psychiatrist (male), and the nursery school teacher (female). The children had known their teacher for approximately 1 month. The interactions took place in a comfortable room containing a small table and chairs and an assortment of toys. The children's mothers remained present during the interactions with the psychiatrist and teacher, and they observed unobtrusively from a chair at the side of the room. During the sections of videotape used in the present study, the adults were told to interact with the children "just as they normally would."

Videotapes were coded using a behavior checklist. During each 15-second interval (an audiotaped "beep" sounded every 15 seconds) a coder recorded the presence of the following operationally defined child behaviors: smile, giggle/laugh, positive squeal, frown, fuss/cry, and negative scream/yell. Each time a behavior was checked it was also categorized as to its relation to the immediate context. The following categories were used: random-unrelated (having no apparent connection to anything in the social or physical environment, solitary-play-related (contingent upon the child's independent play activity), and partner-related (occurring during interaction with the partner). Only those 15-second intervals in which the child's face was visible on the screen were deemed codable. Uncodable intervals were not counted in the total observation time. Five minutes (or 20 15-second intervals) of interaction with each partner were accumulated, resulting in a total of 15 minutes (or 60 15-second intervals) of coded behavior for each child.

RESULTS

For the present study the following composite scores were used: *Total Affect* (total number of 15-second intervals in which one or more of the checklist behaviors occurred, out of a possible total of 20 per partner (5 minutes) or 60 across the three partners (15 minutes); *Positive Affect* (total number of intervals in which one or more of the following behaviors occurred: smile, giggle/laugh, and positive squeal); and *Negative Affect* (total number of intervals in which one or more of the following behaviors occurred; frown, fuss/cry, and negative scream/yell). To determine interrater reliability, a second coder independently recorded the behavior of a subsample of six children (30% of the full sample), yielding reliability coefficients from 0.81 to 1.00, with a mean of 0.92.

Data analysis was oriented toward answering three basic questions: (1) Did the autistic children differ from the developmentally delayed children in overall frequency of affect? (2) Did the frequency of affect vary according to whom the child was interacting with (mother versus psychiatrist versus teacher)? (3) How was affect related to the immediate context (random-unrelated versus solitary-play-related versus partner-related), and did this differ in the two groups of children?

Table 1 displays the means and S.D. of Positive Affect, Negative Affect, and Total Affect (means are based on sums across the three partners, for a possible total of 60 intervals). Results of a multivariate analysis of variance (examining frequency of Positive and Negative Affect across the three partners in the two groups) yielded a significant main effect of "group" ($F = 4.14$, $p < 0.05$), indicating that the Autistic children displayed significantly less affect that did the Delayed children. Separate univariate analyses of variance indicated that this group difference was caused almost completely by a significant difference in Positive Affect ($F = 8.35, p < 0.01$). The Autistic group displayed Positive Affect in only 11 of 60 intervals, whereas the Delayed group displayed more than twice that amount. Negative Affect, in contrast, occurred rarely in both groups and did not differ in frequency between the two groups (F, 0.05; p, N.S.).

Table 1. Number of Intervals of Positive Affect, Negative Affect, and Total Affect, out of a Possible Total of 60

	Autistic		F	Delayed	
	Mean	S.D.		Mean	S.D.
Positive Affect	11.00	10.08	8.35**	27.0	14.68
Negative Affect	2.3	1.95	NS	2.5	3.75
Total Affect	13.3	9.3	4.14*	29.5	15.19

$* p < 0.05$; $** p < 0.01$.

Positive and Negative Affect are broken down according to the three partners in Table 2. Multivariate analysis of variance did not yield a significant main effect of "partner" (mother versus psychiatrist versus teacher) (F, 2.72; p, N.S.), indicating that, in the two groups combined, affect did not vary significantly according to whom the child was interacting with. A significant interaction effect of "group" X "partner" ($F = 4.46, p < 0.05$), however, revealed that the patterns of scores across partners did differ in the two groups. Univariate analyses of variance indicated that this interaction effect was caused not by Positive Affect, which was essentially the same across partners in both groups (F, 0.41; p, N.S.), but to Negative Affect, which was not distributed similarly in the two groups ($F = 6.68, p < 0.01$). Post hoc multiple comparison Bonferoni t tests indicated that, whereas Negative Affect was essentially evenly distributed across partners in the Delayed group, it was not in the Autistic group. The Autistic group displayed significantly more Negative Affect in their interactions with the unfamiliar psychiatrist than they did with either the mother or the teacher (t values > 3.14, p values < 0.05).

Table 3 breaks down the frequency of Positive Affect according to the three categories of contextual relatedness. The overall frequency of Negative Affect was too low for such a subanalysis. Reporting these data as proportions allows us to compare the groups' patterns of contextual relatedness in isolation of differences in actual frequency. The data were subjected to z tests for the significance of differences between two proportions. As can be seen, the Autistic and Delayed groups were very different in terms of the circumstances under which Positive Affect was displayed. The Autistic group displayed a higher percentage of Positive Affect that was Random-Unrelated or Solitary-Play-Related than did the Delayed group. The Delayed children almost never displayed Positive Affect under those conditions. They were significantly more likely than the Autistic children to display Positive Affect during interaction with a partner.

Table 2. Number of Intervals of Positive and Negative Affect, out of a Possible Total of 20

	Positive Affect With:			Negative Affect With:		
	Mother	Psychiatrist	Teacher	Mother	Psychiatrist	Teacher
Autistic	3.50	2.40	5.10	0.10	2.10 *	0.00
Delayed	9.90	9.60	9.50	0.60	0.80	1.10

* $p < 0.05$.

Table 3. Positive Affect: Proportions in Relation to Context

	Autistic		z	Delayed	
	%	Mean Frequency		%	Mean Frequency
Random-unrelated	24%	(2.6)	9.32*	0.3%	(0.1)
Solitary-play-related	28%	(3.1)	5.92*	6%	(0.7)
Partner-related	48%	(5.3)	9.00*	94%	(25.2)

* $p < 0.001$.

DISCUSSION

The present findings lend empirical support to the clinical observation that young autistic children display specific deficits in the area of affective expression. It appears to be the case that these deficits are not simply a result of general developmental immaturity, as the autistic children in the present study differed in a number of significant ways from a matched sample of nonautistic, developmentally delayed subjects.

The autistic children displayed less than half as much positive affect as did the nonautistic, developmentally delayed children. When they did smile or laugh, it was just as likely to be a random, self-absorbed way as it was to be related to social interaction. The delayed children, in contrast, almost never displayed random, self-absorbed smiling and laughing. In fact, their positive affect occurred in a social context 97% of the time.

Although these group differences in positive affect were striking, it may be important to highlight the fact that they do not reflect a polarized, all-or-none phenomenon. The data suggest that it is *not* the case that autistic children are characteristically flat in affect, or that the affect they do express is typically inappropriate or unrelated to the interpersonal context. The autistic children in this study did, on occasion, display clear episodes of smiling and laughing, and these episodes did appear at times to be related to the behavior of their partners. Although it is important to document that the frequency of these episodes is far lower than is the case with nonautistic children with comparable developmental delays, it may be equally important to stress that appropriate, partner-related smiling and laughing does occur in young autists.

Negative affect occurred rarely in both groups of children in this study, and there was no overall differences in frequency. The autistic group, however, differed from the delayed group in terms of their pattern of negative affect across the three partners. The delayed group displayed the same amount of negative affect with each partner, whereas the autistic group was significantly more negative with one partner, the unfamiliar, male psychiatrist. Whether this was caused by something specific about that partner's actual behavior, or to gender or familiarity factors is unclear; however, it is noteworthy that these very young autistic children were able to distinguish among partners in a way that prompted differential negative reactions. This finding is in accord with those of Freitag (1970), who demonstrated differential social responsiveness to different people in autistic children.

The results of this investigation add a new dimension to the existing data on autistic children's understanding of and ability to imitate emotional expression. Studies by Hertzig and Snow (1985), Hobson (1986), Jennings (1973), and Langdell (1978, 1981), although differing somewhat in methodologies and specific findings, all strongly suggest that autistic children have particular difficulty performing tasks that involve analyzing affective cues. This deficit presumably contributes to the relative inability of autistic persons to comprehend the emotional experiences of others. The present data extend these findings by suggesting that autistic children are disordered, not only in their ability to understand and imitate affect, but in their natural, spontaneous expression of affect as well.

It would appear from the results of this study that the area of emotional expression in autism is one worthy of further exploration. Although the present data are likely representative of young autistic children's real-life functioning in brief, nonstressful, one-to-one interactions, they provide only a very limited sample of what the autistic child's full emotional experience consists of. Further investigative work examining autistic children's affect in a wider range of situations, across a broader range of ages, is needed for a more complete, empirically based understanding of the unusual nature of affect in autism.

REFERENCES

Bretherton, I., Fritz, J., Zahn-Waxler, C. & Rigeway, D. (1986), Learning to talk about emotions: a functionalist perspective, *Child Develpm.,* 57:529–548.

Fein, D., Pennington, B., Markowitz, P., Braverman, B. & Waterhouse, L, (1986), Toward a neuropsychological model of infantile autism: are the social deficits primary? *This Journal,* 25:198–212.

Freitag, G. (1970), An experimental study of the social responsiveness of children with autistic behaviors. *J. Exp. Child Psychol.,* 9:436–453.

Hermelin, B. & O'Connor, N. (1970), *Psychological Experiments with Autistic Children,* Elmsford, N.Y.: Pergamon Press.

Hertzig, M. & Snow, M. (1985, October), Affect and cognition in autism. *Proceeding of the 32nd Annual Meeting of the American Academy of Child Psychiatry,* San Antonio, Texas.

Hobson, R. P. (1986), The autistic child's appraisal of expressions of emotion. *J. Child Psychol. Psychiat.,* 27:321–342.

Jennings, W. (1973), A study of the preference of affective cues in autistic children. *Dissertation Abstracts International,* 34:4045–4046.

Kanner, L. (1943), Autistic disturbances of affective contact. *Nerv. Child,* 2:217–250.

Knobloch, H., Stevens, F. & Malone, A. (1980), *Manual of Developmental Diagnosis.* Philadelphia: Harper and Row.

Langdell, T. (1978), Recognition of faces: an approach to the study of autism. *J. Child Psychol. Psychiat.,* 19:255–268.

—————— (1981), *Face perception: an approach to the study of autism.* Unpublished doctoral dissertation, University of London.

Reichler, R. & Schopler, E. (1971), Observations on the nature of human relatedness. *J. Aut. Childh. Schizo.,* 1:283–296.

Rutter, M. (1978), Language disorder and infantile autism. In: *Autism: A Reappraisal of Concepts and Treatment,* ed. M. Rutter & E. Schopler. New York: Plenum Press.

Part VIII

PSYCHOLOGICAL ISSUES WITH PHYSICAL ILLNESS

Many diseases of childhood, which in the past were fatal or disabling, can now be treated with varying degrees of success. How complicated the treatment may be, how intrusive and painful it is to the body, and how long it has to last differs with the disease, depending on its severity and a host of other circumstances.

By now there have developed a host of children who have survived such threatening illnesses—children who have come successfully through chemotherapy, through organ transplants, through other therapeutic manipulations of all types. Some are left free of danger, others have the threat of recurrence hanging over them for a given number of years or for the rest of their lives. Others are left with limitations that change the fabric of what their lives would have otherwise been.

Besides the need for constantly seeking to improve the treatment itself, a new problem has arisen—namely, what is the quality of life for these child survivors? Has the nature of the treatment brought stresses to children and families that now become part of the responsibility of the treatment team? Does treatment of the illness include preventive, concurring, and follow-up measures so that the life that has been saved will be worth living? And if such questions are pertinent, can we lay down general principles for specific diseases and for specific therapeutic procedures? The first step in examining these questions is to find out what has really happened to these child survivors. The papers in this section deal with this issue in regard to a number of serious physical illnesses. Only by having some knowledge of the problems that occur can one begin to plan appropriate psychosocial strategies.

The paper by Wasserman and her co-workers reports 40 subjects with Hodgkin's disease whose treatment achieved complete remission. The follow-up time selected was five years after the completion of therapy. The issues probed included positive as well as problem aspects of therapy, life events during these interim years, and current worries related to possible effects of either the illness or the treatment. The work is carefully done and the data reported are valuable.

Levine and her associates report a study of factors affecting cognitive functioning of hemiplegic children, dividing the 41 cases into three degrees of severity. The authors examine the relatedness of congenital versus acquired brain lesions, size, location, and laterality on various aspects of cognitive functioning. The questions studied also give some information on the functional plasticity of the developing brain. These data add considerably to what has been obtained by other investigators.

Chronic, life threatening diseases of childhood, especially when there is considerable uncertainty about outcome, place stress not only on the child-patient. The family is also placed under severe stress. There is an impact on all family members, but in different ways depending on the nature of the relationship to the patient and on the developmental level of the siblings. In the paper by Fife, 34 families with a child newly diagnosed to have acute lymphocytic leukemia were studied with regard to coping devices, anxieties, and effects on siblings—all extremely relevant issues for the treatment team.

In the final paper of this section by Krener on the psychiatric liaison to liver transplant recipients, we are given a brief but thoughtful clinical discussion that can apply to other types of organ transplants and even to other complicated and hazardous surgical procedures for children.

28

The Psychological Status of Survivors of Childhood/Adolescent Hodgkin's Disease

Abby L. Wasserman, Elizabeth I. Thompson, Judith A. Wilimas, and Diane L. Fairclough
St. Jude Children's Research Hospital, Memphis, Tennessee

To assess psychosocial late effects of childhood/adolescent cancer, semistructured interviews were conducted with 40 subjects who had achieved complete remission from Hodgkin's disease and completed therapy at least five years previously. Mean ages were 12.8 years at diagnosis and 24.7 years at interview. Side effects of treatment were most often mentioned as the "worst thing" about having had Hodgkin's disease. Although subjects had missed a mean of six months of school, and 40% had reported unpleasant school experiences, their educational levels exceeded those expected in sex-, age-, and state-matched populations. Almost all subjects said that they had benefited in some way from the experience of having cancer. In contrast to the female subjects, male subjects expressed little interest in having their reproductive status assessed. Current concerns included discrimination in employment or in obtaining life or health insurance.

Reprinted with permission from the *American Journal of Diseases of Children,* 1987, Vol. 141, 626–631. Copyright 1987 by the American Medical Association.

This investigation was supported in part by a grant from the American Lebanese Syrian Associated Charities, Memphis.

We wish to thank Kit Yatsula and others in The After Completion of Therapy Clinic for assistance in location and recruitment of subjects, Mary Lawler for secretarial assistance, and Christy Wright for editorial assistance.

Based on current cure rates, it is estimated that by the year 1990, one of every 1000 20-year-old persons will be a survivor of childhood cancer.[1] By the year 2000, one in 1000 people between the ages of 20 and 29 years will have survived cancer in childhood.[2] Yet little is known about the late effects on the lives of these long-term survivors, and the perceptions of these individuals regarding their illness and its treatment have received limited research attention.

To address these issues, and to generate hypotheses regarding possible therapeutic interventions and modifications in aspects of current treatment protocols, we studied subjects in remission from Hodgkin's disease who had completed their treatment at least five years previously. Because of the excellent long-term survival rate (approaching 90%)[3] and the age distribution of the illness, Hodgkin's disease provides an ideal model for studying late effects in a population of individuals who have begun to face the challenges of adult life.

By focusing on adolescent and young adult Hodgkin's survivors who had been treated within one institution, namely, St. Jude Children's Research Hospital (SJCRH), Memphis, we were able to obtain a sample in which therapeutic milieu, age, disease factors, survival rates, degree of disfigurement or physical limitations, and differences in treatment protocols were unlikely to present major confounding variables. We were also able to assess the accuracy of patients' memories regarding the extent of their illness and nature of its treatment because hospital protocols require that patients and parents be kept informed regarding the extent and treatment of their disease, side effects, and long-term outlook.

In selecting study variables, we drew as much as possible on the available literature regarding cancer survivors and sequelae of chronic disease with childhood/adolescent onset. Since our goal was to generate hypotheses regarding late effects in this age group, the patients' subjective perceptions of their experience with cancer and its treatment were probed extensively.

SUBJECTS AND METHODS

Subjects

Subjects were eligible for participation if they (1) had completed their treatment for Hodgkin's disease at SJCRH at least five years previously, (2) were under the age of 20 years at the time of diagnosis, and (3) were scheduled for a routine biennial clinic visit during the study period (September 1984 to July 1985). Letters of explanation were sent to all subjects who met these criteria, and interviews were then scheduled at the next clinic visit for those who agreed to participate.

Procedure

The subjects were scheduled for in-depth interviews at their next clinic visit. All interviews were conducted by the same staff psychiatrist to minimize interview bias.

The same 30 open-ended questions were asked in each interview, with follow-up questions as appropriate. Although subjects were encouraged to elaborate on responses, the psychiatrist neither interpreted answers nor suggested possible responses. Questions were grouped in the following categories.

1. Recall regarding extent of disease and nature of treatment. (Responses were checked against hospital records.)
2. Perceptions of the "worst thing" about having Hodgkin's disease.
3. Reactions of schoolmates, friends, and family to the patient's illness.
4. Risk-taking behavior during the illness and treatment period, as well as current behavior.
5. Any perceived benefits of having had cancer.
6. Information on relapse, if any, and concerns regarding recurrence or development of a second malignant neoplasm.
7. Current educational or employment status and level of educational attainment.
8. Current socioeconomic status, based on Hollingshead's Two Factor Index of Social Position.[4]
9. Any current problems viewed as associated with Hodgkin's disease (physical limitations, disfigurement, employment discrimination, etc).

In addition to questions about the specific variables of interest, interviews also included a diagnostic assessment using *Diagnostic and Statistical Manual of Mental Disorders,* ed 3, criteria.[5] Use of these criteria (the standard nosologic system in psychiatry) permits comparison with population incidence figures for specific age groups.

Statistical Analysis

Both means and medians were calculated for continuous data; means are reported herein because the results were found not to differ. Fisher's exact test was used to test independence of responses and sex or age. Normal approximation of the binomial was used to compare data on educational levels and marital status with those from the general population. The analysis is exploratory, and *P* values are descriptive.

RESULTS

All of the 45 subjects eligible for study agreed to participate; five of these subjects could not be included because their travel plans did not allow time for the interview.

To determine whether this sample was representative of the hospital's total population of long-term survivors of Hodgkin's disease (ie, those who met the study criteria but who did not have a routine visit scheduled during the study period [N = 121]), statistical comparisons of sex ratio, stage of disease at diagnosis, type of therapy, percentage of relapses, and residual physical limitations were performed. No significant differences were found for any variable, although the study population was slightly older (mean age, 26 years) than the overall population (mean age, 23 years).

Characteristics of the sample are given in Table 1. Subjects were interviewed a mean of 11.9 years (range, seven to 19 years) after diagnosis. The majority (n = 37) were white; most were from the lower socioeconomic strata, as is true of the hospital's overall patient population. A wide geographic area was represented, with the majority of subjects coming from states in the Southeast and Midwest. All subjects were Karnofsky status 100.[6]

Data on disease stage, treatment, and recurrence are presented in Table 2. Most subjects (n = 33) were able to recall the stage of disease at diagnosis; younger subjects (< 13 years of age at diagnosis) showed less accuracy of recall (*P* = .009), tending to underestimate the extent of their disease. Type of treatment was remembered accurately by all but two subjects. One boy, who was 4 years old at diagnosis, could not remember undergoing a splenectomy; he also did not remember receiving chemotherapy. A male subject who was 11 years old when treated mistakenly thought he had received chemotherapy in addition to radiotherapy.

Concerns During Therapy

Side effects of therapy. All patients reported notable side effects (including radiation burns, nausea and vomiting, and infections requiring prolonged hospitalization); half of the subjects viewed these events as the "worst thing about having Hodgkin's." Female subjects were more likely than male subjects to point to side effects as the most traumatic aspect of their illness. Specifically, significantly more female subjects cited loss of hair (*P* = .03). A

Table 1. Demographic Characteristics of Sample

Characteristic	No. (%) of Subjects
Sex	
M	22 (55)
F	18 (45)
Age at diagnosis, y	
<12	12 (30)
12-19	28 (70)
Age at interview, y	
10-24.9	20 (50)
25-38	20 (50)
Time from diagnosis, y to interview	
7-12.9	23 (57.5)
13-19	17 (42.5)
Social class*	
I, II	5 (12.5)
III, IV, V	35 (87.5)

*According to classification by Hollingshead.[4]

Table 2. Illness History and Treatment

Item	No. (%) of Subjects
Stage at diagnosis	
I	7 (17.5)
II	17 (42.5)
III	15 (37.5)
IV	1 (2.5)
Treatment	
Radiation only	5 (12.5)
Radiation and chemotherapy	35 (87.5)
Splenectomy (as part of staging laparotomy)	26 (65.0)
Relapses	
None	35 (87.5)
One	4 (10.0)
Two or more	1 (2.5)

group of concerns mentioned by 43% of patients (several subjects cited more than one "worst thing") involved complaints associated with their illness itself (eg, lassitude) and with other aspects of treatment (eg, hospitalizations and specific procedures). Other "worst things" included loneliness (17%) and missing a phase of growing up (15%). Fear of dying was cited by only 5% of the subjects.

School and peer experiences. These subjects missed an average of six months of school, with a range of eight weeks (for subjects who received only radiotherapy) to more than a year for those who had developed complications. Subjects who had received both radiotherapy and chemotherapy, without complications, missed an average of six months of school. All subjects had a homebound teacher during their school absences.

Although not cited specifically as a "worst thing" about the illness, unpleasant experiences with classmates were reported by 40% of those subjects who returned to the schools they had attended before their treatment. These subjects noted that peers teased them about their baldness or thinness, avoided them because they might be "contagious," or generally treated them as outcasts. Positive experiences with peers were reported by five subjects (12%) who felt that they had been "spoiled" by friends at school. The remainder felt that they had been treated "normally," although four of these subjects were told of their supposed deaths by schoolmates and neighbors.

Relationships with family and siblings. Almost half of the subjects felt that their parents had spoiled them during their illness. The majority either noticed no change in relationships with siblings (n = 11) or reported positive changes and extra attention (n = 13). Nine patients (24%) felt resentment and jealousy from siblings. Female subjects were more likely than male subjects to state that they had been spoiled by parents ($P = .06$) and siblings ($P = .01$).

Among subjects who had been in their teens at the time of diagnosis, three subjects were engaged and one subject was married. The two engagements involving male subjects were subsequently cancelled by their fiancées, causing both men great distress. The one female subject who was engaged found her fiancé very understanding and the relationship continued as planned. The married female subject reported receiving much support and comfort from her spouse.

Risk-taking behavior. Overall, one third of the subjects reported changes in risk-taking behavior either during their illness or after recovery. Eight subjects (four male and four female subjects) described increased risk-taking during and shortly after treatment but viewed themselves as having "settled down" since then. Six (two male and four female subjects) felt that they had become considerably more cautious since their illness. The remaining subjects described no change in their degree of risk taking; three of these subjects said that they had always been risk takers.

Long-term Adjustment

Education and employment. At the time of interview, all subjects were working, attending school, or both. Table 3 shows that the proportion of high school graduates in this sample is greater than would be expected based on state-specific population statistics (82.5% vs 68%, $P = .07$) (W. V. Grant, PhD, oral communication, August 1985). The seven subjects who dropped out of school gave extended absences due to their cancer therapy as their reason; three of these subjects later obtained a general education diploma. Half of the study group has gone on to postsecondary schooling; another three subjects who are still in high school plan to attend college. Of those who were working, two men and five women are in helping professions.

Physical sequelae. Almost half of the sample said that they had no current physical problems attributable to the disease or therapy. Physical residual effects reported by other subjects (expressed as percentages of the total sample) included disfigurement (30%), neurologic problems (eg, decreased reflexes, incoordination, muscle weakness, and sensory abnormalities) (30%), dyspnea (15%), easy fatigability (5%), and sterility (3%). Ten subjects complained of more than one abnormality. In addition, there were five instances of residual effects that were obvious to the interviewer but not mentioned by the patients: four male subjects had narrow shoulders and short crown-rump length secondary to radiotherapy, and one female subject had scars on her neck from a herpes zoster infection.

Only one subject, a 22-year-old woman, spontaneously mentioned sterility when asked about physical problems. Direct questioning revealed that the majority of subjects—60% of male subjects and 44% of female subjects—did not know whether they were sterile or not. Only two male subjects had had

Table 3. Schooling Completed*

	Male Subjects	Female Subjects	Total No. (%) of Subjects
Quit school/obtained GED later	6/2	1/1	**7** (17.5)
Still in school	2	1	**3** (7.5)
Graduated high school	7	4	**11** (27.5)
Some college	2	8	**10** (25.0)
College degree	5	4	**9** (22.5)

*GED indicates general education diploma.

sperm counts done, although this procedure is routinely suggested at clinic visits; each man underwent testing because he was planning to be married. Another man, who has not had testing, considers himself sterile because he has not fathered any children during eight years of marriage to a woman who had three children previously. Five men believe themselves to be fertile based on wives' or girlfriends' pregnancies. Six of the 18 women consider themselves sterile, four women have had children, and the remaining eight female subjects have normal menstrual cycles but have not attempted to become pregnant. Attitudes toward possible sterility differed dramatically between the sexes. The female subjects expressed far more concern, and several women had sought consultation regarding their childbearing potential. By contrast, many of the men expressed indifference, and several men said that they had not informed potential spouses of the possibility of their own sterility.

Marriage and divorce. At the time of interview, eight men and ten women were married, two women were engaged, and five men and one woman had been divorced. Although the overall proportions of marriage and divorce in the sample are not different from general population statistics, separate analysis of the men indicates a significantly high rate of divorce compared with age- and race-specific statistics for the United States[7] (23% vs 5.4%, *P* = .002). In addition to the six subjects who have had natural children, six other subjects have stepchildren and two subjects have adopted children.

Discrimination and related issues. In general, the subjects were fairly reluctant to discuss their illness with others. Four of the younger subjects (mean age, 17 years) totally refuse to acknowledge their experience with cancer. Eight subjects who had kept their disease a secret when they were younger said that they were now willing to talk about it. The majority were cautious, never volunteering information but responding if confronted with direct questions. Three subjects said that they use their personal experience with cancer to educate other people.

Although most respondents believed that they had not experienced job discrimination, about half of those who had been asked health-related questions on job applications had not revealed their cancer history. Several instances of discrimination were apparent: five male subjects had been denied entry into the armed forces, one subject was refused employment by a state agency, and one subject was transferred from his job in a hotel kitchen for fear that he might "contaminate" the food. One woman lost seniority after her relapse.

Although almost two thirds of these subjects had some form of health insurance coverage, this was clearly an area of concern. One subject's group policy excludes all cancer-related problems. Another man was unable to accept a better position because he would have lost his group coverage. For subjects without the group option, either through their own employment or through spouses or parents, health insurance was expensive or unobtainable; two subjects have individual policies at an exorbitant cost, and the others have no coverage. Only 12 subjects have life insurance policies, two of which exclude cancer.

Recurrence. Thirteen subjects admitted being concerned about the possibility of a recurrence or second malignant neoplasm but said that they "tried not to think about it." More women than men described fears of recurrence ($P =$ .06). Among the 23 subjects who denied fears about recurrence, seven subjects stated that their spouses or parents worry. One of the subjects mentioned that he is trying to protect himself from a relapse by "serving God"; another subject feels that a daily intake of asparagus will protect her. Most of the subjects said that they would definitely undergo therapy again if there should be a recurrence; however, six subjects thought that it would depend on their age and prognosis, and two subjects said that they definitely would not accept therapy. All five patients who have had a recurrence said that they experienced more psychological difficulties the second time. One subject sought psychological counseling to help him during his second course of therapy. All of those subjects who had suffered a relapse feel that now they are cured, but four of the five subjects worry about another recurrence.

Psychiatric status. The frequency of psychiatric diagnosis in the sample (15%) is basically no different from that found in community studies.[8] A depressive disorder (dysthymia) was seen in one male subject, personality disorders (schizoid, antisocial, and borderline) in three male subjects, histrionic personality disorder in one female subject, and adjustment disorder with mixed emotional features in another female subject. Only two of these disturbances could be linked directly with Hodgkin's disease. The woman with adjustment disorder was reacting to feared sterility, and the man with depression dates the onset of symptoms to the death of his mother, whom he is convinced "worried to death" about his illness.

Excessive alcohol use, which did not meet the criteria for a diagnosis of alcoholism, was admitted by three subjects. Twelve subjects said that they had tried marijuana, three of them to reduce the nausea associated with chemotherapy. No other substance abuse was reported.

Perceived benefits. When asked whether any good had resulted from their experience with cancer, 95% of the subjects responded positively. Their specific responses fell into the following categories: increased appreciation of being alive (26%), improved outlook on life (26%), increased involvement with other people (26%), increased religious feelings (18%), greater maturity

(15%), more patience and tolerance (13%), not taking good health for granted (15%), and becoming closer to families (8%).

COMMENT

Children and adolescents with cancer face illness- and treatment-related stresses that have been reported to have a deleterious impact on later functioning.[9,10] Our sample shows that these young adult survivors of Hodgkin's disease have good overall adjustment and are leading essentially normal lives, as did Fergusson's[11] toddler population and Holmes'[12] mixed tumor population. Their educational achievement is statistically better than that of comparable populations, and there is no increased incidence of depression or other psychiatric disorders. Almost all subjects believed that they had benefited in some way from their experience with cancer. The areas of perceived benefit, such as a better outlook on life, an increased appreciation of being alive, and increased maturity, might have facilitated their adjustment to the demands of school, work, and personal relationships.

This is not to say that there were no illness-related problems, either overt or hidden. The most vivid negative memories focused on the physical aspects of the illness and its treatments. As previously described, the relationship of the adolescents to their environment during their illness was not an easy one.[13] Separation from family, friends, and normal daily activities caused extreme feelings of loneliness that were recalled vividly. Missing school and social activities, which are so important for the development of strong peer relations and camaraderie,[14,15] created a void that several subjects still feel. Loss of hair was extremely distressing, especially among female subjects, whose self-image tends to be correlated with their physical appearance.[14] The emotional problems associated with the disease were described by subjects as decreasing over time. Although more than half of the subjects reported residual physical problems common after radiotherapy and chemotherapy for Hodgkin's disease,[16,17] there were few complaints of these disabilities. Interestingly, five subjects failed to mention observable physical deformities, indicating that they had probably incorporated these changes into their body image and no longer considered them abnormalities, which may be indicative of constructive and supportive attitudes regarding their abnormalities from their families.[18]

In contrast to the younger subjects, the ones who were adolescents at the time of diagnosis had excellent recall of the treatment received and the extent of their disease and felt very positive about having been kept informed throughout their diagnosis and treatment. This finding suggests that as younger subjects mature, we should again discuss with them their diagnosis, type of therapy, and possible long-term side effects. Youth seems to have its benefits, for those who were younger at the time of diagnosis felt that their failure to comprehend the seriousness of their illness helped them "get through."

A major area of concern and distress was the manner in which subjects were treated by others; therefore, better education about cancer, its treatment, and its favorable prognosis—whether done within the context of the subject's school and community[13] or on a more global level (eg, television specials)—is necessary to increase the public's understanding of the disease process and the effects of therapy so that children and adolescents treated for cancer will have an easier time reentering school and age-appropriate activities. It has been shown that students in dissonant environments suffer more anguish than do students in consonant environments.[19] The more that can be done to make the school and neighborhood accepting of these patients who may look different due to their cancer treatment, the less suffering the patients will experience. Decreasing the time required for therapy and lessening the severity of the side effects would produce less disruption in the patients' lives and fewer emotional repercussions; of course, these are areas of ongoing research in oncology.

All subjects in our study are either in school or working, in contradistinction to findings in adult patients.[20] One wonders how much the drive to achieve independence accounts for the better working record of this younger population. However, these adolescents and young adults (average of 12 years after discontinuation of therapy) still feel that job discrimination and difficulties obtaining health and life insurance, which have been consistent findings among long-term survivors of cancer,[21-24] are major problems. To avoid potential job discrimination, some subjects do not mention on job applications that they have had cancer. None of them felt that this was wrong since they were cured of the cancer and their health would not adversely affect their work performance. Although the 20% of our subjects who have experienced job discrimination is lower than figures found in other surveys— 42% in the sample of Fobair et al[20] and 54% and 84% reported by Feldman[21]—the effects were still major. The men who were excluded from the armed forces felt that this has had a lasting effect on their lives (eg, being unable to use the GI Bill to help further their educations).

Because a large part of job discrimination is said to result from the increased cost of insurance for survivors of cancer, which can only get worse with prepaid health maintenance insurance contracts,[20] one way of dealing with both problems would be to have federal or state insurance programs for those who have had cancer so that the cost to individuals or their employers would be the same as for those who have not had cancer.

The six women in our sample who consider themselves sterile (absence of menses without exogenous hormones) did not appear to suffer alienation from others and loss of confidence in their own sexuality, as reported in post-Hodgkin's disease sterile women by Chapman et al.[25] It is possible that hormone replacement, which is routinely used at SJCRH for those with absent or extremely irregular menses, may eliminate the emotional distress reported to accompany ovarian failure (this question is under investigation). Even without signs of ovarian failure, one woman was extremely upset because she had been told by (or had misunderstood) her gynecologist that her fallopian tubes or ovaries could not be felt because they had "shriveled up from the radiation." In fact, her ovaries had been moved out of the radiation field at the time of laparotomy. She was calmed after the interview when she was told she did have her reproductive organs and they appeared functional.

Despite the well-documented hypospermia or azoospermia following chemotherapy and radiotherapy for Hodgkin's disease,[16,17,26] of which all male subjects were aware, compliance with sperm testing was poor, even among subjects who were married or engaged. Although some subjects exhibited an attitude of indifference, one man admitted, "I have not gotten the nerve to pursue it." Two men accepted responsibility for the pregnancies of the women they were dating without question. Both of these couples married, and neither of the women has become pregnant again in over five years of unprotected intercourse. Four men said that there was no point in a sperm count because their stepchildren were "enough"; not one has impregnated his wife during their years of marriage with no birth control. These vignettes suggest that for many of these men, the possibility of sterility is so devastating to their self-image that they invoke all types of excuses to avoid having sterility or "unmanliness" confirmed. Social measures of "manliness," such as measured by strength (eg, muscular development of the shoulders and chest) and the ability to procreate, suffered with the cancer treatment. This constellation of findings may in part account for the broken engagements and high divorce rate among the male subjects.

It thus appears important that men be given hope through counseling that they are still masculine and can be fathers even if they have been treated for Hodgkin's disease. All male subjects 15 years of age or older who do not have low sperm counts secondary to active Hodgkin's disease[27] should be encouraged to bank their sperm prior to treatment. Artificial insemination can be suggested if sperm counts are low and sperm has not been banked.

Women, too, need to know that recent advances in the field of infertility allow for hope of conception. We have had the experience of women dependent on exogenous hormones for menses who have discontinued the hormones, ovulated, and become pregnant. For those who do not ovulate and are willing to undergo the time and expense, in vitro fertilization with a donated egg and husband's sperm is a possibility. Adoption is an alternative, but couples must be counseled to place themselves on waiting lists and expect a long wait for a child, especially an infant. Infertility may not even be an issue for some couples, and single adults should be made aware of this fact. On talking to couples in which one member is infertile due to cancer therapy, the partner is usually more concerned that the sterile member is alive and well than able to bear children.

The use of denial appeared extensively in this population and was reflected in attitudes toward recurrence and second malignant neoplasms. The reported incidence of second malignant neoplasms following combined modality therapy for Hodgkin's disease ranges from 5% to 10%,[28-30] yet a majority of the subjects said that they do not worry about recurrences or second malignant neoplasms; the others try not to think of them. It seems that since cancer continues to be a threat to these subjects, the only way of being able to live a normal life is to deny the threat (as do smokers and others at risk for cancer who have not been stricken).[31] It appears that a second cancer is more difficult to handle than the first one. Even if the patient had no major emotional problems during the first treatment for cancer, it is recommended that supportive counseling be offered if a relapse occurs.

Age at the time of diagnosis and treatment appears to have affected the way the subjects coped with the experience. Those who were younger during treatment felt that their failure to comprehend the seriousness of their illness was beneficial. According to the criterion proposed by Mattsson,[32] one fourth of the subjects who were adolescents when treated could be described as risk-taking, defiant adolescents who have poor adjustment to their chronic disorders. However, all of these subjects outgrew this behavior, indicating that recovery from psychosocial problems that accompany cancer in this age group is possible.

Reduction in risk-taking behavior and increased willingness to talk about the experience with cancer indicates that these subjects have been able to incorporate the experience more positively into their self-image and no longer have to "prove themselves" or hide their history of cancer from others (except in relation to job applications, in which case they feel that the information continues to be to their disadvantage). This finding confirms data reported by Koocher et al,[33] ie, increasing time since disease onset is associated with decreases in severity and number of emotional problems related to the disease.

The goal of cancer therapy, particularly in children and adolescents, is to maintain a high cure rate while decreasing treatment toxicity, including potential psychosocial and physical sequelae. Awareness of psychosocial problems by pediatric oncologists could lead to earlier intervention in the form of adolescent groups, peer support, and even referral for supportive counseling. Society as a whole needs to be educated about cancer and its favorable prognosis. Perhaps these children and adolescents would then face less trauma on returning to their communities after treatment, employment discrimination would lessen, and society would be more willing to accept the risk of insuring these long-term survivors of cancer.

REFERENCES

1. Meadows AT, Krejmas NL, Belasco JB: The medical cost of cure: Sequelae in survivors of childhood cancer, in Van Eys J, Sullivan MP (eds): *Status of The Curability of Childhood Cancers.* New York, Raven Press, 1980, pp 263–276.
2. Meadows AT, Hobbie W: The medical consequences of cure. Read before the American Cancer Society National Conference on Advances in the Care of the Child with Cancer, Los Angeles, June 1985.
3. Zittoun R, Audebert A, Hoerni B, et al: Extended vs involved fields irradiation combined with MOPP chemotherapy in early clinical stages of Hodgkin's disease. *J Clin Oncol* 1985;3:207–214.
4. Hollingshead AB: *Two Factor Index of Social Position.* New Haven, Conn, Yale University Press, 1957.
5. American Psychiatric Association, Committee on Nomenclature and Statistics: *Diagnostic and Statistical Manual of Mental Disorders,* ed 3. New York, Biometrics Research Division, New York State Psychiatric Institute, 1977.
6. Mor V, Laliberte L, Morris JN, et al: The Karnofsky performance status scale. *Cancer* 1984;53:2002–2007.
7. Bureau of the Census: *Marital Status and Living Arrangements: March 1984,* US Dept of Commerce publication series P-20, No. 399, 1985.
8. Myers JK, Weissman MM, Tischler GL, et al: Six-month prevalence of psychiatric disorders in three communities. *Arch Gen Psychiatry* 1984;41:959–967:
9. Zwartjes WJ: The psychological costs of curing the child with cancer, in Van Eys J, Sullivan MP (eds): *Status of the Curability of Childhood Cancers.* New York, Raven Press, 1980, pp. 277–284.
10. Pfefferbaum B: Criteria for functional cure of cancer, in Van Eys J, Sullivan MP (eds): *Status of the Curability of Childhood Cancers.* New York, Raven Press, 1980, pp 27–32.
11. Fergusson JH: Late psychologic effects of a serious illness in childhood. *Nurs Clin North Am* 1976;11:83–93.
12. Holmes HA, Holmes FF: After ten years, what are the handicaps and life styles of children treated for cancer? *Clin Pediatr* 1975;14:819–823.
13. Pfefferbaum B: Pediatric oncology: A review of the changing psychological aspects. *Int J Psychiatry Med* 1979;9:289–296.
14. Malmquist CP: Development from 13 to 16 years, in Noshpitz JD (ed): *Basic Handbook of Child Psychiatry.* New York, Basic Books Inc, 1979, vol 1, pp 209–210.

15. Brunstetter RW, Silver LB: Normal adolescent development, in Kaplan HI, Sadock BJ (eds): *Comprehensive Textbook of Psychiatry/IV.* Baltimore, Williams & Wilkins, 1986, pp 1608–1613.
16. Sullivan MP, Fuller LM, Butler JJ: Hodgkin's disease, in Suton WW, Fernbach DJ, Vietti TJ (eds): *Clinical Pediatric Oncology,* ed 3. St Louis, CV Mosby Co, 1984, pp 437–442.
17. Kaplan HS: *Hodgkin's Disease.* Cambridge, Mass, Harvard University Press, 1980, pp 421–441, 469–477.
18. Belfer ML, Lukens PF: Body image: Impacts and distortions, in Levine MD, Carey WB, Crocker AC, et al (eds): *Developmental-Behavioral Pediatrics.* Philadelphia, WB Saunders Co, 1983, pp 623–632.
19. Petersen AC, Offer D: Adolescent development: Sixteen to 19 years, in Noshpitz JD (ed): *Basic Handbook of Child Psychiatry.* New York, Basic Books Inc, 1979, vol 1, p 219.
20. Fobair P, Hoppe RT, Bloom J, et al: Psychosocial problems among survivors of Hodgkin's disease. *J Clin Oncol* 1986;4:806–814.
21. Feldman FL: *Work and Cancer Health Histories: Work Expectations and Experiences of Youth With Cancer Histories (Ages 13–23).* Oakland, Calif, American Cancer Society, 1980.
22. Koocher GP, O'Malley JE: *The Damocles Syndrome and Psychosocial Consequences of Surviving Childhood Cancer.* New York, McGraw-Hill International Book Co, 1981.
23. Brunnquell D, Hall M: Issues in the psychological care of pediatric oncology patients. *Am J Orthopsychiatry* 1982;52:32–44.
24. Anderson JL: Insurability of cancer patients: A rehabilitation barrier. *Oncol Nurs Forum* 1984;2:42–45.
25. Chapman RM, Sutcliffe SB, Malpas JS: Cytotoxic-induced ovarian failure in Hodgkin's disease. *JAMA* 1979;242:1882–1884.
26. Sherins RT, DeVita VT: Effect of drug treatment for lymphoma on male reproduction capacity. *Ann Intern Med* 1973;79:216–220.
27. Chapman RM, Sutcliffe SB, Malpas JS: Male gonadal dysfunction in Hodgkin's disease. *JAMA* 1981;245:1323–1328.
28. Zanini M, Zucali R, Banfi A: Bone and soft-tissue sarcomas in the follow-up of Hodgkin's disease. *Tumori* 1983;69:473–476.
29. Pederson-Bjergaard J, Larsen SO: Incidence of acute non-lymphocytic leukemia preleukemia, and acute myeloproliferative syndrome up to ten years after treatment of Hodgkin's disease, *N Engl J Med* 1982;307:965–971.
30. Door FA, Coltman CA: Second cancers following antineoplastic therapy. *Curr Probl Cancer* 1985;9:1–43.
31. Reed HD, Janis IL: Effects of a new type of psychological treatment on smoker's resistance. *J Consult Clin Psychol* 1974;42:748–750.
32. Mattsson A: Long-term physical illness in childhood: A challenge to psychosocial adaptation. *Pediatrics* 1972;50:801–811.
33. Koocher GP, O'Malley JE, Gogan JL, et al: Psychological adjustment among pediatric cancer survivors. *J Child Psychol Psychiatry* 1980; 21:163–173.

PART VIII: PSYCHOLOGICAL ISSUES
WITH PHYSICAL ILLNESS

29

Factors Affecting Cognitive Functioning of Hemiplegic Children

Susan Cohen Levine and **Peter Huttenlocher**
Wyler Children's Hospital, University of Chicago, Illinois
Marie T. Banich
University of Illinois, Urbana-Champaign
Eugene Duda
Christ Community Hospital, Chicago, Illinois

The results of psychological testing, EEGs and CT scans were examined for 41 children with congenital or early acquired hemiplegia. On average, IQ was depressed and the magnitude of this depression was highly correlated with lesion size, degree of hemiparesis and EEG abnormality, but not with location of lesion. There were no significant effects of lesion laterality on Verbal vs. Performance IQ on Wechsler tests. However, receptive vocabulary, as measured by the Peabody Picture Vocabulary Test, was differentially depressed by left-hemisphere damage. Further, on a variety of verbal tasks, patients with congenital lesions performed better than those with acquired lesions. In contrast, no significant differences were found between the two groups on spatial tasks.

Reprinted with permission from *Developmental Medicine and Child Neurology*, 1987, Vol. 29, 27–35. Copyright 1987 by Mac Keith Press, London.

We are grateful to the Spencer Foundation for supporting this research. We also thank Margaret Koch-Weser for help in the early stages of the research, Jerre Levy for helpful comments and suggestions, and Karen Peterson for preparation of the manuscript for publication.

Unilateral cerebral lesions that occur perinatally or in early childhood have been reported to have different effects on cognitive functioning than later acquired lesions. Most notably, persistent aphasias frequently follow left hemisphere damage in adults, but rarely do so in children (Basser 1962; Lenneberg 1967; Woods and Teuber 1973, 1978; Woods and Carey 1979). Such differences have been ascribed to the plasticity of the developing brain, enabling intact cortical regions to take over functions usually localized in the damaged areas. It is clear, however, that there are limitations to this functional plasticity. Early unilateral brain lesions have been shown to depress over-all level of intellectual functioning. Although occasional single cases with high intelligence have been reported (Smith and Sugar 1975), the average IQ of patients with infantile hemiparesis or early hemispherectomy is about 20 points below normal (Perlstein and Hood 1955, St. James-Roberts 1981). Also, the nature of deficits varies with lesion laterality. Certain language functions are more disrupted after early damage to the left hemisphere (Dunsdon 1952, Annett 1973, Dennis and Kohn 1975, Dennis and Whitaker 1976, Rankin *et al.* 1981), whereas certain spatial functions are more impaired after early damage to the right hemisphere (Wood 1955, Wedell 1960, Nielsen 1966, Kohn and Dennis 1974).

The relationship between early brain damage and cognitive functioning can be examined more closely by the use of computerized axial tomography of the brain (CT). Two recent CT studies have found a correlation between lesion location and IQ. Cortical lesions and lesions extending from the surface of the cortex to the lateral ventricle (true porencephaly) were found to be associated with lower intellectual level than were lesions confined to subcortical white matter and basal ganglia (Cohen and Duffner 1981, Kotlarek *et al.* 1981). However, lesion size was not measured in these studies, and it is possible that differences in the average size of the different types of lesions account for the reported IQ differences.

In addition, several studies suggest that depressed cognitive functioning of hemiplegic children may be due to the effects of abnormal electrical activity or seizure-related cerebral anoxia on the developing brain (Byers 1941, Perlstein and Hood 1955). However, Cohen and Duffner (1981) found EEG abnormalities to have little predictive value for intellectual ability in their group of patients with congenital hemiplegia.

The present study was undertaken to answer some of the remaining questions regarding the effects of lesion location, lesion size, and seizure activity on cognitive functioning of children with hemiplegia of early onset. Our findings are consistent with the hypothesis of considerable functional plasticity of the developing brain, but also indicate significant intellectual deficits related to early unilateral loss of brain tissue.

METHOD

Neurological examinations, psychological testing, EEG readings and CT-scans were obtained for 41 children seen in the Pediatric Neurology Clinic at Wyler Children's Hospital, University of Chicago, between 1976 and 1984. Table I summarizes some of the characteristics of these patients.

Degree of hemiparesis was assigned a grading of 1 to 3, depending on its severity. In all cases the impairment was more severe in the upper than the lower extremities; all the children were ambulatory, without assistance, but with hemiparetic limp. Hand function was most easily gradable and this was used for assignment of severity of hemiparesis, as follows: grade 1 = able to grasp with thumb-forefinger; grade 2 = able to grasp with whole-hand; grade 3 = unable to grasp.

Each child was assigned an EEG and seizure rank from 0 to 4, with 0 = normal EEG and no recurrent seizures (N = 11); 1 = focal slowing on EEG without epileptic foci and without recurrent seizures (N = 9); 2 = normal EEG or focal slowing and recurrent seizures (N = 4); 3 = unilateral focal spikes on EEG and recurrent seizures (N = 8); 4 = bilateral spikes on EEG and recurrent seizures (N = 9). Thus 21 (51 per cent) of the 41 hemiplegic children in this study had epileptic seizures, which compares closely with previous reports (Perlstein and Hood 1955, Ingram 1964).

The CT scans were used to identify the locus of the lesion and also to estimate its size, which was done in two ways. First, the horizontal extent of the lesion was estimated by selecting the slice on which the lesion was largest, and calculating the ratio of the maximal anterior-posterior extent of the lesion to the anterior-posterior diameter of the slice (maximal diameter ratio). Second, the vertical extent of the lesion was estimated from the number of sections in standard CT plane of 1cm thickness on which the lesion was evident. Based on these two estimates, lesions were assigned to one of four size categories, as follows: 0 = no detectable lesion; 1 = lesions visible in only one or two sections and maximal diameter ratio below 0·2; 2 = lesions visible in three or four sections, and maximal diameter ratio between 0·2 and 0·4; 3 = lesions visible in five or more sections and maximal diameter ratios above 0·4. Two cases that did not fit these limits were classified separately; one was a case in which four sections were involved but with a maximal diameter ratio of only 0·14; this was classified as category 2. The other case had five abnormal sections and maximal diameter ratio of 0·32; this was classified as category 3. Cases in which ventricular enlargement was the only

Table I. Summary of patients

Case	Sex	Age at acquisition	Aetiology	Mean age at testing (SD)
Left-hemisphere lesion (right hemiplegia)				
L1-19	9 M, 10 F	Congenital/perinatal	Mostly uncertain	8 yrs 8 mths (4 yrs)
L20	M	11 mths	Astrocytoma	
L21	M	9 mths	Head trauma	
L22	M	1½ mths	Meningitis	
L23	M	7 mths	Embolic stroke during cardiac catheterization	
L24	M	2½ yrs	Stroke	9 yrs 3 mths (4 yrs 4 mths)
L25	M	9 yrs	Head trauma	
L26	F	6 yrs	Chronic focal encephalitis	
L27	F	11 mths	Sickle-cell disease, stroke	
Right-hemisphere lesion (left hemiplegia)				
R1-R6	4 M, 2 F	Congenital/perinatal	Mostly unknown	7 yrs 8 mths (5 yrs 1 mth)
R7	M	3 yrs	Head trauma	
R8	M	9½ yrs	St. Louis encephalitis with stroke	
R9	M	19 mths	Vasculitis	
R10	M	6 yrs	Sickle-cell disease, stroke	7 yrs 7 mths (2 yrs 9 mths)
R11	M	5 yrs	Moya Moya disease, stroke	
R12	F	5 yrs	Sickle cell disease, stroke	
R13	F	7 mths	Stroke with febrile illness	
R14	M	8 mths	Head trauma	

finding were classified according to the number of sections that showed the enlarged portion of the ventricle.

Finally, lesions were classified into one of six grades, based on lesion location, using a method devised by Cohen and Duffner (1981): grade 1 = normal scan; grade 2 = unilateral ventricular enlargement contralateral to the hemiparesis, with preservation of normal ventricular outline, and without shift of structures; grade 3 = unilateral areas of decreased density extending superiorly from the centrum semiovale inferiorly into the basal ganglia (white matter lesions); grade 4 = unilateral areas of decreased density in the periphery of the cortex (gray matter lesions); grade 5 = areas of decreased density extending from the surface of the cerebral hemisphere into the subjacent ventricle (white and gray matter lesions); grade 6 = unilateral small hemisphere with shift of midline structures to that side, with or without increased size of ipsilateral ventricular system.

All the patients were given a psychological test battery including a standardized intelligence test (either the Wechsler Intelligence Scale for Children—Revised [WISC-R] [Wechsler 1974], the Wechsler Preschool and Primary Scale of Intelligence [WPPSI] [Wechsler 1967], the Wechsler Adult Intelligence Scale [WAIS] or the Stanford-Binet, Form L-M [Terman and Merrill 1962], depending on age at testing). The Draw-a-Person Test (Koppitz 1968), the Bender-Gestalt Test of Visuo-Motor Integration (Koppitz 1964), the Peabody Picture Vocabulary Test (Dunn 1965) and the Northwestern Syntax Screening Test (Lee 1969) were also administered.

RESULTS

An exact probability test on the distribution of patients with regard to laterality of lesion and aetiology was marginally significant ($p = 0.085$). There were equal numbers of children with acquired left- and right-hemisphere lesions ($N = 8$), but there were about three times as many with congenital lesions in the left hemisphere ($N = 19$) than in the right ($N = 6$). In addition, a t-test indicated that left-hemisphere lesions tended to be larger than lesions in the right hemisphere ($t = 1.66$, $df = 40$, $p = 0.10$). There was no difference in lesion size between congenital and acquired cases.

Correlational analyses show that both Verbal and Performance IQs decrease with increasing lesion size (Figure 1).* Table II gives the correlation of Verbal IQ (VIQ), Performance IQ (PIQ) and Full-scale IQ (FIQ) in relation to lesion size. The correlation of IQ with lesion size is slightly higher when lesion size is estimated from its maximal diameter on CT-scan than when it is estimated from the number of CT slices on which the lesion appears. However, the correlation of the two lesion size measures is extremely high ($r = 0.92$, $df = 33$, $p < 0.001$).

Further analyses showed that the degree of hemiparesis and EEG grade both increase with increasing lesion size ($r = 0.67$, $df = 39$, $p < 0.01$; $r = 0.36$, $df = 39$, $p < 0.05$, respectively (Figure 2 and 3). The EEG results suggest that the likelihood of seizures is markedly greater for those with the largest lesions (Figure 3). In addition, both degree of hemiparesis and EEG grade are related to cognitive functioning. Degree of hemiparesis correlated significantly with VIQ ($r = -0.51$, $df = 37$, $p < 0.01$) and PIQ ($r = -.46$, $df = 37$, $p < 0.01$) and FIQ ($r = -0.61$, $df = 39$, $p < 0.01$) (Figure 4). EG

---

*Two children are omitted from all figures and analyses of Verbal and Performance IQ since they were administered the Stanford-Binet because of their age.

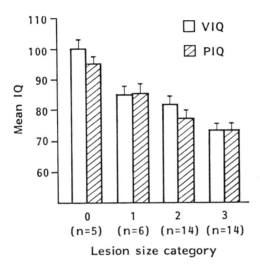

Figure 1. Mean VIQ and PIQ as function of lesion size.

Table II. Correlations of Lesion Size with IQ

	Maximal diameter ratio[1]	Number of CT slices[2]	Lesion size category[3]
VIQ	r = −0·51 df = 30 p < 0·01	r = −0·34 df = 37 p < 0·05	r = −0·47 df = 37 p < 0·01
PIQ	r = −0·42 df = 30 p < 0·02	r = −0·31 df = 37 p < 0·05	r = −0·48 df = 37 p < 0·01
FSIQ	r = −0·46 df = 32 p < 0·02	r = −0·33 df = 39 p < 0·05	r = −0·43 df = 39 p < 0·01

[1]Used to measure horizontal extent of lesion; [2]used to measure vertical extent of lesion; [3]derived from 1 and 2 (see text).

grade also correlated significantly with VIQ (r = −0·37, df = 37, (p < 0·05), PIQ (r = −0·40, df = 37, p < 0·05) and FIQ (r = 0·38, df = 39, p < 0·02). However, a one-way analysis of variance revealed no significant main effect of EEG grade on VIQ, PIQ or FIQ when lesion size was entered as a covariate.

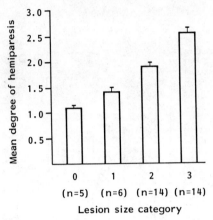

Figure 2. Mean degree of hemiparesis as function of lesion size.

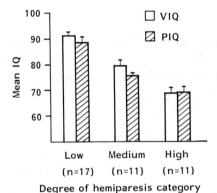

Figure 3. Mean EEG rank as functions of lesion size.

Because degree of hemiparesis, lesion size and EEG grade correlated with each other, as well as with IQ, the question arose as to which of these factors accounted for more of the variance in IQ. A step-wise linear regression revealed that degree of hemiparesis accounted for significantly more of this variance than either lesion size or EEG grade. Moreover, the use of lesion size of EEG data together with hemiparesis data did not significantly increase the amount of IQ variance accounted for, suggesting that all three factors are similar indices of underlying neurological impairment.

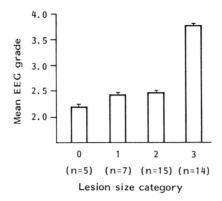

Figure 4. Mean VIQ and PIQ as function of degree of hemiparesis.

Possible effects of lesion location on IQ were also examined. We compared the IQs of patients with damage to cortical regions to those of patients with damage to cortical and subcortical regions (two patients whose lesions were confined to subcortical regions were not included in this analysis). There were no significant differences in VIQ, PIQ or FIQ. We also compared the IQs of patients with temporal and/or parietal lesions, which are likely to impinge on classic language comprehension areas, to those of all other patients: again, no significant differences were found. Finally, the IQs of patients categorized according to the lesion grades of 1 to 6 (Cohen and Duffner 1981) were examined. In agreement with Cohen and Duffner's report, the IQs of patients with grades 4 to 6 (N = 15) were lower than those with grades 1 to 3 (N = 24) (F = 4·07, df = 1, 38, p < 0·05). Degree of hemiparesis was also more severe in patients with lesion grades of 4 to 6 (F = 14·96, df = 1, 38, p < 0·0004). However, when lesion size was entered as a covariate, these effects disappeared (FIQ: F = 0·14, NS; degree of hemiparesis: F = 1·65, NS). Thus the differential effects of type of lesion reported by Cohen and Duffner may be accounted for by differences in the average size of lesions.

Mean VIQ, PIQ and FIQ scores are shown in Figure 5: the scores of all groups are well below the population mean of 100. An analysis of variance was performed with IQ scale score (Verbal, Performance) as a within-subjects factor, lesion laterality (left, right) and aetiology (congenital, acquired) as between-subjects factor, and lesion size as a covariate. No significant main effects or interactions involving lesion laterality or aetiology were found, but lesion size was a significant covariate (F = 7·70, df = 1, 32, p < 0·01).

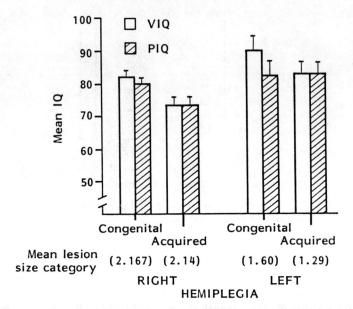

Figure 5. Mean VIQ and PIQ of children with right hemiplegia and left hemiplegia with congenital acquired lesions. Note that lesion size is greater with right and left hemiplegia and with congenital than acquired lesions.

Possible effects of lesion laterality and aetiology on the various WISC-R subtest scores were also investigated. There were no significant main effects or interactions involving lesion laterality. There were marginally significant main effects of aetiology, such that congenital cases performed better than acquired cases on three WISC-R verbal subjects: Vocabulary ($F = 4.12$, df = 1, 31, $p < 0.06$); Information ($F = 3.64$, df = 1, 31, $p < 0.07$); and Comprehension $F = 2.76$, df = 1, 31, $p < 0.11$). Lesion size was a significant covariate on all verbal subtests ($p < 0.03$ or better), except Similarities and Digit Span, and was significant or marginally significant on all Performance subtests ($p < 0.07$ or better).

Separate analyses of variance with lesion laterality and aetiology as between-subjects variables and lesion size as a covariate were performed on patients' scores on the Bender-Gestalt Test, the Peabody Picture Vocabulary Test (PPVT), the Northwestern Syntax Screening Test, and the Draw-A-Person Test. Consistent with their below-average IQ levels, all patient groups scored below average on these tests. The only significant effects occurred on the PPVT. There was a main effect of aetiology in that congenital cases performed better than acquired cases (F $=$ 5·67, df $=$ 1, 27, p $<$ 0·025)(mean Peabody IQ of congenital group 90·0; acquired group 72·4). There was also a main effect of lesion side, in that those with left hemiplegia performed significantly better (90·0) than those with right hemiplegia (72·4)(F $=$ 6·99, df $=$ 1, 27, p $<$ 0·02).

DISCUSSION

In agreement with previous studies *(e.g.* Perlstein and Hood 1955, Annett 1973, St. James-Roberts 1981, Cohen and Duffner 1981), we found that unilateral cerebral lesions in infancy or early childhood resulting in hemiparesis are associated with a significant decrease in IQ. Teuber and Rudel (1962) have suggested that certain tasks show functional plasticity after early brain-damage, while others do not. Tasks that do show plasticity are characterized as those on which adult brain-damaged patients show deficits after damage to specific areas. In contrast, tasks for which no functional plasticity is evident are characterized as those on which adult patients show deficits that are not area-specific. On such tasks, children with more severe (and perhaps larger) lesions are more impaired, and this may apply to many of the tasks included on IQ tests.

The magnitude of IQ depression in children with early unilateral lesions is considerable. Mean IQ in the largest lesion category was 20 to 30 points below the norm. Consistent with previous reports, 49 per cent of our sample obtained FIQ scores about 80 as compared to 51 per cent in the study by Cohen and Duffner (1981) and 90 per cent of normal children (Sattler 1974). The FIQ standard deviation of our sample is 17·8 (variance 316·8) compared to a standard deviation of 15 (variance 225) for the normal population. These variances differ significantly (F $=$ 1·41, df $=$ 40, ∞, p $<$ 0·05). Lesion size (as measured by maximal diameter ratio) was found to account for 21·2 per cent of the between-subject variance in IQ. Removing this percentage from the variance of our sample, the remaining variance no longer differs significantly from the normal population. In fact, after the variance due to lesion size is removed the standard deviation of our sample is 15·8, which is extremely close to that for the normal population. Lesion size therefore appears to account for all of the IQ variation in our sample, aside from the normal population variation related to genetic endowment, education and other environment factors.

Our findings suggest that left-hemisphere lesions tend to be larger than those in the right hemisphere. This may explain the small over-all IQ advantage of left-hemiplegic children in the present study, as well as in previous studies which did not have access to information on lesion size

(Perlstein and Hood 1954, Annett 1973). Our findings also suggest that the left hemisphere is more susceptible than the right to congenital lesions. Perlstein and Hood (1954) suggest that this may be attributable to the higher percentage of babies born with left occiput anterior. Metabolic differences between the left and right hemispheres may also be a factor (Levy, personal communication).

The classification of lesions into different types, as proposed by Cohen and Duffner (1981) and by Kotlarek *et al.* (1981), did not have predictive value for IQ, EEG or degree of hemiparesis that was not accounted for by differences in lesion size. The association of some lesion types with low IQ, in particular grades 4 to 6 of Cohen and Duffner, appears to be due to the fact that such lesions are on average larger than are those in grades 1 to 3. Thus, with respect to IQ level, the immature cerebral cortex appears to have equipotentiality, as proposed many years ago by Lashley (1929).

Significant effects of size of unilateral lesions on cognitive functioning are supported by previous studies of both children and adults. In particular, Woods and Carey (1979) reported no deficits in language production or comprehension in children with partial perinatal damage to the left hemisphere, whereas Dennis and Kohn (1975) report significantly impaired syntactic comprehension in patients with more severe left hemisphere lesions and subsequent hemispherectomy. Similar effects of the extent of lesions have been reported in adults. For example Kertesz *et al.* (1979) found that the degree and speed of recovery of language functions in adults with aphasia was correlated with lesion size.

No significant effect on IQ of EEG abnormalities or of seizures was found in our patients when lesion size was entered as a covariate. Very frequent intractable seizures occurred in only one of our patients. Our data and those of Cohen and Duffner (1981) suggest that seizures are rarely a factor in the depressed IQ of hemiplegic children. The early reports of such an association (Byers 1941, Perlstein and Hood 1955) are limited by the fact that possible correlations between seizures and lesion size were not considered.

The highly significant correlation between lesion size and degree of hemiparesis may be attributable to the increased probability of more severe motor area involvement with larger lesion size. Alternatively, it may indicate that motor functions in childhood are subserved by more widespread areas than in adulthood. Some suggestive evidence supports this latter possibility, in that the only identifiable lesion in three of the hemiparetic patients appeared to be confined to the parietal lobe and in two to the temporal and parietal lobes. It should also be noted that degree of hemiparesis correlated just as highly with VIQ as with PIQ, suggesting that it is an index of general neurological impairment rather than simply motor impairment.

The finding that left and right brain-damage had similar effects on Verbal and Performance IQ is consistent with most previous studies (Annett 1975, St. James-Roberts 1981; but see Kershner and King 1974) and suggests that IQ tests are relatively insensitive measures of the specific deficits associated with lesion laterally. Studies comparing early right *vs.* left hemisphere lesions clearly show that there are limits to equipotentiality. For example patients with early left hemispherectomy are differentially impaired in the understanding of passive sentences ('the girl is pushed by the boy') (Dennis and Kohn 1975, Dennis and Whitaker 1976). In contrast, those with early right hemispherectomy (Kohn and Dennis 1974) are differentially impaired on those visuospatial abilities that normally develop after age 10. Earlier-developing visuospatial abilities showed no effects of lesion laterality. In the present study, children with left hemisphere lesions had a more restricted receptive vocabulary than those with right hemisphere lesions. However, the latter group did not perform more poorly on any of the tests of visuospatial ability. In view of the Kohn and Dennis findings that patients with right hemispherectomy only show differential deficits on spatial tasks that are beyond the 10-year level, the absence of differential visuospatial deficits in our group with left hemiplegia may be attributable to their relatively young age (mean 8 years 4 months).

There is some indication from our data, as well as from other studies (Woods and Carey 1979), that the effects of cerebral lesions on language functions depend on the age at which the lesion is acquired, even during childhood. Our children with acquired lesions performed significantly worse than those with congenital lesions on several WISC-R verbal subtests, as well as on the Peabody Picture Vocabulary Test. Similarly, Annett (1973) and Woods and Carey (1979) reported a higher incidence of language difficulties among children with lesion onset after age one than during the first year of life.

In contrast to our findings for a variety of language tasks, effects of lesion aetiology (congenital/acquired) on visuospatial ability, as assessed by the Performance subtests of the WISC-R and the Bender-Gestalt, were not significant. Considered together, these results suggest that the time-course of functional plasticity may be somewhat different for verbal and spatial abilities. For verbal abilities it appears to be less harmful if the lesion occurs during the first year of life, whereas for spatial abilities the timing of the lesion during the infancy-childhood period seems to be less important (Woods 1980).

The present study suggests that functional plasticity following early, unilateral brain damage has certain limitations. First, the larger the lesion size the greater the depression of over-all intellectual functioning. Second, specific deficits are superimposed on this lower intellectual functioning, and the nature of these deficits depends on lesion laterality. Finally, functional plasticity during development is not an all-or-none phenomenon, and the time-course of plasticity may differ for verbal and spatial tasks. Delineating the factors that affect intellectual functioning following early brain damage, and the extent to which particular functions are spared or impaired, may contribute to our understanding of developmental changes in brain-behavior relations.

REFERENCES

Annett, M. (1973) 'Laterality of childhood hemiplegia and the growth of speech and intelligence.' *Cortex, 9,* 4–33.

Basser, L. S. (1962) 'Hemiplegia of early onset and the faculty of speech, with special reference to the effects of hemispherectomy.' *Brain, 85,* 427–460.

Byers, R. K. (1941) 'Evolution of hemiplegias in infancy.' *American Journal of Diseases of Children, 61,* 915–927.

Cohen, M. E., Duffner, P. K. (1981) 'Prognostic indicators in hemiparetic cerebral palsy.' *Annals of Neurology, 9,* 353–357.

Dennis, M., Kohn B. (1975) 'Comprehension of syntax in infantile hemiplegias after cerebral hemidecortication: left hemisphere superiority.' *Brain and Language, 2* 472–482.

―――― Whitaker, H. (1976) 'Language acquisition following hemidecortication: Linguistic superiority of the left over the right hemisphere.' *Brain and Language, 3,* 404–433.

Dunn, L. M. (1965) *Expanded Manual for the Peabody Picture Vocabulary Test.* Minneapolis: American Guidance Service.

Dunsdon, M. (1952) *The Educability of Cerebral Palsied Children,* London: Newnes.

Ingram, T. T. S. (1964) *Paediatric Aspects of Cerebral Palsy.* Edinburgh: Livingstone.

Kershner, J. R., King, A. J. (1974) 'Laterality of cognitive functions in achieving hemiplegic children.' *Perceptual and Motor Skills, 39,* 1283–1289.

Kertesz, A., Harlock, W., Coates, C. (1979) 'Computer tomographic localization, lesion size, and prognosis in aphasia and nonverbal impairment.' *Brain and Language, 8,* 34–50.

Kohn, B., Dennis, M. (1974) 'Selective impairments of visuospatial abilities in infantile hemiplegics after right cerebral hemidecortication.' *Neuropsychologia, 12,* 505–512.

Koppitz, E. M. (1964) *The Bender Gestalt Test for Young Children.* New York: Grune & Stratton.

―――― (1968) *Psychological Evaluation of Children's Human Figure Drawings.* New York: Grune & Stratton.

Kotlarek, F., Rodewig, R., Brüll, D., Zeumer, H. (1981) 'Computed tomographic findings in congenital hemiparesis in childhood and their relation to etiology and prognosis.' *Neuropediatrics, 12,* 101–109.

Lashley, K. S. (1929) *Brain Mechanisms and Intelligence: A Quantitative Study of Injuries to the Brain.* Chicago: University of Chicago Press.

Lee, L. L. (1969) *Northwestern Syntax Screening Test.* Evanston, IL: Northwestern University Press.

Lenneberg, E. A. (1967) *Biological Foundations of Language.* New York: Wiley.

Nielsen, N. (1966) *A Psychological Study of Cerebral Palsied Children.* Copenhagen: Munksgaard.

Perlstein, M. A., Hood, P. N. (1954) 'Infantile spastic hemiplegia. I: Incidence.' *Pediatrics, 14,* 436–441.

—— Hood, P. N. (1955) 'Infantile spastic hemiplegia. III: Intelligence.' *Pediatrics, 15,* 676–682.

Rankin, J. M., Aram, D. M., Horwitz, S. J. (1981) 'Language ability in right and left hemiplegic children.' *Brain and Language,* 14, 292–306.

St. James-Roberts, I. (1981) 'A reinterpretation of hemispherectomy data without functional plasticity of the brain.' *Brain and Language, 13,* 31–53.

Sattler, J. M. (1974) *Assessment of Children's Intelligence.* Philadelphia: W. B. Saunders.

Smith, A., Sugar, O. (1975) 'Development of above normal language and intelligence 21 years after left hemispherectomy.' *Neurology, 25,* 813–818.

Terman, L. M., Merrill, M. A. *Stanford-Binet Intelligence Scale. Manual for the Third Revision. Form L-M.* Boston: Houghton Mifflin.

Teuber, H.-L. Rudel, R. G. (1962) 'Behaviour after cerebral lesions in children and adults.' *Developmental Medicine and Child Neurology, 4,* 8–20.

Wechsler, D. (1967) *The Wechsler Preschool and Primary Scale of Intelligence Manual.* New York: Psychological Corporation.

—— (1974) *The Wechsler Intelligence Scale for Children—Revised.* New York: Psychological Corporation.

Wedell, K. (1960) 'The visual perception of cerebral palsied children.' *Child Psychology and Psychiatry, 1,* 215–227.

Wood, N. E. (1955) 'A comparison of right hemiplegics and left hemiplegics in visual perception.' *Journal of Clinical Psychology, 11,* 378–380.

Woods, B. T. (1980) 'The restricted effects of right hemisphere lesions after age one: Wechsler test data.' *Neuropsychologia,* 18, 65–70.

—— Carey, S. (1979) 'Language deficits after apparent clinical recovery from childhood aphasia.' *Annals of Neurology, 6,* 405–409.

—— Teuber, H. L. (1973) 'Early onset of complementary specialization of cerebral hemispheres in man.' *Transactions of the American Neurology Association, 98,* 113–117.

—— —— (1978) 'Changing patterns of childhood aphasia.' *Annals of Neurology, 3,* 273–280.

30

The Family's Adaptation
to Childhood Leukemia

Betsy Fife

*Riley Hospital for Children, Indiana University Medical Center,
and Indiana University, Bloomington*

James Norton and Gary Groom

Indiana University School of Medicine, Bloomington

*This baseline study obtained data measuring the specific effects of
childhood leukemia on family life and on the lives of individual
family members. Mothers, fathers, siblings, and patients were
included in the data collection. Specific variables measured were
marital adjustment, anxiety level, dynamics of family interaction,
and the school behavior of patients and siblings. The data were
collected at designated intervals over a one year period beginning at
the time of diagnosis. In addition, the data were utilized to
speculate on those families that appeared to be at risk for the
development of long-term psychosocial problems secondary to, or
aggravated by the illness. Results indicated that patterns of coping
for families, as well as for individual family members, were
relatively constant over time. Families with predominantly stable
relationships and adequate support within the family unit were able
to maintain their usual quality of life over an extended period of*

Reprinted with permission from *Social Science Medicine*, 1987, Vol. 24, No. 2, 159–168.
Copyright 1987 by Pergamon Journals Ltd.

The authors wish to express their thanks to Wm. George McAdoo for his valuable ideas and
contributions to this project. We also wish to thank Robert Baehner, Arthur Provisor, and
Margaret Martin for their support; and Pamela Rappaport, Susan Szabo, Marian Huhman, and
Wanda Lancaster for their technical assistance. We particularly appreciate the families who
shared themselves so willingly with us. This research was funded by PHS grant R01 NU00784.

*time despite the onset of acute stress. However, families with pre-
existing problems prior to diagnosis for the most part experienced
increased deterioration in family life and had difficulty coping.
Results of the Spielberger State-Trait Anxiety Scale, the Locke-
Wallace Marital Adjustment Test, the Moos Family Environment
Scale, the MMPI, and school data supporting these conclusions are
given.*

INTRODUCTION

Effective chemotherapy and radiation treatment have significantly extended the life span of most children with leukemia; consequently, for many it has
become a chronic, life-threatening illness accompanied by the stress and
anxiety of uncertainty [1]. Furthermore, the literature indicates wide
recognition of the fact that the incidence of all forms of childhood cancer and
the ensuing stress have a pervasive impact on family members, and on many
aspects of family functioning [2–4]. The effects of this impact have raised
increasing concern about issues regarding the quality of life, the psychosocial
costs of treatment, and the need to identify those families and individuals who
are at risk for the development of long-term problems secondary to the
illness. Although the scientific rigor of research investigating the problems of
this population is increasing, an insufficient number of studies has incorporated valid and reliable objective measures to obtain quantitative data indicating
the specific effects of the illness on the integrity of the family unit and on the
lives of individual members. In addition, available findings are contradictory.

One of the earlier investigations studying the impact of this catastrophic
disease on the family was carried out by Binger *et al.* in 1969 [5]. This
research was conducted with 20 families whose children had died of
leukemia. Interview was the technique used, and effects of the stress of the
illness on the patient, parents, siblings, and the family system were discussed
with the parents. In 50% of these families at least one member required
psychiatric intervention. One or more siblings in approx. 50% of the families
engaged in behavior patterns that indicated difficulty coping, many parents
manifested such problems as depression, somatization, and overactivity, and
patients expressed feelings of anxiety and loneliness.

Powazek *et al.* [6], conducted a study of families' adaptation to childhood
leukemia that combined the use of interview and psychometric measures, in
which the data was obtained primarily from the mother's perspective. Based
on quantitative measures administered at the time of diagnosis, maternal
profiles indicated more disturbance than those of the patients. Only 8% of the
patients manifested a high level of anxiety; however, 45% of the mothers

were highly anxious, 38% were depressed, and 55% presented signs of neurotic maladjustment. Subsequent testing 6 months following diagnosis showed a decrease in these measures of maternal distress. In addition, according to mothers' reports, 81% of the families had siblings who developed maladaptive behavior changes following diagnosis. The primary difficulties they indicated for fathers were a lack of participation in the treatment process, and an unwillingness to openly discuss the illness and related problems.

On the other hand, the findings of Kupst *et al.* [7], who also utilized quantitative measures in a longitudinal study to directly assess mothers and fathers, and assessment by medical personnel and psychosocial staff to assess family coping, indicated no significant change in the adjustment of family members from the time of diagnosis for a one year period. Moreover, the majority of families and their individual members were evaluated as coping adequately. It is important to note that this research did not include quantitative data directly assessing the coping behaviors of patients or siblings, for example, psychometric measures or school data. In addition, two thirds of the families participating in the project received some form of intervention. A design was utilized that included a control group and two different levels of intervention; however, no statistically significant difference was found among the three groups. These authors also report a two year follow-up study in which the methods and findings remain essentially unchanged [8].

Research comparing the responses of school age patients and their healthy siblings to the diagnosis of childhood cancer was done by Cairns *et al.* [2] utilizing three assessment instruments. The Piers-Harris Children's Self-Concept scale indicated no significant difference between the two groups and both were within normal limits. A family interaction test given to 14 patient-sibling pairs revealed that siblings felt their mothers overprotected and overindulged the patient, while the thematic apperception test disclosed that siblings, like patients, have significant anxiety and fear for their own health, and experience similar feelings of social isolation.

In addition, there has been much concern about the impact of childhood cancer on the marriage relationship, with varying reports about its effects. Kaplan *et al.* [9] in a study conducted by periodically surveying 40 families of children diagnosed with leukemia, beginning at the onset of the illness, reported 5% had divorced, 18% had separated, and an additional 70% had serious marital problems. Lansky *et al.* [10] utilized the Arnold sign indicator analysis of MMPI profiles to measure the level of marital stress in 38 couples who had children diagnosed with cancer, and a comparison group whose children were being treated for hemophilia, along with a normal group, and a group of marital counselees. Data, which indicated findings contrary to those of Kaplan, revealed that parents of children with cancer experienced an increased level of marital stress; however, the mean stress level of these couples was lower than that reported for the marriage counselees, and no greater percentage of them resorted to divorce than couples from the population at large.

This overview of the literature indicates a central concern about all members of families of children with cancer, for individuals belonging to families do not resolve the stresses they experience independently, nor are they immune to the effects of problems experienced by other family members. Therefore the research discussed in this paper, unlike other studies reported in the literature to date, has included each family member over the age of 5 years in the collection of quantitative data. The central purpose has been to investigate patterns of coping behavior that develop throughout the first year of illness as a means of determining when treatment may be indicated for the prevention of secondary psychosocial problems.

Families of children newly diagnosed with acute lymphocytic leukemia provided the focus for this research. The sample was restricted to this single diagnosis to control insofar as it is possible for variability in treatment regimen and course of the illness. A scale designed to measure marital adjustment, an anxiety scale, and the MMPI were used as indicators of the coping behaviors of both mothers and fathers while an anxiety scale and academic records were utilized in conjunction with teachers' reports and parent interviews to determine the effects of the illness on patients and siblings. A family interaction scale measured the impact of the diagnosis on family relationships. The data were collected at scheduled intervals over a one year period. In addition the data were utilized to verify speculations on those families who appeared to be at the greatest risk for the development of long-term psychosocial problems secondary to, or aggravated by the illness.

METHOD

Subjects

The study included 34 families; the patients ranged from 22 months to 16 years of age, with 46% of them being of school age, and a mean age at diagnosis of 6.3 years. Families were approached about participating in the study during the initial hospitalization, 2–3 days following confirmation of the child's diagnosis. The purpose of the study was explained to parents and available children at that time, samples of the questionnaires they would be requested to complete were shared with them, and signed consent was obtained from all participating parents and adolescent patients—siblings were usually not available. A consent rate of 87.5% was obtained from the families interviewed with one of these families consenting to give only school data. During the course of the 12 month investigation one family withdrew. It should also be noted that five children died during the first year following diagnosis, and at that time collection of quantitative data from these families was discontinued, as it was felt to be too intrusive during this stressful period. However, periodic contact was maintained with the families, and school records were obtained for siblings from the two families having remaining children of school age.

A total of 33 mothers, 27 fathers, 31 siblings between the ages of 6 and 17 years of age, and 13 patients of school age were participating subjects. There were six single parent families in the sample, and five families in which one or both parents had previously divorced or remarried. All participating families were Caucasian; incomes ranged from less than 10,000 to $50,000 annually with 58.6% having an income under $15,000 per year, and 57.2% of the primary providers having had no education beyond high school.

Prognosis, a particularly significant variable as it affects the degree of optimism for long-term survival, is defined by the patient's age and white cell count at diagnosis. Prognostic categories for the patients in this sample were as follows: six had a poor prognosis, 24 were in the average group, and prognosis of five patients was above average. The majority of children in the sample spent relatively brief periods of time in the hospital during the first year following diagnosis, they remained in first remission, and had a relatively uneventful course of illness. The number of hospital days ranged from 6 to 118 days, with the median being 20 days.

These families lived between 30 and 185 miles from the treatment center with the mean distance being 104 miles; 11.4% of the families experienced the stress of not feeling they had adequate medical support in case of emergency, due to their lack of confidence in the local physician. In addition, through periodic interview and administration of the Holmes-Rahe Readjustment Rating Scale, it was determined that 55.9% of the families experienced major concurrent stressors in conjunction with the stress of the illness. Events ranged from financial problems and the birth of a new child, to the death of a member of the extended family, to recent widowhood, divorce and remarriage.

Procedure

Data reported in this paper were obtained over a period of one year at scheduled intervals as described in Table 1. A total of four psychometric measures was utilized.

Table 1. Data Collection Schedule

Measure	Period of diagnosis and chemotherapy induction admission (day 10)	Period of radiation therapy (days 14–28)	Period of remission and continued treatment (1 month to 12 months post-diagnosis)
Moos Family Environment Scale	Parents, first week following diagnosis		Parents, 2nd, 4th, 7th, 10th months
Locke-Wallace Marital Adjustment Test	Parents, first week following diagnosis		Parents, 2nd, 4th, 7th, 10th months
Spielberger Anxiety Inventory			
Trait Measure	Patient, parents, siblings, first week following diagnosis		Patient, parents, siblings, 6th, 12th months
State Measure	Patient, parents, siblings, first week following diagnosis	Patient, parents, siblings once during this 14 day period	Patient, parents, siblings, 6th, 9th, 12th months
MMPI			Parents, 3rd, 12th months
Social Readjustment Rating Scale	Parent for family, first week following diagnosis		Parent for family at 12th month

The Moos Family Environment Scale was administered to obtain a measure of patterns of interaction and the social climate of the family. The scale contains ten subscales along three dimensions: relationship, personal growth, and system maintenance. Six specific scales were of particular interest for this research: cohesion, expressiveness, conflict, independence, organization, and control. Item-to-subscale correlations were calculated by Moos [11] to determine internal consistency which ranged from 0.45 to 0.58. Test-retest reliability was also computed and varied from 0.68 to 0.86.

The Locke-Wallace Short Marital Adjustment Test provided an indicator of the level of satisfaction and adjustment within the marriage. Locke and Wallace [12] computed reliability by the split-half technique and corrected by the Spearman-Brown formula, obtaining a coefficient of 0.90. Validity was determined by comparing the mean score of 48 subjects known to be experiencing marital difficulty, with a matched group judged to be well adjusted; the difference in the observed data was significant with the 'critical ratio' being 17.5. This particular scale was selected as it is brief, easily understood, and includes items most pertinent to fundamental aspects of the marital relationship.

The Spielberger State-Trait Anxiety Inventory is comprised of two self-report scales. One form measures state anxiety (A-state), which is conceptualized as a transitory emotional condition characterized by subjective, consciously perceived feelings of tension and apprehension. A-states may vary in intensity and fluctuate over time. The other form measures trait anxiety (A-trait) which refers to relatively stable individual differences in anxiety proness, that is, differences between people in their tendency to respond to situations perceived as threatening with elevations in A-state intensity. The test-retest reliability of the A-trait scale, as calculated by Spielberger [13] is relatively high, ranging from 0.73 to 0.86; however, the coefficient for the A-state scale tends to be low as would be expected for a measure sensitive to the influence of situational factors. A State-Trait Anxiety Inventory was also developed to be used with children 9 to 12 years of age that is a downward extension of the adult form. The trait scale was administered to all parents, and to siblings and patients 9 years of age and above during the diagnostic period, and again at 6 and 12 months post-diagnosis. However, since situational anxiety is an indication of the degree of stress an individual is experiencing, the state scale was given at six different intervals as indicated in Table 1 to determine changes in anxiety levels as treatment progressed.

The MMPI, a 566 item personality test that is extensively used for the diagnosis of psychopathology and research, was administered to the parents to measure defensiveness, somatization, anxiety, and depression. This was first given 3 months post-diagnosis when life had returned to a more normal routine for the majority of subject families, and again at 12 months. Like the other psychometric measures it was given during clinic visits; however, due to inadequate time the forms were usually completed at home and returned by mail within 2 weeks.

Interviews with both parents at the time of diagnosis, and the available parent 6 and 12 months following diagnosis, were utilized to supplement the quantitative data described above. These structured interviews took place during clinic visits, and were approx. 30–45 min long. They included questions regarding the existence of concurrent stressors, the home, school, and social adjustment of the patient and siblings, and changes occurring within the family. They were also conducted with each family 2 years post-diagnosis in the interest of long-term follow-up. Those families whose children died were contacted by telephone.

A further source of data included the records of patients' and siblings' school attendance and academic performance for the year prior to diagnosis, and each succeeding report given throughout the first year of treatment. In addition, a teacher's report form developed specifically for the purposes of this research was obtained for each child of school age immediately following diagnosis and at the conclusion of the 12 month data collection period. Questions pertained to the child's attitude toward authority figures, changes in classroom performance, and poor relationships.

One hundred percent cooperation was obtained from the schools; however, it was not possible to obtain all data requested from each participating family member throughout the one year period. The problem of missing data has been accounted for in the statistical procedures used in analysis (see below). Patients and siblings were the least consistent subjects, therefore a two-dollar payment was given to them immediately following completion of the data, which improved their response rate considerably. Greater cooperation on the part of parents in completing the Locke-Wallace Short Marital Adjustment Test was also noted when the title on the forms was changed to 'Marital Inventory', which apparently had a less evaluative connotation.

RESULTS

Repeated measures analysis of variance was utilized to analyze the statistical findings of the Spielberger Anxiety Scale, the Marital Adjustment Test, and the Moos Family Environment Scale. The data were analyzed for change over time beginning at diagnosis for a 12 month period. In addition, analyses were run according to prognostic category, however, no significant differences were found between them on any of the measures. Because of missing data these analyses had to be performed using 'general linear model' programs: BMD $\times$ 65 [14] or SAS GLM [15]. The times of administration for each measure are indicated in Table 1.

The Spielberger State-Trait Anxiety Scale

Longitudinal analysis of the *state* anxiety measure for both mothers and fathers indicated a continuous decrease in the level of situational anxiety. This change was significant over the 12 month period with the largest decline occurring in the first 2 months following diagnosis for both mothers and fathers; however, initial scores were not as high as would be expected under these stressful circumstances. The results are given in Table 2. Anxiety state scores for both patients and siblings were low from the time of diagnosis and showed no significant change over time. From the perspective of this data, it appears that the use of denial as a coping mechanism may have been operating with both parents and children in this sample, although to a greater extent with patients and siblings. This hypothesis is validated to some extent by both researcher and teacher observations of several children whose questions and behavior indicated a high level of anxiety, although their anxiety state scores were low. In the instance of siblings, it may also be that their low level of underlying anxiety is partially accounted for by a lack of direct involvement in the treatment process. There was no significant change in scores on the anxiety trait scale for any category of family members as would be expected given the stable nature of the measure, and the means were within normal limits.

Locke-Wallace Marital Adjustment Test

Initial scores indicating the level of marital satisfaction for both mothers and fathers in this sample were considerably lower than the score for well adjusted couples; however, they were also above the mean for couples seeking therapy and known to be experiencing marital conflict. Fathers indicated the highest level of dissatisfaction on that aspect of the questionnaire pertaining to general marital happiness, while mothers were most discontent with a lack of consensus in decision making. Longitudinal analysis indicated a steady decline in marital happiness for both fathers and mothers, although it did not reach statistical significance. The sharpest decline occurred approx. 4 months following diagnosis for both parents. Results are given in Table 3.

Table 2. Longitudinal Analysis of Anxiety State Scores

Time point	Mothers ($N = 33$), least squares estimated means*	Fathers ($N = 27$), least squares estimated means*
Diagnostic period	50.59	50.07
Radiation period	44.98	43.48
Three months post-diagnosis	44.69	39.11
Six months post-diagnosis	42.34	40.27
Nine months post-diagnosis	40.46	42.67
Twelve months post-diagnosis	39.16	41.24
Test of overall trend:		
F	8.42	6.58
df	5, 133	5, 94
Probability	($P < 0.0001$)	($P < 0.0001$)

*Highest possible score = 80.

Because of missing data, these analyses were carried out using 'general linear model' programs (see text p. 162). Such programs generate and test for significance among means which are estimated from the least squares fit of the analysis of variance model, rather than the actual means of observed values. (If there were no missing data, these would be the same.) Hence the term 'least squares estimated means.'

Table 3. Least Squares Means of Marital Adjustment Test Indicating Change Over Time

Administration time	Least squares means*, mothers ($N = 28$)	Least squares means* (fathers ($N = 27$)
Time of diagnosis	115.94	115.92
Second month following diagnosis	119.33	113.27
Fourth month following diagnosis	113.22	105.06
Seventh month following diagnosis	114.27	111.87
Tenth month following diagnosis	110.90	108.63
Test of overall trend:		
F	2.12	1.96
df	4, 74	4, 66
Probability	$P = 0.087$	$P = 0.11$

*[12] Mean for adjusted couples = 135.9. Mean for poorly adjusted couples = 71.7.

Moos Family Environment Scale

Longitudinal analysis of the ten subscales on the family interaction measure essentially demonstrated stability over time for the families in this sample despite the stress they were experiencing. However, there were three aspects of family life that parents indicated changed to some extent for them. The first is the issue of the level of control within the family (FES scale no. 10), or the extent to which the family is organized around the enforcement of rules. Both parents indicated an increase in the degree of control maintained within the family approx. 4 months following diagnosis; however, this was followed by a return to the level indicated at the time of diagnosis by the twelfth month. This increase was greater for fathers ($P = 0.017$) than for mothers ($P = 0.168$). This finding is congruent with the need for individuals to increase control in one area of living as a coping behavior, when the stress level is high and control has been lost in another. A feeling of lack of control is particularly characteristic of parents who experience a keen sense of helplessness, and a temporary loss of their parental role when a child incurs a serious illness.

There was also an increase for both parents along the dimension of moral-religious emphasis (FES scale no. 8). This was particularly true for fathers who indicated a steady increase with the overall change being significant at P < 0.01; while the mothers also experienced an increase along this dimension it was not significant ($P = 0.267$). The mean scores for mothers and fathers were approximately equal on this scale at the time of diagnosis, with a difference first occurring 2 months after diagnosis when mothers' scores increased. However, by 4 months the trend had reversed with fathers' scores becoming significantly higher than their spouses by the sixth month ($P = 0.047$). The importance of religious belief for fathers may be partially a result of their frequent lack of direct involvement in the care and treatment of the child, and a subsequent need to find less tangible ways of coping with the stress.

A third change was noted in mothers' indications that the extent of their family's involvement in recreational activities (FES scale no. 7) declined to a low point 4 months following diagnosis, and then gradually returned to the initial level. This overall change was significant at $P = 0.018$. Fathers indicated only a negligible change. This difference in parents' perceptions was significant at $P = 0.012$ and may be accounted for by the decreased activity of many mothers outside of the home during the period of intensive treatment.

Pearson product-moment correlation coefficients were obtained between specified scales of the family interaction measure, and also between certain of these scales and the measure of marital satisfaction. Several interesting findings were obtained. First, moral-religious emphasis appears to contribute to both a sense of cohesion and marital satisfaction for mothers in the sample ($r = 0.50$ and $r = 0.54$), while the relationship between the variables of moral-religious emphasis and marital satisfaction was minimal for fathers. Secondly, there was a significant correlation between a sense of cohesion and marital satisfaction ($r = 0.63$), as well as cohesion and openness in communication for fathers ($r = 0.56$), whereas this was not significant for mothers. Finally, the level of organization within the family was related to the feeling of cohesion and marital satisfaction for both parents ($r = 0.53$ and $r = 0.54$ for mothers, and $r = 0.62$ and $r = 0.48$ for fathers). In summary, the dimensions of cohesion, moral-religious emphasis, and the need for increased organization and control appear to be particularly significant aspects of family dynamics in crisis situations.

The MMPI

This measure was administered 3 and 12 months post diagnosis to parents participating in the study. However, not all parents completed this questionnaire on both occasions; therefore, the data are presented in two different tables. Table 4a summarizes the findings based on all parents taking the MMPI at either time, while Table 4b pertains only to those parents

Table 4a. Proportion of Mothers and Fathers with Scores Above $T = 60$ on Designated MMPI Scales

Scale	Third month				Twelfth month			
	Fraction		Percentage		Fraction		Percentage	
	Mothers	Fathers	Mothers	Fathers	Mothers	Fathers	Mothers	Fathers
A (anxiety)	2/29	3/20	6.9	15	2/24	3/16	8.3	18.8
Pt (psychasthenia)	10/29	9/20	34.5	45	5/24	7/16	20.83	43.8
D (depression)	12/29	6/20	41.4	30	4/24	5/16	16.7	31.3
D-S (subtle depression)	12/29	5/20	41.4	25	13/24	8/16	54.2	50
Hs (hypochondriasis)	6/29	4/20	20.7	20	4/24	7/16	16.7	43.8
Tt (defensiveness)	6/29	5/20	20.7	25	8/24	5/16	33.3	31.3

participating at both administration times. The following discussion is based on the data in Table 4b unless otherwise indicated. The generally accepted cut off points for T-scores on the MMPI are: low—T score of 45 or below; moderate elevation—T score of 60–70; marked elevation—T score of 70 or above [16].

A second measure of anxiety was obtained from the results of the 'A' scale of the MMPI, which indicates overt, short-term, situational anxiety. Like the results of the state anxiety indicator of the Spielberger Scale, the scores were lower than would be expected for these parents, with only 8% of the mothers and 15% of the fathers who took the MMPI registering moderate or higher elevations of conscious anxiety. The scores did not change much between the third and twelfth months following diagnosis (see Table 4a). However, the Psychasthenia Scale that measures anxiety of a long-term nature produced quite different results; 21.4% of the fathers and 28.6% of the mothers had at least moderate elevations on this scale at the third month, while the percentage dropped for mothers at the twelfth month and the percentage for fathers increased. It is interesting to note that scores on this scale are known to increase during times of situational stress, and elevated scores may also indicate a high level of intellectualizing as a defense mechanism [16].

The clinical depression scale, scale 'D', measures the degree of sadness and pessimism the individual fee⸱⸱⸱t the time the MMPI is administered. A relatively high percentage ▮▮▮▮mothers (33.3%) experienced at least a

Table 4b. Proportions of Scores Above $T = 60$ for Mothers and Fathers Having Scores at Both the Third and Twelfth Months

	Third month				Twelfth month			
	Fraction		Percentage		Fraction		Percentage	
Scale	Mothers	Fathers	Mothers	Fathers	Mothers	Fathers	Mothers	Fathers
A (anxiety)	1/21	1/14	4.8	7.1	2/21	3/14	9.5	21.4
Pt (psychasthenia)	6/21	3/14	28.6	21.4	5/21	5/14	23.8	35.7
D (depression)	7/21	3/14	33.3	21.4	4/21	4/14	19	28.6
D-S (subtle depression)	8/21	5/14	38.1	35.7	11/21	7/14	52.4	50
Hs (hypochondriasis)	3/21	2/14	14.3	14.3	4/21	6/14	19	42.9
Tt (defensiveness)	6/21	3/14	28.6	21.4	5/21	5/14	23.8	35.7

moderate degree of depression around the third month following diagnosis, but this dropped to 19% by the twelfth month. Though fewer fathers (21.4%) had feelings of depression about 3 months following their child's diagnosis, this percentage increased by the twelfth month to 28.6%. In addition, results of the 'D-S' scale were analyzed. This particular scale provides a measure of the subtle indications of depression and is particularly useful in differentiating this characteristic in the normal population. These results, like those of the 'D' scale, indicated a notable degree of depression in both mothers and fathers; however, the results differed as there was an increase rather than a decrease in the percentage of mothers as well as fathers experiencing depression at the twelfth month.

A third variable analyzed was the level of somatization shown by these parents. This was measured by the Hypochondriasis Scale that indicates the number of bodily complaints claimed by a person, and the extent that these complaints are used to manipulate others [16]. The number of mothers and fathers scoring moderate elevations was approx. 14% at the third month with a slight increase for mothers at the second administration time, and a marked increase to 42.9% for fathers.

Individuals with elevations on both the Hypochondriasis and Depression Scales tend to be irritable and depressed, and they respond to stress with physical symptoms, resisting psychological explanations [17]. It is worth noting that 100% of the mothers with elevated scores on the Hypochondriasis Scale 3 months following diagnosis also had above average scores on one or both of the depression scales.

In addition to the variables indicating parents' reactions to their child's illness, a measure of defensiveness as manifested by the 'Tt' Scale was obtained. A high score demonstrates caution about revealing oneself. We have assumed that subjects displaying a high degree of defensiveness on this particular scale were also circumspect in responding to other questionnaires they were asked to complete. The results were as follows. On the first administration, 3 months post-diagnosis 28.6% of the mothers and 21.4% of the fathers indicated high levels of defensiveness. On the second administration, 12 months post-diagnosis, 23.8% of the mothers and 35.7% of the fathers indicated an elevated degree of defensiveness.

In addition to these analyses of individual scales, correlations were obtained to determine the relationship between depression and specific scales on the family interaction measure and the level of marital satisfaction. The following relationships were statistically significant for fathers ($P < 0.025$), who indicated that a lack of family cohesion, and marital unhappiness are associated with elevated levels of depression. However, the only significant relationship for mothers was the correlation between the depression and family cohesion ($P = 0.018$) at the third month. It should be noted that the MMPI administered at the third month was correlated with the Family Environment Scale and Marital Inventory from the second month, while the twelfth month MMPI was correlated with findings from the tenth month on the family and marital scales.

Although the number of parents willing to respond to the MMPI was more limited than the other scales utilized in this research, the investigators believe its use was important for several reasons. First, it provided measures of depression and somatization which are significant impediments to functional coping. Second, it gave an indication of the openness with which subjects were willing to respond to questions asked in the study. Third, it provided a means for validating the findings of other measures.

School data. Findings from the school data of patients and siblings are summarized in Tables 5 and 6 respectively. However, a few comments regarding this aspect of the data are necessary. In regard to attendance problems, several mothers indicated during interviews that it was difficult for them to enforce school attendance for the ill child if he/she complained of not feeling well, although their reluctance decreased if the child continued to make satisfactory progress from a medical standpoint. Furthermore, several teachers noted in their comments that when they detected problems with a particular patient or sibling and were aware of the circumstances, they made

Table 5. Summary of Patients' School Data

Problem	N of patients experiencing the problem*	Ages of those patients
Attendance, excessive number of absences that were medically unnecessary for them (more than 70 days)	6 (46.2%)	6 years, 8 years (2), 10 years, 11 years, 12 years
*Decline in academic performance (decrease of 0.5 or more in GPA on 4.0 scale)	6 (46.2%)	8 years, 10 years, 11 years 13 years (2), 17 years
Incidence of behavior problems most commonly mentioned include: withdrawal, lack motivation, poor concentration, anger and rebelliousness, regression	4 (30.8%)	7 years, 11 years, 13 years, 17 years

*Percents shown are percents of the 13 patients of school age.

Table 6. Summary of Siblings' School Data

Problem	N of siblings experiencing the problem*	Ages of those siblings
Attendance, an increased absenteeism of 10 days or more as compared with the year prior to diagnosis	6 (19.4%)	9 years, 10 years, 14 years, 15 years, 17 years (2)
Decline in academic performance (decrease of 0.5 or more in GPA on 4.0 scale)	12 (38.7%)	7 years (2), 10 years (3), 11 years (2), 12 years (1), 13 years (2), 14 years, 17 years
Incidence of behavior problems including: withdrawal, deterioration in self confidence, uncooperative, preoccupied, hostile, anxious, regression, lack motivation, attention seeking	17 (54.8%)	6 years (4), 7 years, 8 years, 9 years (3), 10 years (2), 11 years (2), 12 years, 14 years, 17 years

*Percents shown are percents of the 31 siblings observed.

an effort to help the child. This frequently had positive results, but the willingness of teachers to offer help appeared to be partially dependent on the parents' ability to maintain an effective relationship with the school. For example, teachers of several children from one family who were experiencing difficulty made no effort to extend extra assistance to any of them as they felt the children's problems were due to family dynamics. During interviews the parents in this family expressed hostility toward both the schools and teachers indicating they felt there was a lack of concern, yet they did not take initiative to resolve the problem. This kind of circumstance indicates a need for care givers to intervene.

An analysis of functional vs dysfunctional families. In addition to the data analyses discussed above, which included all subject families, ten families were selected for comparison of their coping ability based solely on interview assessment. Data from these families were then analyzed to determine if it is possible to assess and predict by traditional interview methods those families most vulnerable to the development of secondary psychosocial problems, as validated by objective data from the subjects themselves, by the incidence of psychosocial crises within the family following diagnosis, and by data from teachers. Selection of these families took place one year following diagnosis after ongoing monthly contacts during data collection. The criteria used were the family's history of stress and coping behavior prior to the diagnosis, their ability to cope with the child's illness and its consequences, and the apparent level of marital stability and support. Five of the families were assessed to be effective functional systems who were coping adequately with current circumstances, and five families appeared to be engaging in predominantly dysfunctional transactions. The specific measures included in the analysis to compare these two sets of families were the Marital Adjustment Test; the cohesiveness, expressiveness, and conflict scores of the Family Environment Scale; and state anxiety scores. Major changes occurring in the family following diagnosis were also noted, and content of the school data of both patients and their siblings was included.

The accuracy of the assessment of family functioning through the interview method was confirmed by the data. Repeated measures analysis of variance was utilized to test for differences between the two groups of families on the Marital Adjustment Test, the Family Environment Scale, and the State Anxiety Scale [18]. As before, these analyses had to be carried out using 'general linear model' procedures because of missing data. The findings are given in Tables 7 and 8. Significance was obtained between the overall groups' means on the marital scale, as well as on the cohesion scale of the family interaction measure, which indicates the extent of commitment to and

Table 7. Repeated-measures Analysis of Variance for Scores on Marital Adjustment Test from Functional and Dysfunctional Family Group

Source of variation	df	Mean squares	F	Probability	Least squares* estimates of means
Mothers					
Between groups	1	14943.3	14.54	0.005	133.012 Functional group
Among mothers within groups	8	1027.6			93.542 Dysfunctional group
Time	4	148.1	1.40	0.266	
Time × groups	4	206.8	1.95	0.136	
Time × mothers in groups	23	105.8			
Fathers					
Between groups	1	7610.0	7.33	0.027	119.541 Functional group
Among fathers within groups	8	1038.5			92.695 Dysfunctional group
Time	4	554.5	2.72	0.052	
Time × groups	4	188.4	0.92	0.466	
Time × fathers in groups	26	204.2			

*See note, Table 2.

Table 8. Repeated-measures Analysis of Variance for Scores on Cohesion Scale of the Family Environment Scale from Functional and Dysfunctional Family Groups

Source of variation	df	Mean squares	F	Probability	Least squares* estimates of means
Mothers					
Between groups	1	896.7	13.07	0.007	59.6208 Functional group
Among mothers within groups	8	68.6			49.5881 Dysfunctional group
Time	4	105.0	2.57	0.067	
Time × groups	4	48.7	1.19	0.343	
Time × mothers in groups	22	40.9			
Fathers					
Between groups	1	4611.6	10.86	0.011	61.067 Functional group
Among fathers within groups	8	424.6			38.472 Dysfunctional group
Time	4	41.3	2.96	0.040	
Time × groups	4	43.9	3.16	0.032	
Time × fathers in groups	24	13.9			

*See note, Table 2.

support within the family unit. The significant time $\times$ groups interaction for fathers on the cohesion scale is due to the fact that the level of cohesion for fathers in the functional group changed very little over the year, while that indicated by fathers in the dysfunctional group showed a sharp decline immediately following diagnosis. However, the expressiveness scale that designates the degree to which family members are encouraged to act openly and express feelings directly, and the conflict scale that measures the open expression of anger and aggression, did not indicate a significant difference between these groups, either for mothers or fathers. State anxiety scores also were not significantly different between the two groups of parents. A t-test difference of means procedure used to analyze findings on the MMPI, showed fathers of the dysfunctional group to be significantly more depressed both 3 months and one year following diagnosis than fathers from the functional group (significant at $P = 0.002$ and $P = 0.018$ respectively). In addition, fathers from the dysfunctional group had a higher level of anxiety at 12 months following diagnosis than fathers from the functional group. Results indicated there were no significant differences for mothers.

School data revealed important differences between the groups, particularly that of the siblings. On a GPA scale of 1.0 to 4.0, 4 of 5 siblings from dysfunctional families had a drop in GPA of 0.5 or more when comparing academic performance for the year prior to diagnosis with that of the year following the onset of the illness, whereas only one of six siblings from functional families had a drop in GPA of that magnitude. Interestingly, there were no negative changes in the GPA of patients in either group of families, which could possibly be accounted for by teachers' special allowances for the seriously ill child when assigning grades.

Teachers' responses on the behavioral report form discussed on page 162 also indicated variation, with siblings' data being the most significant. Negative behaviors were reported for four siblings from the dysfunctional family group, including rebelliousness, attention seeking, lack of motivation, anxiety, aggressiveness, and poor peer relationships. Teachers indicated that for all but one of these siblings the behaviors were evident *prior* to diagnosis, but in the instance of two students they became more intense following diagnosis. One adolescent improved markedly with counseling provided by the school. Two siblings from functional families were reported to show passive negative behavior that included withdrawal and a lack of motivation. This behavior was not new for one sibling, and the teacher of the other child reported offering extra time and help to him with improvement following. Again, there were few changes reported for patients, however, the teacher of a child from the dysfunctional group indicated problems of aggressiveness with peers and teachers, anger, and a negative attitude regarding academic work.

It is curious that in regard to attendance, two patients of functional families had extensive medically unnecessary absences of 2 and 3 months before returning to school on a regular basis, while all patients from the dysfunctional family group returned to regular school attendance immediately following radiation therapy. There were no notable changes in attendance patterns for siblings of either group.

Long-term follow-up data obtained by interview 2 years post-diagnosis, indicated a substantial difference in the incidence of psychosocial problems in these two groups of families. Each of the five families in the dysfunctional group reported significant stressful events. Divorce had occurred in one family, and separation with divorce pending had taken place in a second family. Two other families had members under psychiatric care—one sought family therapy for marital problems and poor adjustment of a sibling, while the mother in the other family entered therapy for depression. The adolescent patient of a fifth family refused to complete the recommended course of chemotherapy while still in first remission, and threatened to leave home if forced to do so; an adolescent sibling in this same family began heavy use of drugs and alcohol. However, data from the five families in the functional group indicated life had returned to its usual pattern, none of them had sought psychiatric intervention, there had been no incidence of divorce or marital separation, nor were any significant psychosocial problems reported for either patients or siblings. In other words, it appears likely that families who have difficulty coping prior to the onset of a crisis will have increased problems as a result of the added stress. This was determined using the same variables for pre-crisis and post-crisis assessment. While the sample of this selected group is small, and the results therefore cannot be generalized, the findings present interesting possibilities that warrant consideration for future research.

DISCUSSION AND CONCLUSIONS

Primary objectives of this research were to measure the impact of the stress of childhood leukemia on specific family members and the family unit on a longitudinal basis during the first year following diagnosis. According to the results of this study, patterns of coping for families, as well as for individual family members, appear to be relatively constant over time. Families with predominately stable relationships and adequate support within the family unit appeared to be able to maintain their usual quality of life over an extended period of time in terms of family dynamics, despite the onset of acute stress. However, families having problems existing prior to diagnosis experienced increased deterioration in family life and had difficult coping.

There are several observations that need emphasizing.

1. A certain level of denial appears to serve as a functional coping mechanism that enables families to make necessary adaptations and maintain some sense of equilibrium when they are confronted with acutely stressful situations.

2. A time that change in family dynamics seems most likely to occur is approx. 4–6 months following the child's diagnosis, perhaps a time when the reality of the diagnosis makes its greatest impact, fatigue is present as a result of an intensive treatment regimen, and the flurry of activity has subsided. Even on dimensions of the family interaction measure where the extent of change over the total measurement period did not reach significance, this particular period frequently revealed a trend toward change for both mothers and fathers. It should also be emphasized that this was the time for fathers when the sharpest decline in marital satisfaction occurred.

3. On the other hand, it is interesting to note that no major changes in family structure such as divorce, separation, or an adolescent leaving home occurred in any of the families in this sample until at least 9 months post-diagnosis. Perhaps the acute stress of the initial crisis prevented the incidence of these kinds of events.

4. The notable decline in marital satisfaction for mothers and fathers, along with the increased incidence of depression at the end of the first year for both parents, give cause for concern and consideration of the need for preventive intervention.

To date, the major thrust of research involving this population has emphasized the incidence of psychosocial pathology. However, data from this research, and the findings of Lansky [10] and Kupst and Schulman [7, 8] indicate a need in future work to assess family strengths such as the presence of support and cohesiveness, and capitalize on these resources in planning both preventive and therapeutic intervention. In addition, there is a need to obtain long term data from families to determine the effects of the stress over extended periods of time.

There is also a need for research that makes use of valid and reliable measurements. One reason for the lack of this type of research with this particular population may be a reluctance to risk increasing the stress of families experiencing a major crisis. However, the consent rate of 87.5% which we were able to obtain after providing families with a detailed explanation of what their participation would include, along with the drop out rate of only 2%, indicates the subjects in this sample did not feel it increased their level of stress. In fact, several parents stated that completing the questionnaires for the study enabled them to confront issues they might have otherwise avoided, and served to open communication in their families, which suggests that participation in the study was itself an indirect form of intervention. Our inability to gather complete data for each time period seems to be partially a function of the way individuals coped with the stress that would have been added by their participation in the study at specific time periods.

In summary, reports of research done to evaluate the effectiveness with which families cope with childhood cancer are varied. Therefore, further studies need to be undertaken using objective measures to examine coping patterns and assess those families most vulnerable to the development of secondary psychosocial problems. Carefully planned, replicable intervention must then be provided and its effectiveness must be empirically validated.

REFERENCES

1. Miller D. Acute lymphoblastic leukemia. *Pediat. Clin. N. Am.* 27, 269–271, 1980.
2. Cairns N. U., Clark G. M., Smith S. D. and Lansky S. B. Adaptation of siblings to childhood malignancy. *J. Pediat.* 95, 448–487, 1979.
3. Townes B. D., Wold D. A. and Holmes T. Parental adjustment to childhood leukemia. *J. psychosom. Res.* 18, 9–14, 1974.
4. Fife B. L. Childhood leukemia is a family crisis: A review. *J. psychiat. Nursg,* 198, 29–35, 1980.
5. Binger, C. M., Ablin A. R., Feuerstein R. C., Kushner J. H., Zoger S. and Mikkelsen L. Childhood leukemia: emotional impact on patient and family. *New Engl. J. Med.* 280, 414–418, 1969.
6. Powazek M., Payne J. S., Goff J., Paulson M. and Stagner S. Psychological ramifications of childhood leukemia: one year post-diagnosis. In *The Child with Cancer* (Edited by Schulman Ir. J. and Kupst M. J.), pp. 143–155, Thomas, Springfield, Ill., 1980.
7. Kupst M. J., Schulman J. L., Honig G., Maurer H., Morgan E. and Fochtman D. Family coping with childhood leukemia: one year after diagnosis. *J. Pediat. Psychol.* 7, 157–174, 1982.
8. Kupst M. M., Schulman, J. L., Maurer H., Honig G., Morgan E. and Fochtman D. Coping with pediatric leukemia: a two year follow-up. *J. Pediat. Psychol.* 9, 149–163, 1984.
9. Kaplan D., Grobstein R. and Smith A. Severe illness in families. *Hlth Soc. Work* 1, 72–81, 1976.

10. Lansky S. B., Cairns N. U., Hassanein R., Wehr J. and Lowman J. Childhood cancer: parental discord and divorce. *Pediatrics 62*, 184–188, 1978.
11. Moos R. *Preliminary Manual for Family Environment Scale.* Consulting Psychologists Press, Palo Alto, Calif., 1974.
12. Locke H. and Wallace K. Short marital adjustment and prediction tests: their reliability and validity. *Marriage Family Liv 21*, 251–259, 1959.
13. Spielberger C. Theory and measure of anxiety status. In *Handbook of Modern Personality Theory* (Edited by Cattel R. and Dreger R.), pp. 239–253. Hemisphere/Wiley, Washington, D.C., 1977.
14. Dixon W. *Biomedical Computer Programs, X-series Supplement.* University of California Press, Berkley, 1970.
15. Ray A. (Ed.). *SAS User's Guide: Statistics.* SHS Institute, Cary, N.C., 1982.
16. Duckwork J. *MMPI Interpretation Manual for Counselors and Clinicians,* 2nd edn. Accelerated Development, Muncie, Ind., 1979.
17. Graham J. *The MMPI: A Practical Guide.* Oxford University Press, New York, 1977.
18. Winer B. *Statistical Principles in Experimental Design,* 2nd edn, Chap. 7. McGraw-Hill, New York, 1971.

PART VIII: PSYCHOLOGICAL ISSUES
WITH PHYSICAL ILLNESS

31

Psychiatric Liaison to Liver Transplant Recipients

Penelope G. Krener

University of California, Davis, Medical Center, Sacramento

Child psychiatric consultants perform psychiatric assessment and liaison among various clinical services. Execution of these familiar roles for pediatric liver transplantation recipients exposes unfamiliar and difficult bioethical problems. Administrative problems arise if the recipient's suitability is too narrowly evaluated. Assessment may be time-limited. The intensive care unit environment and the VIP characteristics of child transplantation patients may distort observations and constrain opportunities for preventive preoperative psychologic management. Unnecessary psychiatric complications may ensue, which imperil the transplantation surgery. The primary caretakers may have an extraordinary emotional investment, so liaison is pressured. Three cases are presented to illustrate these points. Medical ethical perspectives and the limitations of medical training to prepare physicians to perceive them are indicated. That these limitations also affect the psychiatrist is acknowledged, and a clinical research approach is suggested.

Contemporary psychiatrists are consentingly sucked into increasingly numerous moral and social vacuums. In consultation to a university hospital transplantation service, the psychiatry liaison team finds itself routinely, often simultaneously, serving in administration, assessment, treatment, liaison, and clinical research roles. These consultant roles will be briefly described in the

Reprinted with permission from *Clinical Pediatrics,* 1987, Vol. 26, No. 2, 93–97. Copyright 1987 by J.B. Lippincott Co.

context of liver transplantation in children, a new clinical territory in which certain older bioethical questions may take unfamiliar forms.

Transplant surgery, described as an "acute traumatic experience superimposed on the problems of adapting to a chronic illness," [1] requires conventional consultation roles, but also demands a sensitivity to ethical issues beyond the usual clinical terrain. When the patient is a child, the urgency felt to employ heroic measures is culturally endorsed by strong beliefs that a child's rights include a life that extends freely and fully before him. This paper describes the experience of the child psychiatry consult liaison team with a new liver transplantation program in a university hospital, focusing particularly on tactical and ethical issues impinging on the child psychiatrist's roles.

ADMINISTRATIVE ISSUES

Although organ transplantation has been within the realm of possibility since 1954, it has only recently become a widely available, plausible treatment option for end-stage disease. Ethical questions were at first concerned with whether to subject patients to high-risk, last-resort procedures. Swept forward by rapid increase of technologic expertise, the transplantation field now must deal with questions of supply, demand, and distribution of organs and secondarily with questions of encouraged voluntary versus presumed consent for organ donation.[2]

Liver transplantation is still uncommon by comparison with other organ transplant programs. The cost of transplantation surgery and postoperative care is too high[3] for all but a minority of patients to afford without a third party or public funds, so criteria must be developed to allocate limited funds. Psychiatric consultation is therefore requested to appraise suitability for benefiting from the surgery, including the stability of the patient's social supports. Psychiatrists thus become expert witnesses for financial guarantors, as state funds cannot be authorized to pay the medical expenses unless it is ascertained that the patient has a "support system" when he leaves the hospital.

ASSESSMENT ISSUES

Clinical assessment of the impact of the illness on the patient's brain, psyche, and family is a fundamental corollary of medical care. A basic psychiatric consultant function is the assessment of the patient's mental status and premorbid functioning. In patients with end-stage hepatic disease, encephalopathy is common, may be insidious and gradual in its development, and may fluctuate in degree. It may be associated with various endocrine and other dysfunctions.[4] Assessment of mild encephalopathy assumes the examiner can calibrate the patient's current functions to his normal functioning,[5] which is more reliable for adult patients than for children. In the child, emotional reactions to illness, hospitalization, and diagnostic overtures by strangers may mimic the irritability and excitability characteristic of clouding of consciousness. A child's drowsiness may be withdrawal behavior; his long reaction time or short attention span or decreased clarity of thinking may be characteristics of his own learning style. Extended illness commonly puts sustained strain on relationships and leads routinely to regression or at least to skewing and delay of timely progression of stages of the child's separation from the parent. Plateauing of development may occur in the chronically ill child,[6] just as diminishing strength may contribute to a long period of lack of effort for the adult patient, long before he or she comes to the point of considering transplantation.

Case 1

A 14-year-old girl from a rural area had developed insidious hepatic failure 6 years earlier. Although transmitted records indicated that she had previously been referred for appropriate speciality care, her parents had understood that there was no medical treatment, so the child became a beloved invalid for whom the family prayed. She developed massive ascites and severe nutritional problems and was referred emergently to the university hospital when her umbilicus ruptured. At this time, the family was offered the hope of a liver transplant, but a long period of medical management was necessary to strengthen her enough to withstand the stress of surgery. This medical necessity allowed time for extended psychosocial assessment and therapeutic support. Initially quite shy, passive, and childish, she blossomed into a sociable young adolescent. During this time, the youngster developed friendships in the hospital, showed increased interest in age-appropriate books, began to develop some independence from her mother, and inaugurated robust relationships with other adults on the treatment team. Her transplant surgery was uncomplicated, and she recovered rapidly. The childlike thought seen earlier only surfaced occasionally, as when she joked postoperatively that she was afraid that her liver, which had been given by the family of a teenage suicide, was still unhappy inside her.

Assessment problems are minimized if the consultation liaison team is able to see the patient before the hospitalization for transplantation surgery and if resources are available to do systematic developmental and psychometric assessments. This lessens the difficulty of separating acute from chronic disease effects. Still, the amount of improvement to be hoped for is unpredictable,[7] as patients vary in the extent of recovery of function.

PSYCHOSOCIAL SUPPORT AND TREATMENT ISSUES

Preoperative psychosocial support for the patient and family is affected by uncertainty of surgical outcome. Outcome for organ transplantation depends on the extent to which technological factors can change the direction of pathophysiological processes. Data about the relationship between the type and severity of liver disease and transplantation success rates is beginning to be gathered.[2] But outcome is affected variously and intangibly by other patient factors more difficult to measure, such as fear, hope and having something or someone to live for.[8] Here the consulting doctor as well as the patient are unsure about what kind of life the patient may hope for after transplantation. When the psychiatrist is involved preoperatively, he may be drawn into what Caplan[2] has called "the charade of consent," consent that may be factually informed but is perhaps touched by desperation. Intense feelings affect interpretation of facts, especially by parents whose consent for their child's surgery offers uncertain hope of recovery in the long run but also guarantees the child certain pain and suffering in the short run. A majority of patients for whom renal transplantation is imminent are found to have organic losses in intellectual functioning.[9] Organic delirium or deficit similarly is expected in patients with hepatic failure. If the patient is a child, the picture of organic delirium or intellectual damage is superimposed on developmental delay and regression, and its history is filtered through the emotional lens of parental feelings.[8]

Postoperative psychosocial support must often be prolonged. Attitude affects outcome.[10] Anxiety and elation buoy the patient and family preoperatively,[1] and the surgeon may share these good feelings. This is a healthy adaptation, but it mitigates against consideration of the perioperative discomforts and threat of postoperative complications. After transplant surgery, patients have a "heightened interest in and attention to details of their medical condition"[11] arising from their awareness of the possibility of transplant rejection, which has been described as "sitting on a powder keg."[12] When the child is in critical stage of recovery, parents may experience a relative feeling of helplessness and uncertainty about which of their own actions are useful for the child. Their coping behavior may have gotten their child to the transplant, but after the surgery, the parent may be at a loss to master the situation, to cope, and to influence the child's outcome favorably. Often parents focus on the outward and visible signs of recovery, such as vital signs, input and output, and laboratory values, to an extent that may cause uneasiness in the surgical team.

Postoperative depression has been described in adult recipients.[13] The child, who may be in a more concrete stage of cognitive development, may have formed extremely specific expectations about how things will go for him after the transplant. To the expectable postoperative exhaustion and depression is added disillusionment when he learns that he can't get a new liver and then go right out and be as vigorous as his age mates.

Case 2

> Consultation was requested to manage depression in a postopera-
> tive child combined with critical, erosive anxiety in his mother.
> The mother scanned all laboratory slips, collared all professionals,
> and restlessly busied herself alongside the nurses but was unable
> to talk to and play with her child. The patient turned toward the
> wall in a fetal position and refused to eat. The staff was
> exasperated with mother who appeared to be challenging their
> competence and with the patient who appeared to be defeating
> their best efforts. Painstaking intervention in conjunction with the
> social worker disclosed the mother's fragile mastery of her own
> emotionally deprived and victimized childhood, which made it
> difficult for her to bear the helpless period of awaiting postopera-
> tive recovery, to trust the treatment team, and to allow herself to
> be strong but still taken care of. After days of reading storybooks
> to the wordless child, the consultant and child life worker were
> rewarded with his drawings depicting that he had believed that he
> would get a new liver and then be able to eat pizza right away,
> beat up his stronger little brother, and go home.

For child patients the comprehension of the illness and of the threat of demise is constrained by their level of cognitive maturation.[14] Children of preschool age do not understand the irreversibility of death. Having less capacity to judge the relative perspectives of their parents' sad feelings they are intensely influenced by them and may thus experience the sad affects associated with the threat of their own death without understanding its "meaning." School aged children may conceptualize death as irreversible, but also as external, and have correspondingly concrete expectations that their parents and doctors will take observable steps to protect them from dying. Adolescents may recognize that death is an ending of internal bodily functions, which is a result of several alterable factors, but inevitable and permanent. These described stages assume typical development, which may be stunted or skewed in the chronically ill child. In the acutely ill child, regression is also characteristic, making assessment of the child's level of comprehension trickier. As noted, the transplant recipient is both acutely and chronically ill.

The meaning to the patient of receiving another person's vital organ[15] is affected by the foreknowledge that one's own chance for life is linked to the donor's sudden death. The child, whose conceptualization of death is evolving developmentally, may be able to comprehend only unevenly the simple facts, let alone the existential implications of being a liver transplant recipient. Perplexed adults ask the child psychiatrist "what do I tell him when he asks where his new liver came from?"

LIAISON ISSUES IN AND BEYOND THE HOSPITAL

In a complex, time-pressured, and hierarchical environment, much communication may be implicit, inviting misinterpretation. An important liaison function is to make explicit the expectations of various services so that the several specialties inevitably involved in the care of a transplant patient communicate more clearly. In the case of highly technical "heroic" treatment, liaison extends beyond the hospital.

The media cannot be excluded as a presence that may become either benevolent or treacherous. Rapid communication of a child's need for a vital organ can be lifesaving. Airing the joy of a successful transplant experience may inspire and fortify potential donors and recipients. But if parents inadvertently disclose their anxiety, distress, or displeasure, or if they are put in a position to represent delicate and detailed medical conclusions, the media and the medical team may become adversaries.

Case 3

A 3-year-old girl experienced smooth, faultless transplant surgery but developed signs of rejection before the end of the first week. On the eve of the transplant and just after it, her mother, energized and euphoric, met with the television crew to tell of the transplant optimistically. She also spoke openly and at length to the consultant about her daughter's development, the expected changes after the transplant, and the ways in which she could help the sibling to understand and adjust to her illness and recovery. When the child's condition began to deteriorate, the surgeon hopefully described possible treatment interventions including a second transplant, but the pediatrician intensivist, who also met with mother daily, was pessimistic and felt he had to prepare her for the worst. The mother's hoped yo-yoed, and she prepared in her distress to go to the medial with her complaints. She developed an insomniac vigil, sitting stiffly near the intensive care unit, responding woodenly to the consultants, her thoughts halting and her previous articulate competence gone. The consultant reported to both the surgeon and the pediatrician the mother's confusion and suggested that mother receive information from one person consistently. This change was implemented. The mother adjusted herself to the guarded prognosis, became more energetic, and coped better as her daughter endured through a second transplant but ultimately died.

DISCUSSION

Liver transplantation for children spans an interface between highly technical medical achievement and exquisite ethical and family support issues. For this group, psychiatric consultation is particularly vital and difficult, because management of pediatric liver recipients exemplifies the need to go beyond a biomedical model to optimize patient survival.

Traditionally, training and roles of the various specialists may interfere with coordinated support to patient and family. Preclinical medical training immerses the student in new factual material. Formal medical ethics training has been offered in medical schools only recently, although individual teachers and mentors guide students informally. The structured, factual preclinical teaching is followed by a sink-or-swim direct experience on core and specialty clerkships. This prepares the medical student to assume a physician identity, to empathize with surgeons, pathologists, internists, or pediatricians. It may not prepare him to see how patients and families perceive the hospital and may not enable him to recognize ways in which all are together affected by larger economic or administrative pressures. The physician is encouraged to dedicate himself individually to patient needs and to respond to those needs with disciplined technical action, often without consideration of broader conceptual ethical systems. Individual physicians carry their own personal style to the bedside and draw on their own life experience to find an explanatory context for phenomena unexplained by the biomedical model.

A psychiatric colleague may be consulted. The training of a psychiatrist, however, is founded on the same basic medical training as is that of the surgeon or pediatrician and is a product of the same medical ethos and milieu. His psychiatric training attunes him to interpersonal and intrapsychic issues, not specifically to systems issues. Tempted to respond to the cultural expectation for doctors to be all things to all people, and for psychiatrists to be clairvoyant, he may rely heavily on interpersonal diagnostic skills but may be no better prepared to arrive at judgments concerning ethical questions. Expected to alleviate psychic pain, he may be able to offer some comfort to the patient and family but may still find himself helplessly sharing the pain his fellow physician experiences when the urge to undo a genetic or infectious tragedy meets with limited success.

Moreover, psychiatric consultation lends itself more to individual variations in professional style and in theoretical orientation than do other specialties with clearer diagnostic and treatment outcome criteria. Reduced federal resources to support consultation liaison services in teaching hospitals, typically the institutions in which organ transplantation programs are found, has destabilized and diversified funding for liaison services. Psychiatry consultant time is impinged upon for activities not directly related to emergency clinical management, such as execution of legal documents, psychiatric holds, and conservatorships. However, necessary and sufficient consultation for pediatric liver transplant recipients requires sustained availability.

Young liver transplant recipients also exemplify challenging biopsychosocial puzzles. Clinical research approaches should include systematic assessment of the family's psychosocial adjustment and the impact on it of the child's illness and treatment. Psychiatric and neuropsychiatric assessment of the child before and after transplantation is necessary to evaluate the cognitive and emotional impact of the initial illness, the improved organ functioning, and the medications used to maintain the transplant.

REFERENCES

1. Buchanan DC. Group therapy for kidney transplant patients. Int J Psychiatry in Medicine 1975;6:523–32.
2. Caplan AL. Organ transplants: the cost of success. Institute of Society, Ethics, and the Life Sciences. The Hastings Center Report. 1983;13(6):23–32.
3. Starzl TE, Shunzaburo I, Van Thief DH, et al. Evolution of liver transplantation. Hepatology 1982;2:614–36.
4. Ahlqvist J. Hormonal influences on immunologic and related phenomena. In Ader R (ed). Psychoneuroimmunology. New York: Academic Press, 1981, pp 355–404.

5. Famularo RA, Kimball CP. Liaison psychiatry considerations in renal hemodialysis patients with acute organic cerebral disorders. In Levy, NB (ed). Psychonephrology 2. New York: Plenum 1983, pp 71–8.
6. Klein SD, Simmons RG. The psychosocial impact of chronic kidney disease on children. In Simmons RG, Klein SD, Simmons RL (eds). Gift of Life. New York: Wiley 1977, pp 89–118.
7. Bernstein DM. Psychiatric assessment of the adjustment of transplanted children. In Simmons RG, Klein SD, Simmons RL (eds). Gift of Life. New York: Wiley 1977, pp 119–48.
8. Eisendrath RM. The role of grief and fear in the death of the kidney transplant patients. Am J Psychiatry 1969;126:381–7.
9. Greenberg RP, Davis G, Massey R. The psychological evaluation of patients for a kidney transplant and hemodialysis program. Am J Psychiatry 1973;130:3.
10. Engel GL, Schmale AH Jr. Psychoanalytic theory of somatic disorder: conversion, specificity and the disease onset situation. J Am Psychoanalytic Assoc 1967;15:344–65.
11. Freyberger H. The renal transplant patient: three-stage model and psychotherapeutic strategies. In Levy NB (ed). Psychonephrology 2. New York: Plenum 1983, pp 259–66.
12. Armstrong S. Children and adolescents on hemodialysis and transplantation programs. In Levy NB (ed). Psychonephrology 2. New York: Plenum 1983, pp 213–22.
13. Penn D, Bunch D, Olenk D, et al. Psychiatric experiences with patients receiving renal and hepatic transplants.. In Castelnuovo-Tedesco (ed). Psychiatric Aspects of Organ Transplantation. New York: Grune and Stratton, 1971.
14. Koocher GP, O'Malley JE. The Damocles syndrome. Psychosocial issues in treatment of childhood cancer. New York: McGraw-Hill, 1981, pp 1–30.
15. Viederman M. The search for meaning in renal transplantation. Psychiatry 1974;37:283–90.

Part IX

CHILD ABUSE

The recognition that child abuse is a frequent and serious phenomenon in our society has led to many studies which have attempted to identify specific characteristics of abusing parents. A number of reports have suggested that abusing parents themselves were victims of abuse as children. The concept that "the abused child becomes an abusive parent" has become widely accepted. Kaufman and Zigler critically review the literature and demonstrate that the unqualified acceptance of this formulation is unfounded and its use may pose many negative consequences. They conclude by challenging researchers to put aside this intergenerational myth and ask, instead, "Under what conditions is the transmission of abuse most likely to occur?"

Only recently have mental health professionals and others begun to expose the shocking fact that child sexual abuse is widespread and can have serious psychological consequences for the victim. In *Annual Progress 1987* we reprinted one of the first systematic studies of this issue, by Browne and Finkelhor, which indicated that research in this area was still in its infancy and suffered from many methodological problems. It was clear, even from these flawed reports, that child sexual abuse can result in significant detrimental effects. In the present section Burgess and her co-workers describe the many specific pathological sequelae to child sexual abuse. Their story is noteworthy because of its long-term follow-up and detailed exposition of the many ways in which socially deviant behaviors can result from such abuse.

It is clear that child physical and sexual abuse constitute a major psychosocial risk to the healthy development of innumerable children. The failure by families, neighbors, and professionals to report such occurrences of abuse when they become aware of them has led to many tragedies and should be considered criminal neglect. But, unfortunately, there is the other side of this problem. It is becoming clear that allegations of child abuse, and especially sexual abuse, are not always valid. For example, a divorced vindictive mother or father may falsely accuse the former spouse of abusing their child. By doing so, the accuser may hope to ruin the other's social or professional status in the community and deny him or her visitation rights with the child. This is, unfortunately, by no means a rare problem, and Wong, in her survey of the literature, estimates that of 1.9 million cases of reported child abuse, 1.2 million were found to be unsubstantiated. Compounding this problem is the difficulty in obtaining clear, objective evidence from children, who are so often confused, intimidated, and anxious when they are required to testify.

The papers by Wong and Benedek and Schetky discuss in detail the problems in validating allegations of abuse, especially sexual abuse, and spell out the techniques that professionals can use in eliciting the facts, with special emphasis on the approach to interviewing the child.

The fact that a report of child abuse may be false, however, in no way diminishes the responsibility of health professionals and the community in taking such reports seriously and investigating them seriously. Otherwise, all too many children will continue to be victims of abuse, with all the serious consequences this can have for their healthy development.

REFERENCE

Browne, A., & Finkelhor, D. (1988). Impact of child sexual abuse: A review of the research. In S. Chess, A. Thomas, and M. Hertzig (Eds.), *Annual Progress in Child Psychiatry and Child Development 1987*, pp. 555–584. (Reprinted from *Psychological Bulletin*, 1986, Vol. 99, No. 1, pp. 66–77.)

32

Do Abused Children Become Abusive Parents?

Joan Kaufman and Edward Zigler

Yale University, New Haven, Connecticut

The belief that abused children are likely to become abusive parents is widely accepted. The authors review the literature cited to support this hypothesis and demonstrate that its unqualified acceptance is unfounded. Mediating factors that affect transmission are outlined and the findings of several investigations are integrated to estimate the true rate of transmission.

The belief that abused children are likely to become abusive parents is widely accepted by professionals and lay people alike. It is noted in introductory psychology text books,[41] and advanced on radio and television commercials that advocate "the report of abuse to avoid the cycle of abuse." Despite the popularity of this belief, there is a paucity of empirical evidence to support the transmission formulation.

Many papers cited in support of the intergenerational hypothesis merely assert its validity without providing any substantive evidence.[3,4,8,15,21,39] The remaining papers derive their data from four primary sources: case study materials, agency records, clinical interviews, and self-report questionnaires. The basic elements of these studies vary greatly, however. They differ in the subjects studied (identified abusers *vs* high risk populations *vs* nationally representative samples), in their definitions of "history of abuse" and "current abuse," in the experimental design employed (retrospective *vs* prospective), and in the type of data sources utilized to substantiate claims of past and current abuse.

Reprinted with permission from the *American Journal of Orthopsychiatry,* 1987, Vol. 57, No. 2, 186–192. Copyright 1987 by the American Orthopsychiatric Association, Inc.

This paper critically reviews the literature cited in support of the intergenerational hypothesis. Throughout, the effects of variations in the research design of different studies are highlighted. A number of mediating factors that affect the likelihood of abuse occurring in successive generations are also briefly outlined. In conclusion, the findings of several studies are integrated to estimate the true rate of transmission. Numerous researchers have questioned the validity of the intergenerational hypothesis;[5,6,13,17,19,28,33,40] this review demonstrates that its unqualified acceptance is unfounded.

LITERATURE REVIEW

Case History Studies

Most papers that used case study materials were based on observations of parents whose children were treated in hospital emergency rooms for nonaccidental injuries.[10,12,22] A strong association between child maltreatment and a parental history of abuse was uniformly reported. The generalizability of these studies is limited, however, by researchers' failure to utilize: *a)* representative samples, *b)* comparison subjects, *c)* observers who were blind to the subjects' maltreatment status, *d)* formal definitional criteria for the terms "history of abuse" and "current abuse," or *e)* descriptive or inferential statistics in reporting research findings. Given these methodological problems, the findings of studies relying on case study materials as their primary data source must be interpreted with a high degree of caution.

Agency Record Studies

Agency record review studies were conducted to investigate the child-rearing practices of abusing families over several generations,[25] and to learn about the childhood experiences of parents whose children were brought to hospital emergency rooms for nonaccidental injuries.[23,27,30] Studies that employed record review procedures possess many of the same methodological problems as those that used case study materials. In addition, the findings of these studies are often difficult to interpret because omissions in agency records are rarely systematically recorded. For example, at the conclusion of one paper, the authors stated[23] "in all cases where information was available, the adults [in their study] had been subjected early in life to emotional deprivations" (p. 907). Since the authors failed to mention the number of cases for which there was information available, the significance of the clause "in all cases" cannot be determined. The reliability and validity of using agency reports to detect a parental history of child maltreatment has been questioned elsewhere.[1] Since information pertaining to child-rearing histories is rarely recorded consistently within agencies, let alone across agencies, findings from record review studies are inevitably limited as well.

Clinical Studies

Of the clinical interview studies, Steele and Pollack's[34] work is probably the most widely referenced, despite the authors' cautionary note that their "study group of parents is not to be thought of as useful statistical proof of any concepts" (p. 90). Steele and Pollack interviewed 60 child abusing parents participating in a psychological treatment program. The authors reported that all the parents in their study were abused as children. In this study, however, a history of abuse was defined as being subjected to "intense, pervasive, and continual demands" from one's parents, a definition far from the legal criteria developed by the Juvenile Justice Standards Project.[38] Without an appropriate comparison group it is impossible to determine whether these experiences are unique to abusive parents, or simply true of most adults receiving psychological services. The number of adults who were subjected to similar childhood experiences and neither abuse their children nor receive psychological services cannot be ascertained from this study.

The findings of other studies[14,24] that used clinical interviews as their primary data source are equally limited. While all these studies were undoubtedly valuable in generating hypotheses about the possible relationship between child maltreatment and abusive parenting, due to methodological problems, their findings simply cannot be considered conclusive evidence in support of the intergenerational hypothesis.

Self-Report Studies

The studies reviewed thus far were guided by the psychiatric model of abuse, which emphasizes aberrant parental characteristics to explain the etiology of child maltreatment. Studies that used self-report questionnaires moved beyond this conceptual approach to include multiple assessments reflective of investigators' broadening understanding of the factors associated with the etiology of abuse. Factors identified by the socio-ecological model of abuse, such as poverty, stress, and isolation, were assessed, as were factors associated with the child-as-elicitor model which includes measures of infant prematurity and child temperament. Unfortunately, while comparison groups were consistently employed in these studies, and analyses conducted to assess the effects of the individual measures collected, the statistical relationships among the various determinants of abuse were rarely explored to determine the relative effects of the various factors examined.

In all the self-report studies reviewed, the dimension "a history of abuse" consistently differentiated the abusers from the comparison subjects.[2,7,9,11,16,18,29,31,32,35] However, considerable overlap between these two groups was always reported. This suggests that, although a history of abuse is more common among parents who maltreat their children, many parents who do not report abusive childhood experiences become abusers and a sizable number of parents who were maltreated as children do not. The research designs of these investigations varied greatly and produced estimates of the rate of intergenerational transmission that ranged from 18% to 70%. The methodology and results of three studies are now detailed to illustrate how variations in basic research elements affected the estimated rates of intergenerational transmission obtained.

The first study was conducted by Hunter and Kilstrom[18] who interviewed 282 parents of newborns admitted to a regional intensive care nursery for premature and ill infants. Information concerning the parents' childhood, the mother's pregnancy, and the family's social networks was collected. In this study, abuse was defined to include incidents of neglect as well as overt abuse. Confirmed reports of abuse or neglect registered in the state central agency during the children's first year of life were used to determine current abuse status. At the time of the initial interview, 49 parents reported a childhood history of abuse or neglect. At the one-year follow-up, ten babies were reportedly maltreated. Nine of them had parents with a history of abuse or neglect; however, 40 parents with comparable childhood histories were not identified as maltreaters. The rate of intergenerational transmission reported in this investigation was 18%, since only nine of the 49 parents who reported a history of abuse were identified as maltreaters.

This study pointedly illustrates how variations in the choice of subjects (identified abusers *vs* high-risk sample) and experimental design (retrospective *vs* prospective) affect the outcome of research findings. If this study had been conducted retrospectively with only the parents who were identified as maltreaters, the link between a history of abuse and subsequent child abuse would have appeared deceptively strong, since nine out of ten of the abusive parents reported a history of maltreatment (90%). By employing a prospective research design, Hunter and Kilstrom were able to identify 40 parents who broke the cycle of abuse (82%).

Parents who did not repeat the cycle of abuse differed from those parents who did in the following ways: they had more extensive social supports, they had fewer ambivalent feelings about the pregnancy, their babies were physically healthier, and they were more openly angry about their earlier abuse and better able to give detailed accounts of those experiences. They were also more likely to have been abused by only one of their parents as children, and were more apt to report a supportive relationship with one of their parents when growing up.

The generalizability of Hunter and Kilstrom's study is restricted, however, because of the nonrepresentative nature of their sample (parents of ill infants), the limitations associated with the data source used to detect current incidents of abuse (agency records), and the fact that the follow-up did not extend beyond one year. Despite these qualifications, this study clearly demonstrates the superiority of prospective research designs and highlights the need to interpret retrospective studies with caution.

The second study was conducted by Egeland and Jacobvitz,[9] who used a semistructured interview to collect information about the childhood histories and current disciplinary practices of 160 high-risk, low-income, predominantly single-parent mothers. In addition, measures of stress, isolation, and child characteristics were also obtained. In this study, a history of abuse was restricted to incidents of severe physical punishment including being thrown against a wall, hit repeatedly with an object, or intentionally burned. Current abusers were subdivided into three categories: a "physical abuse" group who used severe physical punishment tactics, a "borderline abuse" group who administered daily or weekly spankings that did not cause bruises or caused red marks that disappeared, and an "other" group which included women whose children were being cared for by someone else (reasons for the out-of-home care were not specified). The authors reported an intergenerational transmission rate of 70% for mothers with a history of severe physical abuse. This percentage, however, included mothers who physically abused their children (34%), mothers who fell into the borderline abuse category (30%), and mothers whose children were being reared away from the home (6%).

The high-risk nature of Egeland and Jacobvitz's sample confounds the results of this study. The influence of a history of abuse upon subsequent parenting cannot be separated from the effects of poverty, stress, and social isolation. In interpreting the findings it is important to keep in mind the simultaneous effects of these different variables. The results of this study are more appropriately interpreted as the result of multiple determinants on the etiology of abuse (e.g., history of abuse, poverty, stress, isolation), rather than the effect of a single determinant (e.g., history of abuse).

The definition of "current abuse" used also affected the rate of intergenerational transmission obtained. In general, the broader the definitional criteria employed, the greater the apparent link between a history of abuse and current abuse. As noted, Egeland and Jacobvitz included the borderline abuse category in their computation of the rate of intergenerational transmission. They found that 30% of the mothers who reported a history of abuse fell into this category, but an even larger percentage of mothers who reported emotionally supportive childhoods were categorized as borderline abusers (39%). Given the failure of the borderline abuse category to differentiate these two groups, the validity of this category, and the conclusion that aberrant childhood histories "caused" the borderline parenting is questionable. Since a national survey of disciplinary practices reported that 97% of all children in the United States have been physically punished,[36] it appears the borderline abuse group's parenting is more reflective of a cultural norm than a parenting deviation. While on a continuum of parenting, the types of behavior associated with the borderline abuse group are not optimal, they can be understood in light of cultural (*e.g.*, acceptance of corporal punishment as a legitimate means of discipline) and environmental (*e.g.*, stress, isolation) determinants and not developmental (*e.g.*, history of abuse) factors.

Egeland and Jacobvitz also reported a number of mediating factors that affected the likelihood of transmission occurring with the women in their study. They found that nonrepeaters were more likely than repeaters to have one parent or foster parent who provided support and love while growing up, to be involved in a relationship with an emotionally supportive spouse or boyfriend, and to report fewer current stressful life events. They also showed a greater awareness of their history of being abused, and were consciously resolved not to repeat the pattern of abuse with their own children. These characteristics are highly similar to those reported by Hunter and Kilstrom.[18]

Although, for these reasons, the 70% transmission rate reported by Egeland and Jacobvitz is likely to be an overestimation, their study provides a valuable contribution to understanding the interrelationships among the many determinants of abuse. Since the effects of a history of abuse upon subsequent parenting often cannot be separated from the effects of poverty, stress, and social isolation, this study highlights the importance of assessing multiple factors and giving careful thought to the choice of comparison groups used in investigations of this kind.

The last self-report study reviewed was conducted by Straus,[35] who interviewed a nationally representative sample of 1,146 two-parent families with a child between the ages of 3 and 17. Straus obtained an 18% rate of transmission. There are two reasons why this figure is probably an underestimation. First, the definition of a history of abuse used in this study included only experiences of physical punishment or abuse that occurred during adolescence. Since this is an age when physical punishment is least likely to occur,[37] numerous individuals who were mistreated when they were younger, but not as teenagers, were probably omitted from the history of abuse category. Secondly, single parents and parents of children in the 0–2 age range were excluded from this study. This is problematic, since these two groups are at greater risk for abuse than two-parent families with older children. Despite these concerns, this study demonstrates that the link between being maltreated and becoming abusive is far from inevitable.

SUMMARY

The findings of the different investigations reviewed are not easily integrated because of their methodological variations. Nonetheless, the best estimate of the rate of intergenerational transmission appears to be 30% ± 5%. This suggests that approximately one-third of all individuals who were physically abused, sexually abused, or extremely neglected will subject their offspring to one of these forms of maltreatment, while the remaining two-thirds will provide adequate care for their children.

This figure was derived as follows. For the reasons discussed previously, we believe the estimates obtained by Hunter and Kilstrom[18] and Straus[35] are somewhat low. Despite questions about the validity of the borderline abuse category used by Egeland and Jacobvitz,[9] we relied heavily on their finding that only 34% of the severely abused mothers in their study physically abused their children. Since they employed a high-risk sample, it is reasonable to assume that the intergenerational hypothesis will be confirmed in less than one-third of all cases when more representative populations are sampled.

The rate of abuse among individuals with a history of abuse (30 ± 5%) is approximately six times higher than the base rate for abuse in the general population (5%).[26] Although this suggests that being maltreated as a child is an important risk factor in the etiology of abuse, the majority of maltreated children do not become abusive parents. As discussed elsewhere,[20] many mediating factors affect the likelihood of transmission; consequently, unqualified acceptance of the intergenerational hypothesis is simply unwarranted.

CONCLUSION

Although there is some truth to the notion that abuse is cyclical, there are also many factors that diminish the likelihood of abuse being transmitted across generations. Being maltreated as a child puts one at risk for becoming abusive but the path between these two points is far from direct or inevitable.

In the past, unqualified acceptance of the intergenerational hypothesis has had many negative consequences. Adults who were maltreated have been told so many times that they will abuse their children that for some it has become a self-fulfilling prophecy. Many who have broken the cycle are left feeling like walking time bombs. In addition, persistent acceptance of this belief has impeded progress in understanding the etiology of abuse and led to misguided judicial and social policy interventions. The time has come for the intergenerational myth to be put aside and for researchers to cease asking, "Do abused children become abusive parents?" and ask, instead, "Under what conditions is the transmission of abuse most likely to occur?"

REFERENCES

1. Aber, L.A. and Zigler, E. 1981. Developmental considerations in the definition of child maltreatment. New Dir. Child Devlpm.: Devlpm. Persp. Child Maltreat. 11:1–30.
2. Altemeier, W. et al. 1982. Antecedents of child abuse, J. Pediat. 100:823–829.
3. Bleiberg, N. 1965. The neglected child and the child health conference. N.Y. State J. Med. 65:1880–1885.
4. Blue, M. 1965. The battered child syndrome from a social work viewpoint. Canad. J. Pub. Hlth 56:197–198.
5. Burgess, R. and Youngbade, L. The intergenerational transmission of abusive parental practices: a social interactional analysis. *In* New Directions in Family Violence Research, R. Gelles et al, eds. Sage, Beverly Hills, Calif. (in press)
6. Cicchetti, D. and Aber, L.A. 1980. Abused children–abusive parents: an overstated case? Harv. Ed. Rev. 50:244–255.
7. Conger, R., Burgess, R. and Barrett, C. 1979. Child abuse related to life change and perceptions of illness: some preliminary findings. Fam. Coord. 58:73–77.
8. Corbett, J. 1964. A psychiatrist reviews the battered child syndrome and mandatory reporting legislation. N.W. Med. 63:920–922.
9. Egeland, B. and Jacobvitz, D. 1984. Intergenerational continuity of parental abuse: causes and consequences. Presented at Conference on Biosocial Perspectives in Abuse and Neglect, York, Me.
10. Fontana, V. 1968. Further reflections on maltreatment of children. N.Y. State J. Med. 68:2214–2215.
11. Gaines, R. et al. 1978. Etiological factors in child maltreatment: a multivariate study of abusing, neglecting, and normal mothers. J. Abnorm. Psychol. 87:531–540.
12. Galdston, J. 1965. Observations on children who have been physically abused and their parents. Amer. J. Psychiat. 122:440–443.
13. Garbarino, J., Burgess, R. and Carson, B. 1980. Child maltreatment as a developmental issue. (Unpublished manuscript)
14. Green, A., Gaines, R. and Sandgrund, A. 1974. Child abuse: pathological syndrome of family interaction. Amer. J. Psychiat. 131:882–886.
15. Harper, F. 1963. The physician, the battered child, and the law. Pediatrics 31:899–902.
16. Herrenkohl, E., Herrenkohl, R., and Toedtler, L. 1983. Perspectives on the intergenerational transmission of abuse. *In* The Darkside of Families: Current Family Violence Research, D. Finkelhor, et al, eds. Sage, Beverly Hills, Calif.

17. Hertzberger, S. 1983. Social cognition and the transmission of abuse. *In* The Darkside of Families: Current Family Violence Research, D. Finkelhor, et al, eds. Sage, Beverly Hills, Calif.
18. Hunder, R. and Kilstrom, N. 1979. Breaking the cycle in abusive families. Amer. J. Psychiat. 136:1320–1322.
19. Jayartne, S. 1977. Child abusers as parents and children: a review. Soc. Wk 22:5–7.
20. Kaufman J. and Zigler, E. The intergenerational transmission of child abuse. *In* Research on the Consequences of Child Maltreatment, D. Cicchetti and V. Carlson, eds. Cambridge University Press, Cambridge. (in press)
21. Kempe, C. 1973. A practical approach to the protection of the abused child and rehabilitation of the abusing parent. Pediatrics 51:804–812.
22. Kempe, C. et al. 1962. The battered child syndrome. JAMA 181:17–24.
23. Mc Henrey, T., Girdany, B. and Elmer, E. 1963. Unsuspected trauma with multiple skeletal injuries during infancy and childhood. Pediatrics 31:903–908.
24. Morris, M., Gould, R. and Matthews, P. 1964. Toward prevention of child abuse. Children 11:55–60.
25. Oliver, J. and Taylor, A. 1971. Five generations of ill-treated children in one family pedigree. Brit. J. Psychiat. 119:473–480.
26. Parke, R. and Collmer, C. 1975. Child abuse: an interdisciplinary review. *In* Review of Child Development Research, Vol. 5, E. M. Hetherington, ed., Chicago University Press.
27. Paulson, M. and Blake, P. 1969. The physically abused child: a focus on prevention. Child Welf. 48:86–95.
28. Potts, D., Hertzberger, S. and Holland, A. 1979. Child abuse: a cross-generational pattern of child rearing? Presented to the Mid-Western Psychological Association, Chicago.
29. Quinton, D., Rutter, M. and Liddle, C. 1984. Institutional rearing, parental difficulties and marital support. Psychol. Med. 14:107–124.
30. Silver, L., Dublin, C. and Lourie, R. 1969. Does violence breed violence: contributions from a study of the child abuse syndrome. Amer. J. Psychiat. 126:404–407.
31. Smith, S. and Hanson, R. 1975. Interpersonal relationships and childrearing practices in 214 parents of battered children. Brit. J. Psychiat. 127:513–525.
32. Spinetta, J. 1978. Parental personality factors in child abuse. J. Consult. Clin. Psychol. 46:1409–1414.
33. Stark, E. 1985. Women battering, child abuse, and social hereditary: what is the relationship? Marital Violence: Sociol. Rev. Monogr. 31:147–171.
34. Steele, B. and Pollack, C. 1968. A psychiatric study of parents who abuse infants and small children. *In* The Battered Child Syndrome, R. Helfer and C. Kempe, eds. University of Chicago Press.
35. Straus, M. 1979. Family patterns and child abuse in a nationally representative sample. Inter. J. Child Abuse Negl. 3:213–225.
36. Straus, M. 1983. Ordinary violence, child abuse, and wife beating: what do they have in common? *In* the Darkside of Families: Current Family Violence Research. D. Finkelhor et al, eds. Sage, Beverly Hills, Calif.
37. Straus, M., Gelles, R. and Steinmetz, S. 1980. Behind Closed Doors: Violence in the American Family. Anchor/Doubleday, Garden City, N.Y.

38. Wald, M. 1975. State interventions on behalf of 'neglected' children: a search for realistic standards. Stanford Law Rev. 27:985–1040.
39. Wasserman, S. 1967. The abused parent of the abused child. Children 14:175–179.
40. Zigler, E. 1976. Controlling child abuse in America: an effort doomed to failure. *In* Proceedings of the First National Conference on Child Abuse and Neglect, D. Adamovics, ed. DHEW, Washington, D.C.
41. Zimbardo, P. and Ruch, F. 1975. Psychology and Life (9th Ed.). Scott, Foresman, Glenview, Ill.

33

Abused to Abuser: Antecedents of Socially Deviant Behaviors

Ann W. Burgess
University of Pennsylvania School of Nursing, Philadelphia
Carol R. Hartman
Boston College School of Nursing, Chestnut Hill, Massachusetts
Arlene McCormack
University of Lowell, Massachusetts

The authors interviewed 34 young people who had been sexually abused as children 6 or 8 years after the abuse had occurred and compared them with 34 control subjects who had not been abused. They also compared subjects who had been abused for less than 1 year with those who had been abused for more than 1 year. The findings suggest a link between childhood sexual abuse and later drug abuse, juvenile delinquency, and criminal behavior. The authors explore the effects of pretrauma factors of previous childhood physical abuse and parental modeling of aggression and the postdisclosure factors of social and family blaming.

The psychodynamic impact of memories of childhood sexual trauma on symptoms of hysteria was described by Freud in 1896 (1). In 1963 Gleuck (2) uncovered traumatic consequences of incestuous episodes in a clinical population of schizophrenic patients receiving ECT. More recently, research-

Reprinted with permission from the *American Journal of Psychiatry,* 1987, Vol. 144, No. 11, 1431–1436. Copyright 1987 by the American Psychiatric Association.

Support for data collection and analysis was provided by Department of Justice grant 84-JN-AX-K010 from the Office of Juvenile Justice and Delinquency Prevention.

The authors thank Maureen P. McCausland and Patricia Powers for assistance in data collection, Peter Gaccione for computer analysis, and Robert A. Prentky for suggestions on statistics.

ers using retrospective techniques have studied histories of childhood abuse in hospitalized psychiatric patients (3), outpatient psychiatric populations (4), suicidal persons (5), sex offenders (6, 7), juvenile sex offenders (8), and prostitutes (9, 10). In speculating on a link between childhood sexual abuse and internalizing processes, Rieker and Carmen (11) reconceptualized the "victim to patient" process as an interplay among abuse events, family relationships, and other life contexts. They emphasized that a fragmented identity is derived from accommodations to the judgments of others about the abuse and that the patient's original defenses form the core of the survivor's later psychopathology.

Using a prospective sample of children who had been victims of sexual abuse, in this paper we will examine symptoms and behaviors that manifested themselves intermittently and chronically from the initial abuse period through different follow-up periods. We were particularly interested in understanding what may operate in conjunction with sexual abuse that leads to the externalizing behaviors of drug use, juvenile delinquency, and criminal behavior.

METHOD

Sample

Between 1976 and 1978 we studied six instances of multiple child victims sexually abused by one adult (12). These six solo rings involved 36 children. In 1978–1981, we studied five additional instances of multiple child victims sexually abused by several adults who recruited and abused the children, produced pornography, and established a network of customers (13). These five syndicated and/or transitional rings involved 30 children. In 1984, we began to recontact the 66 young people who had been abused and their families. Eleven (17%) of the families could not be located. Of the 55 located, the interview was refused by two state agencies (in one case both the grandparent and the youngster were willing to be interviewed; in the other case the girl had been psychiatrically hospitalized for 3 years), 14 parents (we received no data regarding the youngsters' willingness to be interviewed), and four youngsters (they refused after their parents agreed). Thirty-five (53%) of the original 66 children agreed to participate in the interview. One of these youngsters, who had originally denied being sexually abused in a ring, continued his denial and was not included in the study. Thus, 34 (52%) of the 66 sexually abused youngsters are reported on here.

The present study assesses these young people by comparing them with control groups of nonabused youngsters. We had originally intended to use a single control group of non-sexually-abused siblings for all 34 subjects. However, one of the characteristics of sex rings is that children are used to recruit other children into the ring and children often recruit their siblings. When this had occurred in our sample, we selected another control subject from the school that the victim had attended. We then divided the sample into two studies for analysis on the basis of type of control group and length of time the child had spent in the sex ring. Nonabuse was determined by asking the control subjects if they had ever been pressured or forced to have sex. Oversampling was done to ensure adequate numbers of control subjects; seven control subjects were dropped because they answered yes to the question about sexual abuse (one sibling and six schoolmates).

Study 1 is an 8-year follow-up interview of 17 white adolescents who had been sexually exploited in sex rings for less than 1 year (12). Six were boys and 11 were girls. Their ages ranged from 14 to 20 years (mean = 17.4 years) at follow-up. All had lower- or working-class backgrounds as indicated by both their mother's and their father's education. (The educational level of all of the parents was the high school level or below; 11 (65%) of the mothers and 14 (82%) of the fathers had not completed high school.) Family economic status indicated that 15 (88%) of the family incomes were "approximately the same as all other family incomes in the neighborhood." The 17 adolescents were matched in gender and closest age to 17 siblings who had not been abused. The control group in study 1 constituted a within-family control.

Study 2 is a 6-year follow-up interview of 17 white sexually abused boys who had been exploited in a sex ring for more than 1 year (13). Their ages ranged from 17 to 21 (mean = 19.8 years) at follow-up. All of their parents had lower- or working-class backgrounds as indicated by their mother's and their father's education. (The educational level of all the fathers was less than the high school level.) Their family economic status was judged to be "lower than most in the neighborhood" and welfare was the major source of income. These 17 adolescents were matched in age, race, gender, and family structure with 17 schoolmates who had not been sexually abused.

In both study 1 and study 2, the sexually abused youngsters were compared with non-sexually-abused control subjects in family history, family structure, and previous trauma. We also examined the nature of the sex ring abuse and compared the abused and nonabused subjects in study 1 and study 2 on different outcome behaviors, including symptom expression, substance use, sexual behavior, peer and family interaction, and delinquent or criminal activities.

Data Collection

The 34 youngsters who had been abused took part in a semistructured interview that consisted of three sections. The first section covered the background of their sexual abuse and consisted of descriptions of the sexual contact, the background of the offenders, the sex rings, and the prostitution; reports of abuse; and a summary of what happened in the criminal justice system. The second section was the family interview and covered the subject's family structure, the sociodemographic profile of the family, new incidents of sexual abuse, and the effects of disclosure. The third section was the child interview and included the Piers-Harris Children's Self-Concept Scale (14), the Moos Family Environment Scale (15), beliefs about sexual abuse and exploitation, a life events scale, the Impact of Event Scale (16), a coping checklist, a delinquent behavior checklist, and the subject's sexual behavior status.

The 34 control subjects took part in another semistructured interview that covered any history of sexual abuse and exploitation and included a behavior checklist, a delinquent behavior checklist, the subject's sexual behavior status, a life events scale, the Piers-Harris scale, and the Family Environment Scale. Delinquent or criminal activities for all 64 youngsters were confirmed through school and/or arrest records.

Questions related to the disclosure of the abuse were examined by asking whether the child felt pressured, threatened, rejected, punished, or blamed by his or her parents for telling about the abuse.

The abused youngsters' perceptions of their family environments after disclosure of the abuse were assessed by using subscales of the Family Environment Scale that represent the domain of family relationships (15). Twenty-seven true/false self-report items from this scale made up three subscales—cohesion, expressiveness, and conflict. Family Environment Scale subscales possess adequate internal consistency and test-retest reliability and have been used in a variety of studies of both healthy and distressed families (15, 17). Questions on the cohesion subscale addressed the extent to which the family environment was shared and mutually supportive and included the items "We really get along well with each other," "There is a feeling of togetherness in our family," and "Family members really help and support one another."

Data Analysis

Frequency tabulations were made on the age of the abused child, family history and structure, previous trauma, and nature of abuse. Cross-tabular analysis was used to assess outcome behaviors of the sexually abused subjects and their controls within study 1 and study 2 and between study 1 and study 2. The statistical significance of relationships was assessed by using Fisher's exact test for small samples. The Bonferroni correction was used to adjust for type I error inflation. Because study 1 included both boys and girls, sex was controlled to ensure that the results were not affected by sex.

Conceptual Framework

The study's conceptual framework provides a guide for the interpretation of data. The model uses three critical phases in traumatic experiences and a cognitive-behavioral structure of information processing of traumatic events (18–20). Phase 1, the period before the traumatic event, included the child's age and personality development, the history and structure of the family, and the child's history of previous trauma. Phase 2, the period of activities relevant to the abuse and exploitation of the child, included data on the offender's behavior (e.g., operation and organization of the sex ring), the child's coping and defensive responses, and the "trauma learning," or the stored information regarding the traumatic event. This information is accessed through sensations, perceptions, and cognitions. When the abuse remains undisclosed, encapsulation of the trauma occurs, and the child's life at school and in peer activities parallels the ongoing abuse. Trauma replay is critical here; reenactment, repetition, and displacement of the sexual activity can occur. Phase 3, the period of disclosure of the ring's activities, includes the social responses of others to finding out about the abuse and the behavior of the child following such disclosure.

RESULTS

The small sample sizes, sex distribution, selectivity of the sample (sexually abused children officially recognized through criminal court proceedings), the fact that the abuse was carried out by adults who were not family members, and the complexity of the lives of these young people make it impossible to suggest any causal link between childhood sexual abuse and social deviance. These data and the results of the interviews do, however, suggest trends for hypotheses to be tested on larger, random samples.

Although study 1 had a fairly equal distribution of two-parent (N = 9) and one-parent (N = 8) families, in study 2 the majority (N = 12) were one-parent families; only five were two-parent families. In study 2, more fathers had histories of alcohol abuse (N = 10, 59%), had criminal histories (N = 4, 24%), and had been absent for more than 10 months before the subject was 12 years old (N = 12, 71%) than in study 1 (N = 5, 29%; N = 1, 6%; N = 6, 35%, respectively). Also, more of the subjects had been physically abused as children in study 2 than in study 1: 14 (82%) versus three (18%). Thus, more of the youngsters in study 2 than in study 1 had a parent role model for absence, aggression, and alcoholism and a history of childhood physical abuse before sexual victimization.

In study 1, the perpetrators had access to the children through the neighborhood, the family, or work. Children were in the ring for less than 1 year, reported minimal involvement in pornography, and did not tell anyone about the ring, fearing that they would not be believed. Also, each perpetrator conducted the sexual acts on a one-to-one basis without witnesses, peer sexual activity was not encouraged, alcohol and drugs were available but not imposed, and, although sex may have been discussed, the talk focused on liking and preferences for one another. At disclosure of the sexual abuse, the children in study 1 were under age 12; they continued to attend school.

In study 2, the offender was a volunteer athletic coach, but he had control over the boys by his access to confidential files and family information. The boys were in the sex ring for more than 1 year; older siblings were encouraged to recruit younger siblings; using alcohol and drugs and participating in pornography were expected behaviors; ritualized homosexuality with sadistic features characterized the activities; and threats and acts of violence occurred between older and younger boys. At disclosure of the abuse, the victims were teen-agers; the majority dropped out of school.

In both study 1 and study 2, the symptoms of the abused youngsters after disclosure of the abuse were suggestive of chronic posttraumatic stress and pointed to high levels of anxiety, fears, and intrusive thinking, especially in comparison with the levels of the control groups. There were significant differences (p < .01) between sexually abused young people and their nonabused siblings in study 1. These included a history of stomachaches, fear of being alone, sleep problems, excess energy, nervousness, inhibition of feelings, blanking out, and confused feelings about sex. In study 2, the one significant difference between the sexually abused youngsters and their controls was the presence of flashbacks.

In comparing use of alcohol and drugs in study 1 and study 2, we found a tendency for the abused youth in study 1 to experiment with drugs more than their controls—marijuana, for example. However, alcohol was the only substance the abused youngsters used significantly more often than the nonabused youngsters in study 1 (p = .05), and it was used with parental consent. The abused youngsters in study 2 used amphetamines, heroin, and psychedelics significantly more than did their controls (p < .001).

There were no significant differences in sexual interests and behavior between the sexually abused youngsters and their controls in study 1; however, in study 2 the abused young people differed from their controls on two sexual behaviors—compulsive masturbation (p = .03) and prostitution (p = .03).

The abused youngsters in study 1 reported difficulty in relationships with friends of the opposite sex (p = .007), and the abused youngsters in study 2 reported engaging in physical fights with friends (p = .01). In behavior with parents, the abused youngsters in study 1 did not differ significantly from their controls on any of the five indicators of parental interaction (physical fights, verbal fights, disobeying rules, wanting extra parental attention, or withdrawal or avoidance of parents); however, the abused youngsters in study 2 reported physical fights with their parents (p < .01).

There were significant differences (p < .001) between the abused youngsters in study 1 and study 2 in their families' reactions to disclosure of the abuse. The sexually abused youngsters in study 2 were much more likely to feel pressured, threatened, or rejected for telling about the abuse; to feel punished by their parents for the abuse; and to feel parental blame. Thus, it is not surprising that study 2 victims were more likely to feel sorry that they disclosed the abuse. For example, Jed, age 14, was the oldest boy in a sex ring at the time of disclosure. His father, visibly upset at the disclosure, blurted out, "You pervert; you must have liked it to stay in the troop." Jed's behavior deteriorated; he isolated himself from his friends and dropped out of school. His sexual activities escalated, as did his use of drugs and alcohol. He had numerous encounters with police, and a high-speed car chase culminated in a serious accident. His parents reported him as a runaway in 1982.

Tests of mean difference for each of three family environment dimensions (cohesion, expressiveness, and conflict) indicated no significant differences between the sexually abused youngsters and their controls in study 1. A difference was found, however, in study 2 between the sexually abused youngsters and their controls on the dimension of conflict within family relationships. The sexually abused subjects were less likely than were their controls to have family members who were supportive, and they perceived their families as openly expressing anger, aggression, and conflict.

There were such striking differences between the abused and nonabused subjects in study 2 in the area of delinquent and criminal behaviors that the Bonferroni correction was applied to ensure noninflation of a level of significance (p < .004). There were no differences in study 1 between the abused youngsters and their nonabused controls in delinquent and criminal activities. Abused youngsters in study 2, on the other hand, were significantly more aggressive, unresponsive to authority, and resistive to societal mandates for personal control than nonabused control subjects. They were more likely than their controls to have trouble with the law, run away from home, steal from the family, break and enter homes, purposely destroy property, engage in physical assault without provocation, and use a weapon (table 1). For example, the numbers of abused young people arrested at least once for crimes that resulted in convictions and jail or prison before age 18 were as follow: car theft, 15; breaking and entering, 15; destruction of property, 14; assault and battery, 11; carrying a weapon, six; assault and battery with a dangerous weapon, four; armed robbery, three; statutory rape, one; rape, sodomy, and false imprisonment, one; attempted murder, one; and second-degree murder, one.

DISCUSSION

The present study identifies trauma-related variables and intervening variables that suggest a descriptive link between childhood sexual abuse and the development of socially deviant behaviors in young people. It also extends our understanding of children's informational processing of traumatic events. The findings suggest that delinquent and criminal behaviors are associated with the previous trauma of childhood physical abuse in boys who were in adult and peer sex and pornography rings for an extended time and who, on disclosure, were blamed for their sexual participation, were socially excluded, and dropped out of school. Following disclosure, these boys managed their flashbacks through the extension of drug abuse, and the ring-specific behaviors of compulsive masturbation, prostitution, and aggressive acts continued and escalated. In contrast, youngsters who were molested for a limited time in a sex ring that was not organized around peer exploitation came from more stable and nonblaming families and did not display delinquent or criminal behaviors significantly more than their nonsexually-abused siblings. After disclosure, they continued to attend school with their peers, and they reported general posttrauma symptoms and trauma-specific symptoms of confusion regarding sexual feelings and gender role.

Table 1. Delinquent or Criminal Activity of 17 Young People Who Had Experienced Prolonged Sexual Abuse and 13 Schoolmates Who Had Not Been Abused[a]

Variable	Sexually Abused Subjects		Control Subjects		χ^2 (df=1)	p[b]
	N	%	N	%		
Had trouble with the law	17	100	1	8	12.12	.001
Arrested	17	100	2	15	9.35	.005
Participated in acts of violence	14	82	4	31	3.88	.07
Ran away from home	13	76	1	8	9.37	.003
Took things or money from family	15	88	6	46	4.19	.05
Stole less than $20	17	100	5	38	5.59	.02
Stole more than $20	15	88	3	23	9.21	.004
Participated in breaking and entering	15	88	1	8	14.50	.0001
Purposely destroyed property	17	100	4	31	10.54	.002
Physically assaulted someone without provocation	13	76	0	0	14.83	.0001
Used a weapon	13	76	0	0	14.83	.0001

[a]Validation of delinquent or criminal activity through official records was possible for 13 of the 17 control subjects. The four control subjects who did not report any of the listed activities are not included in this table.
[b]Correction for the Bonferroni type 1 inflation error indicated statistical significance at p<.004.

We will discuss here the dimensions of three critical phases in this 6- and 8-year prospective study within a model of traumatic event processing. The first critical phase is the phase before the trauma. A family history for instability and violence, documented here and by other researchers (21–24), suggests that a parental role model for criminality, substance abuse, and emotional isolation who is also physically abusive in the family may predispose an abused child to feelings of anger and resentment. These feelings, in turn, foster retaliative feelings and fantasy (25), an identification with group aggression (23), and drug use (26–29). The cumulative trauma of previous physical abuse adds to the psychological burden for the child and, as Green (22) emphasized, adversely influences ego defenses, character formation, mastery, and cognitive development.

In the trauma phase, the abused youngsters in study 2 had had an extended period of time to repeatedly experience, witness, and practice the adult-initiated sex, sadism, and pornography. We suggest that the trauma replay through reenactment and repetition of sexual acts on younger and weaker children provided the child a sense of mastery and superiority in not being concerned about the fear, pain, shame, or degradation of another. These children split with their empathic capacities for that part of themselves which was terrified, humiliated, and victimized.

During trauma encapsulation, several levels of defense begin with dissociation. This accommodates alterations in physiological states ranging from numbness, anxiety, and tension to accelerated affects (30, 31). A further level of cognitive and behavioral organization occurs through a splitting of two internalized schemata—an externalizing pattern of aggressive acting out and an internalizing pattern of avoidance and withdrawal (32, 33). Both schemata are present because the child had to either submit, inhibit, or dissociate that part of the self which could be assertive or resist. The combined trauma learning and encapsulation increase the likelihood that the victim will adapt to the overall aggressive victimizing role.

In the third critical phase, the posttraumatic phase, disclosure brings to the surface the child's memories of the traumatic experience and its attendant affects. It is not surprising that use of alcohol and drugs, introduced by the abuser to assist the child in controlling tension, symptoms, and avoidant thoughts associated with the victimizing experience, is extended during this phase as stress develops concerning the response of family, peers, and outsiders. The abused youngsters in study 1 used alcohol with parental permission; however, the selection of drugs by the abused youngsters in study 2 is quite revealing. That these young people reported flashbacks emphasized the visual component of the ring activities (e.g., witnessing and pornography). Although the relationship to imagery and aggressive behavioral responses is not yet clear, there is evidence that some sex offenders are highly visual and employ sexual fantasies in their crimes (26, 34). The selection by abused youngsters in study 2 of psychedelic drugs and amphetamines, known to be stimulants and activators of imagery, and heroin, known as an antithesis for rage and aggression, suggests the need by some of these young people to maintain visual stimulation and to regulate their sensory state for an optimum level of sexually aggressive arousal after disclosure. Our impressions, and as suggested by Khantzian (26) and others (27–29), are that drug choice is not a random phenomenon but, rather, self-medicating for either subduing or heightening tension.

High-quality support and acceptance by family and peers have the potential to mediate a child's anxiety regarding disclosure of sexual abuse. In families that are supportive and nonblaming but unable to confront and discuss directly the abusive situation, the pattern of avoidant behaviors may predispose the child to covert predatory acts within the family or neighborhood. For example, Bill described walking into the room with the offender, pretending he was a "wind-up toy" as he complied with the sexual demands. While Bill was in high school, the activities of the sex ring were disclosed. Bill's mother was terminally ill at the time, and Bill had not disclosed the abuse because he was told by his abuser that it would kill his mother if she found out. Bill sought out the school nurse in an effort to deal with his grief but refused to talk about the abuse. Bill's mother died after the abuse was revealed. Bill graduated from high school, enlisted in the military, and appeared to be functioning adequately. At age 19, however, while he was on leave from a tour in Japan, Bill's father reported that Bill was exhibiting himself at home and that he had attempted to sexually abuse his 12-year-old sister. We do not know what happened in Japan, but Bill's sexual aggression towards his sister suggests two interpretations. 1) Bill's fantasies were activated while he was in Japan because the sexual ritual of the abuse involved the offender's telling stories of his war experiences in that country. On return home, Bill acted out these fantasies on his sister. 2) Bill's return home brought to the surface a delayed posttrauma stress response in which he repeated his own victimization at age 12.

Overt aggressive patterns emerge in families that are disorganized, nonsupportive, and blaming in attitude. For example, 18-year-old Joe had been in consenting sexual relationships with girls since the disclosure of the ring's activities and had continued heavy drug use. When one of his former girlfriends refused his sexual advances and tried to terminate the relationship he hit her repeatedly on the head with a hammer and raped her, which resulted in her emergency hospital admission to the intensive care unit. We speculate that this young man felt a heightened narcissistic entitlement;

during the ring activity he had been a favored boy victim. His girlfriend's rejection and refusal of sex provoked rage and the murderous act.

CONCLUSIONS

When prolonged sexual abuse is compounded as in the witnessing and perpetrating of sexual dominance in a ring, the nature of the experience can have a primary influence on the young person's response pattern. Major cognitive operations necessary to process and manage distress develop. Basic to these is dissociation, which in turn leads to a sealing of the event and the splitting of psychological and sensory experiences. We theorize, for those abused youth who become abusers, that through dissociation there is a massive blocking at a sensory level (e.g., their need to override numbness by seeking extreme states of excitement through drugs), at a perceptual level (e.g., a minimal cue response for interpersonal feelings of tenderness, attachment, and caring paired with a heightened predilection for deviant stimuli), and at a cognitive level (e.g., the condoning of sexual violence by adults and negation of social values). The trauma learning from the sex ring activities interacts with past cumulative childhood trauma and negative social responses to disclosure. The youth's denial of his position of vulnerability and helplessness as a victim enhances identification with aggression. This reformulation of the actual trauma experience creates the link from abused to abuser.

The therapeutic implications of this study are that efforts need to be aimed at 1) identifying and interrupting sexual abuse, 2) understanding the organization of the victim's defensive structure and its relationship to the abuse, 3) modifying the psychological defenses so that the victim can tolerate discussing the abuse, 4) unlinking the trauma at sensory, perceptual, and cognitive levels from dysfunctional behaviors, 5) processing the integrated trauma to past memory, and 6) rebuilding coping behaviors that provide for a positive interaction with the future.

REFERENCES

1. Freud S: The etiology of hysteria (1896), in Collected Papers, vol 1. Edited by Jones E; translated by Riviere J. New York, Basic Books, 1959
2. Gleuck BC: Early sexual experiences in schizophrenia, in Advances in Sex Research. Edited by Biegel H. New York, Harper & Row, 1963
3. Carmen E(H), Rieker PP, Mills T: Victims of violence and psychiatric illness. Am J Psychiatry 1984; 141:378–383
4. Herman J, Russell D, Trocki K: Long-term effects of incestuous abuse in childhood. Am J Psychiatry 1986; 143:1293–1296

5. Briere J, Runtz M: Suicidal thoughts and behaviors in former sexual abuse victims. Can J Behavioral Sciences 1986; 18:413–423

6. Groth AN: Sexual trauma in the life histories of sex offenders. Victimology 1979; 4:6–10

7. Seghorn TK, Boucher RJ, Prentky RA: Childhood sexual abuse in the lives of sexually aggressive offenders. J Am Acad Child Psychiatry (in press)

8. Fehrenbach PA, Smith W, Monastersky C, et al: Adolescent sexual offenders: offender and offense characteristics. Am J Orthopsychiatry 1986; 56:225–233

9. James J, Meyerding J: Early sexual experience and prostitution. Am J Psychiatry 1977; 134:1381–1385

10. Silbert MH, Pines AM: Sexual child abuse as an antecedent to prostitution. Child Abuse Negl 1981; 5:407–411

11. Rieker PP, Carmen E(H): The victim-to-patient process: the disconfirmation and transformation of abuse. Am J Orthopsychiatry 1986; 56:360–370

12. Burgess AW, Groth AN, McCausland MP: Child sex initiation rings. Am J Orthopsychiatry 1981; 51:110–119

13. Burgess AW, Hartman CR, McCausland MP, et al: Response patterns in children and adolescents exploited through sex rings and pornography. Am J Psychiatry 1984; 141:656–662

14. Piers E, Harris D: The Piers-Harris Children's Self-Concept Scale. Nashville, Counselor Recordings and Tests, 1969

15. Moos R, Moos B: Family Environment Scale Manual. Palo Alto, Calif, Consulting Psychologists Press, 1981

16. Horowitz MJ, Wilner N, Alvarez W: Impact of Event Scale: a measure of subjective stress. Psychosom Med 1979; 41:209–218

17. Moos R, Moos B: Adaptation and quality of life in work and family settings. J Community Psychiatry 1983; 11:158–170

18. Hartman CR, Burgess AW: Child sexual abuse: generic roots of the victim experience. J Psychotherapy & the Family 1986; 2:77–87

19. Horowitz MJ: Stress Response Syndromes, 2nd ed. New York, Jason Aronson, 1986

20. Child molestation: assessing impact in multiple victims. Archives of Psychiatric Nursing 1987; 1(1):33–39

21. Straus M, Gelles R, Steinmetz S: Behind Closed Doors: Violence in the American Family. New York, Anchor Press/Doubleday, 1980

22. Green AH: Children traumatized by physical abuse, in Post-Traumatic Stress Disorder in Children. Edited by Eth S, Pynoos RS. Washington, DC, American Psychiatric Press, 1985

23. Hartstone E, Hansen KV: The violent juvenile offender: an empirical portrait, in Violent Juvenile Offenders: An Anthology. Edited by Mathias RA, DeMuro P, Allinson RS. San Francisco, National Council on Crime and Delinquency, 1984

24. Garbarino J, Gilliam G: Understanding Abusive Families. Lexington, Mass, Lexington Books, 1980

25. Burgess AW, Hartman CR, Ressler RK, et al: Sexual homicide: a motivational model. J Interpersonal Violence 1986; 1:251–272

26. Khantzian EJ. The self-medication hypothesis of addictive disorders: focus on heroin and cocaine dependence. Am J Psychiatry 1985; 142:1259–1264

27. Wieder H, Kaplan EH: Drug use in adolescents: psychodynamic meaning and pharmacogenic effect. Psychoanal Study Child 1969; 24:399–431

28. Milkman H, Frosch WA: On the preferential abuse of heroin and amphetamine. J Nerv Ment Dis 1973; 156:242–248
29. Krystal H, Raskin HA: Drug Dependence: Aspects of Ego Functions. Detroit, Wayne State University Press, 1970
30. Stoller R: Splitting: A Case of Female Masculinity. New York, Delta Books, 1973
31. Hartman CR, Burgess AW: Child to child sexual abuse. J Interpersonal Violence (in press)
32. Achenbach TM, Edelbrock CS: The classification of child psychopathology: a review and analysis of empirical effects. Psychol Bull 1978; 85:1275–1301
33. Ross AO: Psychological Disorders of Children: A Behavioral Approach to Theory, Research and Therapy. New York, McGraw-Hill, 1974
34. Abel GG, Rouleau JL, Cunningham-Rathner J: Sexually aggressive behavior, in Modern Legal Psychiatry and Psychology. Edited by Curran W, McGarry AL, Shah SA. Philadelphia, FA Davis, 1985

34

False Allegations of Child Abuse: The Other Side of the Tragedy

Donna L. Wong
Private Practice, Tulsa, Oklahoma

As the incidence of child abuse and neglect has risen, so has the problem of false allegations of abuse. Currently, of the 1.9 million cases reported for child abuse, 1.2 million are found to be unsubstantiated.

After a bitter divorce and custody battle, a father is arrested on a complaint by his ex-wife and charged with the sexual abuse of his 2½-year-old daughter. After a 2-year legal battle, he is acquitted of the charges and has joint legal custody of the child. The victory comes after being denied contact with his daughter for almost 2 years, losing most of his practice as a psychologist, and incurring legal expenses of $70,000.

Although physical and sexual abuse of children are heinous acts, and although failure to report such acts is a tragedy and a crime, it is also tragic to falsely accuse innocent families. Unfortunately, much less attention has been directed to the problem of false accusation and the devastating consequences of misdiagnoses. Children may be needlessly taken from their homes with restricted visits by parents, parental rights may be terminated, alleged offenders may suffer public ridicule, and families may experience great financial strain from loss of employment and/or legal expense in their

Reprinted with permission from *Pediatric Nursing,* 1987, Vol. 13, No. 5, 329–333. Copyright 1987 by Anthony J. Jannetti, Inc.

The author wishes to thank Douglas Besharov, William McIver, Ralph Underwager, and Hollida Wakefield for their reviews of this article.

attempt to regain custody through the courts (Schetky & Boverman, 1985; Schultz, 1986).

Numerous reports of mistaken diagnosis of abuse exist in the medical literature. Some of them involve lack of understanding of cultural traditions, such as the Oriental practices of coin rubbing and cupping, which produces welts or bruises (Asnes & Wisotsky, 1981; Saulsbury & Hayden, 1985) or the use of heat (moxabustion), which causes circular burns that may resemble inflicted wounds (Feldman, 1984). Several diseases may be erroneously attributed to abuse, such as hemophilia, meningitis, sudden infant death syndrome, osteogenesis imperfecta, and erythema multiforme (Adler & Kane-Nussen, 1983; Hurwitz & Castells, 1987; Kirschner & Stein, 1985). Nonintentional injuries may also be wrongly diagnosed as abuse, such as burns from metal buckles on car seats (Schmitt, Gray, & Britton, 1978) or lacerations from seat belts (Baker, 1986).

Despite such reports, the topic of false allegations of abuse appears rarely in the professional literature, although national attention to this problem is mounting (Bailey, 1986; Joyner, 1986; Lacayo, 1987; "The numbers game," 1987). Certainly, no one can deny that child abuse is one of the most pervasive and serious problems in our society. Since the institution of laws to protect children in the early 1960s, the incidence of reported child abuse has risen dramatically. Overall child reporting levels have increased 188% between 1976 and 1985 (American Humane Association [AHA], 1987). However, the statistics reflect only part of the tragic story. In society's attempt to deal with child maltreatment, there have been increasing numbers of families who have been falsely accused of abuse.

STATISTICS

Statistics on the incidence of child abuse are at best estimates of the true severity of the problem. In the United States, statistics on abuse are compiled by the American Humane Association (AHA), which is under contract with the National Center on Child Abuse and Neglect. The AHA's yearly report for 1985, *Highlights of Official Child Neglect and Abuse Reporting,* is considered the most reliable data available and is the source quoted below. However, the latest report that analyzes case files for 1985 is limited to only 5 states in the United States for several categories of information. Consequently, the reported findings may not reflect the true characteristics of abuse in every state.

In 1985, an estimated 1,928,000 children were reported for child abuse and neglect to Child Protective Services. Of these cases, 732,000 (approximately

38%) were substantiated for maltreatment. The definition of "substantiation" varies widely across counties and states but all definitions imply "a degree of certainty that the involved child is in fact at risk, and in many states that some level of intervention is warranted on the child's behalf" (AHA, 1987, p. 9).

A certain level of unsubstantiated reporting is expected when there is mandatory reporting of suspected child maltreatment. However, Douglas Besharov, former head of the National Center on Child Abuse and Neglect, states that in his opinion a 30% to 40% rate is acceptable, but the present rate of over 60% is unacceptable. While the incidence of reported cases of abuse has risen steadily, so has the number of unsubstantiated reporting. In 1975, the unsubstantiated rate was about 35% (Besharov, 1987).

Another important statistic is type of maltreatment. While child abuse is often equated with extreme cruelty, in reality major physical injury occurred in 2.2% of all maltreated children in 1985. The most common type of maltreatment was deprivation of necessities (55.7%) (AHA, 1987).

CHILD ABUSE LAWS

Until Dr. Henry Kempe, a radiologist, first brought attention to the "battered child syndrome" in 1962, there were virtually no laws protecting children from abuse. However, by 1967 all 50 states had mandatory reporting laws and some form of child protective services (CPS) to investigate reports of abuse or neglect. While the laws were legislated to protect the child from further abuse and have been very successful, some important aspects of these laws may be working against the protection of children and families.

All states require professionals to report suspected abuse. Mandatory reporting laws have been highly effective in raising professional awareness of suspected abuse. Such laws provide immunity for professionals who report suspected abuse even if the complaint is found to be unsubstantiated. However, they may impose civil or criminal liability for not reporting should it be discovered that the professional had reasonable knowledge of the abuse (Elvik, 1987). Unfortunately, health professionals may "play it safe" by reporting cases that remotely appear to be abuse or neglect rather than risk the chance of missing a suspected case (Besharov, 1985).

All states have hotlines for people to call and report suspected abuse. Most hotlines take complaints regardless of the circumstances reported and will investigate such anonymous reports even if the caller can cite no specific reason to suspect maltreatment. Of reports by anonymous callers, about 85% are found to be unsubstantiated (Besharov, 1987).

Unfortunately, the result of overreporting causes a severe backlog of reports to child protective services. With such a strain on case workers, it is difficult, if not impossible, to investigate all complaints within 24 hours. With so much time devoted to checking unsubstantiated reports, case workers often do not have the time needed to conduct thorough investigations of bonafide reports. Consequently, children who have been abused may not receive the protection they require (Besharov, 1987).

The definitions of abuse and neglect are broad and vague. There is no one definition for abuse and neglect; rather each state defines child maltreatment differently. The one common characteristic of these definitions, however, is vagueness (Duquette, 1982). For example, one state defines neglect as "failure to provide any other care necessary for the child's well-being." Many definitions include the term "threatened or suspected harm," which implies that before abuse or neglect occurs, a child can be taken from the home (Pride, 1986). Consequently, most complaints can be considered legitimate under these laws. With abuse and neglect so broadly defined, it is impossible to screen out irrelevant complaints, which further burdens the CPS.

The laws may violate "due process" and the accused person's civil rights. The United States Constitution provides that no state shall deprive a person of life, liberty, or property without due process of law. "Due process" refers to the fair treatment of all concerned and generally includes the right of a person to know what actions are prohibited, what charges are made against him, and to have a fair hearing and representation by an attorney. Once a petition is filed in the court, due process requirements apply. However, the majority (80% to 85%) of child abuse and neglect cases referred to CPS never reach the courts and do not receive the protection of due process (Duquette, 1982).

Once a report is made to the CPS, officials can take the potentially abused child from the home, school, day care center, or other place of residence before the case is substantiated. In addition, the accused abuser is not required by law to be informed of the charge at the time of the investigation and no state requires its investigators to limit their investigation to the reported charge (Pride, 1986).

The accused person may also not be allowed to know the identity of his or her accuser or to have access to confidential state records. The defense attorney also may not have the right to see such records, which could include testimony from the accuser, the victim, medical personnel, social services, or the police. The U.S. Supreme Court upheld this decision in a ruling on February 24, 1987 (Pennsylvania vs Ritchie), although some states allow access to records.

Many states have no provisions for removing an unsubstantiated record from official files, such as an abuser registry, or for challenging the information in a report. All that may be needed to place a name on a registry is some credible evidence that abuse occurred, regardless if the actual investigation has been done. For example, an abuser registry may list the name of a person reported to be sexually abusing a child even though the case is eventually found to be unsubstantiated. In future unsolved sex crimes, this person may be questioned because his name remains on the registry (State "abuser registry," 1986).

INVESTIGATIVE TECHNIQUES

One of the most difficult and frustrating aspects of substantiating complaints of child abuse is the collection of reliable and valid testimony. Since the majority of abuse occurs in young children (43% of reported children are 5 years of age or younger), their limited verbal and cognitive ability presents a major challenge to investigation. Currently, two techniques are commonly used, especially in the investigation of sexual abuse of young children. Despite their widespread acceptance, both the use of anatomically correct dolls and drawings have been subjected to minimal research regarding their reliability or validity.

Once children have fairly good verbal skills, interviewing is the principle method of investigation. However, misuse of interrogation techniques can influence a child's testimony and lead to erroneous conclusions. The misuse of any of these investigative techniques increases the likelihood of a false allegation or conviction of abuse.

Anatomically correct dolls. Anatomically correct dolls are usually cloth or plastic dolls that have simulated genitals and breasts and embroidered or printed pubic hair. There may be anal, genital, and oral openings to allow for penetration during play. The dolls are clothed in garments appropriate for their sex with closures that make removal easy. These dolls were originally used in play therapy to help sexually abused children deal with the experience. Currently, however, they are being used as diagnostic tools in investigation of suspected cases of sexual abuse.

Although there have been attempts to standardize the interviewing protocol using these dolls, there is considerable data demonstrating that the suggested protocols are not followed. One suggested protocol strongly advocates that the interviewer not receive information relative to the suspected abuse prior to the interview with the child, avoid leading questions or cueing responses, and interview the child away from the parents. The authors acknowledge that "biased data may well cause an unfair conviction of an innocent person if the child's responses are lead based on prior information of the interviewer" (White, Strom & Santilli, 1985, p. 5). However, a review of hundreds of hours of recordings of interviews using the dolls with children suspected of being sexually abused did not identify one instance where these suggestions were followed (Underwager, Wakefield, Legrand, & Bartz, 1986). Even more disturbing is the finding that the use of the standardized interview protocol was not effective in minimizing the problems with using the dolls (Reamulto, Jensen, Wescoe, & Garfinkel, 1986).

In addition, there is little research on the validity of the dolls in assessing abuse. Gabriel (1985) observed 19 nonabused children ages 3 to 5 years playing with the dolls. He recorded 8 categories of behavior, including actively handling the dolls, play that showed private issues, unusual interaction with the genitals, and overt interest in the genitals. Although the study did not compare these children's behaviors with those of abused children, the author stated that many of the observed activities were similar to those described by examiners in sexual abuse investigations. McIver (1986a) conducted a similar study and videotaped 50 non-abused and 10 sexually abused children's interactions with the dolls. Not only did he find much sexual interest from all of the children with the dolls, but also that the interviewer could easily influence the children to demonstrate sexual acts with the dolls. He concluded that the dolls are not useful in discriminating between abused and non-abused children.

However, Jampole and Weber (1987), in their study of the frequency of sexual behavior among sexually abused and non-sexually abused children's play with anatomically correct dolls, found that significantly more children who had been sexually abused demonstrated sexual behavior in their play than nonsexually abused children. They did acknowledge several limitations to their study, such as the effects on either group to outside influences that shape sexual knowledge, such as television, movies, sex education, family attitudes, and previous interviewing concerning the abuse. Based on these few studies with conflicting findings, the validity of anatomically correct dolls as a diagnostic tool remains unclear.

Drawings. The use of drawings is a commonly used projective technique to help children express their feelings. The content of drawings has been extensively studied and some authorities conclude that the drawing of genitals is very rare (DiLeo, 1980; Koppitz, 1968). From this observation has come the suggestion that the presence of genitalia in drawings is significant and may indicate abuse. Unfortunately, very little research has been conducted to substantiate this claim.

Hibbard, Roghmann, and Hoekelman (1987) investigated the drawings (free drawings and completion drawings) of 52 alleged sexually abused and 52 matched nonabused children ages 3 to 7 years. Although the frequency of genitals in the drawings of abused children was five times greater than in the drawing of the nonabused group, the difference was not statistically significant at the .05 level. In addition, when substantiated and unsubstantiated cases were considered separately, the frequency of genitalia in drawings was almost identical (9% vs 10%, respectively). The authors concluded that "although this study suggests an association between the presence of genitalia in human figure drawings and sexual abuse, it does not imply casuality . . . It is important to caution that, based on these data, this tool cannot be used as an epidemiologic screening test for sexual abuse." (p. 135)

Other researchers have investigated the role of art therapy in facilitating children's verbalization of thoughts and feelings related to the victimization and as an indicator of changes in the emotional status of the child (Kelley, 1985). However, this differs from using drawings to diagnose child abuse. As in the use of anatomically correct dolls, drawings must be interpreted cautiously and subjected to further research before being accepted as a valid diagnostic tool.

Interrogation. Interviewing the child regarding the alleged abuse is the most common form of investigation. Interviewing is based on the premise that the child's testimony always represents the truth. Unfortunately, the types of interrogation techniques used by examiners frequently distorts the truth. In essence, the child may not be telling the truth and may not be lying. Rather, the child may be affirming what the investigator wants to hear.

Underwager, et al. (1986) stated that "to make the question one of whether or not children lie about sexual abuse is a mistake. To lie assumes deliberate, willful, and intentional purpose and malice. Few children, indeed, are likely to have either the competence or the balefulness to embark upon such a course, although some adolescents may do so. Rather, given the plastic and malleable nature of children the question is what degree, kind, and type of influence has been exerted upon them. . .In every exposure to interrogation the child learns more about what the interrogator expects. . .The child learns the tale, and by repetition, may come to experience the subjective reality that it (abuse) happened, when it never did happen" (pp. 29, 33).

Their analysis of transcripts and audio and videotapes from hundreds of cases, as well as the work of others (Coleman, 1986; McIver, 1986b) demonstrated that children can be trained to believe something occurred through systematic manipulation described in Table 1.

Underwager and his group found that potentially leading questions, closed questions (questions requiring yes or no answers), modeling, and the use of aids (dolls, drawings, or photographs) comprised 60% of all the interrogators' behaviors. The interaction was one of relatively active adults and passive children. In two videotaped cases, the adults asked questions or made statements at the rate of one every 2 or 3 seconds.

PREDICTION OF ABUSE

Unlike the investigative techniques that have undergone minimal research, the subject of prediction of abuse has been studied extensively. Many researchers have attempted to identify the characteristics of abusing persons with the hope of compiling a risk index that reliably differentiates the abuser

Table 1. Commonly Used Manipulations in Interviews

- Setting up expectations — using statements that pressure the child to conform, such as, "Good children tell the truth"
- Prodding — using statements that imply doubting the child's story and encourages a change of the facts, such as "It isn't that I do not believe you, but if you think of anything else let me know"
- Pressure and coercion — using statements that imply a threat, such as "If you don't talk to me, your mother will be upset"
- Reinforcement — showing positive attention to children when they say what the investigator wants to hear; through "successive approximations," the child is reinforced or rewarded through smiles, hugs, or statements like "good girl, don't you feel better now," for statements leading up to and finally including those the interviewer wants to hear
- Repetition — asking the same question repeatedly until the child relents and gives the investigator expected answers
- Modeling — using adult descriptions of the events in the alleged abuse

from the nonabuser. Starr (1982a) cited numerous studies that have addressed the issue of false positives generated from predictive instruments.

One of the main difficulties with predicting child maltreatment is a clear definition of abuse and neglect. As Gelles (1982, p. 2) states, "It is extremely difficult to predict a phenomenon if no precise and acceptable definition of the phenomenon can be reached." In his studies of defining and classifying cases of child abuse, he found that among several groups of professionals (child and family physicians, emergency room physicians, school guidance counselors, school principals, private and public social workers, and police officers) there was no clear consensus on what conditions constitute child abuse.

Kotelchuck (1982) and Starr (1982b) both conducted separate studies comparing families where a child was diagnosed with abuse or neglect and a matched control group of families with children admitted to the hospital with medical or surgical illnesses. The families were compared for a wide range of characteristics. Both studies found a lack of differences between the groups on almost all characteristics. The only statistically significant differences in the Kotelchuck study were a greater degree of social isolation and an unhappier maternal childhood in abused families. Starr found evidence for social isolation as well as poorer health in the abused child, less adequate maternal functioning, and greater family violence.

Both researchers used the identified risk index to hypothetically reclassify the studies' subjects as abused or non-abused children. They found a 25% to 30% error rate for false positives (children not abused who are classified as abused). Kotelchuck (1982) demonstrated the implications of this error rate by applying it to a hypothetical screening on a mythical population of 1,000 children with an estimated abuse rate of 10%:

1. 75 actual child abuse and neglect cases would be correctly predicted.
2. 25 true abuse cases (false negatives) would be missed.
3. 675 cases would be correctly identified as nonabuse.
4. 225 cases of false positives would be found.

Both authors concluded that while the predictive accuracy was quite good, the number of false positives was unacceptably high.

SUGGESTIONS FOR PREVENTING FALSE ACCUSATIONS

While every child who is a victim of maltreatment must be protected, the question remains: how high should the cost of protection be? Some professionals maintain that any cost is acceptable. Krugman (1985, p. 868) stated: "I believe that the costs to children of not reporting (abuse) are much higher than the risks of a social evaluation. Henry Kempe emphasized: "No child ever died of a social work evaluation—many have died because we didn't get one." What price is acceptable? Individuals must decide for themselves. Krugman added: "There is no substitute for competence in the diagnosis of either diseases of children or a child's unexpected death." Health professionals must exercise the greatest degree of competence in assessing suspected cases of child abuse.

As the largest group of health care professionals, nurses are likely to come in contact with children who may be victims of abuse or neglect. Often the indications of maltreatment are obvious and the decision to report the family for abuse is well substantiated. However, there are also occasions when the indications are subtle, the parents' story may be plausible, or other facts cast doubt on the possibility of abuse. Table 2 lists suggestions for nurses to minimize the possibility of misdiagnosing abuse.

Table 2. Minimizing Child Abuse Misdiagnosis

1. Be aware that false allegations of abuse are common and can have devastating consequences for the family.
2. Become knowledgeable about the types of cases of mistaken diagnosis of abuse, such as cultural practices and diseases that may mimic inflicted physical injury or the use of sexual abuse charges in custody battles.
3. Be familiar with the child abuse legislation in your state and work for better laws when abuses of the system occur.
4. Remember that there is no diagnostic test for abuse; anatomically correct dolls and drawings are only tools to help in confirming the diagnosis.
5. Give the parents or accused person every opportunity to present their account of the incidents.
6. Document the information obtained in interviews with the child, family, and other significant individuals.

Despite the most careful attention to these guidelines, errors will occur and are part of the cost of protecting children from maltreatment. Families falsely accused of abuse are victims and deserve our compassionate understanding. Such families may also benefit from the services provided by the national organization of Victims Of Child Abuse Laws (VOCAL), P.O. Box 11335, Minneapolis, MN 55411. VOCAL is a support group for persons falsely accused of abuse and an advocacy group with the goal of promoting constructive investigation of abuse reports and legislation that provides due process for the accused.

While the issues of false allegations will undoubtedly generate controversy, it is hoped that attention will be drawn to a problem that deserves as much consideration as child abuse has received. In our zeal to help and protect abused children, the number of casualties among innocent families must be appreciated and minimized.

REFERENCES

Adler, R. & Kane-Nussen, B. (1983). Erythema multiforme: confusion with child battering syndrome. *Pediatrics, 72,* 718–720.

American Humane Association (AHA), (1987). *Highlights of official child neglect and abuse reporting 1985.* Denver, CO: AHA.

Asnes, R.S., & Wisotsky, D.H. (1981). Cupping lesions simulating child abuse. *Journal of Pediatrics, 99,* 267–268.

Bailey, J. (1986, November 19). Grueling child-abuse cases push many prosecutors to their limits. *Wall Street Journal,* p. 29.

Baker, R.B. (1986). Seat belt injury masquerading as sexual abuse. *Pediatrics, 77,* 435.

Besharov, D.J. (1987, Winter). Contending with overblown expectations. *Public Welfare, 45,* pp. 7–11.

Besharov, D.J. (1986). "Doing something" about child abuse: The need to narrow the grounds for state intervention. *Harvard Journal of Law and Public Policy, 8,* 539–589.

Coleman, L. (1986, October 25). Keynote speaker, VOCAL National Convention, Torrance, CA.

DiLeo, J.H. (1980). *Children's drawings as diagnostic aids.* New York: Brunner/Mazel.

Duquette, D. (1982). Protecting individual liberties in the context of screening for child abuse. In Starr, R.H., *Child abuse prediction: Policy implications* (pp. 191–204), Cambridge, MA: Ballinger Publishing Company.

Elvik, S.L. (1987). From disclosure to court: The facets of sexual abuse. *Journal of Pediatric Health Care, 1,* 136–140.

Feldman, K.W. (1984). Pseudoabusive burns in Asian refugees. *American Journal of Diseases of Children, 138,* 768–769.

Gabriel, R. (1985). Anatomically correct dolls in the diagnosis of sexual abuse of children. *Journal of the Melanie Klein Society, 3,* 40–51.

Gelles, R.J. (1982). Problems in defining and labeling child abuse. In R.H. Starr, (Ed.), *Child abuse prediction: Policy implications* (pp. 1–30). Cambridge, MA: Ballinger Publishing Company.

Hibbard, R., Roghmann, K., & Hoekelman, R. (1987). Genitalia in children's drawings: An association with sexual abuse. *Pediatrics, 79,* 129–137.

Hurwitz, A., & Castells, S. (1987). Misdiagnosed child abuse and metabolic diseases. *Pediatric Nursing, 13,* 33–36.

Jampole, L. & Weber, M. (1987). An assessment of the behavior of sexually abused and non-sexually abused children with anatomically correct dolls. *Child Abuse & Neglect, 11,* 187–192.

Joyner, G.P. (1986, May 6). False accusation of child abuse—Could it happen to you? *Woman's Day, 10,* 30–42.

Kelley, S.J. (1985). Drawings: Critical communications for sexually abused children. *Pediatric Nursing, 11,* 421–426.

Kirschner, R.H., & Stein, R.J. (1985). The mistaken diagnosis of child abuse: A form of medical abuse? *American Journal of Diseases of Children, 139,* 873–875.

Koppitz, E.M. (1968). *Psychological evaluation of children's human figure drawings.* New York: Grune & Stratton.

Kotelchuck, M. (1982). Child abuse and neglect: Prediction and misclassification. In Starr, R.H., *Child abuse prediction: Policy implications* (pp. 67–104), Cambridge, MA: Ballinger Publishing Company.

Krugman, R.D. (1985). Where you stand depends on where you sit. *American Journal of Diseases of Children, 139,* 867–868.

Lacayo, R. (1987, May 11). Sexual abuse or abuse of justice? *Time, 129,* 49.

McIver, W. (1986a, October 26). *Behavior of abused and nonabused children in interviews with anatomically correct dolls.* Presented at VOCAL National Convention, Torrance, CA.

McIver, W. (1986b). The case for a therapeutic interview in situations of alleged sexual molestation. *The Champion, 10,* 11–13.

Pennsylvania vs. Ritchie. (1987, February 24). Washington, DC: U.S. Supreme Court.

Pride, M. (1986). *The child abuse industry.* Westchester, IL: Crossway Books.

Realmulto, G., Jensen, J., Wescoe, S., & Garfinkel, B. (1986, October). *Child psychiatrists and other professionals: Assessment of children's play with anatomically complete dolls.* Presented at the American Academy of Child Psychiatric Convention, Washington, DC.

Saulsbury, F.T., & Hayden, G.F. (1985). Skin conditions simulating child abuse. *Pediatric Emergency Care, 1,* 147–150.

Schmitt, B., Gray, J., & Britton, H. (1978). Car seat burns in infants: Avoiding confusion with inflicted burns. *Pediatrics, 62,* 607–609.

Schetky, D., & Boverman, H. (1985, October 10). *Faulty assessment of child sexual abuse: Legal and emotional sequelae.* Annual meeting of the American Academy of Psychiatry and the Law, Albuquerque, NM.

Schultz, L. (1986). *Fifty cases of wrongfully charged child sexual abuse: A survey and recommendations.* Unpublished paper, Morgantown, WV: West Virginia University.

Starr, R.H. (1982a). *Child abuse prediction: Policy implications.* Cambridge, MA: Ballinger Publishing Company.

Starr, R.H. (1982b). A research-based approach to the prediction of child. In Starr, R.H., *Child abuse prediction: Policy implications* (pp. 105–134), Cambridge, MA: Ballinger Publishing Company.

State "abuser registry" may violate due process (1986). *VOCAL National Newsletter, 2,* p. 7.

The numbers game: When more is less (1987, April 27). *U.S. News & World Report,* p. 39.

White, S., Strom, G., & Santilli, G. (1985). *Interviewing young sexual abuse victims with anatomically correct dolls.* American Academy of Psychiatry, San Antonio, TX, October 23–37.

Underwager, R., Wakefield, H., Legrand, R., & Bartz, C. (1986, August). *The role of the psychologist in cases of alleged sexual abuse of children.* American Psychological Association Annual Convention. Washington, DC.

35

Problems in Validating Allegations of Sexual Abuse. Part 1: Factors Affecting Perception and Recall of Events

Elissa P. Benedek
University of Michigan Medical Center and Center for Forensic Psychiatry, Ann Arbor, Michigan
Diane H. Schetky
University of Vermont, College of Medicine at Maine Medical Center, Portland, Maine

Child psychiatrists, pediatricians, and child mental health professionals are concerned by a deluge of referrals requesting evaluation of young children in regard to allegations of sexual abuse. Accurately evaluating an allegation of sexual abuse in a young child is always very difficult and time consuming. This paper explores some of the developmental and emotional factors that influence a child's perception of events. The authors discuss some factors that may lead to a false memory or report of such events. They believe it essential that persons doing these evaluations possess the requisite skills and experience.

Child psychiatrists, pediatricians, and child mental health professionals have recently been concerned by a deluge of referrals requesting evaluation of young children in regard to allegations of sexual abuse. A new cottage industry/profession has evolved, and a group of experts in this specialized

Reprinted with permission from the *Journal of the American Academy of Child and Adolescent Psychiatry,* 1987, Vol. 26, No. 6, 912–915. Copyright 1987 by the American Academy of Child and Adolescent Psychiatry.

examination has emerged to fill a serious need. Many of these experts, although well-meaning, seem to be self-proclaimed and biased, always finding sexual abuse where alleged. They lack training in the fundamentals of child development or requisite specialized interviewing techniques, and they seem to be unaware of the long-term effects a false allegation might have on a child, a parent, or a child/parent relationship. Accurately evaluating an allegation of sexual abuse in a young child is always very difficult and time-consuming. In this paper we explore some of the developmental factors that influence a child's perception of events. We then discuss some factors that may lead to a false memory or report of events and interviewer factors that may influence the child's report of events.

In recent years, sexual abuse of children has received increasing attention in the psychiatric literature and popular press. No longer are children's allegations of sexual abuse presumed to be fantasy as they were in Freud's time. Most professionals look upon such charges as valid distress signals worthy of careful investigation. In our experience in evaluating cases of alleged sexual abuse in children and adolescents, we have found them generally to be truthful. Historically, courts have tended to treat the child witness and his or her memory of events much the way they do an adult witness, with the exception that the competency of a child under age 14 to testify is determined by the judge. Such a determination is most often based upon establishing that the child has a reliable memory and is able to differentiate truth from falsehood and appreciate that lying is morally wrong. As noted by Terr (1980), the legal criteria governing a child's ability to give testimony are often at odds with psychiatric guidelines, which recognize that children have unique ways of perceiving, reacting to, and relating traumatic experiences. Some of the developmental factors that account for these differences will be discussed.

DEVELOPMENTAL FACTORS AFFECTING CHILDREN'S PERCEPTION AND RECALL OF EVENTS

Cognitive Factors

The predominance of primary process thinking. The young child shows a relative weakness of secondary process or logical thinking compared with the strength of his or her impulses and fantasies, as noted by A. Freud (1965). Thus, magical thinking and need for immediate discharge of impulses may prevail until the child starts to enter latency. At about age 6 more logical thinking predominates, the ability to postpone immediate gratification of instincts takes over, and the thinking process matures (Piaget, 1951). Some recent critics of Piagetian theory (Brainerd, 1978) suggest that on many tasks, preschoolers may be less illogical and egocentric in their thinking than suggested by Piaget. Borke (1971, 1973, 1975, 1978) noted that even very young children have the capacity to adopt another's perception and not be egocentric if the task is simple and does not involve the use of language. Borke cautions, however, that young children do not perform well on complex cognitive tasks.

In evaluating the very young child who may have been sexually abused, it is important to determine whether the child can distinguish fact from fantasy and external events from internal psychic ones. Externally derived memories are more likely to contain temporal and spatial information than are dreams or fantasies. They are also more likely to include detail and sensory information. It is useful to inquire about sensual experiences including taste, smell, and touch in attempting to verify sexual abuse. Asking the child hypothetical questions such as "Is this real or pretend?" may also be helpful. For example, a child examining an anatomical doll commented spontaneously that the doll's breasts were pretend—they were really buttons.

Sexual immaturity. Children will interpret sexual events according to where they are in their own sexual development. Thus the young child may interpret sexual abuse not as a sexual activity, per se, but rather as an aggressive attack and violation of his or her body or as a form of affection. Although an accurate knowledge of the origin of babies is not typically reached until age 12, there is some evidence that by age 4 children are aware of sex differences and are willing to speak freely about them. Precocious knowledge about sexual matters beyond the domain of the child's age group should alert the examiner to sexual abuse. Exceptions may include children of physicians and medical students and those with prior exposure to anatomically correct dolls or x-rated movies and the Playboy channel on cable television. Although adolescents are presumed to be knowledgeable about erections and ejaculations and may use those words, such descriptions coming from a 3-year-old should wave a red flag. The Oedipal child may fantasize about sexual activity with the opposite sexed parent, but in normal situations this does not lead to verbal allegations of abuse of graphic descriptions. (For example: A 5-year-old child told the examiner that he and his father engaged in fellatio but could not explain what "fellatio" was. In contrast, a 3-year-old spontaneously volunteered that she and her daddy slept together "in their skins." This description of parental nudity is in the child's language consonant with sexual overstimulation as seen by a 3-year-old.)

Language. Language problems may often lead to confused communications between children and adults. The child's tendency toward concrete thinking may lead to problems in credibility as with the child witness who, when asked if he'd been in the defendant's home, replied "No," because he'd been in his apartment, not his home. Other potential sources of confusion arise from the fact that children often use their own terminology for genitalia. It is important to clarify what they mean before jumping to conclusions. Additional communication problems arise when trying to understand the young child whose speech is immature or who has articulation problems. It is important to obtain from the child his or her own language for genitalia body parts and to use that language in all discussions.

Memory. Studies have shown that children's memories tend to be more fragmented and less complete than those of adults, and that because children lack prior knowledge it is difficult for them to relate one set of events to another and organize disparate elements into a cohesive whole (Johnson and Foley, 1984). Memory tends to improve with age up until adulthood (Brown, 1975). Children make more errors of gross omission than do adults, yet at the same time they may notice seemingly irrelevant items missed by adults (Neisser, 1984). They may also try to fill the gaps in their memories by confabulating. As they mature they learn to screen out irrelevant information and focus on core details or action. Their skills in encoding events into language also improves.

Leading questions are permitted in examining child witnesses in court in attempts to refresh their memories of events. Adults, like children, are also suggestible but attorneys are not permitted as much latitude in leading adult witnesses (Grahm, 1985). Dale et al. (1978) demonstrated that children are influenced by leading questions but did not explain how or why. They further demonstrated that children subjected to a leading question were likely to incorporate the misleading information into their accounts of an event when questioned about it 2 weeks later. Murray (1983), studying 7- to 11-year-olds, arrived at similar findings and concluded that leading questions lowered accuracy compared with neutral questions for all age groups. Cohen and Harnick (1980) also noted the suggestibility of young children under age 12 and reported that leading questions affect children's responses to questions put by a different questioner on a second occasion. Leading questions from a neutral evaluator may thus jeopardize the accuracy of a child's recall of events at the time of an evaluation and in further evaluations.

Another type of memory involves facial recognition and, here again, children, at least under laboratory conditions dealing with recognition of strangers, are far less accurate than adults (Chance and Goldstein, 1984). Further, memory for faces becomes more vague with lapse of time. Thus, one risk of delaying an evaluation or trial is that a young child may not remember or may misidentify the face of an alleged perpetrator.

It should be noted that the above mentioned studies were all done in laboratory situations that were in no way comparable with the trauma experienced by a child who is sexually abused. In an attempt to study recall of traumatic events, Goodman and Hirschman (Goodman, 1987) studied young children getting immunizations in a doctor's office before entering school. They found them to be highly accurate in their recall of events, and any errors made were in the direction of omission. The 5- to 6-year-old children were better able to resist suggestion then were the 3- to 4-year-olds, but the suggestions they responded to were more likely to deal with peripheral details rather than with action or persons involved. They concluded that the weaker a child's memory, the more suggestible the child is. They also studied the children's reactions to a photo line-up of persons involved in administering the immunizations and found that the accuracy of identification among the 3- to 4-year-olds dropped markedly within a week. In another study, Goodman and Rudy (Goodman, 1987) studied children's responses to more neutral events and found them to be quite resistant to suggestions that they might have been abused. It should be noted, however, that suggestions were put to them by a neutral person, and it remains to be seen how these findings would compare with repeated suggestions put to a young child by a trusted parent.

A different research approach to trauma was undertaken by Terr (1979), who studied 26 children involved in the Chowchilla bus kidnapping. She noted that, although not amnestic for the event, several children misidentified the perpetrator. On follow-up 4 years later, the children were able to give fully detailed accounts of their experience, although "accompanying affects had become translated into metaphors, dream-like visualizations, and psychophysiological responses" (Terr, 1983).

In terms of assessing the reliability of children's memories during clinical evaluation, it is helpful to have historical data and a chronological account of the child's allegations and to compare them from one occasion to another. Allegations may change over time as the child becomes more comfortable with the interviewer. One must remain alert to the effect of multiple examinations of the child, however, and the possibility that an examiner may induce a child to elaborate on prior allegations by either giving positive reinforcement or by continued interrogating that the child interprets as a demand for further information, which he or she then confabulates in order to please the examiner.

Time sense. Children do not share adults' sense of time or even units for measuring time, yet they may be quite accurate if allowed to describe events in relation to temporal events such as seasons, holidays or birthdays, television shows, or even meals. An hour may be a meaningless unit to a preschooler, yet the child can grasp the idea if equated to the length of his or her favorite television show. Children have also been shown to be quite accurate with regard to frequency of occurrence or temporal or sequential order of events (Brown, 1975; Hasher and Zacks, 1979), but, often, young children cannot accurately give the frequency of abuse or tell dates, time, or day if they do not yet understand numbers.

Emotional Factors

Dependency on caretaker. Young children are taught to believe their parents and to regard them as authority figures. Given a young child's emotional and physical dependency on his parents and wish to please them, it becomes exceedingly difficult for the young child to challenge his parents' perception of events that may differ from his own. Allen and Newtson (1972) observed in the laboratory situation that adult influence on children's judgment decreased sharply from first to fourth grade and increased again slightly in tenth grade. Thus if a child is repeatedly told that something occurred that did not, she may come to doubt her own perceptions. A 4-year-old child was repeatedly told that her father touched her "private parts." On examination she repeated that allegation but could not point to her private parts or to those of an anatomical doll, although she could identify names of body parts. A parallel situation occurs in false retraction of allegations. As one 11-year-old said regarding her former allegations that her stepfather had tickled her private parts, "My mother says it didn't happen. She must be right. I must have been mistaken." Waiting room conversations may provide valuable clues, as with the little girl who was overheard saying to her mother "I told her everything you told me to. Did I do a good job?"

Regressive pull of divorcing parents. Children in the midst of divorce may have greater dependency needs, a greater fantasy life, and be more susceptible to parental influence, particularly when they are residing with only one parent. Schuman (1984, 1987) noted that adults caught up in domestic litigation also exhibit regressive behavior manifest by heightened focus on sexuality, bitterness, vindictiveness, and faulty perceptions. Such parents may project their fantasies onto the child and, as Schuman noted, the "child's ambiguous report becomes exaggerated and projected back onto the child in a positive feedback loop."

Loyalty conflicts. Children quite naturally feel compelled to protect their parents even when abused by them. They may be forced to take sides, but they still feel guilty at what they might be doing to the other parent. Conflicts intensify when children have been threatened, e.g., by family disruption or the prospect of a parent going to jail. In one case an abused child was told by her father "God wants you to lie in order to keep our family together."

Loyalty conflicts also occur outside of the family as children may identify with the abuser and have positive feelings for him or her in spite of the abuse that has occurred. Thus, a child's obvious affection for an alleged abuser cannot be used as an absolute sign that abuse did or did not occur.

Ego impairment. Terr described misperception as a defense in children who have been severely traumatized (1980). Other studies (Fish-Murray et al., 1987) have demonstrated that cognitive impairment occurs in children who have been physically or sexually abused when they are confronted with affective stimuli that interfere with perception and interpretation of information at hand. These children may demonstrate adequate reality testing in daily life or in the courtroom during voir dire and then lose this ability when placed in a highly charged emotional situation that brings back an earlier trauma, such as confronting an offender in a courtroom.

Occasionally, the question of psychosis may arise in regard to a child's allegations of sexual abuse. Terr (1980) noted that some children who have been severely traumatized may hallucinate. Visual and auditory hallucinations or delusions of a sexual nature are beyond the domain of most young children. Some children, however, may incorporate the language of those around them, be they parents or other disturbed children, into their psychotic productions. Discrete sexual experiences are rarely hallucinations.

Interviewer Problems

Having reviewed factors within children that affect memory perceptions, we will now look at how adults may influence children. All too often, evidence in sexual abuse cases is obtained by police, rape crisis workers, or protective services workers who lack awareness of child development and the training and experience necessary to interview the young child. In addition, court personnel are operating under great time pressure, e.g., the need to get a restraining order or make an arrest. In their efforts to get information, they may (willingly or unwillingly) use suggestive, coercive, or other unprofessional techniques. One of the authors was recently asked by a child protection worker how she could validate sexual abuse in 15 minutes. When told this was impossible she replied, "But that's all the time my department will allot me!" Unfortunately, some clinicians still adhere to the myth that children never lie, despite the fact that they themselves may be parents of normal children who "fib."

Precourt interviews of children by parents, police, and mental health personnel are not generally carried out under supervision or videotaped and often are rife with suggestions to children. We have been told repeatedly by children that authorities will not allow them to go to the bathroom or eat until they "tell what really happened." Such coercive techniques are never appropriate.

Other suggestive, coercive, and deplorable techniques sometimes used include threats to the child that she will not be able to see her parents or return home until she tells "what happened." As reported in the *Miami Herald* on March 21, 1985, one mother went so far as to threaten her 7-year-old son with never seeing his father again, never being able to ride his bike, and having to go to the hospital where they would stick needles in him if he didn't tell his mother that his father had "put his finger in his tushy." After a series of relentless threats and endless interrogations, the child told his mother what she wanted to hear and repeated this story to the authorities. This taped conversation was admitted as evidence in court and the father was sentenced to life in prison.

Other possible sources of contamination include the interviewer's relationship to the child and offender. In one case the questioning officer was a colleague of the alleged offender; in another, the interviewer was having an affair with the child's mother. Obviously, the closer the involvement, the more difficult it is for the interviewer to be objective and for the child not to be influenced by the interviewer's affect and preconceived notions of what actually happened. In addition, even the most experienced clinician is not neutral about allegations of sex abuse; e.g., it is easy to lapse into using terms offender/perpetrator and victim before findings of guilt. How questions are phrased is also of the utmost importance. For instance, in the Jordon, Minnesota sexual abuse scandal reported in the February 18, 1985 issue of *Newsweek,* a child witness confessed that he had made up detailed stories of abuse because "I could tell what they wanted me to say by the way they asked the questions" (p. 75).

Persons conducting child sexual abuse evaluations need to be objective. They also must be skilled at interviewing and building rapport with young children, possess an understanding of the dynamics of child sexual abuse, and have a solid knowledge of child development. Furthermore, the same interviewer should have access to the child on several different occasions. Interviewers need to be comfortable in discussing sex with children and aware of their own feelings and how they might affect the interview process. Although this may seem quite obvious, unfortunately, as noted above, in practice this is often not the case. Interviewers must also be objective and open to the possibility that an accusation may be false and that an "alleged" perpetrator may be an innocent victim.

Although our preference is that mental health clinicians with degrees in child related fields perform these evaluations, we recognize that this is often not feasible and that front line investigators are apt to be police or protective service workers. We would urge the latter to avail themselves of further training in the area of investigating and understanding child sexual abuse and to recognize when to refer these cases to more highly trained professionals.

CONCLUSION

To accurately evaluate an allegation of sexual abuse in a young child, the examiner must understand the cognitive, emotional, and social factors that surround the allegations. Additionally, the evaluator must be sensitive to his or her verbal and nonverbal communication with a child and approach the evaluation in an objective and unbiased manner.

REFERENCES

Allen, V.L. & Newtson, D. (1972), Development of conformity and independence. *J. Pers. Soc. Psychol.,* 22:18–30.

Borke, H. (1971), Interpersonal perception of young children: egocentrism or empathy? *Develpm. Psychol.,* 5:263–269.

―――― (1973), The development of empathy in Chinese and American children between three and six years of age: a cross-cultural study. *Develpm. Psychol.,* 9:102–108.

―――― (1975), Piaget's mountains revisited: changes in the egocentric landscape. *Develpm. Psychol.,* 11:240–243.

―――― (1978), Piaget's view of social interaction and the theoretical construct of empathy. In: *Alternatives to Piaget: Critical Essays on the Theory,* ed. L.S. Siegel & C.J. Brainerd. New York: Academic Press.

Brainerd, C.J. (1978), Learning research and Piagetian theory. In: *Alternatives to Piaget: Critical Essays on the Theory,* ed. L. S. Siegel & C.J. Brainerd. New York: Academic Press.

Brown, A. L. (1975), The development of memory: knowing about and knowing how to know. In: *Advances in Child Development and Behavior,* Vol. 10, ed. H. W. Teese, New York: Academic Press, pp. 103–152.

Chance, J.E. & Goldstein, A. C. (1984), Face-recognition memory: implications for children's eyewitness testimony. *J. Soc. Issues,* 40:69–85.

Cohen, R. & Harnick, M. S. (1980, The susceptibility of the child witness to suggestion. *Law Hum. Behav.,* 4:201–210.

Dale, P.S., Loftus, E.F. & Rathburn, E. (1978), The influence of the form of the question on the eyewitness testimony of preschool children. *J. Psycholinguist. Res.,* 7:269–277.

Fish-Murray, C., Koby, E. & Van der Kolk, B. (1987), *Evolving Ideas: The Effect of Abuse on Children's Thoughts in Psychological Trauma,* ed. B. Van der Kolk. Washington, D. C.: American Psychiatric Press.

Freud, A. (1965), *Normality and Pathology.* New York: International Press, p. 59.

Goodman, G. (1987, March) *Child sexual abuse and the law: new research on children's memory.* Paper presented at Conference on Child Sexual Abuse, sponsored by Appellate Division, 1st Judicial Division, and Fordham University School of Law, New York.

Graham, M.H. (1985), Indicia of reliability and face-to-face confrontation: emerging issues in child sexual abuse prosecuting. *U. Miami Law Rev.,* 40:19–95.

Hasher, L. & Zacks, R.J. (1979), Automatic and effortful processes in memory. *J. Exp. Psychol.,* 108:356–388.

Johnson, M.K. & Foley, M.A. (1984), Differentiating fact from fantasy: the reliability of children's memories. *J. Soc. Issues,* 40:33–50.

Murray, S. (1983), *The effect on post-event information on children's memory for an illustrated story.* Unpublished manuscript.

Neisser, U. (1984), The control of information pickup in selective looking. In: *Perception and Its Development: A Tribute to Eleanor Gibson,* ed. A. D. Pick. Hillsdale, N. J.: Lawrence Erlbaum. pp. 201–219.

Piaget, J. (1951), *The Origin of Intelligence in Childhood.* New York: Norton.

Schuman, D. (1984), False accusations of physical and sexual abuse. *Bull. Amer. Acad. Psychiat. Law,* 14:5–21.

_____ (1987), Psychodynamics of accusation: positive feedback in family system. *Psychiat. Annals,* 17:242–247.

Terr, L. (1979), Children of Chowchilla: a study of psychic trauma. *The Psychoanalytic Study of the Child,* 34:532–623.

_____ (1980), The child as a witness. In: *Child Psychiatry and the Law,* ed. E.P. Benedek & D.H. Schetky. New York: Brunner/Mazel.

_____ (1983) Chowchilla revisited: the effects of psychic trauma ten years after a school bus kidnapping. *Amer. J. Psychiat.,* 140:1543–1550.

Part X
ADOLESCENT ISSUES

The first article in this section, by Kashani and coworkers, utilizes an epidemiological frame to examine the relationship among adolescent personality profiles, psychiatric disorders, and parenting styles among adolescents living in a midwestern college town. The study is unique in that it utilizes an instrument specifically designed for adolescents, the Millon Adolescent Personality Inventory, to assess personality attributes. Similarities between adolescents with psychiatric disorders and those adolescents who perceived their parents as less caring were found. The group of adolescents with psychiatric disorders were noted to be discontented, pessimistic, and unpredictable, while those who described their parents as caring were characterized by a sociable, confident, serious-minded, rule-conscious personality profile. Recognizing that it is impossible to determine causality, the authors discuss a number of possible developmental models to account for the relationship between personality, parental attitudes, and psychopathology. Of particular interest is the proposal that neither parental attitudes nor personality cause psychopathology. According to this model, there are no bad parental attitudes or personality patterns, there is only a mismatch between the two constructs. This interactionist view is similar to and consistent with the goodness of fit model proposed to account for the relationship found between temperament and psychiatric disorder among the subjects of our New York Longitudinal Study.

The next two papers in this section address a problem of increasing social and clinical importance—adolescent suicide. The study reported by Spirito and co-workers compared 71 adolescents admitted to a general pediatrics unit following a suicide attempt and requiring medical treatment to a matched sample of adolescents referred for psychiatric consultation while hospitalized for a variety of other medical conditions. Measures included self-report scales of hopelessness and depression, as well as clinical examination and review of past medical and psychiatric history. Only past psychiatric history significantly differentiated suicide attempters from controls. The authors conclude that medically hospitalized adolescent suicide attempters have a history of risk factors that are very similar to those associated with general emotional difficulties in adolescents.

Similar conclusions were reached by Khan, who studied a group of 120 emotionally and behaviorally disturbed adolescents, composed of suicidal adolescents who were hospitalized on a psychiatric service; hospitalized nonsuicidal adolescents; and never-hospitalized nonsuicidal adolescents. Those who were suicidal could not be distinguished on the basis of age, sex, social class, type of peer and family relationship, academic achievement, or early loss of a parent by death or divorce. Similarly, clinical diagnoses failed to differentiate between the suicidal and nonsuicidal adolescents. The results of these two studies of very different populations of suicidal adolescents suggest that environmental, demographic, and diagnostic factors shed little light on the cognitive and emotional responses of an adolescent in the face of a perceived, overwhelming stress and suggest, as does Kahn in a thoughtful discussion, that in order to predict the suicidal potential of an adolescent, more attention needs to be paid to the "coping style" of the individual adolescent under stressful situations.

36

Personality, Psychiatric Disorders, and Parental Attitude Among a Community Sample of Adolescents

Javad H. Kashani, Edwin W. Hoeper, Niels C. Beck, Colleen M. Corcoran, Carolyn Fallahi, Jeanne McAllister, Tomas J. K. Rosenberg, and John C. Reid

University of Missouri-Columbia

This community study reports on the relationship among adolescent personality profiles, psychiatric disorders, and parenting styles. A group of adolescents with psychiatric disorders was found to be discontented, pessimistic, and unpredictable. Adolescents who described their parents as caring were characterized by a sociable, confident, serious-minded, rule-conscious personality profile.

Currently, there is no universally accepted definition of personality, and there is dissatisfaction with the concept of personality as no more than a collection of personality traits (Rutter, 1985). The general agreement, however, is that "personality is that which gives order and congruence to all the different kinds of behavior in which the individual engages" (Hall and Lindzey, 1978). In other words, a specific individual usually responds to a specific situation in a characteristic manner; similar situations, both present and future, tend to result in fairly predictable behavioral patterns (Costa et al., 1980; Eysenck and Eysenck, 1980). These behavioral patterns apply not only to actions but also to thought patterns and attitudes. Therefore, personality seems to describe a consistent response pattern by which an

Reprinted with permission from the *Journal of the American Academy of Child and Adolescent Psychiatry*, 1987, Vol. 26, No. 6, 879–885. Copyright 1987 by the American Academy of Child and Adolescent Psychiatry.

individual carries out the activities of daily living and deals with unique and disruptive situations (Rutter, 1985).

According to DSM-III, personality traits are enduring patterns of perceiving, thinking about, and relating to other persons (and ourselves); they are exhibited in a wide range of important social and personal contexts. When these traits become inflexible and maladaptive, causing significant occupational and social impairment or subjective distress, they are referred to as personality disorders. By definition, personality traits become manifest during childhood or adolescence and continue throughout adult life.

An association in adults between personality disorders and psychiatric disorders, especially affective disorders, has recently been described (Costa et al., 1980; Hirschfeld, 1983a, b; Shea, 1985). Few studies have explored the link between personality and psychiatric disorders in adolescence, however. For instance, McManus et al. (1984), using the Diagnostic Interview for Borderlines, observed that 25% of an adolescent inpatient sample with borderline personality disorder had a coexisting major depressive disorder. Also, Friedman et al. (1982) found that the prognosis of adolescents with major depressive disorder may be poorer for those with a coexisting borderline personality disorder. Other studies addressing this issue have used personality inventories designed primarily for adults, such as the Minnesota Multiphasic Personality Inventory (Hartocollis, 1982; Marks et al., 1974; Sutker et al., 1984). Such an approach, although acceptable at that time because of the lack of an inventory specifically designed for adolescents, is now inappropriate.

The publication of DSM-III and the Millon Adolescent Personality Inventory (MAPI) (Millon et al., 1982) have facilitated studies exploring the relationship between adolescent personality traits and psychopathology, as well as other related issues. The MAPI is a reliable and valid inventory specifically designed for adolescents (*Appendix*). Considering the dearth of knowledge about adolescent psychiatric disorders and personality dimensions, the present study reports the most common traits, concerns, and behavioral correlates of personality as they relate to adolescents with psychiatric disorders. We predict that the personality profiles of subjects with psychiatric disorders differ from those of individuals with no psychiatric disorders. We also hypothesize that a caring parental attitude will have a positive relationship with adolescent personality adjustment.

METHOD

The method has been described in detail elsewhere (Kashani et al., 1987). In brief, subjects for this study consisted of 150 adolescents, 14 to 16 years old, who represented 7% of all adolescents in this age group attending public school in a college town. The names of the subjects were drawn in a systematic manner from a pool of approximately 1,700 students. To maintain group homogeneity, only adolescents whose ages did not change during the 5-month data collection phase of the study were selected. There were an equal number of boys (75) and girls (75) with an equal number of boys (25) and girls (25) in each age group.

Subjects' participation was solicited by phone. Adolescents and their parents were interviewed in their homes by three clinicians, each with a master's degree in psychology. Extensive training of the interviewers led to an interrater agreement rating of at least 95%. Ongoing supervision and retraining exercises were held every 30 to 50 interviews to minimize rater drift (Paul et al., 1977).

Because the subjects were not clinic referred and because the local institutional review board required consent of not only the adolescent but also of both parents, every effort was made to minimize the refusal rate, including conducting the interview at the home of the participants. In addition, a stipend was offered to compensate them for their time. These efforts led to a rate of acceptance of 72.4%. Information with which to calculate socioeconomic status (SES) scores was obtained for 69%. Mean score for the refusal group was 2.9, and the mean SES for the 150 participants was 2.7 (Mann-Whitney U test), p = NS. The SES of the entire sample was as follows: 10.7% class I, 31.3% class II, 29.3% class III, 27.3 % class IV, and 1.4% class V (Hollingshead and Redlich's Social Class, 1958). The adolescents consisted of 142 whites, 6 blacks, and 2 orientals.

Adolescents and their parents were interviewed by a structured interview schedule, the Diagnostic Interview for Children and Adolescents (DICA). Parents were interviewed using the DICA-P (Herjanic et al., 1975, 1982).

Two additional major instruments used in this study were the Parental Bonding Instrument (PBI) (Parker et al., 1979) and the MAPI (Millon, 1982). The PBI measures the type of bonding between the child and his or her parents, based on two dimensions of parental attitude: care and overprotection.

RESULTS

Of 150 adolescents, 28 (18.7%) were considered to be "cases" on the basis of the following criteria: the presence of at least one DSM-III diagnosis, impaired functioning, and demonstrated need for psychiatric treatment. The details of how impaired functioning and need for psychiatric treatment as well as the diagnoses for the entire sample have been reported elsewhere

(Kashani et al., 1987). In this paper, we report the breakdown of the specific diagnoses that occurred in the case group (Table 1).

To determine whether personality scores were sex-dependent, we first contrasted boys and girls regardless of diagnostic grouping. The results showed that girls had lower inhibited trait scores ($F = 5.09$, $p = 0.03$), higher sociable trait scores ($F = 5.97$, $p = 0.2$), lower expressed concern regarding self-concept ($F = 3.93$, $p = 0.05$), higher sexual acceptance expressed concern ($F = 4.02$, $p = 0.05$), and lower scholastic achievement behavioral correlate ($F = 7.61$, $p = 0.007$) (see *Appendix* for description of MAPI).

Because these findings indicated that some sex dependence existed, we examined differences in cases and noncases for boys and girls separately. All comparisons for case differences by gender were done with Mann-Whitney U tests. The only differences in personality for cases that were consistent across gender were the following: less introversive (boys, $p = 0.02$; girls, $p = 0.95$); less respectful (boys, $p = 0.0001$; girls, $p = 0.02$); more sensitive (boys, $p = 0.0001$; girls, $p = 0.03$); higher family rapport expressed concern (boys, $p = 0.0001$; girls, $p = 0.03$); higher impulse control behavioral correlate (boys, $p = 0.0001$; girls, $p = 0.01$); higher societal conformity behavioral correlate (boys, $p = 0.0001$; girls $p = .01$).

In addition, male "cases" were less inhibited ($p = 0.004$), less confident ($p = 0.01$), more forceful ($p = 0.0007$), had more self-concept expressed concern ($p = 0.0004$), more personal esteem expressed concern ($p = 0.01$), more academic confidence expressed concern ($p = 0.0001$), higher scholastic

Table 1. Breakdown of the Specific Diagnoses Occurring in the Cases

Diagnosis	Percentage of Cases With the Diagnosis
Anxiety disorder	46.4
Conduct disorder	46.4
Depression	42.9
Oppositional disorder	32.1
Drug abuse	28.6
Alcohol abuse	17.9
Attention deficit disorder	10.7
Somatization disorder	7.1
Enuresis	3.6
Mania	3.6

achievement behavioral correlate ($p = 0.0001$), and higher attendance consistency behavioral correlate ($p = 0.0003$). On the other hand, the female cases were less cooperative ($p = 0.02$).

The purpose for this study was to look at the relationship among the three constructs of personality, parental attitudes, and psychopathology. Therefore, it was felt that treating the case group as a single entity, disregarding sex differences, was appropriate for the purpose of initial exploration. The characteristics of this combined group are summarized in Table 2.

Among the various psychiatric disorders, the sensitive scale of the MAPI was the only personality trait consistently present in all types of diagnoses, that is, as a specific "personality trait" that coexisted with all psychiatric disorders studied in this investigation.

The second goal of the study was to investigate the effect of caring and overprotection (a term used by Parker) on the adolescent personality profiles. The instrument used was the PBI, which was factor-analyzed into two factors using principal axis and varimax rotation. Two factors were chosen because that was the number of factors used by Parker et al. (1979), who developed the instrument, and because a screen test indicated that two factors were reasonable for the present data. The adolescents were then divided into five groups: (1) a central group, defined as having estimated factor scores on both factors within $\pm$ 0.5 of zero; (2) a high care/high overprotection group, defined as having factor scores on both factors < 0.0 and not being in the center group; (3) a high care/low overprotection group, defined as having a factor score on the case factor as < 0.0 and on the overprotection factor of < 0.0 and not being in the center group; (4) a low care/high overprotection group, and (5) a low care/low overprotection group, defined analogously. Twenty-three people in the center group plus seven people with incomplete data were deleted; therefore, comparisons between groups (Tables 3 and 4) on estimated factor scores were based on 120 people for this second part of the study.

Analysis of estimated factor scores on the care and overprotection factors was also done for boys and girls separately, but in general, the findings for each sex separately paralleled those of the group as a whole, and therefore are not reported.

Two contrasts, using Dunn's procedure with Student's t distribution, were run to compare the two high care groups, as determined by estimated factor scores, with the two low care groups, and two high overprotection groups with the two low overprotection groups on each of the 20 Millon scores. The results of the analysis comparing the group of adolescents with high caring parental attitude factor scores versus the group with low care are illustrated in Table 3. Adolescents who rated their parents as caring were less inhibited,

Table 2. Comparison of Personality Profiles of Adolescents with Psychiatric Disorders, Cases (N = 28) and Noncases (N = 132)

Millon Variables	Cases		Noncases		p
	Mean	S.D.	Mean	S.D.	
Personality styles[a]					
Introversive	29.3	20.0	44.1	21.5	0.002
Inhibited	52.4	28.4	41.6	25.5	0.05
Cooperative	35.5	20.4	47.5	25.0	0.01
Sociable	62.9	28.8	64.2	26.4	0.76, NS
Confident	52.8	25.6	59.9	24.0	0.17, NS
Forceful	68.7	22.5	53.4	25.2	0.004
Respectful	35.6	17.6	56.2	23.3	0.0001
Sensitive	73.5	22.7	47.4	25.9	0.0001
Expressed concerns[b]					
Self-concept	62.5	24.2	48.9	23.4	0.01
Personal esteem	70.0	16.4	56.8	22.5	0.007
Body comfort	54.6	20.5	54.2	24.5	0.87, NS
Sexual acceptance	57.4	20.0	52.9	18.2	0.35, NS
Peer security	57.5	20.5	53.2	21.0	0.33, NS
Social tolerance	54.2	26.2	45.2	24.2	0.12, NS
Family rapport	78.9	21.5	50.9	30.0	0.0001
Academic confidence	63.7	25.8	45.0	21.7	0.0002
Behavioral correlates[c]					
Impulse control	68.3	19.1	45.6	20.4	0.0001
Societal conformity	66.0	16.9	45.0	20.2	0.0001
Scholastic achievement	56.5	22.3	37.2	20.3	0.0001
Attendence consistency	56.6	16.3	39.9	19.9	0.0001

Note: Tests were Mann-Whitney *U* tests.

[a] A higher score indicates a dominant personality trait.

[b] A higher score indicates more concerns and problems.

[c] A higher score indicates more problems with that particular behavior.

less forceful, less sensitive, more sociable, more confident, and more respectful than the control subjects. They were also less concerned about self-concept, personal esteem, social tolerance, family rapport, and academic confidence. In addition, they had significantly fewer problems with behavioral correlates such as impulse control (Table 3).

On the other hand, adolescents who rated their parents as highly overprotective were more inhibited, more sensitive, and less confident than the control subjects (Table 4). They also had significantly more concern with

Table 3. Analysis of High Care Versus Low Care Parental Bonding Factors in 120 Adolescents, for the 20 Millon Personality Variables[a]

Millon Variables	High Care (N = 73)		Low Care (N = 47)		tD	p
	Mean	S.D.	Mean	S.D.		
Personality styles						
Introversive	41.0	19.3	39.8	21.9	0.0	NS
Inhibited	34.4	25.4	57.2	23.8	−4.47	0.0001
Cooperative	48.2	24.2	40.3	23.6	1.89	NS
Sociable	69.6	25.5	55.8	27.0	2.57	0.02
Confident	66.1	25.1	48.7	21.9	3.53	0.001
Forceful	50.2	23.6	65.0	25.2	−3.11	0.004
Respectful	61.8	23.3	38.8	18.0	5.48	0.0001
Sensitive	41.8	23.8	68.3	25.8	−5.30	0.0001
Expressed concerns						
Self-concept	43.2	24.1	62.2	22.0	−4.00	0.0002
Personal esteem	53.9	23.8	67.4	20.5	−2.84	0.01
Body comfort	52.8	25.3	56.3	24.2	−0.53	NS
Sexual acceptance	52.2	18.2	56.7	21.5	−0.98	NS
Peer security	52.8	22.2	56.4	19.2	−0.61	NS
Social tolerance	38.6	21.4	58.4	25.6	−4.25	0.0001
Family rapport	43.0	27.5	76.2	27.2	−6.03	0.0001
Academic confidence	37.9	21.9	62.5	21.2	−5.74	0.0001
Behavioral correlates						
Impulse control	42.0	19.2	61.8	21.3	−5.06	0.0001
Societal conformity	40.6	18.2	62.3	20.3	−5.81	0.0001
Scholastic achievement	29.2	18.4	56.9	19.4	−7.50	0.0001
Attendance	37.7	21.1	51.2	18.2	−3.19	0.003

[a] Twenty-three people in the center group not considered, and seven subjects' responses were deleted because of missing data.

Table 4. Analysis of High Overprotection Versus Low Overprotection Parental Bonding Factors Scores in 120 Adolescents, for the 20 Millon Personality Variables[a]

Millon Variables	High OP (N = 59)		Low OP (N = 61)		tD	p
	Mean	S.D.	Mean	S.D.		
Personality styles						
Introversive	39.8	19.9	41.3	20.8	−0.34	NS
Inhibited	53.0	27.9	33.9	22.8	3.45	0.002
Cooperative	46.7	24.6	43.5	23.9	0.99	NS
Sociable	59.2	27.5	69.0	25.5	−1.45	NS
Confident	51.8	24.7	66.5	23.9	−2.51	0.02
Forceful	58.1	24.4	54.0	25.9	0.51	NS
Respectful	49.4	24.5	56.0	23.5	−0.82	NS
Sensitive	60.1	26.7	44.6	26.8	2.72	0.01
Expressed concerns						
Self-concept	58.4	24.3	43.2	23.4	2.66	0.02
Personal esteem	66.7	20.8	51.9	23.6	2.85	0.01
Body comfort	58.3	22.3	54.3	26.7	1.38	NS
Sexual acceptance	56.7	19.9	51.2	19.1	1.34	NS
Peer security	58.2	23.0	50.3	18.5	1.80	NS
Social tolerance	50.6	25.7	42.2	23.8	1.42	NS
Family rapport	64.9	29.9	47.4	31.4	2.58	0.02
Academic confidence	57.4	20.5	38.0	24.8	3.92	0.0003
Behavioral correlates						
Impulse control	52.5	20.0	47.0	24.2	0.59	NS
Societal conformity	52.9	20.4	45.4	22.5	1.18	NS
Scholastic achievement	47.6	21.1	32.7	22.8	3.10	0.004
Attendance	48.7	22.6	37.6	17.9	2.44	0.03

[a] Twenty-three people in the center group not considered, and 7 subjects' responses were deleted because of missing data.

self-concept, personal esteem, family rapport, and academic confidence. Finally, this group had more problems with scholastic achievement and school attendance (Table 4).

The question as to whether a difference existed between the cases and noncases in terms of their care and the overprotective factor of PBI was investigated. In other words, was the parental attitude in the cases perceived differently than the parental attitude in the noncases? With regard to overprotection, there was no significant difference between the two groups, and the case to overprotection correlation was $+ 0.16$. With regard to caring, the children in the case group reported that their parents were significantly less caring, $f = 13.88, p < 0.0003$ (ANOVA with 1,143 df), and the case to caring correlation was -0.30. We also looked at the relative importance of the Millon personality variables and the PBI subscores in relation to the caseness grouping. A logistical regression that looked at the eight personality variables and the two PBI variables showed that only the Millon Sensitive Scale provided a significant contribution to a model attempting to replicate caseness (model $\kappa = 19.79, p < 0.0001$). A discriminant analysis that looked at the same variable also indicated that only the Millon Sensitive Scale was significant, with $f = 22.649, p < 0.0001$.

Because Parker has postulated that certain combinations of the two PBI dimensions yield pathogenic parental "styles," we made an attempt to find out if the various parental styles were indeed differentially pathogenic. In other words, was there a relationship between these styles or quadrant grouping and being diagnosed as a case? A κ analysis crossing quadrant grouping and caseness was not significant. When styles are derived by using the two subscores (caring and overprotection) as coordinate, it implies that the impact of both subscores on psychopathology are roughly equivalent. Our data, however, show that the caring dimension appears to have a greater impact upon psychopathology than does overprotection. This would indicate that the use of the quadrant grouping might not be appropriate.

The overall picture drawn from these results is that there are similarities between those adolescents with psychiatric disorders and those adolescents who perceived their parents as less caring.

DISCUSSION

The results of this study support the hypothesis that there was a relationship among adolescent personality, parental attitudes, and the existence of psychopathology. Although it is impossible to determine causality, the study provides data for exploration of the relationship among these constructs. The adolescent's personality was tapped by the dimensional scales of the MAPI; adolescent perceptions regarding parental attitudes were measured by PBI subscores; and psychopathology was defined by extraction of those adolescents with a DSM-III diagnosis of psychiatric disorder who were dysfunctional. In addition to the examination of the various dyadic relationships, an overall association was investigated.

The composite personality of a case may be described as follows: The individual is easily excited (less introverted); he or she is not rule-conscious and does not strive to do the right and proper things; life is neither orderly nor well-planned (less respectful); he or she is discontented, pessimistic, and unpredictable, sometimes exhibiting an outgoing and enthusiastic attitude but quickly reverting to the opposite (more sensitive). Additionally, the troubled adolescent is most concerned with the area of family and the perception of what his or her relationship to the family should be. Indeed, among eight expressed concerns, family rapport was rated as most frequently illustrating the pivotal role of the family for the dysfunctional adolescent.

From the behavioral correlates of the MAPI, it was found that impaired impulse control and lack of societal conformity were the most potentially acted-upon behaviors in the cases. Millon (1982) noted that impulse behavior is frequently expressed differently in boys than in girls. Whereas boys tend to be more aggressive, girls frequently act out sexually. This is consistent with the finding of significantly more sexual relationships in cases than in noncases (Kashani et al., 1987). In regard to societal conformity, the troubled adolescent has more disregard for ordinary societal constraints. The personality profile described above is so characteristic of dysfunctional adolescents that it holds true regardless of sex and therefore may be considered a definitive profile.

As pointed out previously, the results of this study indicate that personality, parental attitudes, and psychopathology are interrelated. In Figure 1, we suggest some of the possible models of the construct's interrelationship as a potential guide for future research. The first four models assume that parental attitudes are stable and form the basis for changes in the other two constructs. The second four models assume that personality is the causative factor and the other two constructs are affected by it. The last model represents an interactionist approach and makes no assumptions regarding different stabilities between parental attitudes and personality. Parental attitudes and personality interact with psychopathology resulting from a mismatch between the two. Schematic representations of these hypotheses are presented in Figure 1. It is assumed that there is a certain amount of feedback in all of the relationships; arrows therefore indicate the direction of most influence.

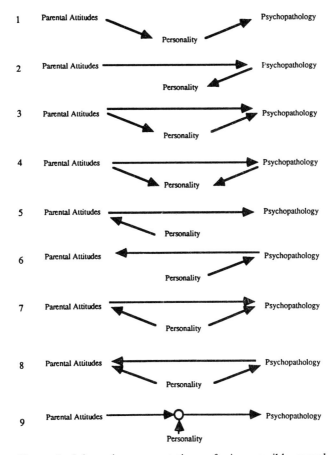

Figure 1. Schematic representations of nine possible causal models describing the relationship among parental attitudes, personality, and psychopathology.

The first four models (the parental attitude base) are as follows: (1) parental attitudes influence the development of personality, which in turn affects the occurrence of psychopathology; (2) parental attitudes affect the likelihood of psychopathology occurrence—psychopathology then modifies personality; (3) parental attitudes influence personality and psychopathology directly, and in addition, parental attitudes have an indirect effect on psychopathology (this is because they affect personality, which then affects psychopathology); (4) like the third model, parental attitudes affect personality and psychopathology directly, but in this model, parental attitudes have an additional, indirect effect on personality because of its effect on psychopathology.

The second four models (the personality base) are as follows: (5) personality influences the development of parental attitudes—parental attitudes then affect the occurrence of psychopathology; (6) personality affects the likelihood of psychopathology occurrence—psychopathology then modifies parental attitudes; (7) personality influences parental attitudes and psychopathology directly, and in addition, personality has an indirect effect on psychopathology (this is because of personality affecting parental attitudes, which then affect psychopathology); (8) similar to the seventh model, personality affects parental attitudes and psychopathology directly, but in this model personality has an additional, indirect effect on personality because of its effect on psychopathology.

The ninth model postulates that, by themselves, neither parental attitudes nor personality cause psychopathology. Psychopathology is caused by the interaction between parental attitudes and personality. According to this model, there are no bad parental attitudes or personality patterns, there is only mismatch between the two constructs. This idea is similar to the goodness of fit model proposed for temperament by Thomas and Chess (1984).

The next question is whether any of these models are stronger or weaker than the others. We believe that arguments can be made for and against some of the models. Because personality is not fully formed in adolescence and hence is malleable to influence by the other constructs, this would weaken the probabilities of models 5 through 8. This is because these models present personality as being the most stable and least malleable of the three constructs. To verify this assumption, more data on the constancy or lack of constancy in personality are needed.

In addition, if parental attitudes can be shown to be stable and not influenced by personality changes or psychopathology, this would further weaken the likelihood of models 5 through 8. Long-term data on the stability of parental attitudes are lacking, however.

Given the commonly held view that most pathology usually occurs after the child has developed a certain amount of personality, it is feasible to assume that psychopathology is a result and not a cause of personality. This is not to say that personality characteristics are not influenced by psychopathology but that the basic pattern of the personality remains intact. It can be hypothesized that the existing aspects of personality are either enhanced or attenuated. If this reasoning is correct, then it would weaken models 2 and 4.

Validation of this reasoning awaits evidence on the stability of personality before and after the occurrence of psychopathology.

The results from the present study show a similarity in personality between the adolescents with low caring parents and the adolescents with psychopathology. This, combined with the assumption of parental attitude, stability, and personality malleability, may support models that show parental attitudes affecting personality and personality affecting psychopathology. The two models that fit this requirement are models 1 and 3; however, the interactionist model, model 9, also fits this requirement. The results from this study that show the relative importance of personality as compared with parental attitudes tend to support a model more similar to model 3.

In conclusion, it appears that the most likely models are models, 1, 3, and 9. As mentioned previously, we do not intend to say that these are the only possible models. In addition, we omit the effect of other factors, such as genetic, social, peers, etc., upon the various constructs. Any model that tried to encompass all of the relevant variables would become so unwieldy as to be nearly useless as a research base. The models presented are an attempt to clarify one small section of the interrelationship among the three constructs and to provide fairly easy to operationalize hypotheses for future research. Much more research and theoretical construction is needed to determine if the assumptions above are valid and, ultimately, which pathway is correct.

APPENDIX

Description of the Millon Adolescent Personality Inventory

The MAPI is a 150-item inventory designed to assess a variety of personality traits, psychological concerns, and problematic behaviors of adolescents. Analysis of the inventory yields 20 subscales including eight personality traits, eight expressed concerns, and four behavioral correlates. The eight personality traits are based on Millon's (1982) theoretical schema. The degree to which an individual characteristically displays each of these personality traits is expressed in a profile configuration. These configurations have been found to be associated with psychological dysfunctions.

The eight personality scales are briefly described as follows:

Scale 1: Introversive. High scorers tend to keep to themselves, appearing rather quiet, and are not easily excited. They often do not feel strongly about things, and although they do not avoid others, they seem indifferent about having them around.

Scale 2: Inhibited. High scorers tend to be ill at ease socially. They have learned it is better to maintain emotional distance with others, often fearing rejection.

Scale 3: Cooperative. High scorers tend to be kind toward others. They are very reluctant to assert themselves and prefer to let others take the lead. They often play down their own achievements and underestimate their abilities.

Scale 4: Sociable. High scorers are talkative, socially charming, and emotionally expressive. They tend to develop strong, albeit brief, relationships with others, and may get bored with routine and longstanding relationships.

Scale 5: Confident. High scorers are often confident of their abilities. They rarely doubt their own self-worth, and they act in a self-assured manner. These individuals tend to take others for granted and tend not to concern themselves with the needs of others with whom they relate.

Scale 6: Forceful. High scorers are strong-willed and tend to dominate others. They frequently question the ability of others and are impatient with the problems or weaknesses of others.

Scale 7: Respectful. High scorers are very serious-minded, rule-conscious persons who tend to keep their emotions in check. They prefer to live their lives in an orderly and well-planned fashion.

Scale 8: Sensitive. High scorers tend to be discontented and pessimistic, often behave unpredictably, and often feel guilt about their moodiness.

Eight expressed concern scales are also included, which focus on feelings and attitudes the adolescent may experience about issues that seem relevant to adolescents. These eight scales are briefly described below:

Scale A: Self-concept. This scale contains items that pertain to the identity issue.

Scale B: Personal esteem. This scale contains items that pertain to the struggle to resolve the disparity between the self the child feels he or she is and the ideal self that child would like to be.

Scale C: Body. This scale contains items that pertain to how an adolescent has integrated the reality of his or her physical growth in puberty, self-attitudes, and family's attitude toward this growth.

Scale D: Sexual acceptance. This scale contains items that pertain to the integration of sexual impulses within the framework of one's self-image.

Scale E: Peer security. This scale contains items that pertain to the intensity of need for group approval.

Scale F: Social tolerance. This scale contains items that pertain to the degree and manner in which the adolescent deviates from appropriate social attitudes and behavior and how this affects his or her interpersonal interactions.

Scale G: Family rapport. This scale contains items that pertain to the adolescent's feelings and perceptions toward his or her family, along with perceptions of what his or her relationship to the family should be.

Scale H: Academic confidence. This scale assesses the degree of academic concern reported by either (1) those adolescents who use others as a comparison group, and (2) those adolescents who use an inner gauge to tell them if they are performing as they should.

The four remaining scales, behavior correlates, focus on acted-upon behaviors or behaviors that may pose serious difficulties for the adolescent. They do not provide direct evidence that the adolescent has or is likely to exhibit these behaviors but gauge how similar the adolescent's answers are compared with those who have exhibited these problem behaviors. The four scales are as follows:

Scale SS: Impulse control. This scale assesses the degree to which an adolescent deviates from the norm in expressing feelings and controlling impulses.

Scale TT: Societal conformity. This scale assesses the extent to which an adolescent "is a problem," that is, the extent to which the adolescent causes distress to others and shows disregard for ordinary societal constraints.

Scale UU: Scholastic achievement. This scale assesses those adolescents whose intelligence appears to be average or above, yet who perform academically below their level of intelligence ability.

Scale WW: Attendance consistency. This scale assesses how similar the adolescents' responses are to those who miss school excessively. It does not indicate the motivation responsible for the absences.

In regard to the psychometric property, the internal reliability of the instrument, measured by the Kudder-Richardson Formula 20, averaged 0.74 with a range from 0.67 to 0.84. The test-retest reliability averaged 0.67 with a range from 0.45 to 0.82. Although it would be better to use objective nontest criteria, the correlation of the MAPI to other instruments measuring the same domain is the best available validity method. Previous results show significant correlations between the MAPI and the 16 Personality Factors instrument, the California Personality Inventory, and the Edwards Personal Preference Survey.

REFERENCES

Costa, P. T., McCrae, R. R., & Arenberg, D. (1980), Enduring dispositions in adult males. *J. Pers. Soc. Psychol.,* 38:793–800.

Eysenck, M. & Eysenck, H. J. (1980), Mischel and the concept of personality. *Brit. J. Psychol.,* 71:191–204.

Friedman, R., Clarkin, J., Corn, R., Arnoff, M., Hurt, S. & Murphy, M. (1982), DSM-III and affective pathology in hospitalized adolescents. *J. Nerv. Ment. Dis.,* 170:511–521.

Hall, C. S. & Lindzey, G. (1978), *Theories of Personality,* 3rd Ed. New York: Wiley.

Hartocollis, P. (1982), Personality characteristics in adolescent problem drinkers: a comparative study. *This Journal,* 21:348–353.

Herjanic, B., Herjanic, M., Brown, F. et al. (1975), Are children reliable reporters? *J. Abnorm. Child Psychol.,* 3:41–48.

———— Reich, W. (1981), Development of a structured psychiatric interview for children: agreement between child and parent on individual symptoms. *J. Abnorm. Child Psychol.,* 10:307–324.

Hirschfeld, R. M., Klerman, G. L., Clayton, P. J. et al. (1983a), Assessing personality: effects of the depressive state on trait measurement, *Amer. J. Psychiat.,* 140:695–699.

———— ———— ———— Keller, M. B. (1983b), Personality and depression: empirical findings, *Arch. Gen. Psychiat.,* 40:993–998.

Hollingshead, A. B. & Redlich, F. C. (1958), *Social Class and Mental Illness.* New York: Wiley.

Hyler, S. E. & Frances, A. (1985), Clinical implications of axis I-axis II interactions. *Compr. Psychiat.,* 26:345–351.

Kashani, J., Beck, N. C., Hoeper, E. W., et al. (1987), Psychiatric disorders among a community sample of adolescents. *Amer. J. Psychiat.,* 144:584–589.

McManus, M., Lerner, H., Robbins, D. et al. (1984), Assessment of borderline symptomatology in hospitalized adolescents. *This Journal,* 23:685–694.

Marks, P. A., Seeman, W. & Haller, D. L. (1974), *The Actuarial Use of the MMPI with Adolescents and Adults.* Baltimore, Md.: Williams & Wilkins.

Millon, T. (1969), *Modern Psychopathology.* Philadelphia, PA.: W. B. Saunders.

——— (1981), *Disorders of Personality: DSM-III-Axis II.* New York: Wiley Interscience.

——— Green, C. J., & Meagher, R. B. (1982), *Millon Adolescent Personality Inventory Manual.* Interpretive Scoring Systems.

Parker, G., Tupling, H. & Brown L. B. (1979), A parental bonding instrument. *Brit, J. Med. Psychol.,* 52:1–10.

——— (1982), Researching the schizophrenogenic mother. *J. Nerv. Ment. Dis.,* 170:452–461.

——— (1984), The measurement of pathogenic parental style and its relevance to psychiatric disorder. *Soc. Psychiat.* 19:75–81.

Paul G. L. & Lentz, R. J. (1977), *Psychosocial Treatment of Chronic Mental Patients.* Cambridge, Mass.: Harvard University Press.

Rutter, M. (1985), Psychology and development: links between childhood and adult life. In: *Child and Adolescent Psychiatry,* Ed. 2, Chapter 45. London: Blackwell Scientific.

Shea, T., Docherty, J. D., Pilkonis, P. A. et al. (1985), *Personality disorders in NIMH treatment of depression collaborative study.* Paper presented at the annual meeting of the American Psychiatric Association, Dallas, Texas.

Sutker, P. B., Moan, C. E., Goist, K. C. & Allain, A. N. (1984), MMPI subtypes and antisocial behaviors in adolescent alcohol and drug abusers. *Drug Alcohol Depend.,* 13:235–244.

Thomas, A. & Chess, S. (1984), Genesis and evolution of behavioral disorders: from infancy to early adult life. *Amer. J. Psychiat.* 141:1–9.

37

Adolescent Suicide Attempters Hospitalized on a Pediatric Unit

Anthony Spirito, Lori Stark, Mary Fristad, Kathleen Hart, and Judy Owens-Stively

Rhode Island Hospital/Brown University Program in Medicine, Providence

Adolescent suicide is becoming of increasing concern. Many adolescent suicide attempters are admitted to a general pediatric medical center for immediate medical treatment. During such an admission, decisions regarding the patients' emotional status and appropriate disposition must be made. Unfortunately, there are few empirical data to guide the clinician in making these decisions. The present study is an attempt to identify important characteristics and psychological status of suicide attempters hospitalized on a pediatric floor. Seventy-one adolescents admitted to a general pediatrics unit following a suicide attempt requiring medical treatment were compared to a matched sample of adolescents referred for psychiatric consultation while hospitalized for a variety of conditions. The patients were compared on historical risk factors believed associated with adolescent suicide attempts and self-report measures of depression and hopelessness. A significant difference was found only on past psychiatric history. Further analyses according to the suicide attempter's toxicity of overdose, psychiatric history, and disposition status also revealed few significant differences. Results are discussed in terms of the need to select appropriate

Reprinted with permission from the *Journal of Pediatric Psychology,* 1987, Vol. 12, No. 2, 171–189. Copyright 1987, by Plenum Publishing Corporation.

The authors thank Paula Meinel, Jayna Halverson, Janet Grace, Lisa Wood, Terry Bosworth, Beverly Meyers, Gregory Fritz, David DeLawyer, and David Guevremont, for their participation in this project as members of the research team in Child Psychiatry at Rhode Island Hospital, and Sue Rosenfield for preparation of the manuscript.

control groups for studies on adolescent suicide attempters and differences between attempters hospitalized in pediatric versus psychiatric settings.

In the past 24 years the United States suicide rate among people 15 to 24 years of age has tripled and suicide has now become the third leading cause of death in this age group (U.S. Monthly Vital Statistics, 1982). This pattern remains whether cross-sectional or cohort analysis is used (Murphy & Wetzel, 1980). In addition, it has been estimated that there may be from 50 to 100 suicide attempts for each completed suicide (McIntire, Angle, Wikoff, & Schlicht, 1977). This high rate of suicide attempts among adolescents is of great concern. Studies have shown that 10% of adolescent suicide attempters make further attempts within 1 year (Haldane & Haider, 1967; Hawton, O'Grady, Osborn, & Cole, 1982), whereas other studies report a 31% recurrence rate within 2 years of the attempt (McIntire et al., 1977). The most likely time for repeated attempts for adolescents is in the 3 months after the previous episode (Hawton & Osborn, 1984). Of even more concern is the association that has been found between prior unsuccessful suicide attempts and eventual completed suicide (Barraclough, Bunch, Nelson, & Sainsbury, 1974; Kreitman, 1977; Otto, 1972). Otto (1972) found that the overall death rate of adolescent suicide attempters was three times as high as that of a carefully matched control group in a sample of 1,547 Swedish adolescent suicide attempters followed-up 10 to 15 years after their initial attempt.

Adolescents who attempt suicide are often admitted to a general pediatric setting for immediate medical treatment and stabilization following an attempt. Physicians working in the general pediatric setting often do not have the expertise to evaluate the emotional status of such an adolescent and frequently seek a psychiatric consultation. Thus, one of the roles a pediatric psychologist and other psychiatric personnel play in such a setting is crisis assessment and disposition management of the adolescent suicide attempter. The ability of pediatric psychologists to make a useful and valid contribution in this regard is dependent on several factors. These factors include knowledge of characteristics associated with patients at risk for a repeated attempt in the immediate and short-term future (0–3 months) and the ability to assess these characteristics and the emotional status of the adolescent patient in an expedient and timely manner.

While a great deal of research has investigated factors associated with attempted and completed suicide among adolescents, most of these studies have examined adolescents on inpatient psychiatric units (McManus, Lerner, Robbins, & Barbour, 1984; McIntire et al., 1977; Robbins & Alessi, 1985), those presenting in emergency rooms (Deykin, Alpert, & McNamarra, 1985;

Garfinkel, Froese, & Hood, 1982), or normal adolescents who, in a survey, report having made a suicide attempt (Riggs, Alario, McHorney, DeChristopher, & Crombie, 1986). Inpatient psychiatric subjects may differ from the patients in pediatric settings in a number of ways including the fact that they are often evaluated many days or weeks following the attempt, are often admitted to psychiatric facilities due to other factors than simply risk for future suicide attempts, and third-party reimbursement policies. Thus, characteristics believed to be important risk factors in evaluating an attempter may not be as applicable in the general pediatric setting. Such background risk factors include family break up and conflict (Dorpat, Jackson, & Ripley, 1965; Garfinkel et al., 1982; McArnarney, 1979; McIntire et al., 1977); history of child abuse (Adams-Tucker, 1982; Deykin et al., 1985; Green, 1978; Riggs et al., 1986); history of substance abuse (Garfinkel et al., 1982; Riggs et al., 1986); personality disorders (Friedman et al., 1982; McManus et al., 1984); and depression (Carlson, 1983; Robbins & Alessi, 1985). Also, it is unclear how adolescents referred for psychological evaluation following a suicide attempt differ on these variables from adolescents referred for evaluation for other psychological difficulties in a general pediatric setting (Gispert, Wheeler, Marsh, & Davis, 1985; Hawton et al., 1982; Marks, 1979). Thus, one of the goals of the present study was to examine the prevalence of these background risk factors in medically hospitalized adolescents referred for evaluation following a suicide attempt and adolescents referred for evaluation of other psychological difficulties.

Clinicians must also evaluate the current emotional status of the adolescent suicide attempter and recommend an appropriate disposition following discharge. Unfortunately, empirical data describing the psychological status of adolescent suicide attempters on medical floors are lacking. The data available are usually on adolescents hospitalized in an inpatient psychiatric setting (McManus et al., 1984; Robbins & Alessi, 1985) who may not be representative of the attempter on a medical floor. Data-based guidelines for disposition decision making (i.e., predicting who would likely be a repeat attempter, who would benefit from individual or family therapy on an inpatient or outpatient basis, etc.), as yet, do not exist, leaving the clinician to render decisions regarding level of follow-up care without adequate empirical data. Prior research with psychiatrically hospitalized children and adolescents suggests a number of areas of psychological functioning, including, but not limited to, depression, hopelessness, impulsivity, hostility, social competence, family conflict, coping style, and life stress (see Pfeffer, 1986, for review), which might prove fruitful in determining such disposition guidelines.

Depression and related constructs, such as hopelessness, attributional style and suicidal ideation, appear to be an appropriate area of initial inquiry in an attempt to understand different types of attempts and to establish disposition guidelines (Carlson, 1983; Pfeffer, 1986). Indeed, Robbins and Alessi (1985) found a strong relationship between depressed mood and suicidal behavior in hospitalized adolescent psychiatric inpatients. Beck, Steer, Kovacs, and Garrison (1985) reported "hopelessness" to be predictive of successful suicide attempts in adults, whereas others have found that child psychiatric inpatients who attempted suicide or evinced suicidal ideation had greater hopelessness scores than psychiatric patients without suicidal ideation and/or attempts (Kazdin, French, Unis, Esveldt-Dawson, & Sherrick, 1983).

In addition to describing the characteristics of adolescent suicide attempters on a pediatric medical unit, the present study evaluated the clinical utility of measures of depression, and the related constructs of hopelessness and attributional style, in differentiating subgroups of adolescent suicide attempters and aiding in disposition planning for attempters. Because of the importance of rapid but appropriate disposition planning for adolescent suicide attempters, widely used self-report measures were chosen for this study. These scales are particularly relevant for the pediatric medical setting because they are brief and can be administered by psychometrists.

METHOD

Subjects

Suicide attempters. Suicide attempters consisted of 71 consecutive admissions to a pediatric medical unit following a suicide attempt. Patients were admitted to the pediatric service following a medical evaluation in the Emergency Room that indicated that additional medical care was necessary. Medical care ranged from observation to intensive care management. Evaluations for each of these patients were requested of the Child Psychiatry Consultation Service to determine individual psychological functioning and disposition recommendations. There were 16 males (23%) and 55 females (77%) in the suicide attempter group. Ages ranged from 13 to 18 years in the group, with a mean age of 15.3 years ($SD = 1.4$ years). Eighty-seven percent of the sample was white, with the remaining 13% being black. Of the methods of suicide 82% ($n = 58$) consisted of drug overdoses, with 45% involving only over-the-counter drugs and 55% prescription drug needs as Valium, Percodan, Phenobarbital, etc. The remainder of the suicide attempt methods included hangings (3), jumpings (2), wrist slashing (4), and four other methods.

Comparison group. These subjects consisted of 71 consecutive adolescents who were also referred to the Child Psychiatry Consultation Service while receiving medical treatment on the same adolescent medical unit for reasons other than suicide attempt. This group was matched by sex and age with the attempter group and comprised 15 males and 55 females whose ages ranged from 13 years to 18 years (mean age = 15.4, *SD* = 1.4 years). A *t* test did not reveal a significant difference in age between the attempters and controls (*t* = 0.45). Reasons for psychiatric referral were various, including fainting spells, depression without suicidal ideation, anorexia nervosa, seizure disorders, conversion disorders, tics, headaches, somatic complaints without organic basis and anxiety. On clinical interview, all patients in the comparison group denied suicidal ideation or plans nor had any made a suicide attempt in the past. This group of patients was believed to be a particularly appropriate control group to compare risk factors in this study since they constitute the majority of cases typically referred to child pschiatry consultation services.

Data on the characteristics of both suicide attempters and the comparison group were obtained by systematically reviewing medical records and extracting data on the various characteristics under study. Approval for this portion of the clinical research protocol and the self-report assessment procedures discussed below were obtained from the hospital human investigations committee. Data were obtained primarily by reading consultation reports written by the attending psychiatrist and social work interviews conducted with the parents. A protocol was developed to gather specific information about the various risk factors described in Table I. These characteristics were chosen because they reflect current thinking regarding important risk factors found in adolescent suicide attempters. The suicide attempters were also rated on psychiatric history, toxicity of overdose attempts, and disposition status.

Psychiatric history. A broad classification schema was used to classify psychiatric history as "acute" or "chronic." On the basis of patients and parent reports, as well as other historical data, the suicide attempters were rated as having long-standing emotional (chronic) problems if they had past contact with mental health professionals and a history of dysfunctional behavior in school, peer relations, or family. A suicide attempt that was made by a patient without a history of such problems was classified as an acute response.

Toxicity of overdose. Since the majority of suicide attempts involved overdoses, information regarding agents ingested and dosage units for each agent were given to two members of the local Poison Control Center. They rated each ingestion on the basis of expected outcome if the overdose was untreated. Using these criteria, they rated the overdoses as mild, moderate, or

Table I. Risk Factors of Suicide Attempters and Control Patients Referred to Consultation/Liaison Service

Risk factor	Suicide attempters ($n = 71$) %	Consultation/liaison referrals ($n = 71$) %	χ^2
Family consultation			0.89
Intact	74.6	77.8	
Not intact	25.4	22.2	
Psychiatric history			4.27[a]
Yes	33.8	25.0	
No	66.2	75.0	
Alcohol/drug misuse			0.02
Yes	31.0	23.6	
No	69.0	76.4	
Physically abused			0.19
Yes	18.3	15.3	
No	81.7	84.7	
Sexually abused			2.36
Yes	5.6	12.5	
No	94.4	87.5	
Marital conflict reported			0.16
Yes	21.1	31.9	
No	78.9	68.1	
Alcohol abuse by parents			0.02
Yes	22.5	16.7	
No	77.5	83.3	

[a] $p < .05$.

severe. Since there were relatively few mild overdoses, for the purposes of the analyses discussed below, the mild and moderate overdoses were combined into one group.

Discharge status. Since discharge status was associated with perceived risk for future attempts, we also divided our sample into those who were discharged to outpatient or inpatient psychiatric care.

Instruments

Instruments chosen for investigation in this study were commonly used measures of depression, hopelessness, and suicidal ideation. The measures are described below:

Children's Attributional Style Questionnaire (CASQ). This 48-item instrument lists both good and bad events. Each subject is requested to pick, from a pair of possible causes, the reason that best describes why the event occurred. The causes listed on these questions are designed to tap two of the three attributional dimensions (internal, stable, and global), described by Abramson, Seligman, and Teasdale (1978) to be associated with depressive symptoms. Sixteen questions pertain to each of the three dimensions, with half of the questions describing good events and half of the questions describing bad events. A score of 1 is assigned to each internal, stable, or global response and 0 to each external, stable, or specific response. Appropriate subscales are then formed by summing each score across the three causal dimensions separately for good events and for bad events. Although the CASQ is a relatively new instrument with limited research findings, several studies have been reported that suggest it is a valid instrument (e.g., Seligman et al., 1984).

Children's Depression Inventory (CDI). The CDI (Kovacs 1980/1981) was designed to assess the severity of a variety of symptoms of childhood depression. Each of the 27 items consist of three alternatives, of which the child chooses one. Each set of sentences describes a symptom of childhood depression, such as sleep and appetite disturbance, dysphoria, etc. Items are scored from 0 to 2, resulting in a range of scores of 0 to 54. The CDI has been reported to have high internal consistency with normal and clinical samples of children. Test-retest reliability ranges from .38 to .87, depending on interval length and population (cf. Saylor, Finch, Spirito, & Bennett, 1984).

Suicide Ideation Questionnaire. The Suicide Ideation Questionnaire (Reynolds, 1985) is a self-report measure designed to assess thoughts about suicide in junior and senior high school students. The questionnaire consists of 30 items which are scored on a 0- to 6-point scale with 0 assigned to "never having had the thought" and 6 reflecting "having the thought almost every day." The scale was developed on field testing with over 2,400 adolescents. Coefficient alpha internal consistency measures have been reported at .97. Construct validity has been demonstrated by correlations with highly related constructs such as depression (.59) and hopelessness (.48). The Suicidal Ideation Questionnaire has been found useful for individual assessment and as a screening measure for large group identification of suicidal adolescents (Reynolds, 1985).

Reynolds Adolescent Depression Scale. The Reynolds Adolescent Depression Scale (Reynolds, 1986) consists of 30 items and utilizes a 4-point Likert scale with responses ranging from "almost never" to "most of the time." This scale was developed specifically for adolescents and covers a number of symptoms felt to be indicative of depression including somatic, behavioral, cognitive, mood, and vegetative signs. Internal consistency estimates have ranged from .92 to .96. Six-week test-retest reliability coefficients of .84 was determined with a sample of 126 adolescents. Construct validity of the measure has been assessed by examining the relation of the measure to other self-report and interview measures of depression. In addition, normative data have been collected on over 6,000 adolescents from a variety of socioeconomic levels (Reynolds, 1984).

Hopelessness Scale for Children. The Hopelessness Scale for Children (Kazdin et al., 1983) is a scale on which children indicate whether each of 17 items is true or not true. The scale measures feelings of hopelessness, which have been found to be an important variable related to suicide attempts. Adequate internal consistency (alpha = .97) has been demonstrated as well as test-retest reliability following a 6-week interval. Construct validity has been assessed by examining the relationship of the scale to measures of depression, self-esteem, and social behavior. The scale correlated positively (r = .58) with depression, and negatively with measures of self-esteem (r = −.61) and social skills (r = −.39) in a sample of 262 child psychiatric inpatients (Kazdin et al., 1983; Kazdin, Rodgas, & Colbus, 1986).

Procedure

Although demographic characteristics were available for 71 of the adolescent suicide attempters in the study, self-report measures were not available for all of these subjects. A total of 59 attempters were assessed using self-report measures. Not all patients received all self-report measures and the breakdown by measure can be found below. Suicide attempters were evaluated on the self-report battery within 24 to 36 hours following admission to the hospital. Comparison group subjects were evaluated within 24 to 36 hours of receipt of the consult. Patients in the comparison group were administered self-report measures less consistently and primarily as a function of the individual clinician's interest in using such self-report measures rather than a tendency for more disturbed patients to complete such measures.

Adolescent suicide attempters were evaluated by two separate examiners. One examiner conducted a clinical interview and completed rating scales on suicidal intent and level of depression. The second examiner independently assessed the patient using self-report measures. In order to ensure cooperation and validity of the ratings, all the scales reported in this study were read to the patient and completed by the examiner. These scales are part of a larger battery currently used as a comprehensive assessment protocol for adolescent suicide attempters hospitalized on a pediatrics unit.

RESULTS

Comparing attempters to the consultation/liaison patients, a t test did not reveal any difference by age (t = 0.45). Chi-square analyses did not reveal any differences by sex (χ^2 = 1.71) or race (χ^2 = 1.31).

Attempters Versus Comparison Group: Risk Factors

Table I lists the percentages of attempters and controls on seven background variables. Chi-square analyses revealed only one significant difference between the two groups: The suicide attempters had a larger percentage of patients with a history of psychiatric difficulties than the comparison group ($\chi^2 = 4.27$, $p < .05$).

Attempters Versus Comparison Group: Self-Report Measures

Where clinically appropriate, a number of comparison group patients were administered The Children's Depression Inventory (CDI) and Hopelessness Scale for Children. Twenty patients were administered the CDI and obtained a mean score of 19.0 ($SD = 10.7$). The entire sample of suicide attempters ($N = 53$) obtained a mean score of 18.0 ($SD = 10.4$). These mean scores meet or approach the cutoff score of 19 often used to determine clinically significant levels of depression (Kovacs, 1982). However, a t test did not reveal a significant difference ($t = 0.36$) between the two groups. On the Hopelessness Scale, the comparison group obtained a mean score of 7.8 ($SD = 5.1$) while the attempters ($n = 58$) obtained a mean score of 6.8 ($SD = 4.5$). A t test did not reveal a significant difference ($t = 0.70$) between the two groups.

Suicide Attempters: Psychiatric History

Suicide attempters, as discussed previously, were classified as having chronic psychiatric difficulties or an acute psychiatric episode on the basis of criteria previously described. Forty of the attempters were rated as having chronic difficulties and 31 were rated as having acute difficulties. Chi-square analysis did not reveal any differences between the two groups on risk factors nor were differences detected between the acute and chronic groups on toxicity rating of the overdose or disposition status.

Table II presents the means, standard deviations, and univariate F values for the various self-report measures by psychiatric history. Only two variables were found to discriminate the groups. The acute group had a significantly higher total score on the Reynolds Adolescent Depression Scale ($F = 6.27$, $p < .05$) and a higher score on the Suicide Ideation Questionnaire ($F = 8.59$, $p < .01$).

Suicide Attempters: Toxicity Rating of Overdose

The suicide attempters who took drug overdoses were divided according to the toxicity of their attempt by criteria stated above. Using this criteria, the Poison Control Center classified 26 patients as having made a mild/moderate

Table II. Means, Standard Deviations, and F Values for Dependent Measures in Adolescent Suicide Attempters by Past Psychiatric History (Acute Vs. Chronic)

Measure	Acute			Chronic			
	M	SD	n	M	SD	n	F
Hopelessness scale	6.2	3.3	25	7.3	5.3	33	0.77
Reynolds Adolescent Depression Scale	80.9	11.5	15	68.8	14.0	13	6.27[a]
Children's Depression Inventory Total score	19.2	10.7	30	16.1	10.7	23	1.11
Children's Attributional Style Questionnaire[c]							
GI	3.5	1.7	21	3.7	2.0	18	0.11
GS	3.4	1.4	21	3.6	1.5	18	0.15
GG	4.8	1.6	21	4.5	1.4	18	0.17
BI	3.9	1.6	21	3.7	1.3	18	0.24
BS	3.2	1.7	21	3.0	1.9	18	0.11
BG	2.5	1.6	21	2.6	1.4	18	0.03
Suicide Ideation Questionnaire	109.1	38.6	10	53.5	43.5	10	8.59[b]

[a]$p < .05$.
[b]$p < .01$.
[c]GI = attributional style for good outcome-internality; GS = good outcome-stability; GG = good outcome-globality; BI = attributional style for bad outcome-internality; BS = bad outcome-stability; BG = bad outcome-globality.

attempt, whereas 32 patients made a severe attempt. Chi-square analyses examining the background characteristics of mild/moderate attempters versus severe attempters indicated only one significant difference among the variables. A significantly greater percentage of patients ($\chi^2 = 4.71, p < .05$) who made a severe attempt had a history of substance abuse. No differences were detected between the mild/moderate and severe groups on disposition status nor past psychiatric history.

Table III presents the means, standard deviations, and F values for the various self-report measures by toxicity rating of overdose. Severe attempters had a significantly higher score on the CDI ($F = 5.17, p < .05$). The severe attempters were also noted to be more likely to attribute bad events to stable causes on the CASQ ($F = 8.14, p < .01$) than the mild/moderate group.

Suicide Attempters: Disposition Status

Chi-square analyses conducted by disposition status did not reveal any significant differences on the various background characteristics between those suicide attempters referred for outpatient treatment upon discharge or inpatient psychiatric treatment. No differences between inpatient or outpa-

Table III. Means, Standard Deviations, and F Values for Dependent Measures in Adolescent Suicide Attempters by Toxicity Rating of Overdose

Measure	Mild/moderate attempt			Severe attempt			F
	M	SD	n	M	SD	n	
Hopelessness scale	6.2	4.6	23	7.2	4.3	28	0.70
Reynolds Adolescent Depression Scale	72.0	14.8	12	74.5	12.5	12	0.20
Children's Depression Inventory Total score	14.4	10.3	22	21.2	10.1	25	5.17[a]
Children's Attributional Style Questionnaire							
GI	3.9	2.0	16	3.1	1.5	18	1.87
GS	3.7	1.4	16	3.3	1.3	18	1.00
GG	5.2	1.6	16	4.3	1.4	18	3.20
BI	3.7	1.3	16	4.1	1.4	18	0.79
BS	2.2	1.2	16	3.8	1.9	18	8.14[b]
BG	2.8	1.9	16	2.1	1.0	18	1.95
Suicide Ideation Questionnaire	82.6	52.4	9	76.8	51.8	9	0.05

[a] $p < .05$.
[b] $p < .01$.

tient referrals were found on psychiatric history or toxicity rating of the overdose. Table IV presents the means, standard deviations, and F values for dependent measures of the suicide attempters by disposition status. Although there were several trends ($p > .05$ and $p < .10$) in the expected direction, no significant differences were noted between the two groups on these dependent measures.

DISCUSSION

Over the last two decades, clinicians and researchers have discussed a number of risk factors believed to be, if not predictive of, strongly associated with adolescent suicide attempts. The majority of the research to date has been conducted on psychiatric inpatients or has not utilized appropriate comparison groups which would allow conclusions to be drawn about the generalizability of the importance of these characteristics to suicide attempters hospitalized in a pediatric setting. In the present study, risk factors of adolescent suicide attempters admitted to a pediatric setting are compared to those of medical patients referred for psychological evaluation and hospitalized on the same floor. Such a comparison reveals few significant differences. For example, family disruption has been noted by a number of authors to be a

Table IV. Means, Standard Deviations, and *F* Values for Dependent Measures in Adolescent Suicide Attempters by Disposition Status

	Outpatient			Inpatient			
Measure	*M*	*SD*	*n*	*M*	*SD*	*n*	*F*
Hopelessness scale	6.0	4.2	35	8.1	4.8	24	2.95
Reynolds Adolescent Depression Scale	76.2	12.4	16	73.9	15.6	13	0.20
Children's Depression Inventory	16.2	10.1	32	20.3	10.8	22	2.01
Children's Attributional Style Questionnaire							
GI	4.2	1.9	13	3.4	1.7	27	2.08
GS	4.1	1.6	13	3.2	1.2	27	3.99
GG	4.3	1.6	13	4.8	1.5	27	0.82
BI	3.8	1.6	13	3.8	1.4	27	0.01
BS	3.1	1.6	13	3.0	1.9	27	0.01
BG	2.9	1.8	13	2.3	1.3	27	1.50
Suicide Ideation Questionnaire	89.7	45.7	10	77.1	51.2	10	0.30

very significant factor in adolescent suicide attempters. Previous studies have indicated quite low percentage of intact families among suicide attempters: Gispert et al. (1985) reported 24% intact families in a lower SES sample of attempters in a general medical setting; Garfinkel et al. (1982) found less than 50% of their emergency room sample came from an intact family. Yet, in our sample, approximately 75% of both the suicide attempters and the comparison group came from intact families at the time of the attempt. Similarly, if one looks at past history of child abuse in our group of attempters, there is no difference in rate of child abuse (physical or sexual) when compared to our comparison group. However, the percentage of physical abuse reported by our suicide attempters (18.3%) is similar to that reported by a group of high school students who said they had attempted suicide in the past (22%; Riggs et al., 1986). Consequently, it does not appear that our sample is unusual in the rate of occurrence of child abuse but that a history of child abuse is a risk factor for a variety of emotional difficulties in adolescence. Interestingly, reported rate of sexual abuse was less, although not statistically different, among suicide attempters than our comparison group. Again, this finding underscores the need to take a thorough history when examining adolescent patients because sexual abuse may play a significant role in the symptom presentation of a variety of patients seen on a pediatric unit.

The suicide attempters differ from the comparison patients on only one of the risk factors: past psychiatric history. This finding is most likely accounted for by the fact that although over half of the suicide attempters reported previous emotional difficulties and contact with mental health professionals, the majority of comparison patients had been primarily involved in medical evaluations in the past. Comparison patients may have had a history of past emotional difficulties that presented as somatic complaints and thus had not led to psychological intervention.

The present findings indicate the importance of using appropriate comparison groups in clinical research and not generalizing beyond the limitations of the data. Our findings suggest that medically hospitalized adolescent suicide attempters have a history of risk factors that are very similar to those associated with general emotional difficulties in adolescents and are not particular to suicide attempters. These findings are, at least in part, a reflection of the diverse group of suicide attempters evaluated on a pediatric floor as opposed to a psychiatric floor. However, it is interesting to note that a similar conclusion was drawn by researchers over 16 years ago (Stanley & Barter, 1970) when comparing adolescents hospitalized on a psychiatric floor for suicide attempt versus other patients hospitalized in the same setting.

In evaluating the differences in levels of depression and hopelessness found in suicide attempters versus our comparison group, the findings are similar to the risk factor data. Adolescents hospitalized on a pediatrics unit following a suicide attempt did not report significantly greater amounts of depression or hopelessness than the consultation liaison patients. This was not a uniform finding by any means as there was a great deal of variability in the scores obtained on these measures among the adolescent suicide attempters. However, the percentage of patients scoring in the clinically significant range (CDI > 19) was somewhat higher for the attempters (54%) than the comparison group (38%). As others have noted (e.g., Garfinkel et al., 1982; Gispert et al., 1985) depression is not a necessary prelude to a suicide attempt among either adults or adolescents. Although our findings might be used to support such statements, it is not appropriate to draw conclusions about affective state prior to a suicide attempt using data obtained following an attempt. For example, it may be that the adolescents had been depressed but were becoming less so as psychological help became available following a suicide attempt (Spirito, Faust, Myers, & Bechtel, 1986). It is also interesting to note that the level of depression rated by the consultation liaison patients is fairly substantial. The depression noted in these patients might be related to a number of factors such as a reaction to hospitalization or depression underlying somatic complaints.

Examining the clinical utility of self-report measures of depression and related constructs in adolescent suicide attempters, the findings are mixed. The adolescent suicide attempters rated as having an acute reaction without prior psychiatric difficulties reported a higher degree of suicide ideation and depression than the group with chronic difficulties. These high rates of depression and suicidal ideation suggest an acute stress response but do not appear to suggest a group at any greater risk than other attempters since they are not more frequently referred to inpatient treatment. In fact, they can often be worked with quite effectively using crisis intervention strategies. It would be interesting to examine the range of depression and suicide ideation in a large sample of such "acute" suicide attempters to determine if there are differences within the group. Unfortunately, our sample was not large enough to conduct such an analysis.

Medical ratings by toxicity of attempt indicate that adolescents who take highly toxic overdoses are more distressed, as reflected by their high CDI scores, than the mild/moderate overdose group and more likely to attribute bad events to stable causes. Patients who make such severe overdoses may be persons who experience acute discomfort in response to events in their lives but who do not see the potential for positive change in the future. Thus, a more serious suicide attempt may be made since the future looks bleaker to these adolescents. Such a finding would make clinical sense to those who have worked extensively with this population. Of course, access to certain types of drugs that can result in a serious overdose would have to be a mediating factor.

Another factor, not typically discussed in the literature, is the factual basis of the stated suicide attempt method. An adolescent's account of the number and type of drug ingested can be quite unreliable, but medical care is predicated on the stated number and dosage of drugs. This ambiguity has led the current authors to undertake a study examining the relationship between severity of the attempt as defined by the patient's historical account and severity rated by required medical intervention and clinical course while hospitalized. Other clinicians refute such a finding and state that the adolescent's perception of the lethality of the attempt is much more important in determining psychological status and future risk than the actual drugs taken. McIntire et al. (1977) found this to be true among a group of psychiatrically hospitalized patients. However, only eight of our suicide attempters, upon questioning in a clinical interview, actually said that they wanted to die when they made the overdose. This is much lower percentage than reported in other studies. Consequently, lethality of intent may be more helpful in establishing risk among psychiatrically hospitalized adolescent suicide attempters than adolescents hospitalized on a pediatrics unit. The small number of subjects who did in fact state they had wanted to die when they made an attempt makes it impossible to conduct statistical analyses with our data. However, it should be noted that six of these patients were eventually referred for psychiatric hospitalization upon discharge. Thus, an adolescent's stated desire to die is important diagnostically, but not likely to be found in many cases in a pediatric setting.

The lack of findings on the Hopelessness Scale is surprising. This scale was specifically included in our evaluation since a good deal of research has been conducted examining the relationship between hopelessness, depression, and suicidal intent in both adults (Beck, et al., 1985; Wetzel, Marguiles, Davis, & Karam, 1980) and children (Kazdin et al., 1983). These studies point to hopelessness as a more important construct than depression in determining future risk in suicide attempters. The difference found between severe and moderate overdose groups on the CASQ (i.e., the severe group attributed bad events to stable causes more than the moderate group) might reflect hopelessness despite the fact that the specific scale used in this study did not discriminate groups. It should be noted, however, that the average scores found in our suicide attempters ($M = 6.8$) are only slightly higher than those found in a sample of 1,360 high school students in the same geographic region as our attempters ($M = 4.9$; Ashworth, Spirito, Colella & Benedict-Drew, 1986).

Other factors are needed to predict severity of attempt and adolescents to be considered high risk. Similar to the hopelessness results, attributional style is not useful, for the most part, in discriminating amongst the adolescent suicide attempters. It had been hypothesized that the attempters with a history of chronic difficulties would demonstrate greater dysfunctional attributions, but this is found on only one dimension. It may be that if a comparison group were employed a difference would be evident. Studies with adults (e.g., Ellis & Ratliff, 1986) have shown differences in attributional style among suicidal and nonsuicidal adults hospitalized on a psychiatric unit. We are not able to compare our group of attempters with control data on the CASQ so we cannot evaluate this question.

The findings appear generalizable to other pediatric settings since age, sex, and method of suicide appear similar to other studies. For example, the male (23%)/female (77%) ratio is similar to that found in a study of attempters hospitalized on a pediatric floor (Marks, 1979). In other studies, the percentage of females has varied from 61% (Gispert et al., 1985) to 90% (Hawton et al., 1982). Our mean age (15.3) is similar to Gispert et al. (1985; 15.3) but is slightly younger than that found by Marks (1979) and Hawton et al. (1982). Hawton et al. (1982) had a similar percentage of white adolescents (82%) in their sample of overdose patients on a pediatrics floor as in the current sample (87%). Previous studies have also had a similar number of drug overdoses, ranging from 71% (Gispert et al., 1985) to 95% (Marks,

1979), as the 82% found in the sample reported here. Hawton et al. (1982) found 66% of their sample ingested nonopiate analgesics, which is similar to the percentage in this study (55%).

Discharge status was selected as the final variable to examine among our attempters since referral to inpatient hospitalization is felt to be a marker of increased risk. Our findings suggest that depression and related constructs are not the key factors in the clinician's determination of who is at high risk following an attempt since no differences are found on measures for patients referred to inpatient or outpatient treatment. Perhaps other individual factors may play more of a role in such a disposition. Anger, for example, has been discussed as an important variable in adolescent suicidal behavior (Cohen-Sandler, Berman, & Keene, 1982; Gispert et al., 1985; Kosky, 1983). It may be that some clinician rating of hostility combined with certain other mediating factors, such as family support system, would better predict ultimate discharge status. It is not likely that inpatient dispositions were made on the basis of serious psychiatric disturbance, such as psychosis, since very few adolescents seen in our setting were diagnosed as such. Finally, disposition decisions may be more related to differences in clinician judgments than any particular clinical indicator. If this is true then research is certainly needed to help guide clinical judgment in a more empirical fashion. Since special funding through state agencies was available for children without insurance coverage deemed in need of inpatient psychiatric care, the findings do not appear to be a factor of socioeconomic status or insurance coverage.

The failure to find more substantial differences among suicide attempters on measures of depression and related constructs is somewhat surprising. Although it would be easy to fault self-report measures as a primary culprit for a lack of findings, the fact that these scales were read to patients to ensure more accurate responding helps negate such criticism. Two other factors might be more appropriately implicated. First, the relatively small sample and the substantial variability in scores certainly may have affected the ability to detect statistical differences. Such sample size limitations are inherent in clinical research with relatively rare populations. If larger comparison groups were available, clearer and more consistent differences might emerge between suicide attempters and other clinical groups. However, the wide variability in scores encountered in both patient groups does not make this prospect seem likely. Instead, studies with larger numbers might help in identifying cohesive subgroups within the apparently heterogeneous group of suicide attempters on a pediatric floor. Such subgrouping may lead to refined diagnostic and treatment recommendations.

Second, it may well be that there are more important factors to examine in attempting to assess risk factors and determine the appropriate dispositions in adolescent suicide attempters. For example, some researchers have begun to look at life events over developmental stages among suicidal children and have found some significant differences when compared to a control group of children with other psychiatric difficulties (Cohen-Sandler et al., 1982). In our own work, we were able to find few differences on social adjustment (Spirito, Halverson, & Hart, 1985) and observed behavior on the pediatrics floor (Spirito, Stark, Fristad, & Hart, 1986). However, on a coping scale specifically developed for suicide attempters and other pediatric populations, adolescent suicide attempters were found to have significantly fewer coping strategies than normal adolescents (Spirito, Stark, & Williams, 1986). For example, adolescents who said that break up with a boyfriend/girlfriend resulted in the suicide attempt were compared to normals who reported break up with a boyfriend/girlfriend as the most significant stress they had experienced in the prior month. Data analyses indicate that the suicide attempters had significantly poorer problem-solving skills, sought social support less often, and used active avoidance of the stressor much less often than the normals. These preliminary findings with this scale are quite encouraging and may point to a clinically useful tool with this population.

Beyond simply examining new constructs, clinicians and researchers working with adolescent suicide attempters also need to conduct follow-up research with this group since long-term adjustment is certainly the more crucial reflection of appropriate disposition recommendations. (Following the comparison group to determine if any of these patients later attempt or complete suicide would also be interesting.) Knowing who is likely to follow through with treatment recommendations in and of itself would be a significant advancement for the clinician working in a pediatric setting. In addition, the measures we employ to assess depression and related constructs may be important in determining who is likely to be at risk for future emotional difficulties and further suicide attempts in the year following a hospital admission. Thus, a research strategy that focuses on a comprehensive assessment of psychological variables coupled with routine follow-up of suicide attempters appears to be our best means of advancing the kinds of knowledge important to the clinician making treatment and disposition recommendations on a pediatric unit.

REFERENCES

Abramson, L.Y., Seligman, M. E. P., & Teasdale, J. D. (1978). Learned helplessness in humans: Critique and reformulation. *Journal of Abnormal Psychology, 87,* 49–74.

Adams-Tucker, C. (1982). Proximate effects of sexual abuse in childhood: A report in twenty-eight children. *American Journal of Psychiatry, 139,* 1252–1256.

Ashworth, S., Spirito, A., Colella, A., & Benedict-Drew, C. (1986). Implementation and assessment of a pilot suicidal awareness, identification and prevention program. *Rhode Island Medical Journal,* in press.

Barraclough, B., Bunch, J., Nelson, B., & Sainsbury, P. (1974). A hundred cases of suicide: Clinical aspects. *British Journal of Psychiatry, 125,* 355–373.

Beck, A. T., Steer, R. A., Kovacs, M., & Garrison, B. (1985). Hopelessness and eventual suicide: A 10-year prospective study of patients hospitalized with suicidal ideation. *American Journal of Psychiatry, 142,* 559–563.

Carlson G. A. (1983). Depression and suicidal behavior in children and adolescents. In D. P. Cantwell & G. A. Carlson (Eds.), *Affective disorders in childhood and adolescence.* New York: SP Medical and Scientific.

Cohen-Sandler, R., Berman, A. L., & King, R. A. (1982). Life stress and symptomatology: Determinants of suicidal behavior in children. *Journal of the American Academy of Child Psychiatry 21,* 178–186.

Deykin, E. Y., Alpert, J. J., & McNamarra, J. J. (1985). A pilot study of the effect of exposure to child abuse or neglect on adolescent suicidal behavior. *American Journal of Psychiatry, 142,* 1299–1303.

Dorpat, T. L., Jackson, J. K., & Ripley, H. S. (1965). Broken homes and attempted and completed suicides. *Archives of General Psychiatry, 12,* 213–216.

Ellis, T. E., & Ratliff, K. G. (1986). Cognitive characteristics of suicidal and nonsuicidal psychiatric inpatients. *Cognitive Therapy and Research,* in press.

Friedman, R. C., Clarkin, J. F., Korn, R., Aronoff, M. S., Hurt, S. W., & Murphy, M. C. (1982). DSM-III and affective pathology in hospitalized adolescents. *Journal of Nervous and Mental Diseases, 170,* 511–521.

Garfinkel, B. D. Froese, A., & Hood, J. (1982). Suicide attempts in children and adolescents. *American Journal of Psychiatry, 139,* 1257–1261.

Gispert, M., Wheeler, K., Marsh, L., & Davis, M. S. (1985). Suicidal adolescents: Factors in evaluation. *Adolescence, 20,* 753–762.

Green, A. H. (1978). Self-destructive behavior in battered children. *American Journal of Psychiatry, 135, 579–582.*

Haldane, J. D., & Haider, I. (1967). Attempted suicide in children and adolescents. *British Journal of Clinical Practice, 21,* 587–589.

Hawton, K., O'Grady, J., Osborn, M., & Cole, D. (1982). Adolescents who take overdoses: Their characteristics, problems, and contacts with helping agencies. *British Journal of Psychiatry, 140,* 118–123.

Hawton, K., & Osborn, M. (1984). Suicide and attempted suicide in children and adolescents. In B. B. Lahey & A. E. Kazdin (Eds.), *Advances in clinical child psychiatry (Vol. 7).* New York: Plenum Press.

Kazdin, A. E., French, N. H., Unis, A. S., Esveldt-Dawson, K., & Sherrick, R. B. (1983). Hopelessness, depression and suicidal intent among psychiatrically disturbed children. *Journal of Consulting and Clinical Psychology, 51,* 504–510.

Kazdin, A. E., Rodgas, A., & Colbus, D. (1986). The Hopelessness Scale for Children: Psychometric characteristics and concurrent validity. *Journal of Consulting and Clinical Psychology, 54,* 241–245.

Kosky, R. (1983). Childhood suicidal behavior, *Journal of Child Psychology and Psychiatry, 24,* 457–468.

Kovacs, M. (1980/1981). Rating scales to assess depression in school-aged children. *Acta Paedopsychiatry, 46,* 305–315.

Kovacs, M. (1982). *The Children's Depression Inventory: A self-rated depression scale for schoolaged youngsters.* Unpublished manuscript, University of Pittsburgh.

Kreitman, N. (Ed.). (1977). *Parasuicide.* Toronto: Wiley.

Marks, A. (1979). Management of the suicidal adolescent on a nonpsychiatric adolescent unit. *Journal of Pediatrics, 95,* 305–308.

McArnarney, E. R. (1979). Adolescent and young adult suicide in the U.S.-A reflection of societal unrest? *Adolescence, 14,* 765–773.

McIntire, M. S., Angle, C. R., Wikoff, R. L., & Schlicht, M. L. (1977). Recurrent adolescent suicidal behavior. *Pediatrics, 60,* 605–608.

McManus, M., Lerner, H., Robbins, D., & Barbour, C., (1984). Assessment of borderline symptomatology in hospitalized adolescents. *Journal of the American Academy of Child Psychiatry, 23,* 685–694.

Murphy, G., & Wetzel, R. D. (1980). Suicide risk by birth cohort in the United States, 1949–1974. *Archives of General Psychiatry, 37,* 519–523.

Otto, U. (1972). Suicidal acts by children and adolescents: A follow-up study. *Acta Psychiatrica Scandinavia Supplement* 233.

Pfeffer, C. (1986). *The suicidal child.* New York: Gilford.

Reynolds, W. M. (1984). Depression in children and adolescents: Phenomenology, evaluation and treatment. *School Psychology Review 13,* 171–181.

Reynolds, W. M. (1985). *Suicide Ideation Questionnaire.* Unpublished manuscript, University of Wisconsin, Madison.

Reynolds, W. M. (1986). Assessment of depression in adolescents: Manual for the Reynolds Adolescent Depression Scale. *Psychological Assessment Resources,* Odessa, Fl.

Riggs, S., Alario, A., McHorney, C., DeChristopher, J., & Crombie, P. (1986). Abuse and health related risk taking behaviors in high school students who have attempted suicide. *Journal of Developmental Behavioral Pediatrics, 205,* (Abstract).

Robbins, D. R., & Alessi, N. E. (1985). Depressive symptoms and suicidal behavior in adolescents. *American Journal of Psychiatry, 142,* 588–592.

Saylor, C. F., Finch, A. J., Spirito, A., & Bennett, B. (1984). The Children's Depression Inventory: A systematic evaluation of psychometric properties. *Journal of Consulting and Clinical Psychology, 52,* 955–967.

Seligman, N. E. P., Peterson, C., Kaslow, N. J., Tanenbaum, R. L., Alloy, L. D., & Abramson, L. Y. (1984). Attributional style and depressive symptoms among children. *Journal of Abnormal Psychology, 93,* 235–238.

Spirito, A., Faust, D., Myers, B., & Bechtel, D. (1986). *Clinical utility of the MMPI in the evaluation of adolescent suicide attempters.* Manuscript submitted for publication.

Spirito, A., Halverson, J., & Hart, K. (1985, November). *Relationship between social skills and depression in adolescent suicide attempters.* Paper presented at the Association for the Advancement of Behavioral Therapy, Houston.

Spirito, A., Stark, L. J., Fristad, M., & Hart, K. (1986, November). *Behavioral observations of adolescent suicide attempters hospitalized on a general pediatrics floor.* Paper presented at The Association for the Advancement of Behavior Therapy, Chicago.

Spirito, A., Stark, L. J., & Williams, C. (1986). *Differential coping styles in adolescent suicide attempters versus normal adolescents experiencing similar life stress.* Unpublished manuscript.

United States Monthly Vital Statistics. (1982). Vol. 31.

Wetzel, R. D., Margulies, T., Davis, R., & Karam, E. (1980). Hopelessness, depression and suicidal intent. *Journal of Clinical psychology,* 41, 159–160.

38

Heterogeneity of Suicidal Adolescents

Aman U. Khan

Southern Illinois University School of Medicine, Springfield

One hundred twenty adolescents who were divided into three groups: 40 hospitalized suicidal adolescents (first time attempters); 40 hospitalized nonsuicidal adolescents; and 40 never-hospitalized nonsuicidal adolescents from an outpatient psychiatric clinic. Comparisons of the three groups revealed no significant differences in age, race, social class, type of peer and family relationship and academic achievement. Similarly, clinical diagnoses on Axis I and Axis II (DSM-III) failed to differentiate between the suicidal and nonsuicidal adolescents. It appears that, in order to predict the suicidal potential of an adolescent, more attention needs to be paid to the "coping style" of the adolescent under stressful situations. Most suicidal adolescents in this study experienced a great difficulty in coping with their angry and sad feelings. They also manifested a diminished capacity to think through the consequences of their actions.

All suicide attempters are potentially at risk for actual suicide. The risk for suicide, however, varies with age, sex, psychiatric diagnosis and a large number of socioeconomic variables (Tishler and McKendry, 1981; Tuckman and Youngman, 1968). The national statistics indicate that current suicidal rate in the 15–24-year-old age group is 12.8 per 100,000 population. Although no definite data are available, a few estimates indicate that the ratio of attempted suicide to completed suicide in adolescent population may be as high as 120 to 1 (Dorpat and Riley, 1967; McIntire et al., 1977). The female

Reprinted with permission from the *Journal of the American Academy of Child and Adolescent Psychiatry, 1987, Vol. 26, No. 1, 92–96.*

adolescents attempt suicide 3–5 times more than male adolescents, but the number of successful suicides is 3–4 times higher in male than in female adolescents (Silverman, 1968). Suicide rates for nonwhites are lower than those for whites, with two important exceptions: (1) nonwhite females between the ages of 15 and 19 have a slightly higher rate than white females of the same age and (2) there has been a striking increase in suicide rate among nonwhite males of 15–24 years of age.

The current literature seems to focus largely on the family dynamics of the suicidal adolescents. Williams and Lyons (1976) found that families of suicidal adolescents evidenced less effective productivity, specificity, adaptive interaction and a higher rate of conflict. Wenz (1978, 1979a, 1979b) noticed that the families of suicidal adolescents exhibited a lower degree of "normalness" and a greater degree of "powerlessness." Garfinkle et al. (1982) found more psychiatric illness (primarily drug and alcohol abuse), suicide, paternal unemployment and absence of one parent in the families of suicidal adolescents than in the families of normal adolescents. Wenz (1979a, 1979b) reported that suicidal adolescents had more conflict in relationships with parents and peers, more broken romances and academic achievement problems. Kosky (1983) concluded that suicidal adolescents experienced more significant personal losses, academic underachievement, marital disintegration among the parents, past intrafamilial violence and physical abuse than the psychiatrically ill nonsuicidal adolescents.

The studies of the premorbid personality of suicidal adolescents display variable findings. Crumley (1981) reported borderline personality disorder as the most common personality diagnosis in his group of suicidal adolescents. Garfinkel et al. (1982) found that the most suicidal adolescents had a past history of psychiatric illness and that they engaged in more substance abuse.

The nature of the psychopathology in suicidal adolescents is also surrounded by a great deal of controversy. Although most investigators acknowledge that suicidal adolescents are emotionally disturbed, the nature and the extent of the disturbance remains controversial. Some authors (Jacob, 1971) consider suicidal attempts as resulting from minor adjustment problems in the family and peer relationships, while others regard suicidal attempts as a symptom of severe psychopathology. Hudgens (1974) asserted that a psychiatric disorder is a necessary precondition for a suicidal attempt. Tishler and McKenry (1981), in a study of an emergency room population of 46 suicidal attempters matched with 46 nonattempters, found that the suicide attempters were significantly more distressed than the nonattempters. The attempters manifested more anxiety, depression, hostility and lower self-esteem. Schlebusch and Minnaar (1980), in a South African study, found conduct disorder to be the most frequent diagnosis for suicidal adolescents.

In a sample of 40 suicidal adolescents selected retrospectively from a private psychiatric practice, Crumley (1979) labeled 80% of the sample as affective disorders on Axis I (DSM-III). Some investigators (Goldberg, 1980) make little distinction between the suicidal attempts of most adults resulting from major depression and those of adolescents.

Our experience with suicidal adolescents has indicated that a suicide attempt is a symptom, albeit a very serious one, occurring in a heterogeneous population of adolescents with different premorbid personalities and different intrapsychic conflicts. Regarding suicidal adolescents as a single group with a unitary underlying psychopathology is unproductive. A better understanding of the emotional and cognitive responses of each suicidal adolescent is more helpful in planning a suicide prevention program.

METHOD

This is a study of 120 adolescents between the ages of 14 and 17. They are divided into three groups: 40 hospitalized suicidal adolescents, 40 hospitalized nonsuicidal adolescents, and 40 never hospitalized adolescents treated in the Outpatient Psychiatric Clinic. The suicidal group included most of the adolescents who were brought to the emergency room of a large University hospital over a period of 2 years after a suicidal attempt. Many of the adolescents were first admitted to the pediatric service. Only first-time attempters were selected for this study. This criterion was used because (in our experience) repeaters tend to have different motivation and dynamics underlying their second and subsequent suicidal attempts. None of the adolescents in this group were married or pregnant or suffered from a life-threatening physical condition. All of the adolescents were of average or above average intelligence. The duration of stay in the psychiatric service ranged from 3 to 6 weeks.

The hospitalized nonsuicidal group included adolescents who were hospitalized in the same psychiatric service for other reasons during the same period of time. The third group of never hospitalized adolescents was selected randomly from the outpatient psychiatric clinic patient pool treated during the same period.

The hospitalized adolescents were studied and treated intensively by a treatment team with individual, group and milieu therapy. Suicidal adolescents were evaluated on the Hamilton Rating Scale for depression and Beck's Depression Self Inventory. In addition to a routine laboratory workup, clinically depressed adolescents received a dexamethasone suppression test. Data were collected from the adolescents and their families in several structured interviews carried out by the author, psychiatric residents and the other professional staff separately and sometime jointly. The data derived from these interviews were discussed in team meetings to arrive at a consensus with regard to the diagnosis, nature of the family and peer relationships, dynamic process and other measurements used in this study.

RESULTS

The three groups were compared with regard to age, sex, racial background, social class, peer relationship, family relationship, academic achievement, loss of a parent by death or divorce before the teenage years and incidence of sex abuse in childhood. Chi square analysis of the data (Table 1) did not reveal any significant differences in age, social class and racial background. The ratio of male and female varied widely in the three groups. Females comprised 85% of the suicidal group, 30% of the nonsuicidal hospitalized group, and 47% of the outpatient group.

The *family relationship* of each adolescent was evaluated as good, satisfactory or poor both from the perspective of the adolescent and that of the family. Dimensions considered in evaluating this relationship included degree of meaningful communication between the parents and the adolescents, understanding of each others feelings and problems, overt or covert rejection and parental demands and restrictions. For example:

> A 15-year-old white female subject reported that her life for the past 1 year had been miserable. She dreaded coming home because of facing her mother's wrath. She said, "We used to be very close. We could share all kinds of information and laugh. Mother started worrying about me when I began going out with friends in the evenings. She began accusing me of having sex with boys and using drugs . . . . I dread coming home. We always get into bad arguments. She never asks me about the good things I do . . . . My father does not say much but he takes her side when she wants to ground me."

Seventy-four to 86% of the adolescents in all three groups perceived their relationship with families as poor; that is, the parents were overly demanding, not understanding, unloving and engaged in little meaningful communication. However, more parents than adolescents felt that there was meaningful communication between them.

Peer relationship was also evaluated as good, satisfactory or poor. The nature of peer relationship was judged from the adolescent's own account and the parents' observation of the adolescent's social contacts. The number of

Table 1. Characteristics of the Three Groups.

Characters	Suicidal Hospitalized Group 1 (N = 40)		Nonsuicidal Hospitalized Group 2 (N = 40)		Nonsuicidal Outpatient Group 3 (N = 40)	
	N	%	N	%	N	%
Sex						
Female*	34	85	12	30	19	47.5
Male*	6	15	28	70	21	52.5
Race						
White	27	67.5	33	82.5	31	77.5
Black	13	32.5	7	17.5	9	22.5
Social Class						
Middle class	9	22.5	8	20	11	27.5
Lower middle	24	60	20	50	21	52.5
Lower class	7	17.5	12	30	8	20
Family Relations						
Good	3	7.5	8	20	11	27.5
Satisfactory	2	5	3	7.5	6	15
Poor	35	87.5	29	72.5	33	82.5
Academic Achievement						
Good	3	7.5	0	0	2	5
Satisfactory	8	20	10	25	8	20
Poor	29	72.5	30	75	30	75
Parental Loss (Death or Divorce)**						
Present	28	70	29	72.5	16	40
Absent	12	30	11	27.5	24	60
Sexual Abuse						
Present	6	15	1	2.5	3	7.5
Absent	34	85	39	97.5	37	92.5

* $p < 0.001$; ** $p < 0.01$.

friends, type of friendship, closeness and frequency of contact were taken into consideration for this evaluation. The parents expressed more concern about unsatisfactory peer relationships than did the adolescents themselves. However, when questioned specifically about the nature of peer relationship and closeness with friends, 72–87% of the adolescents reported not having a close friend that they could trust and talk to openly.

Academic achievement was judged on the basis of historical information and the test reports provided by the schools. The school records of children with learning difficulties were fairly elaborate in describing their past and current achievement. The judgment about the current level of achievement was based on the comparison of the past with the present performance. None of the children in this study were retarded. The "falling grades" was the most common complaint. Seventy-five percent of the adolescents in all three groups showed a drop in their grades and/or they were failing in one or more subjects in the past 6–9 months prior to the suicidal attempt. The adolescents were inclined to attribute their lower achievement to a chance happening. Those with better insight blamed family problems and felt that their preoccupation with the problems had brought their grades down. Approximately one-third of the adolescents had a history of learning problems of several years duration and had received some form of assistance from special education.

Early loss of a parent by death or divorce has been reported by several studies (Goldberg, 1980) as a significant factor in suicidal adolescents. The loss of a parent from divorce was considered only in those cases in which there had been no contact with the separated parents for 5–9 years. In this study, at least 70% of the adolescents in both hospitalized groups suffered a loss of a parent by death or divorce in the preteen years. However, the outpatient group had significantly more intact families than the hospitalized groups.

Sexual abuse: In evaluating past sexual abuse in childhood, we depended entirely on the information given by the adolescents and the parents in response to a direct inquiry about any incidence of sexual abuse. In our experience, parents and children initially suppress the history of sexual abuse and may report such incidences only after the development of a positive relationship with their therapists. There were six female adolescents in the suicidal group who reported sexual abuse in childhood by a relative, stepfather, a family friend or a boy in the neighborhood. The accounts of the sexual abuse were related to "sexual play" with exposed genitals. None of the cases were brought to judicial inquiry. In fact, in three of the six cases, the parents were not aware of the incidence as the children had never shared the information with them. There was only one female adolescent in the nonsuicidal hospitalized group who reported sexual abuse and none in the outpatient group.

Psychopathology: Tables 2 and 3 list primary (Axis I) and personality (Axis II) diagnoses. It is apparent from the tables that the suicidal group is a heterogeneous group with regard to psychopathology and only about one-third of this group was clinically depressed. Although there is a greater variety of diagnoses among the two nonsuicidal groups, there is no significant difference among the three groups with regard to the frequency of depression and conduct disorders.

Dexamethasone suppression test (DST): The test was completed on 11 of the 14 depressed suicidal adolescents and only two of the results were positive (cortisol values equal or greater than 5 $\mu g/dl$ in either of the two samples taken at 4 p.m. and 11 p.m.).

Dynamic process: Structured interviews were carried out to elicit the details of the circumstances preceding the suicidal attempts. The interviews were focused on determining the emotional and cognitive responses of the adolescents leading to the suicidal attempts. Efforts were also made to determine the "coping style" of each adolescent, both in relation to the suicidal attempt and to other overwhelming situations in the past. In the absence of recall of an actual situation, adolescents were asked to respond to a hypothetical overwhelming situation (i.e., breaking up with a boyfriend or a girlfriend, suspension from school, punishment by parents, etc.). The nature of these data is entirely qualitative and our conclusions are at best preliminary.

The circumstances reported by the suicidal adolescents preceding their suicidal attempts did not seem very different, more serious or catastrophic than the circumstances frequently encountered by the nonsuicidal adolescents. The main difference between the suicidal and nonsuicidal adolescents appeared to be in two areas: (1) ability to cope with anger and sad feelings and (2) cognitive capacity to think through the consequences of their action. Many adolescents in the nonsuicidal groups had had suicidal thoughts but they had not considered suicide as a serious alternative to other ways of dealing with their problems.

Almost all suicidal adolescents reported feeling overwhelmed, helpless and hopeless before attempting suicide. Cognitive abilities to weigh the consequences of their act were rarely utilized. It seemed that overwhelming emotions had taken complete hold of the adolescent and had paralyzed the cognitive abilities. A few suicidal adolescents reported a brief period of partial amnesia just before the suicidal act.

Most adolescents experienced anger and frustration when faced with an overwhelming situation. Many of them displaced these emotions on their

Table 2. Comparison of the Three Groups for Axis I Diagnoses

AXIS I Diagnosis	Suicidal Hospitalized Group 1 (N = 40)		Nonsuicidal Hospitalized Group 2 (N = 40)		Nonsuicidal Outpatient Group 3 (N = 40)	
	N	%	N	%	N	%
Major Depressive Disorder	7	17.5	3	7.5	1	2.5
Bipolar Affective Disorder	0	0	1	2.5	1	2.5
Cylothymic Disorder	0	0	1	2.5	1	2.5
Dythymic Disorder	7	17.5	4	2.5	8	20
Schizophrenic Disorder	0	0	8	10	0	20
Conduct Disorder	10	25	19	47.5	15	37.5
Attention Deficit Disorder	0	0	0	0	2	5
Eating Disorders	0	0	1	2.5	1	2.5
Anxiety Disorders	0	0	1	2.5	2	5
Somatoform Disorders	0	0	1	2.5	3	7.5
Impulse Control Disorder	1	2.5	1	2.5	1	2.5
Functional Encopresis	0	0	0	0	1	2.5
Oppositional Disorder	0	0	0	0	1	2.5
Adjustment Disorders	15	37.5	0	0	3	7.5

Table 3. Comparison of the Three Groups for Axis II Diagnosis

AXIS II Diagnosis	Suicidal Hospitalized Group 1 (N = 40)		Nonsuicidal Hospitalized Group 2 (N = 40)		Nonsuicidal Outpatient Group 3 (N = 40)	
	N	%	N	%	N	%
Paranoid Personality	0	0	1	2.5	0	0
Schizoid Personality	3	7.5	6	15	1	2.5
Histrionic Personality	6	15	0	0	2	5
Narcissistic Personality	9	22.5	1	2.5	3	7.5
Antisocial Personality	4	10	17	42.5	12	30
Borderline Personality	11	27.5	3	7.5	1	2.5
Avoidant Personality	0	0	1	2.5	1	2.5
Dependent Personality	5	12.5	5	12.5	7	17.5
Passive-Aggressive Personality	1	2.5	2	5	4	10
No Diagnosis	1	2.5	4	10	9	22.5

younger siblings, parents, picked a fight with peers or acted out by antisocial activities, drinking and substance abuse. Others were able to channel their anger into more constructive activities or sports. More adolescents in the suicidal group than the nonsuicidal group seemed unable to cope with their anger successfully. The suicidal adolescents perceived their environment as more threatening, arousing in them feelings of helplessness and hopelessness.

As the suicidal adolescents settled in the hospital and began to talk more about themselves, various life-styles emerged. Several adolescents had intense feelings of self-accusation. When they were young, their parents blamed them for whatever went wrong in the families. One adolescent described these feelings: "I have been made to believe that it is always my fault. I started hurting myself as I grew up." There were other adolescents who felt that the adolescent years were too much of a change for them. In the adolescent years, parents became more demanding, less giving and less trusting. This change in parental attitude was interpreted as rejection which aroused anger and frustration in the adolescents. Many adolescents reported having negative and hostile feelings towards their parents before the suicidal attempt, wanting to hurt them and get back at them.

DISCUSSION

Our results indicate that in a group of 120 emotionally and behaviorally disturbed adolescents, suicidal adolescents could not be distinguished on the basis of age, sex, social class, type of peer and family relationship, academic achievement and early loss of a parent by death or divorce. Similarly clinical diagnoses on Axis I and Axis II (DSM-III) fail to differentiate between the suicidal and nonsuicidal adolescents.

Our findings, however, are not surprising. Previous studies have, in part, supported as well as contradicted these conclusions. Stanley and Barter (1970), for example, found that suicidal adolescents did not differ from a matched control group with respect to family and peer relationship. This study, however, reported a greater incidence of parental loss in the suicidal group before the age of 12 and more threatened parental loss through talk of divorce or separation. Topol and Reznikoff (1982) found that suicidal adolescents experienced significantly more problems in peer and family relationships. Similarly, studies of premorbid personalities and clinical diagnoses, as discussed in our introductory review, report variable findings.

These variable findings may be attributed to differences in the selection of patients, the methods of evaluation, the diagnostic criteria, the duration of observation and the nature of the control groups. Many adolescents tend to deny the significance of their suicidal attempts soon after the act and refuse to cooperate with mental health professionals. Removal of the adolescent from his family and social environment into a therapeutic milieu helps him acknowledge his problems and the significance of his suicidal attempt. If the information is gathered during the stage of early denial, a great deal of valuable information is lost.

If our findings are correct, then the question arises: what makes some adolescents commit or attempt suicide under the same social and familial circumstances which are also experienced by nonsuicidal adolescents? It is not surprising that environmental and demographic factors do not distinguish suicidal adolescents from the nonsuicidal groups. Relationship with one's family and peers, the emotional meaning of a loss and the importance of precipitating circumstances are difficult dimensions to quantify. A conflict with one's parents about going out or about clothes, failure on school tests or disappointment in love are ordinary everyday events that occur in the lives of adolescents. In fact, it would be difficult to find an adolescent who has not experienced one of these events. It would be illogical to treat these events as suicidogenic factors. Similarly, personality and psychiatric diagnoses (Axis I and Axis II) are relatively static concepts. They shed little light on the cognitive and emotional responses of an adolescent in the face of a perceived overwhelming stress.

Farberow (1984) pointed out that many problems exist in assessing and predicting suicide. He said, "It's only the odds that can be estimated, which in turn determine the amount of attention that will be applied to the person being evaluated, both immediately and in the long run. What is necessary is a continuous effort to sharpen and delineate the list of variables so that predictions can approximate the goal as closely as possible." We may emphasize that many variables suggested in previous studies require validation and refinement. Our study assigns a low predictive value to psychiatric classification and demographic variables. We suspect that a comprehensive analysis of "coping style" in future studies of adolescents may reveal better predicting variables for suicidal potential. Although the term "coping style" is not clearly defined, we consider it here to include various emotional and cognitive variables such as "cognitive style" (which refers to problem solving approaches that an individual may exercise), social cognition (which broaches the area of interpersonal rather than impersonal problem solving), and dominant emotional reactions to stress (feelings of helplessness, hopelessness, denial, etc.).

REFERENCES

Crumley, F. E. (1979), Adolescent suicide attempts. *J. Amer. Med. Assn.* 241:2402–2407.

_____ (1981), Adolescent suicide attempts and borderline personality disorder: clinical features, *South. Med, J.,* 74:546–549.

Dorpat, J. L. & Ripley, H. S. (1967), Relationship between attempted suicide and committed suicide. *Compr. Psychiat.,* 8:74–79.

Farberow, N. (1984), Suicide risk, not actual occurrence, said predictable. *Psychiat. News* (April 6), p. 54.

Garfinkel, B. D., Froese, A. & Hood, J. (1982), Suicide attempts in children and adolescents, *Amer. J. Psychiat.,* 139:1257–1261.

Goldberg, E. L. (1980), Suicide ideation in the young adult. *Amer. J. Psychiat.,* 138:35.

Hudgens, R. W. (1974), *Psychiatric Disorder in Adolescents,* Chap. 5. Baltimore: Williams & Wilkins.

Jacob, J. (1971), *Adolescent Suicide,* New York: Wiley-Interscience.

Kosky, R. (1983), Childhood suicidal behavior. *J. Child Psychol. Psychiat.,* 24:457–468.

McIntire, M. S., Angle, C. R. & Schlict, M. L. (1977), Suicide and self-poisoning in pediatrics. *Adv. Pediat.,* 24:291–309.

Schlebusch, L. & Minnaar, G. K. (1980), The management of parasuicide in adolescents, *South Afr. Med. J.,* 57:81–84.

Silverman, C. (1968), *The Epidemiology of Depression.* Baltimore: Johns Hopkins University Press, pp. 157–202.

Stanley, J. E. & Barter, J. T. (1970), Adolescent suicidal behavior. *Amer. J. Orthopsychiat.,* 40:87–96.

Tishler, C. L. & McKenry, P. C. (1981), Intrapsychic symptom dimensions of adolescent suicide attempters. *J. Family Pract.,* 16:731–734.

Topol, P. & Reznikoff, M. (1982), Perceived peer and family relationship, hopelessness and locus of control as factors in adolescent suicide attempts. *Suicide Life Threat. Behav.,* 12:141–150. Tuckman, J. & Youngman, W. (1968), Assessment of suicide risk in attempted suicides. In *Suicide Behaviors: Diagnosis and Management,* ed. H. H. Resnik. Boston: Little Brown, pp. 190–197.

Wenz, F. V. (1978), Economic status, family anomie and adolescent suicide potential. *J. Psychol.,* 98:45–47.

_____ (1979a), Self-injury behavior, economic status and the family anomie syndrome among adolescents. *Adolescence,* 14:387–398.

_____ (1979b), Sociological correlates of alienation among adolescent suicide attempts. *Adolescence,* 14:19–30.

Williams C. & Lyons, C. (1976), Family interaction and adolescent suicidal behavior: a preliminary investigation. *Aust. N.Z. Psychiat.* 10:243–252.